Epilepsy and
Developmental
Disabilities

Epilepsy and Developmental Disabilities

Edited by

Orrin Devinsky, M.D.

Professor, Department of Neurology, New York University School of Medicine;
Director, New York University Comprehensive Epilepsy Center

Lauren E. Westbrook, Ph.D.

Adjunct Assistant Professor of Neurology, New York University School of
Medicine

With 56 contributing authors

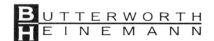

Boston   Oxford   Auckland   Johannesburg   Melbourne   New Delhi

Every effort has been made to ensure that the drug dosage schedules within this text are accurate and conform to standards accepted at time of publication. However, as treatment recommendations vary in the light of continuing research and clinical experience, the reader is advised to verify drug dosage schedules herein with information found on product information sheets. This is especially true in cases of new or infrequently used drugs.

Library of Congress Cataloging-in-Publication Data

Epilepsy and developmental disabilities / edited by Orrin Devinsky, Lauren E. Westbrook, with 56 contributing authors.
      p. ; cm
   Includes bibliographical references and index.
   ISBN 0-7506-7273-0
      1. Epilepsy—Congresses. 2. Developmental disabilities—Congresses. I. Devinsky, Orrin. II. Westbrook, Lauren E.
   [DNLM: 1. Epilepsy—complications—Congresses. 2. Developmental Disabilities—complications—Congresses. 3. Developmental Disabilities—therapy—Congresses. 4. Epilepsy—diagnosis—Congresses. 5. Epilepsy—therapy—Congresses. WL 385 E6025 2002]
   RC372.A2 E645 2002
   616.8'53—dc21

                                                                          2001035524

British Library Cataloguing-in-Publication Data
A catalogue record for this book is available from the British Library.

The publisher offers special discounts on bulk orders of this book.
For information, please contact:

Manager of Special Sales
Butterworth–Heinemann
225 Wildwood Avenue
Woburn, MA 01801-2041
Tel: 781-904-2500
Fax: 781-904-2620

For information on all Butterworth–Heinemann publications available, contact our World Wide Web home page at: http://www.bh.com.

10 9 8 7 6 5 4 3 2 1

Printed in the United States of America

There are human spirits that are not of this world. They glide above, land briefly, and return to flight. They may be camouflaged behind frail and bent frames, mute voices. They go unrecognized or unseen by many. Yet their vision is larger, their heart is purer, and their song is richer and sweeter.

Anna-Katrina Lehrer, Jennifer Millens, and Christopher Smith were three such spirits. They had all known physical disability, stigma, seizures, and numbing numbers and doses of medications. The social, medical, and mental walls appeared enormous to the "normal" outside world but could never contain these souls. Each one intensely expressed their love and joy for life in their own way. Each knew much about life and living. Three brilliant flames of human spirit.

Sadly, those flames were extinguished very early. Their love and their spirit lives on.

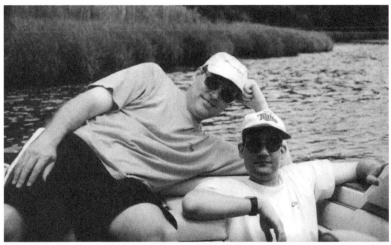

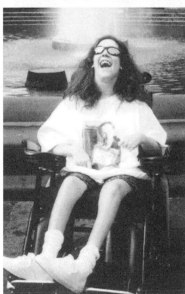
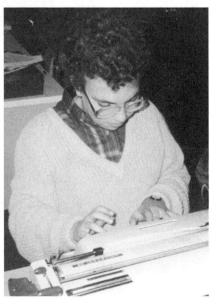

Contents

Contributing Authors

Karen Ballaban-Gil, M.D.
Associate Professor of Clinical Neurology and Clinical Pediatrics, Department of Neurology, Albert Einstein College of Medicine, Bronx, New York; Associate Professor, Department of Neurology, Montefiore Medical Center, Bronx

William B. Barr, Ph.D.
Chief of Neuropsychology, New York University Comprehensive Epilepsy Center, Mount Sinai–New York University Health System, New York

John J. Barry, M.D.
Assistant Professor of Psychiatry and Neurology, Department of Psychiatry, Stanford University School of Medicine, Stanford, California

Vicky Bassi, B.S.
Medical Student, University of Florida College of Medicine, Shands Medical Center, Gainesville

Christine Baudin, M.S., C.C.C./S.L.P., T.S.H.H.
Augmentative Communication Specialist, UCP-GHI Augmentative Communication Center, United Cerebral Palsy of New York City

Brian D. Bell, Ph.D.
Associate Research Scientist, Department of Neurology, University of Wisconsin, Madison

Blaise F. D. Bourgeois, M.D.
Professor of Neurology, Harvard Medical School, Boston; Director, Department of Neurology, Division of Epilepsy and Clinical Neurophysiology, Children's Hospital, Boston

Carol S. Camfield, M.D., F.R.C.P.C.
Professor of Pediatrics, Dalhousie University Medical School, Halifax, Nova Scotia, Canada; IWK Grace Health Centre, Halifax

Peter Camfield, M.D.
Professor and Chair, Department of Pediatrics, Dalhousie University Medical School, Halifax, Nova Scotia, Canada; Child Neurologist, IWK Grace Health Centre, Halifax

Joyce A. Cramer, B.S.
Lecturer, Department of Psychiatry, Yale University School of Medicine, New Haven, Connecticut; Project Director, VA Connecticut Health Care System, West Haven

Marco D'Amelio, M.D.
Department of Neurology, University of Palermo, Palermo, Italy

Orrin Devinsky, M.D.
Professor, Department of Neurology, New York University School of Medicine; Director, New York University Comprehensive Epilepsy Center

Werner K. Doyle, M.D.
Assistant Professor of Neurosurgery, New York University School of Medicine; Attending Physician, Department of Neurosurgery, New York University Medical Center

Daniel L. Drane, Ph.D.
Assistant Clinical Professor, Department of Neurology, Medical College of Georgia, Augusta; Neuropsychologist, The Rehabilitation Institute, Northeast Georgia Medical Center, Gainesville

Michael Duchowny, M.D.
Clinical Professor in Neurology and Pediatrics, University of Miami School of Medicine; Director, Neuroscience Program, Miami Children's Hospital

Alan B. Ettinger, M.D.
Associate Professor of Clinical Neurology, Department of Neurology, Albert Einstein College of Medicine, Bronx, New York; Director, Long Island Jewish Comprehensive Epilepsy Center, New Hyde Park, New York; Director, Huntington Hospital Seizure Monitoring Program, North Shore–Long Island Jewish Health System, New Hyde Park

David S. Feldman, M.D.
Assistant Professor, Department of Orthopedic Surgery, New York University School of Medicine; Chief of Pediatric Orthopedic Surgery, New York University Medical Center, Hospital for Joint Diseases

Ross B. FineSmith, M.D.
Clinical Instructor, Department of Neurology, New York University School of Medicine; Attending Physician, Department of Pediatric Neurology, Saint Barnabas Medical Center, Livingston, New Jersey

Eric B. Geller, M.D.
Director, Adult Comprehensive Epilepsy Center, Saint Barnabas Institute of Neurology and Neurosurgery, Saint Barnabas Medical Center, Livingston, New Jersey

Tracy A. Glauser, M.D.
Associate Professor, Department of Pediatrics, Division of Neurology, University of Cincinnati College of Medicine; Director, Comprehensive Epilepsy Program, Children's Hospital Medical Center, Cincinnati

Anna Gross, B.A.
Medical Student, Mount Sinai School of Medicine, New York

W. Allen Hauser, M.D.
Professor of Neurology and Public Health, College of Physicians and Surgeons, Columbia University, New York; Attending Physician, Department of Neurology, New York Presbyterian Hospital

Bruce P. Hermann, Ph.D.
Professor, Department of Neurology, University of Wisconsin Medical School, Madison

Glenn S. Hirsch, M.D.
Assistant Professor of Psychiatry, New York University School of Medicine; Deputy Director, New York University Child Study Center, New York University School of Medicine

Gregory L. Holmes, M.D.
Professor of Neurology, Harvard Medical School, Boston; Director, Center for Research in Pediatric Epilepsy, Children's Hospital, Boston

Nga Huynh, Pharm.D.
Clinical Pharmacist, Inpatient Pharmacy, Stanford University Hospital, Stanford, California; Clinical Pharmacist, Inpatient Pharmacy, Valleycare Health System, Pleasanton, California

Nancy Lenhart Jones, M.S., C.C.C./S.L.P., A.T.P.
Augmentative Communication Specialist, Manhattan Clinic, United Cerebral Palsy of New York City

Charles A. Kincaid, Ph.D.
Vocational Consulting Group, Springfield, New Jersey

Mariko Kita, M.D.
Director, Department of Neurology, Virginia Mason Multiple Sclerosis Center, Virginia Mason Medical Center, Seattle

Edwin H. Kolodny, M.D.
Bernard A. and Charlotte Marden Professor and Chairman, Department of Neurology, New York University School of Medicine; Attending Physician, Department of Neurology, New York University School of Medicine

Harold S. Koplewicz, M.D.
Arnold and Debbie Simon Professor of Child and Adolescent Psychiatry and Director, New York University Child Study Center, New York University School of Medicine

Ruben Kuzniecky, M.D.
Professor and Director, Department of Neurology, University of Alabama at Birmingham Epilepsy Center, University of Alabama at Birmingham

Josiane LaJoie, M.D.
Pediatric Neurology Fellow, Department of Neurology, Albert Einstein College of Medicine, Montefiore Medical Center, Bronx, New York; Resident, Department of Neurology, Albert Einstein College of Medicine, Montefiore Medical Center, Bronx

David J. Leszczyszyn, M.D., Ph.D.
Assistant Professor of Neurology, Division of Child Neurology, Virginia Commonwealth University Health System, Richmond

Edwin Liu, M.D.
Department of Neurology, Miami Children's Hospital

Daniel J. Luciano, M.D.
Assistant Professor of Clinical Neurology, Department of Neurology, New York University School of Medicine; Director, Clinical Epilepsy Program, New York University Comprehensive Epilepsy Center, Mount Sinai–New York University Health System, New York

Kimford J. Meador, M.D.
Professor, Department of Neurology and Pharmacology/Toxicology, Medical College of Georgia Hospital, Augusta

Diego A. Morita, M.D.
Clinical Fellow, Department of Pediatrics, Division of Neurology, Children's Hospital Medical Center, Cincinnati

Solomon L. Moshe, M.D.
Professor of Neurology, Neuroscience, and Pediatrics, Department of Neurology, Albert Einstein College of Medicine, Bronx, New York; Attending Physician, Department of Neurology, Montefiore Medical Center, Jacobi Medical Center, Bronx

Anjanette A. Naga, B.A.
Research Coordinator, Department of Neurology, New York University Comprehensive Epilepsy Center

Ruth Nass, M.D.
Professor of Clinical Neurology, Department of Neurology, New York University School of Medicine; Director, Learning Diagnostics Program, New York University School of Medicine; Attending Physician, Department of Neurology, New York University Medical Center

Steven V. Pacia, M.D.
Assistant Professor, Department of Neurology, New York University School of Medicine; Director, Neurophysiology Laboratory, New York University Comprehensive Epilepsy Center

John M. Pellock, M.D.
Professor and Chairman, Division of Child Neurology, Medical College of Virginia, Virginia Commonwealth University, Richmond

A. James Rowan, M.D.
Professor of Neurology, Mount Sinai School of Medicine, New York; Chief, Neurology Service, Bronx VA Medical Center, Bronx, New York; Attending Neurologist, Mount Sinai Hospital, New York

Lawrence M. Samkoff, M.D.
Associate Professor of Clinical Neurology, Department of Neurology, New York Medical College, Metropolitan Hospital Center, New York

Steven C. Schachter, M.D.
Associate Professor of Neurology, Harvard Medical School, Boston; Medical Director, Office of Clinical Trials and Research, Beth Israel Deaconess Medical Center, Boston

Michael Seidenberg, Ph.D.
Professor, Department of Psychology, Finch University of Health Sciences, The Chicago Medical School, North Chicago, Illinois

Debra Shabas, M.D.
Assistant Professor of Clinical Neurology, New York University Medical Center; Premier Health Care, Young Adults Institute/National Institute for People with Disabilities, New York

Shlomo Shinnar, M.D., Ph.D.
Professor of Neurology and Pediatrics, Albert Einstein College of Medicine, Bronx, New York; Director, Comprehensive Epilepsy Management Center, Montefiore Medical Center, Bronx

Sanford P. Solomon, M.D.
Assistant Professor of Clinical Psychiatry, Department of Psychiatry, Albert Einstein College of Medicine, Bronx, New York; Staff Psychiatrist, North Shore–Long Island Jewish Health System, New Hyde Park, New York

Vicki Sudhalter, Ph.D.
Head, Clinical Psycholinguistics Laboratory, Department of Psychiatric and Psychological Services, New York State Institute for Basic Research in Developmental Disabilities, Staten Island

Andrew Tarulli, B.A.
Medical Student, New York University School of Medicine

Renée Toueg, M.S.
Lecturer and Speech/Language Pathologist, Department of Linguistics and Communication Disorders, Queens College, City University of New York, Flushing

Eileen P. G. Vining, M.D.
Associate Professor of Neurology and Pediatrics, The Johns Hopkins University School of Medicine, Baltimore

Thaddeus Walczak, M.D.
Associate Clinical Professor, Department of Neurology, University of Minnesota School of Medicine, Minneapolis; Attending Physician, Department of Neurology, Abbott Northwestern Hospital, Minneapolis

Linda Watson, B.Sc.
Research Assistant, Western Australian Cerebral Palsy Register, TVW Telethon Institute for Child Health Research, Perth, Western Australia, Australia

Preface

Epilepsy and developmental disabilities, when combined, create some of the most serious and complex neurologic disorders. Behavior, intellect, movement and sensation, communication, and social and psychological experience may all be affected in a single individual. The medical professionals who care for people with epilepsy and developmental disabilities are usually experienced in caring for one component of these multifaceted disorders. Whereas some neurologists' practices are primarily composed of people with seizures (a proportion of whom also have developmental disabilities), others are primarily composed of people with developmental disabilities (a proportion of whom also have seizures).

The call to find ways to better integrate these distinct yet overlapping areas of expertise is a formidable challenge, but the voices of parents, teachers, psychologists, social workers, physical and occupational therapists, communication specialists, and, perhaps most persuasively, the voices and nonverbal communications of affected individuals themselves, cannot be ignored.

In the fall of 1999, we organized a conference at New York University Medical Center entitled Epilepsy and Developmental Disabilities. We invited specialists from all over North America representing a wide range of fields to present on their area of expertise. This book is a compilation of the presentations by medical and medically related professionals. We hope, that by providing an integrated source of knowledge, we can foster increased interest, greater understanding, better care, and, not least, more compassion for people who live with epilepsy and developmental disabilities.

Orrin Devinsky
Lauren E. Westbrook

Acknowledgments

This conference and book *Epilepsy and Developmental Disabilities* was made possible by unrestricted educational grants from the Fight Against Childhood Epilepsy and Seizures (F.A.C.E.S.), the American Epilepsy Society, the New York University Comprehensive Epilepsy Center, Cyberonics, Inc., Novartis, Pfizer, Inc., Ortho-McNeil Pharmaceutical, UCB Pharma, Abbott Laboratories, Glaxo Wellcome, Inc., and Shire Richwood, Inc.

The following organizations participated and provided valuable input and resources: Epilepsy Foundations of New York City, Long Island, Southern New York, and New Jersey; Epilepsy Institute; the Arc of New Jersey; United Cerebral Palsy of New York City; Young Adults Institute/National Institute for People with Disabilities; and Saint Barnabas Institute of Neurology and Neurosurgery.

Finally, and most important, we acknowledge the individuals and families that are touched by epilepsy and developmental disabilities for all they have taught us.

Orrin Devinsky
Lauren E. Westbrook

Epilepsy and Developmental Disabilities

Part I

Epilepsy and Developmental Disabilities:
Causes and Consequences

Chapter 1

Epilepsy in Children with Mental Retardation and Cerebral Palsy

Marco D'Amelio, Shlomo Shinnar,
and W. Allen Hauser

In children, epilepsy is one of the most prevalent major neurologic disorders, affecting 4–10 children per 1,000.[1–4] The association between epilepsy and cerebral palsy (CP) or mental retardation (MR) is well recognized. Approximately 15–30% of epilepsy cases in childhood are associated with these conditions. In this chapter, we will review the epidemiologic features of both CP and MR and discuss the complex interaction with epilepsy. For purposes of this discussion, we will limit ourselves to CP and MR due to antenatal and perinatal causes that are presumed to be present from birth. We have excluded cases of acquired neurologic deficits associated with such postnatal central nervous system insults as central nervous system infections, hypoxic injury, trauma, and stroke. These deficits are considered also to be risk factors for epilepsy and, in fact, when associated with MR and CP, may carry an even higher risk of epilepsy development than do MR and CP from antenatal and perinatal etiology.[5] However, the epidemiology and epilepsy risks for these latter conditions are distinct from those of neurologic handicaps present from birth.

Epidemiology of Mental Retardation

MR is the condition of a significant deficit in intelligence and adaptive skills necessary for communication, self-care, social interaction, leisure, and work. Our discussion will be limited to deficits presumed to be present at birth, though, in many cases, the intellectual deficit may not be identified for several years.

MR may be classified into four grades of severity, which are defined in terms of intelligence quotient (IQ): mild (IQ, 50–70), moderate (IQ, 35–49), severe (IQ, 20–34), and profound (IQ, <20). Most epidemiologic studies collapse the last three categories into the single category of severe MR, thereby merely distinguishing it from the mild form.

The overall prevalence of MR varies according to the severity of the disability and the country in which it has been evaluated. In developed countries, the prevalence of severe MR in children has consistently been found to range from 3 to 5 per 1,000, whereas wider ranges of prevalence rates have been reported for mild MR (2.5–40.0 per 1,000).[6–8] Few estimates are available from countries with emerging economies, although prevalence rates generally are higher than those in developed countries (5.0–25.0 per 1,000), especially for mild MR which may be more influenced by social and environmental factors than is severe MR.[9–12]

For both severe and mild MR, prevalence increases with increasing age in childhood and tends to decline with advancing age throughout adulthood. Mild MR commonly is recognized when children enter school, whereas severe MR is much more commonly diagnosed during infancy and early childhood.

Chromosomal abnormalities are the leading known cause of severe MR in developed countries.

3

These abnormalities include chromosomal duplication, such as trisomy 21 in Down syndrome, or abnormalities of chromosome structure, such as X-linked trinucleotide repeats (amplification of CGG triplet in the fragile X syndrome), autosomal dominant inherited deletions (e.g., chromosome 9/16 in tuberous sclerosis, chromosome 17 or 22 in neurofibromatosis types 1 and 2), or autosomal recessive substitutions (e.g., chromosome 12 in phenylketonuria).

In developed countries, genetic causes are responsible for 30% or more cases of severe MR. In less developed countries, MR more often is attributed to nutritional deficiencies (folate or iodine) and traumatic, intrauterine, and postnatally acquired infectious diseases.[13] Whether such perinatal events as preterm birth, low birth weight, and birth asphyxia are associated with increased risk of impaired mental development in infancy or childhood remains unclear. These factors seem to be associated with MR only when MR is accompanied by CP.[14-16]

Epidemiology of Cerebral Palsy

CP is defined as a chronic, nonprogressive cerebral disorder in young children that results in impaired motor function.[17] It is classified according to the nature of symptoms (spastic, extrapyramidal, mixed) or the distribution of maximal disability (hemiplegia, 25–40%; diplegia, 10–33%; and quadriplegia, 9–43% of CP cases) or in terms of severity (description of severity). Despite variability in methods, most of the studies indicate a prevalence of 1.2–2.5 per 1,000 children of early school age.[14]

In the past, traumatic delivery was considered a risk factor for CP, but systematic studies fail to show a high correlation with this adverse event.[14,15,18,19] Low birth weight and reduced gestational age at birth are conditions considered to be associated with a high risk for CP. Progress made in neonatal critical care has improved survival of children with these characteristics, and so these children now constitute a large and increasing fraction of all CP cases. Three other factors that contribute to the risk of CP, regardless of birth weight, include congenital malformations, inflammation of the placenta, and twinning. A nonspecific association exists between spastic quadriparesis with movement disorder and birth asphyxia. CP has been attributed to intrauterine toxic exposures (methyl mercury, exogenous thyroid hormone, and estrogens) and intrauterine infections (rubella, toxoplasmosis, and cytomegalovirus). In population-based studies, most cases of CP (80%) show no clinical evidence of birth asphyxia or other adverse events.[14,15,18–20] Although motor dysfunction is the defining characteristic in patients with CP, the disorder often is associated with other problems, including epilepsy and MR.

Risk of Epilepsy among Children with Developmental Disabilities

The reported frequency of epilepsy among children with MR or CP varies widely. This variation can be explained by differences in the definition of epilepsy (inclusion of single or complex febrile seizures as well as a single seizure), sources for case ascertainment (hospitals, private doctor's offices, services for children with mental disabilities), and differences in the severity of MR or CP in children involved in the studies.

Current knowledge of the risk of epilepsy in mentally retarded children derives basically from three different sources: (1) studies of MR that report information about epilepsy; (2) studies of CP that include information about epilepsy and MR; and (3) studies of epilepsy that report information about MR or CP.

Epilepsy in Children with Mental Retardation

Population-Based Studies

The Metropolitan Atlanta Developmental Disabilities Study is a large, population-based, cross-sectional study in which data were collected on 10-year-old children who were born from 1975 through 1977 in the metropolitan Atlanta area and who had one or more of five developmental disabilities: MR, CP, epilepsy, visual impairment, and hearing impairment. Data were collected through educational, medical, or social services for children with disabilities.[21,22] Overall, 15% of children with MR who were enrolled in the Metropolitan Atlanta

Developmental Disabilities Study also had epilepsy. The proportion who experienced seizures increased with increasing severity of MR. Thirty-two percent of children with an IQ lower than 50 had epilepsy, as compared to 8% of those with an IQ between 50 and 70. The highest proportion of children with epilepsy (59%) was among those with profound MR (IQ lower than 20). CP occurred significantly more frequently in children with MR and coexisting epilepsy (52%) as compared to those with MR without epilepsy (6%).

Organizations that provide social, educational, and training and rehabilitation services are a common source of information on the frequency and nature of associated disabilities in children with MR. These services are not only inexpensive sources of information but, in countries where registration is mandatory for all individuals with one of these disabilities, they are reliable sources for large, population-based studies. However, children who exhibit multiple disabilities are more likely to be referred to these services than are children with only one disability. Thus, it is likely that these services enroll children with particularly severe forms of MR, CP, or epilepsy, resulting in an exaggerated association between these disorders.

In Sweden, all individuals with MR are registered to the Board for Provisions and Services to the Mentally Retarded (BPSMR), which supplies services to individuals with MR, whether they reside within institutions or in the community. Forsgren et al.[23] examined the medical records of individuals reported to have epilepsy who were registered with the BPSMR. Information also was obtained from medical records from departments of neurology, pediatrics, and obstetrics. The study adopted the definition of seizures used by the World Health Organization ("transient dysfunction of part or all of the brain due to excessive discharge of a hyper-excitable population of neurons, causing sudden and transitory phenomena of a motor, sensory, or psychic nature"). Neonatal seizures and all afebrile, unprovoked seizures were included. Epilepsy was considered active if an individual was on any antiepileptic drug (AED) or if the last seizure occurred not more than 5 years before the prevalence day.

Twenty percent of the individuals registered to the BPSMR had epilepsy. Epilepsy was more common in individuals with severe to profound MR (IQ <40; 32%) as compared to those with mild to moderate MR (40 <IQ <70; 11%). CP was the most common associated impairment (33.4%). MR was significantly more severe among patients with epilepsy and CP as compared to those without CP.

The BPSMR was the main source of information in another study, which limited its investigation to 6- to 13-year-old children with MR residing in the city of Goteborg, Sweden.[24] The search for children with MR was extended to pediatric clinics, child neuropsychiatric clinics, rehabilitation centers, and electroencephalography laboratories. The frequency of active epilepsy and other associated disabilities on the prevalence day was determined. Epilepsy was defined as the occurrence of two or more unprovoked epileptic seizures and was considered to be active if the child experienced one or more epileptic seizures during the five-year period prior to the prevalence day.

The authors reported the proportion of children with MR and active epilepsy to be 26%. The study, consistent with that of Forsgren et al.,[23] showed an increased risk of epilepsy among children with an IQ lower than 50 (45%), as compared to the group of patients with an IQ between 50 and 70 (15%). In this study, CP was associated with MR and epilepsy in 43% of children. CP was more common in those with severe MR (59%) as compared to those with moderate MR (14%).

Goulden et al.[5] investigated the cumulative risk of seizures and epilepsy in a prospectively identified cohort of 221 children with MR born between 1951 and 1955 in Aberdeen, Scotland. By age 22 years, 33 (15%) had epilepsy. An additional 16 (7%) had experienced at least one seizure but did not meet the criteria for epilepsy. In children with MR and no associated disabilities, the cumulative risk of epilepsy was only 5.2% at 22 years, as compared with a 38% risk in children with both MR and CP.

Nevo et al.[25] reviewed the records of children evaluated in the Tel Aviv Child Development Center between 1981 and 1990. This location serves as primary center for evaluation of all children 0–5 years old who live in the metropolitan area of Tel Aviv and who have one of the following developmental disabilities: speech and language problems, motor and psychomotor delay, and behavior problems. Given the nature of the national health care system in Israel, all

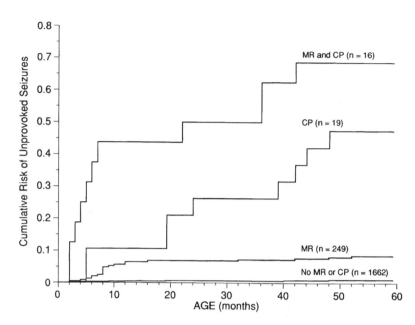

Figure 1-1. Cumulative risk of developing unprovoked seizures in 1,946 children referred to the Tel Aviv Child Development Center: effect of presence of mental retardation (MR) and cerebral palsy (CP) on risk of unprovoked seizures. Kaplan-Meier curves. In this figure, the diagnostic groups are mutually exclusive (i.e., MR is MR without CP, etc.). (Adapted from Y Nevo, S Shinnar, E Samuel, et al. Unprovoked seizures and developmental disabilities: clinical characteristics of children referred to a child development center. Pediatr Neurol 1995;13:235–241.)

children within the geographic area would be referred to the Child Development Center. The authors classified seizures and epilepsy according to the guidelines for epidemiologic studies on epilepsy issued by the Commission on Epidemiology and Prognosis of the International League against Epilepsy in 1993.[26] MR was defined as an IQ of less than 68. Seizures were not the cause of referral to the center. Most of the children (92%) who experienced a seizure were referred to the center after seizure onset. The study showed a higher risk for seizure in children with more severe brain dysfunctions. The observed cumulative risk of seizures in children by 5 years of age was 8% in those with MR only, 47% in those with CP, and up to 68% in those with MR and CP. The results of this study are shown in Figure 1-1. Interestingly, in this study, the risk of seizure disorders by age 5 years in children referred to the Child Development Center for evaluation of disabilities other than MR or CP was not different from that in the general population.

Clinical Series

As compared with population-based studies, higher frequencies of epilepsy have been reported among children admitted to the R. F. Kennedy Center (Bronx, New York) for the evaluation of MR or CP (or both).[27,28] Medical records of 400 children were reviewed to determine the influence of possible prenatal, perinatal, and postnatal clinical factors on the risk for epilepsy. Children's birth records, if available, also were reviewed. The study evaluated the frequency of one or more afebrile, unprovoked seizures in these children. Thirty percent of children with MR or CP (or both) had experienced at least one unprovoked seizure. The risk of seizures increased with increasing severity of handicap. In the group with MR, the rate of unprovoked seizures was more than doubled in the group with an IQ of less than 50 as compared to those with an IQ between 50 and 69. Similarly, in those with CP, the frequency of epilepsy increased from 19% in those with mild motor deficits to more than 50% in those with severe deficits. When the frequency of seizures was evaluated within subtypes of CP, patients with diplegia were unique in that their risk was low overall and within MR strata.

More recently, Eriksson et al.[29] studied epilepsy in children with MR registered to a public organization that provides various services for mentally retarded people in the city of Tampere,

Finland, and several other rural communes. Epilepsy was defined as a "chronic condition in which epileptic seizures tend to occur repeatedly without any detectable extracerebral cause." At the time that the study was conducted, more than 1,500 clients, 197 of whom were no older than 16 years, were enrolled at the organization. Forty percent (78) of these 197 children also had epilepsy. Among the children with epilepsy, mild to moderate MR was present in 32% (35 ≤IQ ≤70), whereas 60% had severe to profound MR (IQ ≤34). The degree of MR of six children was not classified. CP was present in 56% of the children with MR (n = 110); the majority of the childhood CP patients (72%) also had severe or profound MR (IQ ≤34). The high rate of epilepsy reported in the study might be explained, in part, by the fact that the authors evaluated only those children registered with the organization, so that those with milder forms of MR (and fewer service needs) may not have been included.

Epilepsy in Children with Cerebral Palsy

Epilepsy is one of the most common disorders associated with CP. Studies reporting the frequency of epilepsy in children with CP describe the coexistence of the two disorders in up to 50% of children. The reported frequency varies widely (more than for MR) because different sources of information are used and because of the great clinical heterogeneity of CP. Some of the studies dealing with the risk of epilepsy in children with both MR and CP were reviewed in the previous section. The following sections focus on studies that emphasize children with CP.

Population-Based Studies

The feasibility of identifying all cases of a given disorder over several decades makes the population of Rochester, Minnesota, ideal for many epidemiologic studies. Kudrjavcev et al.[30] identified 63 individuals born in Rochester between 1950 and 1976 in whom CP had been diagnosed before their sixteenth birthday. The authors investigated the presence of associated handicaps (MR and epilepsy) and divided patients with CP into two groups: those with mild to moderate CP and those with severe to very

severe CP. Classification by CP severity was based on the function of the most affected limb and, in most cases, was defined by the ability to walk. Patients with mild CP were able to walk without marked difficulty in the absence of any mechanical aids. Patients with CP of moderate severity required no mechanical assistance but ambulated with difficulty. Those with severe CP were able to walk only with the assistance of mechanical aids, and the function of the most affected limb was completely lost even in the presence of mechanical aids. Epilepsy was defined as two or more afebrile seizures occurring after 28 days of life.

Overall, 33% of the children in this study had epilepsy. Epilepsy was twice as common among children with severe CP (52%) as compared to those with mild to moderate CP (23%). None of the children with mild to moderate MR or with severe CP and normal intelligence had epilepsy. More than 65% of patients with severe to very severe CP had an IQ of 35 or less, as compared to 5% of those with mild to moderate CP. Because more than half of those with severe to very severe CP had epilepsy, we can assume that epilepsy was more common in children with CP when accompanying MR was severe as compared to mild to moderate.

Clinical Series

Sussova et al.[31] investigated the frequency of epilepsy in children with the hemiparetic form of CP who were seen at a Prague pediatric neurology center or were registered to an institute caring for all "educable" children with CP. Thirty-seven percent of the children included in the study developed epilepsy. However, this study is characterized by several limitations. Children were highly selected owing to the source used for case ascertainment: Children considered totally uneducable were excluded. As a result of such restriction, only 3 of the 51 children involved had an IQ of less than 85. No clear definition of epilepsy was given. The authors' conclusion that "epilepsy was significantly associated with the probability of intellectual impairment" likely is correct, although their study does not address the question. No children with MR (according to usual definitions) were included in the study: Children were considered intellectually impaired if the IQ was no higher than 94. According to this definition, 63% of the children with epilepsy had an abnormal IQ.

Mrabet et al.[32] determined the frequency of epilepsy in children with CP who were admitted to a specialized center for rehabilitation. Only children with mild forms of MR (IQ, 60–80) were registered to the center. Overall, 26% of children with CP had epilepsy. Moderate to severe MR was significantly more frequent in children with epilepsy and CP (38.8%) than in those with CP and no epilepsy (17.6%).

When children with more severe MR are included, higher rates of epilepsy are reported in children with CP. In a study of children who were inpatients or outpatients of a pediatric department or outpatients of four rehabilitation centers in Athens, epilepsy, defined as the occurrence of at least two unprovoked seizures, was present in 42% of children with CP.[33] Patients with moderate to severe MR (IQ <50) had more than a twofold increased risk of developing epilepsy when compared to patients with normal IQ level (IQ >70). The identification of children from physiotherapy and rehabilitation programs suggests that milder forms of CP probably were not included in the study. This might explain the high proportion of epilepsy found in the study.

Of all children with CP registered to a university referral center (Department of Developmental Medicine and Child Neurology), 36% had concomitant epilepsy,[34] defined as the occurrence of two or more unprovoked seizures. MR (IQ ≤70) was significantly more common among children with CP and epilepsy (54.5%) as compared to those with CP alone (32.4%).

Mental Retardation and Cerebral Palsy in Children with Epilepsy

To determine the extent of the association between seizures and MR or CP, investigators have also looked at the frequency of these disabilities in children with epilepsy.

Population-Based Studies

To obtain information on morbidity and development, children born in 1966 in two Finnish prov-inces were followed to the age of 14.[35] A combination of information sources was initiated during the mother's pregnancy in 1965. Data were available for 96% of all children born in those provinces during that year. Among children who experienced at least "one episode of paroxysmal disturbance of consciousness, sensation, or movement not associated with acute febrile episodes," the reported proportion with MR (IQ ≤70) was 21.2%, and the proportion with CP was 15.9%. Among children with MR, epilepsy was more common in children with an IQ lower than 50 (15.4%) as compared to those with an IQ between 50 and 70 (5.8%).

An unselected population of children aged 4–15 years and residing in the province of Turku, Finland, was investigated to identify those who had experienced at least two unprovoked seizures.[36] More than 31% of all children with epilepsy also had MR, defined as an IQ of less than 70.

Murphy et al.[7] determined the frequency of MR among 10-year-old children with epilepsy who were enrolled in the Metropolitan Atlanta Developmental Disabilities Study. The identification of children with epilepsy was extended to a review of records from electroencephalography laboratories in hospitals, clinics, and private physician's offices serving children of the Atlanta area. Epilepsy was defined as a history of two or more afebrile epileptic seizures diagnosed by a physician. MR (IQ ≤70) was present in 30% of the children with epilepsy, whereas CP was present in 18% of the children with epilepsy. Among the children with epilepsy and MR, 34% had an IQ between 50 and 70, whereas 66% were severely retarded, having an IQ of less than 50.

Steffenburg et al.[37] reported that 38% of children aged 6–13 years who had active epilepsy (at least one epileptic seizure during the 5-year period preceding the prevalence day, regardless of AED treatment) also had MR. In the incidence series of epilepsy in Rochester, Minnesota, 8% of all patients had MR or CP (or both). These were codiagnoses in nearly 15% of children younger than 15 years who had newly diagnosed epilepsy.[38] The National Collaborative Perinatal Project, which examined the incidence of MR, CP, and seizures in a cohort of approximately 50,000 infants followed from conception to age 7 years, also found a substantially increased rate of MR and CP in children with seizure disorders, especially among those with minor motor seizures.[16]

Clinical Series

Braathen and Theorell[39] evaluated the frequency of MR alone or in combination with other disabilities in an unselected population of newly diagnosed childhood epilepsy cases. The study included all children younger than 16 years who had epilepsy, defined as "recurrent unprovoked seizures of cerebral origin," and who started treatment with AEDs during a 2-year period (1990–1992) in the catchment area of a general hospital of Southern Stockholm. Seventy-nine children with epilepsy were identified, 19 (24%) of whom had MR alone or in combination with other disabilities.

More recent community-based series have reported significant neurologic disability in a smaller proportion of children. Berg et al.[40] identified a community-based, unselected cohort of 613 children (age 1 month to 15 years) in Connecticut, who presented with newly diagnosed epilepsy between 1993 and 1997. Eighteen percent of this cohort was classified as having a remote sympathetic etiology, on the basis of the International League Against Epilepsy classification for epidemiologic purposes.[26] The majority of these symptomatic patients had MR or CP.

Factors Predictive of Epilepsy in the Context of Cerebral Palsy and Mental Retardation

The factors associated with the development of epilepsy in children with neurologic deficits from birth are not simple. In a study evaluating prenatal and perinatal characteristics of children affected by CP alone, CP and MR, or CP, MR, and epilepsy found that patients with a combination of the three disabilities were more likely to have a history of neonatal convulsions (a reflection of severity of insult?) and a family history of epilepsy in first-degree relatives.[41] CP, MR, and epilepsy were less likely to occur in children of mothers older than 32 years at delivery, in children with a gestational age of less than 32 weeks, or in children with a birth weight of less than 1,500 g. Similar findings were observed in a

clinic-based cohort from the Kennedy Center in the Bronx.[27,28] In this series, mean birth weight was greater and gestational age longer in the children with CP and epilepsy. Neonatal seizures were more frequent in children with MR and CP without epilepsy. Familial predisposition to epilepsy in children with CP was noted by Aksu,[42] who found a history of epilepsy in parents or siblings of 16% of patients with CP, as compared to only 8% of children with epilepsy without CP.

The findings of these studies suggest that the nature of insults that occur in preterm low-birth-weight infants may differ from the insults that occur in full-term babies and may be less likely to be associated with subsequent epilepsy. They also indicate that a family history of epilepsy may be an additive risk factor for the development of epilepsy, even in children who are already at risk because of neurologic disability. This has been reported in children with febrile seizures for whom a family history of epilepsy is a risk factor for the development of subsequent epilepsy even in children who are neurologically abnormal.[16]

Clinical Characteristics of Seizures in Children with Mental Retardation and Cerebral Palsy

Age of Onset

The age of onset of epilepsy is earlier in children with MR or CP than in children without these conditions. Among children who present with a first unprovoked seizure before age 20, this first seizure occurred earlier than age 3 years in only 27%.[43] In the study of new-onset epilepsy, defined as two or more unprovoked seizures, in children younger than 15 in Connecticut, 14% experienced their first episode before age 1 year.[40] This contrasts with age of onset of epilepsy in a prevalence cohort of people with MR and epilepsy of all ages, in which almost 27% of patients with MR experienced seizures during the first year of life.[23] Seizures occurred at between 1 and 7 years in another 59% of patients. Overall, the first seizure occurred before age 17 in 84% of individuals.

In the population-based series from Goteborg, Sweden, of children between ages 6 and 13 years with active epilepsy and MR, the median age at seizure onset was 1.3 years.[37] Children with severe MR had a significantly earlier seizure onset (median age, 0.8 years) than those with moderate MR (median age, 3.1 years). The onset of epilepsy occurred before age 1 year in 43% of cases, a statistic that is higher than that reported in the previously described population-based study of all childhood epilepsy in Sweden, in which 27% of all children with active epilepsy experienced onset before age 1.[44]

In the Finnish series from the Tampere region, 54% of children with MR and epilepsy experienced onset of epilepsy before the age of 1 year, and 85% had experienced their first seizures by the age of 3 years.[29] Among those who experienced the first seizure in the first year of life, 71% also had CP, whereas CP was present in only 39% of patients who had the first seizure after the first 12 months of life.

Zafeiriou et al.[34] compared two series of patients with epilepsy (with and without CP) whose epilepsy had been diagnosed according to identical criteria. The age of onset was significantly earlier in the group with CP. Onset of epilepsy in the first year of life occurred in 71% of children with CP as compared to 5.3% of children without CP.

Among children with intractable epilepsy with onset before the age of 13 years, the first seizure occurred significantly earlier (2.1 years) in mentally retarded children (IQ <70) as compared to those children with a normal IQ (IQ ≥70, 5.0 years).[45]

Although children with MR experience an earlier onset of epilepsy, onset clearly is not restricted to the very young. The risk of developing epilepsy remains elevated in children with MR at least through the second decade of life.[5,27,28] Goulden et al.[5] found a cumulative risk for epilepsy of 9%, 11%, 13%, and 15% by age 5, 10, 15, and 22 years, respectively. Among those with MR only, the risk did not differ between those with severe MR and moderate MR. The cumulative risk was highest in the group of children with MR and CP. In all groups, new cases appeared in the second decade of life. Similarly, the clinic-based series from the Children's Evaluation and Rehabilitation Center in the Bronx, New York, also found new cases of epilepsy occurring well into the second decade of life.[5,27,28]

As do children with MR, children with CP develop epilepsy in early childhood, 39%[42] to nearly 70%[34] of such children experiencing their first seizure in the first 12 months of life. The median age of onset of epilepsy in children with associated CP (18 months) was substantially younger than in children with epilepsy without CP (84 months). In the study by Hadjipanayis et al.,[33] the first seizure occurred in 58% of children with tetraplegia and epilepsy, as compared to 29.6% of patients with diplegia and 19.6% of those with hemiplegia. Only 6.3% of the epilepsy population without CP experienced their first seizure in the first 12 months of life.

Seizure Types and Frequency

Multiple seizure types, frequent seizures, and intractable seizures characterize epilepsy in children with MR. In the Atlanta Developmental Disabilities Study,[21] multiple seizure types occurred in 25% of children with profound MR, whereas none of the children with mild MR had multiple seizure types. In the population-based study of children with MR and epilepsy from Goteborg, 46% of the children exhibited more than one seizure type.[37] In this study, 30% had a combination of two and 16% had three or more seizure types. The most common seizure types were tonic-clonic, myoclonic, atypical absence, and partial complex seizures.

MR and CP, when present in children with epilepsy, are factors that predict therapeutic resistance to AEDs. In a study of children with MR and epilepsy, 27% of children with MR[23] experienced more than 50 seizures, and 11% experienced more than 300 seizures the year before they were included in the study. Among mentally retarded patients with epilepsy, 5% were being treated with AEDs and, of these, more than 33% were on two AEDs, 15% on three AEDs, and 1% on four AEDs. Huttenlocher and Hapke[45] found that among children with seizures refractory to medical therapy, 61% of children had mild to moderate MR.

Hosking et al.[46] evaluated the frequency of MR or CP in children with epilepsy who were seen at a pediatric center. As compared to those without any neurologic disability, children with CP or severe intellectual impairment had three times the number of admissions to a hospital because of difficulties with seizure control and four times the number of changes in medication for lack of control or the occurrence of side effects. Children with neurologic abnormality also were more likely to remain on two or more AEDs (50%) as compared to those without such abnormality (34%).

Children with CP were more often on AED polytherapy than were children without CP.[29] Zafeiriou et al.[34] found that 53% of patients with epilepsy and CP were on polytherapy as compared to 30% of those with epilepsy without CP. High seizure frequency also was observed in children with CP (52%) as compared to those without CP (31%).[34] In addition, children with CP were more likely to experience prolonged seizures and to require multiple medications to control those seizures.[29] The increased susceptibility of children to very prolonged seizures, including status epilepticus, is well known.[2,47–53] Children are also at increased risk for recurrent episodes of prolonged seizures.[53–55]

Prognosis of Seizures in Children with Developmental Disabilities

Remission

Prognosis of epilepsy is influenced strongly by many factors. Most individuals who develop epilepsy have a high likelihood of achieving remission and, eventually, many patients successfully discontinue the use of medications.[56–60] Frequency of seizures, type of seizure, and number of seizure types are important predictors of outcome. Children with MR, CP, or both have lower remission rates than do children in the general population.[57,58] An overall 5-year seizure-free remission rate of 56% was observed by age 22 years in patients with epilepsy who had MR but no CP.[5] Remission rates were lower (47%) in patients with both MR and CP.

Sillanpaa et al.[60] followed a population-based cohort of 245 patients with childhood-onset epilepsy. Of the 176 survivors available for follow-up in 1992, 30 years or more after the onset of their epilepsy, 143 (81%) had attained 5-year remission at some point, and 112 (64%) were in terminal 5-year remission on or off medications. However, only 45% of the remote symptomatic cases (the majority of whom had MR, CP, or both) were in 5-year terminal remission, as compared with 68% of those with epilepsy of cryptogenic etiology and 92% of those with idiopathic epilepsy. When one limits classifica-

tion of remission status to remission free of AED use, the differences are even more striking. Of the cohort, 47% were in 5-year terminal remission off medications. However, only 19% of those with a remote symptomatic etiology met this criterion, as compared with 57% of those with epilepsy of cryptogenic etiology and 86% of those with idiopathic epilepsy (Figure 1-2). Remission could be achieved even many years after seizure onset.

So that the prognosis of seizures in children with CP could be determined, children referred to a neuropediatric center for seizure disorder were divided in two groups according to the presence or absence of a delayed motor development.[42] AEDs were discontinued if no seizures had occurred for at least 2 years. This end point—seizure freedom off medication—occurred more commonly in patients with epilepsy without CP (52%) than in patients with epilepsy and CP (14%). Seizures recurred after drug withdrawal in 62.5% of patients with CP, whereas only 24.6% of patients without CP experienced relapses. Similar findings were reported by Hosking et al.[46]: Only 5% of children with CP or intellectual impairment reached "ultimate freedom" from seizures, as compared with 44% of children with epilepsy only.

Zafeiriou et al.[34] determined the rates of relapse after discontinuation of AEDs after a 3-year seizure-free period in patients with epilepsy with and without CP. The relapse rate in patients with epilepsy without CP was 4.7%, as compared to 24.7% in the CP group. Interpretation of the results of this study is difficult as the relapse rate in children without CP was lower than in any other series of medication withdrawal in children or adults.[57,61,62]

In studies focusing on medication withdrawal, the presence of MR or CP has consistently been associated with an increased risk of relapse after medication withdrawal.[57,61,62] Shinnar et al.[62] withdrew medications from 264 children who were seizure-free for 2 or more years. Recurrence risk was higher (rate ratio, 1.81) in those with epilepsy of remote symptomatic etiology (almost all of whom had MR or CP) than in those with cryptogenic or idiopathic epilepsy. Etiology remained a significant predictor of relapse on multivariable analysis. Although children with MR or CP had an increased risk of recurrence after medication withdrawal, approximately 50% remained seizure-free, indicating that medication withdrawal is feasible even in this group if they become seizure-free. In

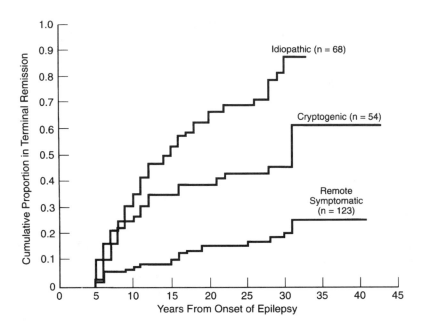

Figure 1-2. Cumulative probability of attaining 5-year terminal remission off antiepileptic drugs in a Finnish childhood-onset epilepsy cohort as a function of etiology. Kaplan-Meier curves. (Reprinted with permission of M Sillanpaa, M Jalava, O Kaleva, S Shinnar. Long-term prognosis of seizures with onset in childhood. N Engl J Med 1998;338:1715–1722.)

No. of Events/No. at Risk (No. Alive and in Follow-Up)

	Years 0–9	**Years 10–19**	**Years 20–29**	**Years 30–39**
Idiopathic	20/68 (68)	19/44 (64)	8/20 (59)	3/6 (51)
Cryptogenic	13/54 (54)	7/39 (51)	3/30 (49)	4/22 (44)
Remote symptomatic	8/123 (123)	9/103 (112)	2/77 (98)	3/46 (84)

children with remote symptomatic epilepsy, presence of moderate to severe MR, but not mild MR or CP, was an additional risk factor for recurrence.

In a meta-analysis of the studies of medication withdrawal in both children and adults available up to 1993, Berg and Shinnar[57] examined the effect of MR or CP on relapse rate. The presence of a remote symptomatic etiology (pooled relative risk, 1.55), of MR (pooled relative risk, 1.66), or of CP (pooled relative risk, 1.79) increased the relapse rate after medication withdrawal, as compared with patients with cryptogenic or idiopathic epilepsy.

Intractability

Children with developmental disabilities who have epilepsy are not only less likely to achieve remission but also are more likely to develop medically refractory, intractable epilepsy.[63–65] In a general hospital population of children with epilepsy,[38] 23% were considered to have intractable epilepsy, defined as the occurrence of more than one seizure per month despite adequate AED plasma levels. Among those with a therapy-resistant epilepsy, 72% were children with neurologic disability (MR and CP). Fois et al.[66] observed that 82% of children with epilepsy who did not respond to treatment were mentally retarded. These children experienced from several seizures per day to at least one seizure per month while being treated with three major AEDs. Conversely, of those who achieved complete clinical control of seizures on medications, only 38% had MR.

In children with MR and epilepsy, the number of seizure types and the frequency of seizures, together with the severity of MR, the occurrence of status epilepticus, and the occurrence of tonic seizures, all were independent predictive factors for intractable epilepsy.[63–65] Early age at onset of epilepsy and the occurrence of infantile spasms have also been associated with intractability in this population.[63]

Mortality

People with epilepsy have an increased mortality when compared with the general population.[67,68] The increased mortality is related to the etiology of the epilepsy.[60,67,68] Both seizure frequency and the presence of another neurologic impairment have a strong influence on mortality risk.[60,69]

Few studies have evaluated mortality in patients with epilepsy and MR or CP (or both). In a population-based study of children with epilepsy,[70] no increase in mortality was noted in children who showed no signs of neurologic impairment, but mortality was increased in children with MR or CP. Because children with MR have increased mortality even without epilepsy, interpreting these findings is difficult. Significantly increased mortality has been observed in persons with MR (standardized mortality ratio [SMR], 1.6) as compared to the general population.[71] Mortality was even higher when MR was associated with epilepsy (SMR, 5.0) and with epilepsy and CP (SMR, 5.8) as compared to the general population. The increase was more pronounced in the youngest in all groups (MR, MR plus epilepsy, MR plus epilepsy plus CP). In individuals with MR and epilepsy, mortality was increased for all seizure types but was more pronounced in persons with generalized seizures. Mortality increased with increasing number of seizures per year (SMR, 4.7 in those with 1–50 seizures per year; SMR, 16.8 in those with >50 seizures per year). Whether mortality was directly correlated to the presence of epilepsy was impossible to determine. A detailed analysis of the circumstances at the time of death of patients with epilepsy showed that none died of a seizure.

Sillanpaa et al.[60] examined the mortality in a cohort of 245 subjects with childhood-onset epilepsy who were followed up for 30 years. Among these patients, 44 deaths occurred, all but 5 in patients either who were not in seizure remission or who had remote symptomatic epilepsy. Thirty-three of the deaths occurred in the 123 subjects with remote symptomatic epilepsy, as compared with 11 deaths in the 122 subjects with cryptogenic or idiopathic epilepsy (p <.001). In the remote symptomatic group, death was definitely or probably related to seizures in 14 cases and to the underlying neurologic disorder in 19, including pneumonia in 12.

Among children with CP and epilepsy, 78% of those who died during a 5-year follow-up period (12% of all children) had severe or profound MR.[29] It has been suggested that prognosis, including intellectual impairment, is determined largely by the underlying origin of seizures and not by the seizures per se.[72,73]

Conclusion

Epilepsy, MR, and CP are manifestations of structural or functional central nervous system disorders. The risk of epilepsy in children with MR or CP is substantially higher than that seen in the general population and is related to the number of disabilities and their severity. The risk remains elevated at least through the first 20 years of life. Among individuals with MR or CP, epilepsy is characterized by (1) early onset of seizures; (2) high initial seizure frequency; (3) presence of multiple seizure types; (4) an increased rate of drug resistance (i.e., a need for polytherapy), especially when MR and CP are associated; (5) lower remission rates; (6) higher recurrence of seizures after treatment is interrupted; (7) higher rates of intractable epilepsy; and (8) increased mortality as compared to that of the general population or patients with epilepsy only.

More studies are necessary to determine whether epilepsy is merely a reflection of an increased severity of the two disabilities or whether epilepsy occurring in the context of MR and CP is a manifestation of additional risk factors. The contribution of epilepsy to adverse outcomes, including mortality, in this population also requires further clarification. The role of genetic susceptibility, which appears to be important in all three conditions, and its interactions with other factors must be explored. Finally, clinicians caring for children with MR and CP need to be familiar with the diagnosis and management of epilepsy in this population, as it is a frequent and serious comorbidity to these disorders.

References

1. Berg AT. The Epidemiology of Seizures and Epilepsy in Children. In S Shinnar, N Amir, D Branski (eds), Childhood Seizures. Basel: S Karger, 1995;1–10.
2. Hauser WA, Hesdorffer DC. Epilepsy: Frequency, Causes and Consequences. New York: Demos Publications, 1990;2–51.
3. Hauser WA, Annegers JF, Kurland LT. Prevalence of epilepsy in Rochester, Minnesota: 1940–1980. Epilepsia 1991;32:429–445.
4. Hauser WA. The prevalence and incidence of convulsive disorders in children. Epilepsia 1994;2[Suppl 35]:1–6.
5. Goulden KJ, Shinnar S, Koller H, et al. Epilepsy in children with mental retardation: a cohort study. Epilepsia 1991;32:690–697.
6. Kiely M. The prevalence of mental retardation. Epidemiol Rev 1987;9:194–218.
7. Murphy CC, Yeargin-Allsopp M, Decoufle P, Drews CD. The administrative prevalence of mental retardation in 10-year-old children in metropolitan Atlanta, 1985 through 1987. Am J Public Health 1995;85(3):319–323.
8. Blomquist HK, Gustavson KH, Holmgren G. Mild mental retardation in children in a northern Swedish county. J Ment Defic Res 1981;25[Pt 3]:169–186.
9. Hasan Z, Hasan A. report on a population survey of mental retardation in Pakistan. Int J Ment Health 1981;19:23–27.
10. Narayanan HS. A study of the prevalence of mental retardation in Southern India. Int J Ment Health 1981;10:28–36.
11. Zaman SS, Khan NZ, Durkin MS, Islam S. Childhood Disabilities in Bangladesh. Dhaka: Protibondi Foundation, 1992.
12. Durkin MS, Hasan ZM, Hasan KZ. Prevalence and correlates of mental retardation among children in Karachi, Pakistan. Am J Epidemiol 1998;147(3):281–288.
13. Stein ZA, Durkin MS, Belmont L. Serious mental retardation in developing countries: an epidemiological approach. Ann N Y Acad Sci 1986;477:8–21.
14. Susser M, Hauser WA, Kiely JL, et al. Quantitative Estimates of Prenatal and Perinatal Risk Factors for Perinatal Mortality, Cerebral Palsy, Mental Retardation and Epilepsy. In JM Freeman (ed), Prenatal and Perinatal Factors Associated with Brain Disorders.

NIH Publ. No. 85-1149. Bethesda, MD: National Institutes of Health, 1985;359–439.
15. Nelson KB, Ellenberg JH. Obstetric complications as risk factors for cerebral palsy or seizure disorders. JAMA 1984:251:1843–1848.
16. Nelson KB, Ellenberg JH. Antecedents of seizure disorders in early childhood. Am J Dis Child 1986;140:1053–1061.
17. Bax MCO. Terminology and classification of cerebral palsy. Dev Med Child Neurol 1964;6:295–297.
18. Nelson KB, Ellenberg JH. Antecedents of cerebral palsy: I. Univariate analysis of risk. Am J Dis Child 1985;139:1031–1038.
19. Nelson KB, Ellenberg JH. Antecedents of cerebral palsy. Multivariate analysis of risk. N Engl J Med 1986;315:81–86.
20. Nelson KB, Ellenberg JH. The asymptomatic newborn and risk of cerebral palsy. Am J Dis Child 1987;141:1333–1335.
21. Trevathan E, Yeargin-Allsopp M, Murphy CC, Ding G. Epilepsy among children with mental retardation. Ann Neurol 1988;28:321.
22. Murphy CC, Trevathan E, Yeargin-Allsopp M. Prevalence of epilepsy and epileptic seizures in 10-year-old children: results from the Metropolitan Atlanta Developmental Disabilities Study. Epilepsia 1995;36:866–872.
23. Forsgren L, Edvinsson SO, Blomquist HK, et al. Epilepsy in a population of mentally retarded children and adults. Epilepsy Res 1990;6:234–248.
24. Steffenburg U, Hagberg G, Viggedal G, Kyllerman M. Active epilepsy in mentally retarded children: I. Prevalence and additional neuro impairments. Acta Paediatr 1995;84:1147–1152.
25. Nevo Y, Shinnar S, Samuel E, et al. Unprovoked seizures and developmental disabilities: clinical characteristics of children referred to a child development center. Pediatr Neurol 1995;13:235–241.
26. Commission on Epidemiology and Prognosis, International League Against Epilepsy. Guidelines for epidemiologic studies on epilepsy. Epilepsia 1993;34:592–596.
27. Benedetti MD, Shinnar S, Cohen H, et al. Risk factors for epilepsy in children with cerebral palsy and/or mental retardation. Epilepsia 1987;27:614.
28. Hauser WA, Shinnar S, Cohen H, et al. Clinical predictors of epilepsy among children with cerebral palsy and/or mental retardation. Neurology 1987;37[Suppl 1]:150.
29. Eriksson K, Erila T, Kivimaki T, Koivikko M. Evolution of epilepsy in children with mental retardation: five-year experience in 78 cases. Am J Ment Retard 1998;102:464–472.
30. Kudrjavcev T, Schoenberg BS, Kurland LT, Groover RV. Cerebral palsy: survival rates, associated handicaps, and distribution by clinical subtype (Rochester, MN, 1950–1976). Neurology 1985;35:900–903.

31. Sussova J, Seidl Z, Faber J. Hemiparetic forms of cerebral palsy in relation to epilepsy and mental retardation. Dev Med Child Neurol 1990;32:792–795.

32. Mrabet A, Bouteraa M, Gouider R. Epilepsy and cerebral palsy. Epilepsia 1993;34[Suppl 2]:19.

33. Hadjipanayis A, Hadjichristodoulou C, Youroukos S. Epilepsy in patients with cerebral palsy. Dev Med Child Neurol 1997;39:659–663.

34. Zafeiriou DI, Kontopoulos EE, Tsikoulas I. Characteristics and prognosis of epilepsy in children with cerebral palsy. J Child Neurol 1999;14:289–294.

35. von Wendt L, Rantakallio P, Saukkonen AL, Makinen H. Epilepsy and associated handicaps in a 1 year birth cohort in northern Finland. Eur J Pediatr 1985;144:149–151.

36. Sillanpaa M. Epilepsy in children: prevalence, disability, and handicap. Epilepsia 1992;33:444–449.

37. Steffenburg U, Hagberg G, Kyllerman M. Characteristics of seizures in a population-based series of mentally retarded children with active epilepsy. Epilepsia 1996;37:850–856.

38. Hauser WA, Annegers JF, Kurland LT. Incidence of epilepsy and unprovoked seizures in Rochester, Minnesota: 1935–1984. Epilepsia 1993;34:453–468.

39. Braathen G, Theorell K. A general hospital population of childhood epilepsy. Acta Paediatr 1995;84:1143–1146.

40. Berg AT, Shinnar S, Levy SR, Testa FM. Newly diagnosed epilepsy in children: presentation at diagnosis. Epilepsia 1999;40:445–452.

41. Arpino C, Curatolo P, Stazi MA, et al. Differing risk factors for cerebral palsy in the presence of mental retardation and epilepsy. J Child Neurol 1999;14:151–155.

42. Aksu F. Nature and prognosis of seizures in patients with cerebral palsy. Dev Med Child Neurol 1990;32:661–668.

43. Shinnar S, Berg AT, Moshe SL, et al. The risk of seizure recurrence after a first unprovoked afebrile seizure in childhood: an extended follow-up. Pediatrics 1996;98:216–225.

44. Sidenvall R, Forsgren L, Heijbel J. Prevalence and characteristics of epilepsy in children in northern Sweden. Seizure 1996;5:139–146.

45. Huttenlocher PR, Hapke RJ. A follow-up study of intractable seizures in childhood. Ann Neurol 1990;28:699–705.

46. Hosking G, Miles R, Winstanley P. Seizures in patients with cerebral palsy. Dev Med Child Neurol 1990;32:1026–1027.

47. DeLorenzo RJ, Towne AR, Pellock JM, et al. Status epilepticus in children, adults and the elderly. Epilepsia 1992;33[Suppl 4]:S15–S25.

48. Gross-Tsur V, Shinnar S. Convulsive status epilepticus in children. Epilepsia 1993;34[Suppl 1]:S12–S20.

49. Hauser WA. Status epilepticus: epidemiologic considerations. Neurology 1990;40[Suppl 2]:9–13.

50. Maytal J, Shinnar S, Moshe SL, Alvarez LA. Low morbidity and mortality of status epilepticus in children. Pediatrics 1989;83:323–331.

51. Dodson WE, DeLorenzo RJ, Pedley TA, et al. The treatment of convulsive status epilepticus: recommendations of the Epilepsy Foundation of America's working group on status epilepticus. JAMA 1993;270:854–859.

52. Shinnar S, Pellock JM, Moshe SL, et al. In whom does status epilepticus occur? Age-related differences in children. Epilepsia 1997;38:907–914.

53. Sillanpaa M, Jalava M, Shinnar S. Status epilepticus in a population based cohort with childhood onset epilepsy in Finland. Epilepsia 1998;39[Suppl 6]:219–220.

54. Driscoll SM, Towne AR, Pellock JM, DeLorenzo RJ. Recurrent status epilepticus in children (abstract). Neurology 1990;40[Suppl 1]:297.

55. Shinnar S, Maytal J, Krasnoff L, Moshe SL. Recurrent status epilepticus in children. Ann Neurol 1992;31:598–604.

56. Annegers JF, Hauser WA, Elveback LR. Remission of seizures and relapse in patients with epilepsy. Epilepsia 1979;20:729–737.

57. Berg AT, Shinnar S. Relapse following discontinuation of antiepileptic drugs: a meta-analysis. Neurology 1994;44:601–608.

58. Berg AT, Hauser WA, Shinnar S. The Prognosis of Childhood-Onset Epilepsy. In S Shinnar, N Amir, D Branski (eds), Childhood Seizures. Basel: S Karger, 1995;93–99.

59. Cockerell OC, Johnson AL, Sander JW, Shorvon SD. Prognosis of epilepsy: a review and further analysis of the first nine years of the British National General Practice Study of Epilepsy, a prospective population-based study. Epilepsia 1997;38:31–46.

60. Sillanpaa M, Jalava M, Kaleva O, Shinnar S. Long-term prognosis of seizures with onset in childhood. N Engl J Med 1998;338:1715–1722.

61. Berg AT, Shinnar S, Chadwick D. Discontinuing Antiepileptic Drugs. In J Engel Jr, TA Pedley (eds), Epilepsy: A Comprehensive Textbook. Philadelphia: Lippincott–Raven, 1997;1275–1284.

62. Shinnar S, Berg AT, Moshe SL, et al. Discontinuing antiepileptic drugs in children with epilepsy: a prospective study. Ann Neurol 1994;35:534–545.

63. Berg AT, Levy SR, Novotny EJ, Shinnar S. Predictors of intractable epilepsy in childhood: a case control study. Epilepsia 1996;37:24–30.

64. Berg AT, Shinnar S, Testa FM, et al. Prediction of early intractability in childhood-onset epilepsy. Epilepsia 1999;40[Suppl 7]:160.

65. Steffenburg U, Hedstrom A, Lindroth A, et al. Intractable epilepsy in a population-based series of mentally retarded children. Epilepsia 1998;39:767–775.

66. Fois A, Tomaccini D, Balestri P, et al. Intractable epilepsy: etiology, risk factors and treatment. Clin Electroencephalogr 1988;19:68–73.

67. Hauser WA, Annegers JF, Elveack LR. Mortality in patients with epilepsy. Epilepsia 1980;21:339–412.

68. Cockerell OC, Johnson AL, Sander JWAS, et al. Mortality from epilepsy: results from a retrospective population-based study. Lancet 1994;344:918–921.

69. Henriksen PB, Juul-Jensen P, Lund M. The Mortality of Epileptics. In: RDC Brackenridge (ed), Proceedings of the Tenth International Congress of Life Assurance Medicine. London: Putnam, 1970.

70. Brorson LO, Wranne L. Long-term prognosis in childhood epilepsy: survival and seizure prognosis. Epilepsia 1987;29:324–330.

71. Forsgren L, Edvinsson SO, Nystrom L, Blomquist HK. Influence of epilepsy on mortality in mental retardation: an epidemiologic study. Epilepsia 1996; 37:956–963.

72. Berg AT, Shinnar S. The contributions of epidemiology to the understanding of childhood seizures and epilepsy. J Child Neurol 1994;9[Suppl 2]:19–26.

73. Dreifuss FE. Prognosis of childhood seizure disorders: present and future. Epilepsia 1994;35[Suppl 2]:S30–S34.

Chapter 2

Metabolic and Genetic Disorders

Edwin H. Kolodny

Metabolic and genetic disorders are a major diagnostic consideration whenever the physician is confronted with cognitive impairment, developmental disabilities, and epilepsy. At the first appearance of developmental delay or seizures, rarely are the clinical signs so specific that the diagnosis is obvious. Even after some months and progression of the disease, the diagnosis often is still in doubt. A biochemical, molecular DNA, or chromosomal anomaly or cerebral malformation can remain hidden, to be discovered only after the appropriate tests are carried out.

As hundreds of metabolic and genetic diseases can be associated with developmental disabilities and epilepsy,[1,2] how can a clinician keep track of this field and know which tests are indicated in a particular case? The aim of this chapter is to describe the approach that the author has found useful in meeting this challenge.

Family History

We generally start by obtaining a family history. Parental consanguinity can raise the presumption of an autosomal recessive disease. More than one affected sibling or close relative in a family also is suggestive of a familial disorder. A maternal inheritance pattern may be a clue to an X-linked disorder, such as Menkes' syndrome, or to the transmission of a defect in mitochondrial DNA, as in mitochondrial encephalomyopathy, lactic acidosis, and strokelike episodes (MELAS). Phe-

notypic heterogeneity can occur even within the same family, so that differences in symptomatology and time course of the illness can be found among siblings receiving the same diagnosis, as in adrenoleukodystrophy and globoid cell leukodystrophy. Availability of a family pedigree provides an opportunity to counsel unaffected family members concerning their own risk for having the disease or for carrying the abnormal gene.

Physical Examination

The physical appearance of the patient can be very helpful in determining a diagnosis. A high forehead is suggestive of a peroxisomal disorder (e.g., Zellweger syndrome or neonatal adrenoleukodystrophy), of lissencephaly, or of the fragile X syndrome. Frontal bossing may suggest Hurler's syndrome, GM_1 gangliosidosis, mucolipidosis II (I-cell disease), or multiple sulfatase deficiency. Microcephaly is characteristic of Angelman's syndrome, Cockayne's syndrome, Smith-Lemli-Opitz syndrome, and Rett syndrome. Other causes of craniofacial deformities associated with epilepsy include pyruvate dehydrogenase deficiency, Lowe syndrome, molybdenum cofactor deficiency, and glutaric aciduria type II (Table 2-1).

Defects in hair and skin are also important clues. Loss of hair occurs in biotinidase deficiency and Cockayne's syndrome, whereas other anomalies of hair typically are found in the muco-

Table 2-1. Cerebral and Somatic Dysmorphism with Epilepsy

Angelman's syndrome
Cockayne's syndrome
Glutaric aciduria type II
Hypomelanosis of Ito
Lissencephaly
Lowe syndrome
Molybdenum cofactor deficiency
Pyruvate dehydrogenase deficiency
Rett syndrome
Smith-Lemli-Opitz syndrome
Tuberous sclerosis
Zellweger syndrome

polysaccharidoses, Menkes' syndrome, and argininosuccinic aciduria. Examination of the skin can reveal nodular lesions on the face and depigmented macules in tuberous sclerosis; café au lait spots and neurofibromas in neurofibromatosis; streaked, whirled, and mottled areas of hyperpigmentation in hypomelanosis of Ito; and thin, atrophic skin in Cockayne's syndrome. A Wood's lamp examination of the skin for hypopigmentation is, therefore, a routine part of our workup of a child who is experiencing seizures.

Growth failure is a common feature of many hereditary metabolic diseases. Short stature is found in patients with the mucopolysaccharidoses and mucolipidoses and in mitochondrial encephalopathies such as Leigh disease, MELAS, and myoclonic epilepsy with ragged red fibers (MERFF).

Hepatomegaly with liver dysfunction may be a sign of Wilson's disease, the Alpers-Huttenlocker syndrome, or Niemann-Pick disease type C. The liver is enlarged early in the course of Niemann-Pick disease types A and B, but liver failure occurs only as a late sequela. Liver failure is found also in certain mitochondrial disorders and in Zellweger syndrome. Splenomegaly in an infant with seizures will suggest type 2 Gaucher's disease, whereas a later onset with seizures and myoclonus is typical of type 3 Gaucher's disease.

Neurologic Examination

Assessment of the very young child with seizures is hampered by the very limited repertoire of

which the nervous system is capable. Nevertheless, one can acquire a good estimate of the child's capabilities by observing his or her level of alertness and interaction with the surroundings and the child's vocalization, feeding habits, motor activity, and muscle tone. Severe hypotonia at birth and progressive spasticity are common to many neurodegenerative diseases.

Vision loss accompanies several neurodegenerative diseases, including the leukodystrophies (e.g., Krabbe's disease and Canavan's disease) and neuronal storage diseases (e.g., GM_1 and GM_2 gangliosidoses, sialidosis type I, and the neuronal ceroid-lipofuscinoses). Findings in the retina may include optic atrophy in the leukodystrophies and Menkes' syndrome, a cherry-red macula in the gangliosidoses and sialidosis type I, and retinal pigmentary degeneration in Cockayne's syndrome, the neuronal ceroid-lipofuscinoses, and mitochondrial encephalopathies. Cortical blindness as an early sign prompts consideration of adrenoleukodystrophy or juvenile globoid cell leukodystrophy and often is part of the clinical picture of MELAS. Disturbances in ocular motility with gaze initiation failure occur in type 2 Gaucher's disease and Niemann-Pick disease type C. Supranuclear palsies of conjugate gaze are also a feature of Leigh disease and Huntington's disease.

Cerebellar ataxia may be noted after the child begins to reach for objects, to sit, and to stand. It may be progressive, as in the sphingolipidoses and in cerebrotendinous xanthomatosis or episodic, as in the aminoacidopathies and organic acidopathies. Rigidity, dystonia, chorea, bradykinesia, athetosis, and tremor are useful extrapyramidal signs of metabolic disease. Among the metabolic diseases that should be considered are Wilson's disease, juvenile Huntington's disease, dentatorubral-pallidoluysian atrophy, and glutaric aciduria type I.

The involvement of peripheral nerves can assist in making a diagnosis of neurometabolic disease. Demyelinating neuropathy occurs in Krabbe's disease, metachromatic leukodystrophy, and Cockayne's syndrome. Schindler's disease and Lowe syndrome are distinguished by an axonal neuropathy. A peripheral neuropathy may also occur in some of the mitochondrial disorders, in Sanfilippo's syndrome, and in neonatal adrenoleukodystrophy.

Age of Onset

The age of onset of seizures is another important element in arriving at a diagnosis. Cerebral malformations such as lissencephaly give rise to frequent seizures as early as the neonatal period. Hypoglycemia, hypocalcemia, intracranial hemorrhage or infection, and drug withdrawal must also be considered when seizures occur in the neonate. Among the hereditary metabolic diseases, seizures in the neonatal period can include biotinidase deficiency,[3] vitamin B_6 dependency,[4] a urea cycle disorder, and Menkes' syndrome (Table 2-2).

Intractable seizures in the period of early infancy can result from Alpers' disease, glucose transporter protein deficiency,[5] and the Haltia-Santavuori variant of neuronal ceroid-lipofuscinosis (CLN1). Biotinidase deficiency and, occasionally, vitamin B_6 dependency may present at this time and not in the neonatal period. The child with Krabbe's disease begins by age 6 months to have seizures and, by 1 year, children with classic Tay-Sachs disease will manifest seizure activity.

The progressive myoclonic epilepsies are associated with clinical onset in later childhood and adolescence. Unverricht-Lundborg disease (Baltic myoclonus) is an autosomal recessive neurodegeneration in which myoclonic jerks and generalized tonic-clonic seizures are associated with progressive mental deterioration and ataxia. This disease has been identified with alterations in the *cystatin B (Stefin B)* gene. Lafora's disease, another autosomal recessive condition exhibiting myoclonus and dementia, is distinguished by periodic acid–Schiff–positive intracellular inclusion bodies in neurons and other tissues. The majority of patients have mutations in the *EPM2* gene on chromosome 6q23-q25.[6] Other familial forms of juvenile myoclonic epilepsy have been linked to chromosomes 6p21.2-p11 and 15q14.

Seizures are a frequent presenting feature in cases of juvenile neuronal ceroid-lipofuscinosis (CLN3), type 3 Gaucher's disease, and sialidosis type I. Later, in young adults, one may encounter seizures as a sign of mitochondrial disease such as MERFF. MERFF is a maternally inherited encephalomyopathy, in most cases due to an A8344G

Table 2-2. Inherited Metabolic Disease and Epilepsy

Neonatal period to early infancy
Pyridoxine dependency, biotinidase deficiency
Amino acidopathies, organic acidopathies
Urea cycle disorders
Menkes' syndrome, Alpers' disease
Glucose transporter protein deficiency
Molybdenum cofactor deficiency
Peroxisomal and mitochondrial diseases
Late infancy to early childhood
Lysosomal storage diseases
Neuronal ceroid-lipofuscinoses, Haltia-Santavuori-variant (CLN1)
Leigh disease
Cockayne's syndrome
Childhood and adolescence
Type 3 Gaucher's disease
Juvenile GM_2 gangliosidosis
Multiple sulfatase deficiency
Sanfilippo's syndrome
Sialidosis
Neuronal ceroid-lipofuscinosis, juvenile (CLN3)
MELAS, MERFF
Unverricht-Lundborg disease
Lafora's disease

MELAS = mitochondrial encephalomyopathy, lactic acidosis, and strokelike episodes; MERFF = myoclonic epilepsy with ragged red fibers.

transition in the tRNA *Lys* gene of mitochondrial DNA.

The familial occurrence of several rare forms of epilepsy has provided geneticists using linkage analysis the opportunity to assign a chromosomal locus to the defective gene, and, in a few instances, the gene itself has been cloned and mutations identified.[7,8] Examples of these are shown in Table 2-3. In the syndrome of benign familial neonatal convulsions, the seizures remit spontaneously by 6 weeks without treatment. Two loci for this autosomal dominant disorder have been found, each of which contains a potassium channel gene (*KCNQ2, KCNQ3*) in which mutations have been identified. Another familial disorder, termed *generalized epilepsy with febrile seizures plus*, has been described with mutations in a sodium channel gene (*SCN1B*). This gene, coded on chromosome 19, was considered a likely candidate because of the

Table 2-3. Genetic Forms of Epilepsy[a]

Epilepsy Type	Chromosomal Locus (+ Gene)
Benign familial neonatal convulsions	20q13.3 ($KCNQ2^b$); 8q24 ($KCNQ3^b$)
Childhood absence epilepsy with tonic-clonic seizures	8q24 ($KCNQ3^b$)
Familial adult myoclonic epilepsy	8q24 ($KCNQ3^b$)
Generalized seizures with febrile seizures plus	19q13.1 ($SCN1B^c$); ($SCN1A^c$)
Benign familial infantile convulsions syndrome	19q13.1 ($SCN1B^c$)
X-linked infantile spasms syndrome	Xp11.4-Xpter
Febrile seizures	8q13-21; 19p13.3; 2q23-24; 5q14-15
Idiopathic generalized epilepsy	3p14.2-12.1
Rolandic epilepsy, paroxysmal exercise-induced insomnia	16p12-11.2
AD infantile convulsions and paroxysmal choreoathetosis	
AD nocturnal frontal lobe epilepsy	20q13.2 ($CHRNA\ 4^d$); 10q, 15q24 ($CHRNA/CHRNA\ 5/ CHRNB\ 4$)
AD lateral temporal epilepsy	10q
Auditory partial epilepsy	10q22-24
Juvenile myoclonic epilepsy	6p21.2-11; 15q14
Unverricht-Lundborg type progressive myoclonic epilepsy	21q22.3
Lafora's disease	6q23-25
MERRF	mtDNA A8344G
Neuronal ceroid-lipofuscinosis	1p32 (CLN1); 16p22.2 (CLN3); 13q21-32 (CLN5)
Progressive epilepsy with mental retardation	8p

AD = autosomal dominant; MERRF = myoclonic epilepsy with ragged red fibers.
[a]Affected gene shown in parentheses.
[b]Voltage-gated potassium channels.
[c]Voltage-gated sodium channels.
[d]Nicotinic acetylcholine receptor alpha$_4$ subunit.

existence of ion channel defects in other paroxysmal disorders and the recognition that the anticonvulsants phenytoin and carbamazepine block sodium channels. The existence of rodent models of epilepsy involving other ion channel genes suggests that additional human epilepsies caused by channelopathies are likely to be discovered.

Ryan[9] has suggested that children with Angelman's syndrome who have a deletion in chromosome 15q11-13 may have more severe epilepsy than those with other causes of Angelman's syndrome because the deleted region includes the gene *GABRB3*, which codes for a GABA receptor–chloride ionophore β subunit.

Etiologic Classification

In planning the approach to diagnosis of developmental disability and seizures in a child, it is useful to consider the major categories of genetic and hereditary metabolic disease. These will guide the types and sequence of testing (Table 2-4).

First, the clinician should determine whether a nongenetic explanation exists for the symptoms. Recent trauma, child abuse with shaking and rupture of bridging veins, a brain tumor, and vascular malformation are considerations. Therefore, a brain imaging study is high on the list of useful tests whenever a progressive disorder is being evaluated. A magnetic resonance imaging scan might reveal a neuronal migration disorder, a leukodystrophy, an abnormality of the basal ganglia (e.g., striatal necrosis), or calcifications. In considering cerebral dysgenesis, we look for pachygyria, schizencephaly, polymicrogyria, heterotopias, and other forms of cortical dysplasia.[10] If a leukodystrophy is found, magnetic resonance spectroscopy might be used to demonstrate the elevation in *N*-acetyl aspartic acid characteristic of Canavan's disease.

Next, screening is performed using blood to determine the complete blood cell count and electrolytes, calcium, magnesium, glucose, lactic acid, pyruvic acid, ammonia, and biotinidase levels. Assessment of blood amino acids and very long-chain fatty acids for peroxisomal diseases and chromosomes (fluorescent in situ hybridization analysis) for Angelman's syndrome also may be undertaken, depending on the clinical findings. If a disorder of fatty acid oxidation is being considered, acylcarnitines are evaluated.

Urine can be examined for its content of *N*-acetyl aspartate (Canavan's disease), mucopolysaccharides (Sanfilippo's syndrome), ligosaccharides (sialidosis), and organic acids. A skin biopsy may be obtained to examine dermal nerves under the electron microscope for storage, as in the lysosomal diseases, Lafora's disease, and neuroaxonal dystrophy. The skin biopsy can also be used for fibroblast cell culture to conduct enzymatic and DNA mutation analyses.

A child's electroencephalogram may be abnormal even before the clinical appearance of seizures, as in Rett syndrome and Angelman's syndrome. For this reason, we examine the electroencephalogram as part of our routine study of the child with cognitive delay. Other neurophysiologic tests that can help to localize seizure pathology include evoked potentials, electromyography, and the study of sensory and motor nerve conduction.

Seizure Frequency and Types

Seizures are only an occasional event in the course of most inherited diseases. However, they may be the predominant symptom, as in lissencephaly, tuberous sclerosis, hypomelanosis of Ito, Zellweger syndrome, Menkes' syndrome, Alpers' disease, neuronal ceroid-lipofuscinosis, Lafora's disease, and Baltic myoclonus. Generally, inherited disease onset in infancy is associated with a greater frequency of seizures than is the appearance of such a disease in juvenile or adult life.

The seizure pattern in infancy generally is mixed, consisting of atypical absence, atonic, and myoclonic phenomena, but generalized seizures with prolonged postictal lethargy also occur. The mitochondrial encephalopathies are associated with myoclonic jerking and, in the case of MELAS, focal twitching.

Table 2-4. Laboratory Assessment

Blood
  Complete blood cell count, electrolytes, calcium, magnesium
  Uric acid
  Liver function tests, ammonia
  Lactic acid, pyruvic acid
  Acylcarnitines, amino acids
Urine
  Organic acids, mucopolysaccharides
  Sialic acid, oligosaccharides
  Purines and pyrimidines
Cerebrospinal fluid
  Glucose, protein, cells, catecholamines
Neurophysiology
  Electroencephalography, evoked potentials
Neuroradiology
  Brain magnetic resonance imaging
Tissue biopsies
  Skin
  Muscle

Treatment

The treatment of seizures due to inherited metabolic disease, chromosomal defects, and brain malformations is notoriously difficult. Pyridoxine-dependent epilepsy and biotinidase deficiency can be effectively managed by supplementation with vitamin B_6 or biotin, respectively. For some of the amino acid, organic acid, and urea cycle disorders, dietary manipulation may be helpful.

Selected cases of certain leukodystrophies (i.e., globoid cell leukodystrophy, metachromatic leukodystrophy, or adrenoleukodystrophy) in the early stage of illness may be amenable to bone marrow transplantation. However, for most genetically determined disorders, polypharmacy may be needed. Valproic acid, clonazepam, lamotrigine, and vigabatrin are the therapeutic mainstays. Controlling stimuli such as noise may reduce the frequency of seizures in patients with stimulus-sensitive myoclonus. Background music in the nursery may also help to raise some children's seizure threshold. Avoidance of metabolic stresses such as fever is important also, and frequent small feedings can help patients with mitochondrial disorders to circumvent their deficits in energy production.

Conclusion

The occurrence of seizures in a child with developmental delay can be an important clue to the presence of an inherited metabolic disease or other genetically determined disorder of the nervous system. As the actual cause may be occult, a systemic approach is needed in the investigation of these youngsters. Biochemical screening, electroencephalography, and brain magnetic resonance imaging are essential. Additional studies are determined by the family history, age of onset, the presence or absence of any distinguishing physical features, and the nature of the neurologic findings. In the management of any child with a developmental disability, the guiding principle should always be to uncover the primary etiology, as this will determine available treatment options, prognosis, and opportunities for preventing a recurrence of the disease in future family members.

Treatment should be tailored to correcting the metabolic error whenever possible. In many of the neurodegenerative disorders involving seizures, however, judicious use of anticonvulsants is the primary treatment modality. If a biochemical or DNA marker is available and the condition is serious enough to warrant prenatal diagnosis, the family should be informed about the availability of this option.

References

1. Lyon G, Adams RD, Kolodny EH. Neurology of Hereditary Metabolic Diseases of Children (2nd ed). New York: McGraw-Hill, 1996.
2. Anderson VE, Hauser WA. Genetics of Epilepsy. In AG Bearn, AG Motulskey, B Childs (eds), Progress in Medical Genetics: VI. Genetics of Neurological Disorders. New York: Praeger, 1998;9–52.
3. Pomponio RJ, Reynolds TR, Cole H, et al. Mutational hotspot in the human biotinidase gene causes profound biotinidase deficiency. Nat Genet 1995;11:96–98.
4. Plecko B, Stockler-Ipsiroglu S, Paschke E, et al. Pipecolic acid evaluation in plasma and cerebrospinal fluid of two patients with pyridoxine-dependent epilepsy. Ann Neurol 2000;48:121–125.
5. Seidner G, Alvarez MG, Yeh J-I, et al. GLUT-1 deficiency syndrome caused by haploinsufficiency of the blood-brain barrier hexose carrier. Nat Genet 1998;18:188–191.
6. Minassian BA, Ianzano L, Delgado-Escueta AV, Scherer SW. Identification of new and common mutations in the EPM2A gene in Lafora disease. Neurology 2000;54:488–490.
7. Szepetowski P, Monaco AP. Recent progress in the genetics of human epilepsies. Neurogenetics 1998;1:153–163.
8. Berkovic SF, Genton P, Hirsch E, Picard F. Genetics of Focal Epilepsies. London: John Libbey, 1999.
9. Ryan SG. Ion channels and the genetic contribution to epilepsy. J Child Neurol 1999;14:58–66.
10. Altman N, Palasis S, Pacheco-Jacome E. Advanced magnetic resonance imaging of disorders of neuronal migration and sulcation. Int Pediatr 1995;10[Suppl 1]:16–25.

Chapter 3

Childhood-Specific Epilepsies Accompanied by Developmental Disabilities: Causes and Effects

Gregory L. Holmes

Although they can occur at any age, seizures are far more common in children than adults. Among children, the highest incidence occurs during the first few years of life.[1,2] Animal studies have suggested that the increased excitability in the developing brain is secondary to a developmental imbalance between maturation of excitatory and inhibitory circuits.[3–8] The main inotropic receptors (γ-aminobutyric acid type A [GABA(A)], N-methyl-D-aspartate [NMDA], and alpha-amino-3-hydroxy-5-methyl-isoxazole-4-propionic acid [AMPA]) display a sequential developmental pattern of participation in neuronal excitation in the neonatal hippocampus.[6] GABA, the main *inhibitory* transmitter in the adult, provides the main *excitatory* drive to hippocampal neurons at early stages of postnatal development, owing to a chloride gradient that leads to depolarization of young neurons (as opposed to the hyperpolarization observed in adults).[7] The other major postsynaptic inhibitory system—postsynaptic GABA(B), adenosine, and 5-hydroxytryptamine–G protein–coupled potassium channels—also experiences delayed maturation, suggesting that the neonatal circuit operates without transmitter-gated inhibition. In contrast, presynaptic inhibition, mediated by adenosine, GABA(B), or other metabotropic receptors, is fully operational at birth, providing evidence that the major form of inhibition in the neonatal circuit is the control of transmitter release.[3]

Children with developmental disabilities are at even higher risk for seizures than is the general population.[9–11] In most children, the pathologic process responsible for the disability is responsible also for the epilepsy. The risk of epilepsy in children with developmental disabilities varies considerably. As a general rule, the more severe and extensive the cerebral pathology, the higher is the likelihood of epilepsy. For example, among children with cerebral palsy, those with quadriplegia, also termed *double hemiplegia*, have the highest incidence of epilepsy, whereas children with diplegia have the lowest incidence.[11–13]

In other situations, the epilepsy itself may be responsible for the disability. In such disorders as Landau-Kleffner syndrome, continuous spikes and waves during slow sleep (also known as *electrical status epilepticus of sleep*), Lennox-Gastaut syndrome, and infantile spasms, the seizures, epileptiform activity, or both either substantially contribute to or result in the disability. The term *epileptic encephalopathy* frequently is used to describe these conditions.[14]

In this chapter, infantile spasms is presented as an example of a syndrome in which the epileptic condition is responsible for all or part of the disability. Using infantile spasms as a backdrop, the

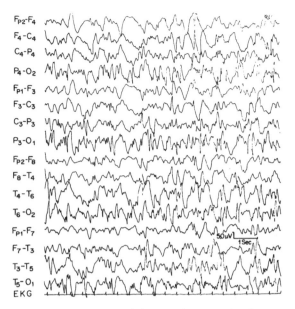

Figure 3-1. Electroencephalogram demonstrating hypsarrhythmia in an infant with infantile spasms. (EKG = electrocardiogram.)

biological effects of seizures on the developing brain are reviewed.

Infantile Spasms

Infantile spasms is a unique, and frequently malignant, epileptic syndrome confined to infants. The usual characteristic features of this syndrome are brief tonic seizures, hypsarrhythmic electroencephalograms (EEGs), and mental retardation.[15,16] The triad of infantile spasms, hypsarrhythmic EEG, and mental retardation is referred to as *West's syndrome.* Not all infants with infantile spasms conform strictly to this definition. Infantile spasms are an age-specific disorder beginning in children during the first 2 years of life. The peak age of onset is between 4 and 6 months of age. Most infantile spasms begin before 12 months of age, clustering between 4 and 7 months. It is unusual for infantile spasms to begin after 18 months.

Some seizures are characterized by brief head nods, whereas others consist of violent flexion of the trunk, arms, and legs. Infantile spasms can be classified into three major groups: flexor, extensor, and mixed flexor-extensor types.[17] Flexor spasms

consist of flexion of the neck, trunk, arms, and legs. Spasms of the muscles of the upper limbs result either in adduction of the arms in a self-hugging motion or in abduction of the arms to either side of the head with the arms flexed at the elbow. Extensor spasms consist of a predominance of extensor muscle contractions, producing abrupt extension of the neck and trunk, with extensor abduction or adduction of the arms, legs, or both. Mixed flexor-extensor spasms include flexion of the neck, trunk, and arms and extension of the legs, or flexion of the legs and extension of the arms with varying degrees of flexion of the neck and trunk. Asymmetric spasms occasionally occur and consist of maintenance of a "fencing" posture. Variability of infantile spasms occurs frequently, with the majority of patients having more than one seizure type.

Infantile spasms frequently occur in clusters, and the intensity and frequency of the spasms in each cluster may increase to a peak before progressively decreasing. The seizures are very brief, and single seizures may be missed by the casual observer. The number of seizures per cluster varies considerably, with some clusters consisting of as many as 150 seizures. The number of clusters per day also varies, with some patients having as many as 60 clusters per day. Clusters can occur rarely during sleep but frequently are seen shortly after awakening. Crying or irritability during or after a flurry of spasms is commonly observed. The number of infantile spasms occurring at night is similar to the number occurring during the day.

Infantile spasms are associated with markedly abnormal EEGs. The most commonly found EEG pattern is hypsarrhythmia,[18] which consists of a high-voltage, slow record dominated by delta activity with frequent and multifocal spikes, sharp waves, and spike and slow wave complexes (Figure 3-1). Variations of hypsarrhythmia include hypsarrhythmia with interhemispheric synchrony, hypsarrhythmia with a consistent focus of abnormal discharge, hypsarrhythmia with episodes of attenuation, and hypsarrhythmia consisting primarily of high-voltage slow activity with few sharp waves or spikes.[18] During sleep, especially rapid-eye-movement sleep, a marked reduction or total disappearance of the hypsarrhythmic pattern may be noted. Although the hypsarrhythmic or modified hypsarrhythmic pattern is the most common type of interictal abnormality seen in infantile spasms, it is not seen in all patients who have this disorder.

A high association exists between infantile spasms and developmental delay.[19–21] In a population-based epidemiologic study of infantile spasms, Trevathan et al.[20] found that 83% of children with a history of infantile spasms had mental retardation at 10 years of age. Profound mental retardation (intelligence quotient <20) was present in 56%. Of a total of 79 children with profound mental retardation living in the Atlanta, Georgia, area, 10% had a history of infantile spasms. Other authors have found infantile spasms to be a significant risk factor for subsequent mental retardation.[19,21–23] In a case-control analysis of 106 patients with tuberous sclerosis, Jozwiak et al.[23] found that the presence of infantile spasms was the only analyzed risk factor that showed a consistent and independent association with poor mental outcome.

The majority of infants who develop infantile spasms has developmental delay prior to the onset of the seizures, with both the developmental delay and spasms resulting from the same symptomatic etiology. However, infants who are normal prior to the onset of their spasms are at substantial risk for developing delays with the onset of the spasms.[24] Likewise, infants with developmental delay may regress after the onset of the spasms, with declines in attention, alertness, eye contact, and activity level. Unless this process can be reversed quickly, permanent impairment of the child is highly likely. Because early cessation of spasms is of prognostic significance, early diagnosis and treatment are essential.[25–28]

The degree of developmental regression that occurs in relation to the severity of the seizures is surprising. Although seizures may be frequent, spasms are relatively brief, lasting for only seconds, and rarely are associated with cyanosis or postictal sleep. Like Landau-Kleffner syndrome and continuous spikes and waves during slow sleep, the interictal EEG activity may be the primary cause of cognitive impairment. Hypsarrhythmia is a severely abnormal pattern, and this dysfunctional state probably prevents normal development. Developmental improvement in a child whose EEG remains so abnormal is unusual.

The reason that seizures during early development can be so detrimental remains undetermined.

Possibly, the combination of a severely chaotic EEG and spasms occurring at a critical developmental stage results in the affected child's unfortunate state. However, seizures occurring during early development display clinical and EEG features different from those seen in seizures in older children and adults, and so comparing the consequences of seizures in infants and adults is difficult. Infantile spasms and hypsarrhythmia will never occur de novo in an adult. Therefore, whether the developmental consequences of infantile spasms are unique to the patient's age or to the specific clinical and EEG features of this syndrome is unclear.

Mechanisms of Seizure-Induced Damage

The reasons that seizures during development can be harmful are myriad. The developing brain is highly plastic, and seizures during early development could have pronounced effects on brain development, perturbing a wide range of phenomena that is activity-dependent, including cell division, migration, sequential expression of receptors, formation and strengthening of synapses, and myelination. Much of the early work on seizure-induced brain damage has concentrated on cell death. Only recently has it been demonstrated that seizures can alter brain development through mechanisms other than necrosis and programmed cell death.

Brain Damage in Status Epilepticus

Animal studies have demonstrated that significant differences exist between the type and extent of seizure-induced brain damage in young and adult animals. Although seizures can induce changes in multiple areas of the brain, the hippocampus has been particularly well studied. In addition to its importance in memory and learning, the anatomy and physiology of the hippocampus are well known, making this neuronal structure an ideal focus of study. In the adult animal, status epilepticus causes neuronal loss in hippocampal fields CA-1, CA-3, the dentate granule cell layer, and the dentate hilus.[29–31] If sufficiently long, a seizure probably can result in damage at any age,[32,33] but a single, prolonged seizure in an immature animal results in less cell loss.[34–40]

In addition to the cell loss, prolonged seizures can cause synaptic reorganization with aberrant growth (sprouting) of granule cell axons (the so-called mossy fibers) in the supragranular zone of the fascia dentata[41,42] and the infrapyramidal region of CA-3.[42] Seizures also activate the trk subtype of neurotrophin receptor in the mossy fiber pathway[43] and alter the expression of certain glutamate subreceptors.[44]

Because the mossy fibers develop primarily in the early postnatal period, the development of these axons may be particularly prone to seizure-induced changes. In studies from our laboratory,[45] we evaluated the effects of seizures induced by kainic acid (KA) during development on synaptic reorganization, using the expression of growth-associated protein-43 (GAP-43), a marker for synaptogenesis, and the Timm stain, which detects the presence of zinc in granule cell axons (Figure 3-2). Age-specific doses of KA, a glutamate agonist and potent convulsant, were used to induce seizures of similar intensity in rats varying in age from postnatal day 12 (P12) to P60. Until age P25, no differences were noted in either Timm or GAP-43 staining between animals with KA seizures and control animals. In P25 and older KA-treated rats, Timm staining was found in the supragranular layer of the dentate gyrus. This staining increased with age at the time of KA injection. Seizures in adult (P60), but not younger, rats also exhibited

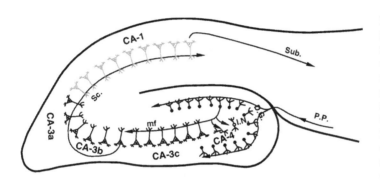

A

B

Figure 3-2. A. Anatomy of the hippocampus. Afferents enter the hippocampus from the entorhinal cortex via the perforant path (P.P.). The axons terminate on the dentate granule (D.G.) cells, which send axons, termed *mossy fibers* (mf), to the interneurons (I.N.) and CA-3 neurons. The CA-3 neurons send axons, termed *Schaffer* (Sc.) *collaterals*, to CA-1. **B.** Example of Timm stain. The mossy fibers of the dentate granule cells are stained black. The axons terminate on the dendrites of the CA-3 in the stratum lucidum. In this example from a rat that had experienced status epilepticus, some mossy fiber terminals are seen in the CA-3 pyramidal cell layer (pcl). In the photomicrograph, the stratum oriens (so), stratum radiatum (sr), and stratum lucidum (sl) also are marked.

increased staining in the suprapyramidal layer of the CA-3 subfields. Changes in GAP-43 were delayed as compared to the Timm staining, with no differences between KA-treated animals and controls until age P35, when a band of GAP-43 immunostaining appeared in the supragranular inner molecular layer, progressively increasing in intensity and thickness over time.

This study confirmed the observations of Sperber et al.,[46] that the degree of sprouting after status epilepticus is age-related. Why status epilepticus does not result in detectable synaptic reorganization in rats younger than P25 is not clear. However, these findings suggest that reactive synaptogenesis benefits from a mature neuronal circuit in the hippocampus. By P21–P25, an adult pattern of mossy terminals has developed[47] and, by P21, the adult pattern of GAP-43 immunostaining has been achieved, as demonstrated in this study. Only after these adult levels are reached does seizure-induced reactive synaptogenesis occur. Like cell loss, mossy fiber changes after seizures clearly are age-related, with younger animals demonstrating less sprouting than older animals after experiencing seizures of similar intensity.

Behavioral consequences after status epilepticus also are related to the age of the animal at the time of the status: Adult animals surviving status epilepticus show deficits in learning, memory, and behavior,[38] whereas young rats experiencing status epilepticus experience comparatively fewer deficits in learning, memory, and behavior.[38,48] Likewise, spontaneous recurrent seizures after status epilepticus are more likely to occur in adult animals than in young animals.[39,49,50]

Multiple reasons may exist for the age-related differences in seizure-induced damage after status epilepticus. Cellular damage occurs from excessive excitatory neurotransmitter release, which activates NMDA receptors, thereby allowing calcium to enter the cell. Calcium results in a cascade of biochemical changes that eventually result in cell death.[51] The immature brain appears to be more "resistant" to the effects of glutamate than does the mature brain.[52–55] Marks et al.[55] found that the degree of calcium entry into the hippocampal subfield CA-1 and subsequent damage was directly related to age. In P1–P3 neurons, glutamate increased intracellular calcium minimally, whereas in P21–P25 neurons, glutamate resulted in marked increases in intracellular calcium

and caused considerable swelling, blebbing, and retraction of dendrites into the soma of the neuron.

The immaturity of the neuronal network also may provide the immature brain with some protection. As noted earlier, reactive synaptogenesis of the mossy fibers appears to occur only when the mossy fibers have reached the mature state.

Neurotrophins have also been demonstrated to offer some protection from seizure-induced injury. Tandon et al.[56] blocked the synthesis of brain-derived neurotrophic factor (BDNF) by the infusion of an 18-mer antisense oligodeoxynucleotide to BDNF in the right ventricle of immature (P19) rats using micro-osmotic pumps and then subjecting the rats to status epilepticus. Rats in whom BDNF synthesis was blocked experienced more cell loss in the hippocampus after status epilepticus than did control rats that did not receive oligodeoxynucleotide. These results suggest that BDNF is involved in providing protection against seizure-induced neuronal loss in the developing brain.

Recurrent Seizures

Although the study of status epilepticus is important in understanding the biological basis for brain damage after seizures, children with epileptic encephalopathies experience recurrent seizures, and the effects of recurrent seizures on the developing brain differ from those occurring after a prolonged seizure. Kindling, a process by which recurrent electrical stimulations initially result in only brief electrical discharges and mild behavioral changes but progressively result in more prolonged and intense electrical and behavioral seizures, occurs at all ages.[57,58] Adult rats that underwent kindling during the first weeks of life have a reduced seizure threshold when studied as adults.[59] This enduring alteration in seizure susceptibility occurs in the setting of no discernible cell loss in young rats.

Despite the lack of cell loss with recurrent seizures, synaptic reorganization does occur in this setting. Using two models of neonatal seizures, pentylenetetrazol and flurothyl, we recently demonstrated seizure-induced changes in the mossy fiber distribution in the hippocampus in mature rats that had experienced neonatal seizures.[60–62] Using both models, we have demonstrated that recurrent

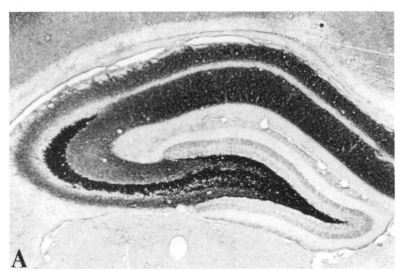

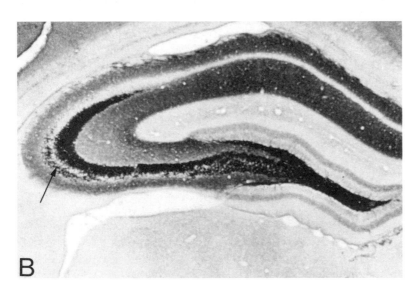

Figure 3-3. A. Example of Timm staining in the hippocampus from a control animal. Normally, little staining is seen in the pyramidal cell layer.
B. Example of Timm staining in an animal with a history of neonatal seizures. Note the increase in staining in the pyramidal cell layer (*arrow*).

seizures during the neonatal period result in subsequent increases in mossy fiber growth in both the supragranular region and the CA-3 hippocampal subfield (Figure 3-3). The terminal sprouting in CA-3 appears to represent new growth of axons and synapses, as opposed to a failure of normal regression of synapses. To determine whether recurrent seizures cause cell loss, we counted principal neurons in the hippocampus. No cell loss was detected after the neonatal seizures.

In addition to altering mossy fiber plasticity, we have found that recurrent seizures result in alterations of neuronal pathways activated during seizures.[62] We subjected immature rats to 50 flurothyl-induced seizures between ages P11 and P23. Immunostaining for c-*fos* immunoactivity was performed to characterize the pattern of neuronal activity after the recurrent seizures. Recurrent seizures progressively activated more brain structures, as revealed by a dramatic increase in both the extent and intensity of c-*fos* immunostaining after the recurrent seizures; mild c-*fos* immunostaining was observed after the twenty-fifty recurrent seizure, whereas extensive c-*fos* immunostaining was observed after the fiftieth seizure. These findings demonstrate that recurrent seizures have a progressive effect on the extent of neuronal activation. Taken together, recent studies clearly demonstrate that immature animals undergo changes in neuronal organization after recurrent seizures, with mossy fiber sprouting in both the CA-3 subfield and supragranular region despite the lack of demonstrable hippocampal cell loss.

These in vivo studies suggest that the excessive excitability associated with recurrent seizures can alter the plasticity of mossy fiber synapses. In a novel approach to the same problem, Ikegaya[63] used organotypic slice cultures and picrotoxin, a GABA(A) channel blocker, to study the effects of prolonged excitability on mossy fiber innervation. He found that prolonged hyperexcitability caused ectopic innervation of the mossy fibers to the stratum oriens and the dentate molecular layer. Furthermore, brief, repetitive stimulation elicited epileptiform discharges in the CA-3 region that were inhibited by an NMDA receptor antagonist. Significantly, picrotoxin did not affect synaptic responses of the Schaffer collaterals, which were fully developed at the time of hippocampal slice preparation.

The aberrant network set up by recurrent seizures may make the brain vulnerable to future injury. Schmid et al.[64] subjected to status epilepticus, using either KA or perforant pathway stimulation, adolescent rats who experienced 25 seizures during the first 4 days of life. The authors found no cell death in animals that had experienced only neonatal seizures. However, animals in which neonatal seizures had occurred had significantly more severe brain injury after both KA and perforant pathway stimulation than did animals without a history of neonatal seizures. Although the mechanism by which this enhanced susceptibility to injury is not yet known, the study provides further evidence that neonatal seizures alter the brain in a maladaptive manner.

Recurrent neonatal seizures are associated with impairment in cognition and behavior. Immature rats exposed to a series of 25 flurothyl-induced seizures and tested as adults demonstrated significant abnormalities in the water maze, a test of spatial memory, and the open-field test, a test of activity level.[60] As compared to control animals, the rats with neonatal seizures had increased CA-3 and supragranular mossy fiber sprouting.

Whether the morphologic changes seen with recurrent seizures are directly responsible for the reduced seizure threshold and cognitive dysfunction is not known. However, the degree of CA-3 mossy fiber projections correlates with learning. Lipp et al.[65] compared the number of trials required for rats to learn to avoid a 10-second electrical shock by moving from one compartment to another after a conditioning stimuli (two-way avoidance learning) and the magnitude of the stratum pyramidal projections of mossy fibers. Learning proved to be directly related to the extent of mossy fiber projections to the pyramidal layers of CA-3, the animals having more CA-3 mossy fiber terminals performed less well than animals with fewer terminals. These authors also found an inverse relationship between the extent of infrapyramidal mossy fiber projections and two-way avoidance learning in rats treated with L-thyroxine.[65] The relationship between the size of the hippocampal mossy fiber projections and learning and memory may be task-dependent.[66] For example, recurrent seizures during the first weeks of life result in impairment in rats' ability to succeed in the water maze and in auditory location but not in a quality discrimination task.[67]

Although the brain's response to neonatal seizures may differ from the response to seizures in the mature brain, that seizures alter the developing brain is becoming increasingly clear.

Conclusion

Substantial evidence now supports the view that, in some situations, frequent seizures or epileptiform discharges result in substantial cognitive decline in children. In addition, animal studies have convincingly demonstrated that seizures during early development can lead to damage. Whether the changes noted in animal models are applicable to humans is not yet clear. However, one could speculate that infantile spasms, through activity-dependent mechanisms, result in the establishment of aberrant neuronal connections. This may explain the observation that children with intractable infantile spasms may continue to have tonic seizures that display the clinical and EEG features of infantile spasms. Although teenagers and adults without a history of infantile spasms never develop such spasms, intractable infantile spasms may lead to changes in connectivity that permit this seizure type to continue.

All the clinical and animal data support the caution that clinicians should make every attempt to diagnose quickly and aggressively treat infantile spasms. Delays in the recognition of infantile spasms or the use of inappropriate therapies may be very detrimental to the child.

Acknowledgments

This research was supported by the National Institutes of Health (NS27984).

References

1. Hauser WA. Seizure disorders: the changes with age. Epilepsia 1992;33[Suppl 4]:S6–S14.
2. Hauser WA, Hersdorffer DC. Epilepsy: Frequency, Causes and Consequences. New York: Demos, 1990.
3. Gaiarsa J-L, Tseeb V, Ben-Ari Y. Postnatal development of pre- and postsynaptic GABA$_B$-mediated inhibitions in the rat CA3 hippocampal region of the rat. J Neurobiol 1994;73:246–255.
4. Cherubini E, Gaiarsa J-L, Ben-Ari Y. GABA: an excitatory transmitter in early postnatal life. Trends Neurosci 1991;14:515–519.
5. Moshé SL, Shinnar S, Swann JW. Partial (Focal) Seizures in Developing Brain. In PA Schwartzkroin, SL Moshé, SL Noebels, JW Swann (eds), Brain Development and Epilepsy. New York: Oxford University Press, 1995;34–65.
6. Ben-Ari Y, Khazipov R, Leinekugel X, et al. GABA$_A$, NMDA and AMPA receptors: a developmentally regulated "ménage à trois." Trends Neurosci 1997;20:523–529.
7. Leinekugel X, Medina I, Khalilov R, et al. Ca^{++} oscillations mediated by the synergistic excitatory actions of GABA$_A$ and NMDA receptors in the neonatal hippocampus. Neuron 1997;18:243–255.
8. Holmes GL, Ben-Ari Y. Seizures in the developing brain: perhaps not so benign after all. Neuron 1998; 21:1–20.
9. Walsh CA. Genetic malformations of the human cerebral cortex. Neuron 1999;23:19–29.
10. Kuzniecky RI, Jackson GD. Developmental Disorders. In J Engel Jr, TA Pedley (eds), Epilepsy: A Comprehensive Textbook. Philadelphia: Lippincott–Raven, 1997;2517–2532.
11. Stephenson JBP. Cerebral Palsy. In J Engel Jr, TA Pedley (eds), Epilepsy: A Comprehensive Textbook. Philadelphia: Lippincott-Raven, 1999;2571–2577.
12. Edebol-Tysk K. Epidemiology of spastic tetraplegic cerebral palsy in Sweden: I. Impairment and disabilities. Neuropediatrics 1989;20:192–197.
13. Uvebrant P. Hemiplegic cerebral palsy. Aetiology and outcome. Acta Paediatrica Scand 1988;345 [Suppl]:1–100.
14. Genton P, Dravet C. Lennox-Gastaut and other childhood epileptic encephalopathies. In J Engel Jr, TA Pedley (eds), Epilepsy: A Comprehensive Textbook. Philadelphia: Lippincott–Raven, 1997;2355–2366.
15. Dulac O. Infantile Spasms and West Syndrome. In J Engel Jr, TA Pedley (eds), Epilepsy: A Comprehensive Textbook. Philadelphia: Lippincott–Raven, 1997; 2277–2283.
16. Holmes GL, Vigevano F. Infantile Spasms. In J Engel Jr, TA Pedley (eds), Epilepsy: A Comprehensive Textbook. Philadelphia: Lippincott–Raven, 1997;627–642.
17. Kellaway P, Hrachovy RA, Frost JD Jr, Zion T. Precise characterization and quantification of infantile spasms. Ann Neurol 1979;6:214–218.
18. Hrachovy RA, Frost JD Jr, Kellaway P. Hypsarrhythmia: variations on the theme. Epilepsia 1984;25:317–325.
19. Rantala H, Putkonen T. Occurrence, outcome, and prognostic factors of infantile spasms and Lennox-Gastaut syndrome. Epilepsia 1999;40:286–289.
20. Trevathan E, Murphy CC, Yeargin-Allsopp M. The descriptive epidemiology of infantile spasms among Atlanta children. Epilepsia 1999;40:748–751.
21. Lombroso CT. A prospective study of infantile spasms: clinical and therapeutic considerations. Epilepsia 1983;24:135–158.
22. Steffenburg U, Hagberg G, Kyllerman M. Characteristics of seizures in a population-based series of mentally retarded children with active epilepsy. Epilepsia 1996;37:850–856.
23. Jozwiak S, Goodman M, Lamm SH. Poor mental development in patients with tuberous sclerosis complex. Clinical risk factors. Arch Neurol 1998;55:379–384.
24. Bednarek N, Motte J, Soufflet C, et al. Evidence of late-onset infantile spasms. Epilepsia 1998;39:55–60.
25. Fois A, Malandrini F, Balestri P, Giorgi D. Infantile spasms—long term results of ACTH treatment. Eur J Pediatr 1984;142:51–55.
26. Riikonen R. A long-term follow-up study of 214 children with the syndrome of infantile spasms. Neuropediatrics 1982;13:14–23.
27. Riikonen R. Infantile spasms: modern practical aspects. Acta Paediatr Scand 1984;73:1–12.
28. Singer WD, Rabe EF, Haller JS. The effect of ACTH therapy upon infantile spasms. J Pediatr 1980;96:485–489.
29. Nadler JV, Perry BW, Cotman CW. Intraventricular kainic acid preferentially destroys hippocampal pyramidal cells. Nature 1978;271:676–677.

30. Olney JW, Fuller T, De Gubareff T. Acute dendrotoxic changes in the hippocampus of kainate-treated rats. Brain Res 1979;176:91–100.

31. Sloviter RS, Dean E, Sollas AI, Goodman JH. Apoptosis and necrosis induced in different hippocampal neuron populations by repetitive perforant path stimulation in the rat. J Comp Neurol 1996;366:516–533.

32. Sankar R, Shin DH, Liu H, et al. Patterns of status epilepticus-induced neuronal injury during development and long-term consequences. J Neurosci 1998;18:8382–8393.

33. Thompson K, Wasterlain C. Lithium-pilocarpine status epilepticus in the immature rabbit. Dev Brain Res 1997;100:1–4.

34. Albala BJ, Moshé SL, Okada R. Kainic-acid-induced seizures: a developmental study. Dev Brain Res 1984;13:139–148.

35. Berger ML, Tremblay E, Nitecka L, Ben-Ari Y. Maturation of kainic acid seizure-brain damage syndrome in the rat: III. Postnatal development of kainic acid binding sites in the limbic system. Neuroscience 1984;13:1095–1104.

36. Nitecka L, Tremblay E, Charton G, et al. Maturation of kainic acid seizure-brain damage syndrome in the rat: II. Histopathological sequelae. Neuroscience 1984;13:1073–1094.

37. Tremblay E, Nitecka L, Berger ML, Ben-Ari Y. Maturation of kainic acid seizure-brain damage syndrome in the rat: I. Clinical, electrographic and metabolic observations. Neuroscience 1984;13(4):1051–1072.

38. Stafstrom CE, Chronopoulos A, Thurber S, et al. Age-dependent cognitive and behavioral deficits following kainic acid-induced seizures. Epilepsia 1993;34:420–432.

39. Stafstrom CE, Thompson JL, Holmes GL. Kainic acid seizures in the developing brain: status epilepticus and spontaneous recurrent seizures. Dev Brain Res 1992;65:227–236.

40. Hirsch E, Baram TZ, Snead OC III. Ontogenic study of lithium-pilocarpine-induced status epilepticus in rats. Brain Res 1992;583:120–126.

41. Tauck D, Nadler JV. Evidence of functional mossy fiber sprouting in the hippocampal formation of kainic acid-treated rats. J Neurosci 1985;5:1016–1022.

42. Represa A, Tremblay E, Ben-Ari Y. Aberrant growth of mossy fibers and enhanced kainic acid binding sites induced in rats by early hyperthyroidism. Brain Res 1987;423:325–328.

43. Binder DK, Routbort MJ, McNamara JO. Immunohistochemical evidence of seizure-induced activation of trk receptors in the mossy fiber pathway of adult rat hippocampus. J Neurosci 1999;19:4616–4626.

44. Friedman LK. Selective reduction of gluR2 protein in adult hippocampal CA3 neurons following status epilepticus but prior to cell loss. Hippocampus 1998;8:511–525.

45. Yang Y, Tandon P, Liu Z, et al. Synaptic reorganization following kainic acid-induced seizures during development. Dev Brain Res 1998;107:169–177.

46. Sperber EF, Haas KZ, Stanton PK, Moshé SL. Resistance of the immature hippocampus to seizure-induced synaptic reorganization. Dev Brain Res 1991;60:88–93.

47. Ribak CE, Navetta MS. An immature mossy fiber innervation of hilar neurons may explain their resistance to kainate-induced cell death in 15-day-old rats. Dev Brain Res 1994;79:47–62.

48. Liu Z, Gatt A, Mikati M, Holmes GL. Long-term behavioral deficits following pilocarpine seizures in immature rats. Epilepsy Res 1995;19:191–204.

49. Cronin J, Obenaus A, Houser CR, Dudek FE. Electrophysiology of dentate granule cells after kainate-induced synaptic reorganization of mossy fibers. Brain Res 1992;573:305–310.

50. Cronin J, Dudek FE. Chronic seizures and collateral sprouting of dentate mossy fibers after kainic acid treatment in rats. Brain Res 1988;474:181–184.

51. Lipton SA, Rosenberg PA. Excitatory amino acids as a final common pathway for neurologic disorders. N Engl J Med 1994;330:613–622.

52. Bickler PE, Gallego SM, Hansen BM. Developmental changes in intracellular calcium regulation in rat cerebral cortex during hypoxia. J Cereb Blood Flow Metab 1993;13:811–819.

53. Carmant L, Liu Z, Werner SJ, et al. Effect of kainic acid–induced status epilepticus on inositol-trisphosphate and seizure-induced brain damage in mature and immature animals. Dev Brain Res 1995;89:67–72.

54. Liu Z, Stafstrom CE, Sarkisian M, et al. Age-dependent effects of glutamate toxicity in the hippocampus. Dev Brain Res 1996;97:178–184.

55. Marks JD, Friedman JE, Haddad GG. Vulnerability of CA1 neurons to glutamate is developmentally regulated. Dev Brain Res 1996;97:194–206.

56. Tandon P, Yang Y, Das K, et al. Neuroprotective effects of brain-derived neurotrophic factor in seizures during development. Neuroscience 1999;91:293–303.

57. Racine RJ. Modification of seizure activity by electrical stimulation: I. After-discharge threshold. Electroencephalogr Clin Neurophysiol 1972;32:269–279.

58. Racine RJ. Modification of seizure activity by electrical stimulation: II. Motor seizures. Electroencephalogr Clin Neurophysiol 1972;32:281–294.

59. Moshé SL, Albala BJ. Kindling in developing rats: persistence of seizures into adulthood. Dev Brain Res 1982;4:67–71.

60. Holmes GL, Gaiarsa J-L, Chevassus-Au-Louis N, Ben-Ari Y. Consequences of neonatal seizures in the rat: morphological and behavioral effects. Ann Neurol 1998;44:845–857.

61. Holmes GL, Sarkisian M, Ben-Ari Y, Chevassus-Au-Louis N. Mossy fiber sprouting following recurrent

seizures during early development in rats. J Comp Neurol 1999;404:537–553.

62. Liu Z, Yang Y, Silveira DC, et al. Consequences of recurrent seizures during early brain development. Neuroscience 1999;92:1443–1454.

63. Ikegaya Y. Abnormal targeting of developing hippocampal mossy fibers after epileptiform activities via L-type Ca^{2+} channel activation in vitro. J Neurosci 1999;15:802–812.

64. Schmid R, Tandon P, Stafstrom CE, Holmes GL. Effects of neonatal seizures on subsequent seizure-induced brain injury. Neurology 1999;53:1754–1761.

65. Lipp H-P, Schwegler H, Heimrich B, Driscoll P. Infrapyramidal mossy fibers and two-way avoidance learning: developmental modification of hippocampal circuitry and adult behavior of rats and mice. J Neurosci 1988;8:1905–1921.

66. Crusio WE, Schwegler H, Brust I. Covariations between hippocampal mossy fibers and working and reference memory in spatial and non-spatial radial maze tasks in mice. Eur J Neurosci 1993;5:1413–1420.

67. Neill J, Liu Z, Sarkisian M, et al. Recurrent seizures in immature rats: effect on auditory and visual discrimination. Dev Brain Res 1996;95:283–292.

Chapter 4

Cerebral Palsy in Children with Epilepsy

Carol S. Camfield, Peter Camfield,
and Linda Watson

The association of epilepsy and cerebral palsy has long been noted. Millions of people in the world have cerebral palsy, and more than one-third of these also have epilepsy.

Many different types and etiologies of both epilepsy and cerebral palsy exist. When the two disorders coexist, it is reasonable to assume that the etiology also is related—that is, that the same brain injury responsible for causing cerebral palsy also has caused the epilepsy. When a child with cerebral palsy develops epilepsy, only detailed knowledge of the type and etiology of the cerebral palsy and the type of epilepsy can prepare the practitioner to respond properly to parents' concerns. Unfortunately, this information is lacking in most cases.

This chapter addresses the epidemiology of epilepsy and cerebral palsy and the association of the two disorders. The interaction among clinical characteristics, type, and severity of this dual handicap is discussed. The pathophysiology of cerebral palsy as it relates to epilepsy is reviewed, as are the clinical course and remission rates of epilepsy and the impact of epilepsy on families of children with cerebral palsy.

Children with cerebral palsy often are multihandicapped. The association of mental retardation with cerebral palsy, which is found commonly in those with epilepsy and cerebral palsy, is addressed in Chapter 1.

Causes and Pathologic Features of Epilepsy and Cerebral Palsy

Cerebral palsy can be divided into four broad types: hemiplegia, diplegia, tetraplegia, and dys-tonic or athetoid (i.e., extrapyramidal). Each type is characterized by its own pathologic process and causes. Epilepsy is a disorder of cerebral cortex, and, therefore, the relevant issue in each type of cerebral palsy is the way in which the cortex is affected.

Hemiplegic cerebral palsy typically follows an unremarkable term pregnancy and is noted only as the corticospinal tracts begin to myelinate after the second to third month of life. The most common pathology is a porencephaly or loss of brain volume in the vascular territory of a major cerebral artery, most usually the middle cerebral artery. The amount of cortical involvement is determined by the size of the infarct. The associated epilepsy is most typically partial and arises from the border of a porencephalic cyst or from the "scar" of a less severe infarct. Therefore, partial epilepsy can arise from any lobe but usually does not arise from the occipital or inferior temporal cortex, as these structures are perfused by the posterior cerebral artery.

Very low-birth-weight infants (<1500-g birth weight) are at high risk for neurologic disability: 1 in 20 survivors has disabling cerebral palsy.[1] *Spastic diplegia* is most clearly associated with prematurity. The cerebral insult occurs at 26–32 weeks of gestation, when the periventricular white matter is especially vulnerable. Periventricular leukomalacia results from ischemia and interrupts the descending corticospinal tracts more from the cortical leg areas than the arm areas. Therefore, many of these children have no cortical lesion, and the relatively low rate of epilepsy is not surprising. If the ischemia has been more severe, then cortical struc-

tures may be impaired, but predicting which cortical areas will be most vulnerable is not easy. The
epilepsy may be partial, but, if there is global
injury, then symptomatic generalized epilepsy may
occur.

Interestingly, spastic diplegia sometimes occurs
in a term infant. Presumably, this condition is
caused by an intrauterine insult at approximately
28–32 weeks. Sometimes, a cotwin is known to
have died at about this time. It has also been suggested that significant proportions of singletons with
spastic cerebral palsy of unknown etiology are the
result of a cotwin death, the so-called vanishing
twin syndrome.[2]

Tetraplegic cerebral palsy has many causes. Sometimes, it is the result of global ischemia, but often it is
related to severe global brain malformation. Typically,
the cortex is widely involved, and the epilepsies often
are of the secondary generalized type.

Dystonic or *athetoid cerebral palsy* has a variety
of causes but usually is believed to result from a
brain injury in the last trimester of gestation or the
perinatal period. The pathologic process centers on
the basal ganglia, and the cortex may be completely
spared. Etiologies include kernicterus and hypoxic-
ischemic damage. The basal ganglia disorder may
be very disabling, especially for tongue and mouth
movements; however, intelligence may be normal
despite severe disability. Sparing of the cortex
means that epilepsy usually is not associated unless
the insult has been global and severe. The presence
of epilepsy therefore reflects global cortical dysfunction, and, again, symptomatic generalized epilepsies prevail.

Epidemiology of Epilepsy in Childhood

Epilepsy is said to occur when an individual has
two or more unprovoked seizures. It appears
sometime during life in 1% of the general population. Hauser and Hesdorffer[3] estimate that 0.4–
0.8% of children will have epilepsy by the age of
11 years. Early studies found that the incidence
of childhood epilepsy in industrialized populations was 50–100 per 100,000 population.[4] However, more recent studies have found the overall
incidence of childhood epilepsy to be 40 per
100,000 children per year.[5,6] The incidence of
epilepsy is highest in the first year of life (120/
100,000) and falls dramatically between 1 and

10 years of age to 40–50 per 100,000. It then
drops even further in the teenage years to 20 per
100,000.

A critical issue when considering epilepsy and
cerebral palsy is understanding whether the epilepsy
is idiopathic or symptomatic. Idiopathic epilepsy,
which appears suddenly with no underlying cause,
often is characterized by a family history of similar
seizures, normal neurologic and intellectual development at the time of onset of the disorder, good
response to the appropriate antiepileptic drug
(AED), and spontaneous remission of seizures later
in life. It often involves generalized seizures. In contrast, symptomatic epilepsy may be the result of an
acquired insult or an indication of an underlying
process, such as abnormal, prenatal neuronal development and migration or the result of a problem
within the developing brain due to intrauterine disease. Symptomatic epilepsy, commonly seen in
those with cerebral palsy, frequently has characteristics opposite those of idiopathic epilepsy: no family
history of a seizure disorder, impairment of neurologic or intellectual abilities, longer need for medication, and a lower spontaneous rate of remission of
the epilepsy. In addition, the seizures often are focal
but can be generalized.

In most large studies of persons with epilepsy
only, 20% of seizures are considered to be symptomatic and the remainder either idiopathic (30%) or
cryptogenic (50%; no identifiable underlying etiology, and the epilepsy does not take the form of one
of the specific idiopathic syndromes).[7] It would
seem intuitively obvious that most epilepsy accompanying cerebral palsy would be symptomatic; however, no sufficiently large or notable studies of
seizure type and linkage with a specific area of
motor deficit exist.

Because we expect children with focal motor
deficits to experience a focal epilepsy and those with
tetraplegia caused by global brain abnormalities to
have generalized seizures, we should be able to refer
to population-based studies of epilepsy to discern
the frequency of seizure type. According to the literature, generalized seizures account for 45% of all
seizure types, whereas focal seizures with secondary
generalized seizures are present in 55% of cases.[5,7]
Unfortunately, these studies note the presence of
only "neurologic abnormality" rather than the specific type of problem (e.g., cerebral palsy, visual
impairment, deafness). Therefore, through the use of

population-based studies of epilepsy alone, we are unable to determine the number of children with epilepsy who also have cerebral palsy and which cortical area is involved.

The importance of a genetic predisposition to epilepsy in those also having cerebral palsy is impressive. The National Collaborative Perinatal Project demonstrated that the incidence of cerebral palsy in offspring was associated with a maternal history of epilepsy.[8] The incidence of nonfebrile seizures in offspring of women with epilepsy but without cerebral palsy was associated with a history of motor deficits in siblings, implying a shared genetic susceptibility to epilepsy and cerebral palsy. When a first-degree relative of a child with cerebral palsy and mental handicap had epilepsy, Curatolo et al.[9] reported that epilepsy was 17 times more frequent in those children than in normal controls. Asku[10] described a cohort of children with cerebral palsy and epilepsy in whom 16% of first-degree relatives also had epilepsy, as compared to 8% of first-degree relatives of the normal controls. Others have found similar results.[3,11] The elevated frequency of epilepsy in first-degree relatives of children with cerebral palsy implies that genetic factors play an important part in both of these chronic disabilities.

Epidemiology of Cerebral Palsy

Cerebral palsy is a term of convenience applied to a heterogeneous group of nonprogressive motor disorders of central origin covering a wide range of cerebral dysfunctions occurring early in life.[12] Often included in the case-finding method is an age of at least 3 years, as the diagnosis of cerebral palsy is occasionally difficult at younger ages.

Incidence of Cerebral Palsy

Population-based data delineating the incidence of cerebral palsy are available from numerous large, longitudinal registers.[1,13–16] These registers yield incidence figures of approximately 2.5 cases per 1,000 live births (Figure 4-1). British versus western Australian registers yield rates of cerebral palsy in singletons (2.3 vs. 1.6 cases per 1,000), twins (12.6 vs. 7.3 cases per 1,000), and triplets (44.8 vs. 27.9 cases per 1,000).[17,18] The Swedish register reports a comparable rate of 2.5 per 1,000 live births among singletons in 1993.[15]

Etiology and Types of Cerebral Palsy

The etiology of cerebral palsy is thought to be multifactorial and is incompletely understood. Early descriptions indicated that birth injury was responsible, which gave rise to a whole generation of pregnancy and delivery interventions. Despite these interventions, the incidence of cerebral palsy has not declined, and recent information indicates that only 2–10% of cases are caused by intrapartum hypoxia.[8,19,20] In addition, a small percentage (perhaps 15%) may occur owing to postneonatal difficulties. Therefore, evidence favors a prepartum origin for most cases of cerebral palsy. Poor intrauterine growth is an important risk factor for cerebral palsy in infants with a gestational age greater than 33 weeks.[21] Approximately 40% of infants who develop cerebral palsy weigh less than 2,500 g at birth, and one study of spastic cerebral palsy found nearly 50% of these infants to have associated prenatal factors, as compared with approximately 20% of those infants weighing more than 2,500 g. Overall, however, 50% of cerebral palsy patients were shown not to have experienced any of the prenatal, perinatal, or neonatal factors.[22] Further in-depth studies are needed to elucidate causal pathways to cerebral palsy.

The predominant types of cerebral palsy identified in 756 children within the western Australia registry (1975–1990) include hemiplegia (36%), diplegia (32%), quadriplegia (16%), extrapyramidal (ataxia, hypotonia, and dyskinesia) (16%).[14] A marked increase in the number of children with quadriplegia and extrapyramidal cerebral palsy has been noted in this register since 1975. This may be due to the increased survival of low-birth-weight and premature infants or, perhaps, better recognition of extrapyramidal cerebral palsy. Other registers have similar information.

Epidemiology of Epilepsy and Cerebral Palsy: The Dual Handicap

Incidence of Epilepsy and Cerebral Palsy

The population-based study by Hagberg et al.[15] found that 28% of persons with cerebral palsy also had epilepsy, and the Danish Cerebral Palsy

Figure 4-1. Incidence of cerebral palsy per 1,000 live births from population-based registers from the United Kingdom, Sweden, and western Australia, 1959–1992. Note that data for the Mersey region of the United Kingdom are for 1967–1989 only; Swedish data are to 1990 only. Rates exclude cerebral palsy due to postneonatal causes.

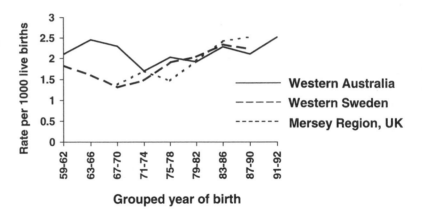

Register reported 27.1% of patients born with cerebral palsy between 1979 and 1986 also had epilepsy.[16] In addition, data from western Australia from 1975 through 1994 include information on the presence of epilepsy in 618 of 1,664 (37%) of patients with cerebral palsy.[14] The type of seizure associated with each type of cerebral palsy is not described within these registers. However, the rate of combined epilepsy and cerebral palsy of 0.8 per 1,000 live births has remained constant over 25 years. With improvements in neonatal care during the last 20 years, the number of surviving premature and low-birth-weight babies has increased, with a concomitant increase in the rate of cerebral palsy.

It is our clinical impression that children severely affected by cerebral palsy have a greater likelihood of developing epilepsy. This aspect was studied in Rochester, Minnesota, between 1950 and 1976, when 64 cases of cerebral palsy were identified.[23] Fifty-two percent of patients with severe cerebral palsy (defined as function limited to mechanical aids and characterized by marked difficulty) also developed epilepsy. Conversely, epilepsy was present in 23% of those with mild to moderate cerebral palsy. Although the sample is small and spans the years before modern prenatal care, more recent data from western Australia support these findings. Watson and Stanley (personal communication) found that 65% of children with severe cerebral palsy born between 1975 and 1994 developed epilepsy, as compared with 24% of children with minimal, mild, or moderate cases of cerebral palsy.

The frequency of occurrence of epilepsy varies according to cerebral palsy type (Table 4-1).

Aicardi[24] combined data from several studies (Ingram, 1964; Hagberg, 1975; Kyllerman, 1982; and Uvebrandt, 1998) and found the frequency of epilepsy associated with various forms of cerebral palsy to be as follows: tetraplegia, 50–90%; hemiplegia, 34–60%; diplegia, 16–27%; and athetoid and dystonic (i.e., extrapyramidal), 23–26%. In a clinic-based group of 323 children with cerebral palsy from Greece, Hadjipanaysis et al.[25] found that 41.8% of children with cerebral palsy had epilepsy and that epilepsy was more common in those with tetraplegia (50%) or hemiplegia (47%) than in those with diplegia (27%) or extrapyramidal types of cerebral palsy. Kwong et al.[26] in Hong Kong found very different epilepsy frequency statistics among 32 children with these dual handicaps, depending on the type of cerebral palsy present: tetraparetic, 71%; hemiparetic, 21%; diplegic, 6%; extrapyramidal, 8%; and mixed with one or more seizure types, 54%.

Referral and diagnostic criteria for all these studies differed, and all had small sample sizes. Therefore, the studies are unlikely to represent the true incidence of epilepsy according to cerebral palsy type. Nonetheless, it is generally believed that patients with tetraplegia and hemiplegia develop epilepsy more often than do those with diplegia. Extrapyramidal cerebral palsy has had the lowest rate of associated epilepsy, probably approximately 10%.

Age at onset of the epilepsy has a close relationship with the type of cerebral palsy. In children with tetraplegia, epilepsy starts significantly earlier (median age, 6 months) than in those with hemiplegia (18 months) or diplegia (24

Table 4-1. Types of Cerebral Palsy Associated with Frequency of Occurrence of Epilepsy

Cerebral Palsy Type	Frequency of Epilepsy Occurrence (%)			
	Zafeiriou[27]	**Hadjipanaysis**[25]	**Aicardi**[24]	**Kwong**[26]
Tetraparetic		50	50–90	71
Hemiparetic	37	47	34–60	21
Diplegic		27	16–27	6
Extrapyramidal		15	23–26	8
Mixed				54

months).[26] Similar results were described from another Greek referral center[27] following up 178 children with epilepsy and cerebral palsy: The prevalence of epilepsy in this clinic was 36%, and the onset of seizures was early, occurring in the first year of life in 73% of the children.

Prognosis of Epilepsy in Children with Cerebral Palsy

Determining the prognosis of epilepsy in children with cerebral palsy is difficult. It undoubtedly depends on the type of cerebral palsy, its cause, and severity. No population-based studies reflecting lengthy follow-up are available. Most prognostic studies are case series that intermix many types of cerebral palsy and lead to the following essential conclusions: (1) The more severe the cerebral palsy, the more likely the child is to develop epilepsy, and seizures usually begin at an earlier age than in children without cerebral palsy; (2) the clinical course and ease of seizure control appear to be related to the severity of the cerebral palsy; and (3) fewer children with cerebral palsy are able to discontinue AEDs than are children with epilepsy without cerebral palsy. Regarding the latter conclusion, however, the child with cerebral palsy plus epilepsy who becomes seizure-free for 1–2 years has a good chance of remaining seizure-free when medication is withdrawn.[28]

Discontinuation of Antiepileptic Drugs in Children with Epilepsy Only

Berg and Shinnar[29] completed a meta-analysis of 25 AED discontinuation studies, in which the number of years that a patient had to be seizure-free before drug discontinuation was not addressed. However, the standard of practice at the time that most studies were conducted required 2–5 seizure-free years. Most of the reviewed studies did not specifically indicate a diagnosis of cerebral palsy. Therefore, the authors were able to consider only the effect of a more ill-defined term, *motor deficits*. In general, the relapse rate for epilepsy patients after 2 years of medication cessation was 30%. However, for children with "motor deficits" (neurologic abnormality), the relative risk of relapse increased to 1.79 (confidence interval, 1.13–2.83), as compared to those whose epilepsy had an idiopathic cause (i.e., no neurologic or cognitive problems).

In a study of 97 consecutively evaluated children who had been seizure-free for 1 year, regardless of seizure type or cause, AEDs were withdrawn over 4–8 weeks.[28] Overall, 39% experienced relapse within the next 24 months (mean follow-up, 32 months). If a child had a significant neurologic abnormality (one that interfered with activities of daily living), the risk of recurrence increased to 51%, as compared to 32% for those with no neurologic abnormality. In addition, those with remote symptomatic epilepsy (59% recurrences) faired worse than those with idiopathic etiology (34% recurrences). Cerebral palsy was not specifically identified in this study, but more than 90% of children who were reported to be "neurologically abnormal" most likely had cerebral palsy.

In our Nova Scotia cohort, 383 children became seizure-free on medication for a long enough period that withdrawal of medication was attempted.[30] Of the 293 without neurologic handicap, 90 had recurrent seizures within 2 years (31%); however, of the 56 children with significant neurologic handicap, 30 (54%) had recurrent seizures, an appreciably higher proportion.

Additional studies by Hollowach-Thurston et al.,[31] Peters et al.,[32] and Matricardi et al.[33] have also found neurologic dysfunction to be an adverse risk factor for relapse.

Discontinuation of Antiepileptic Drugs in Children with Epilepsy and Cerebral Palsy

The control of epilepsies associated with cerebral palsy generally is difficult, especially when the lesions are large or related to specific syndromes such as West or Lennox-Gastaut syndrome. However, in the majority of children (40–60%), a state of seizure freedom will eventually be reached.

Early studies, such as that of Roger and Bureau[34] in 1982, found that 30% of patients with epilepsy and cerebral palsy entered long-term remission after 5–15 years of follow-up, as compared to 70% who had epilepsy only. Eventually, 50% had complete seizure control with 60% off AEDs. In another study, the Marseilles group described 97 children with severe cerebral palsy.[35] The eventual outcome, good or bad, was known within the first 3 years of life. Forty percent were seizure-free by 14 years of age, and half of this latter group no longer required medication. Asku[10] was able to discontinue AEDs in 40% of 174 children who were seizure-free for at least 2 years. Sillanpaa et al.[36] followed through 1992 a cohort of 245 children with active epilepsy in 1961–1964. Of those with remote symptomatic epilepsy, 45% were in remission, and 24% were also off all medication.

Although referral sources, types of follow-up, and results of studies by Delgado et al.[37] and Zafeiriou et al.[27] differed from those of the aforementioned studies, these investigators also found that a significant percentage of children with this dual handicap eventually became seizure-free and could discontinue use of AEDs. In the Delgado et al. study,[37] after 2 seizure-free years, AEDs were discontinued in children with epilepsy and cerebral palsy. During the next 2 years, 42% of those with spastic cerebral palsy experienced relapses. Those with hemiparesis had the highest rate (62%), whereas those with diplegia had the lowest (14%). In the Zafeiriou et al. study,[27] after 3 seizure-free years, AEDs were discontinued, and only 18 of 134 patients experienced relapse over a follow-up period of 5.8 ± 1.2 years. Specifically, 11 (61%) had hemiplegic cerebral palsy, 4 (22%) had dystonic cerebral palsy, and 3 (16%) had diplegia. These numbers are surprisingly low and may reflect a small sample or referral bias.

Overall, children with cerebral palsy and epilepsy take longer than those without this dual handicap to become seizure-free for a period of 1–2 years. However, once they do so, a large number of these handicapped children will remain seizure-free for a significant period after medication withdrawal.

Impact of Epilepsy and Cerebral Palsy on Children and Their Families

What is the impact of epilepsy on children and their families as compared to epilepsy plus cerebral palsy? We have recently developed and validated a brief questionnaire that measures the impact of neurologic chronic disease in children.[38] In families of children with epilepsy only (no behavioral, cognitive, or other neurologic problems), a strong impact was noted only if the children experienced uncontrolled seizures. Otherwise, life was described as fairly normal. In contrast, for families of children with both epilepsy and neurologic motor deficits, the neurologic deficit had a greater impact on family and on the child's life in general—whether at home, in school, or with friends and activities—than did epilepsy alone. In fact, problems identified in any of the three domains—behavioral, cognitive, and neurologic—were more influential than were problems related to epilepsy (Camfield, unpublished data).

Conclusion

The motor disabilities of children with cerebral palsy often are associated with other handicaps, and epilepsy is among the most common of these associated disorders. The dual handicap of epilepsy and cerebral palsy occurs in 1 in 1,000 live births, and the type of cerebral palsy present is related to the epileptic seizure type. In addition, the severity of the cerebral palsy correlates directly with the severity of the epilepsy and its eventual control. For many children with this combined disorder, antiepileptic medication can eventually be discontinued. Not surprisingly, the impact on the family of a child with epilepsy and cerebral palsy is significant, particularly when the epileptic seizures are uncontrolled, but it appears that the motor deficit may actually have a greater overall impact on the family than the presence of epilepsy.

References

1. Cummings SK, Nelson KB, Grether JK. Cerebral palsy in four northern California counties, births 1983 through 1985. J Pediatr 1993;123:230–237.
2. Pharaoh PO, Cooke RW. A hypothesis for the aetiology of spastic cerebral palsy—the vanishing twin. Dev Med Child Neurol 1997;39:292–296.
3. Hauser WA, Hesdorffer DC. Epilepsy, Frequency, Causes, and Consequences. New York: Demos, 1990;18–21.
4. Hauser WA. The prevalence and incidence of convulsive disorders in childhood. Epilepsia 1994;35[Suppl 2]:S1–S6.
5. Camfield CS, Camfield PR, Wirrell E, et al. Incidence of epilepsy in childhood and adolescents: a population based study in Nova Scotia from 1977–1985. Epilepsia 1996;37:19–23.
6. Hauser WA, Annegers JF, Kurland LT. Incidence of epilepsy and unprovoked seizures in Rochester, Minnesota: 1935–1984. Epilepsia 1993;34:453–458.
7. Berg AT, Shinnar S, Levy SR, Testa FM. Newly diagnosed epilepsy in children: presentation at diagnosis. Epilepsia 1999;40:445–452.
8. Nayae RL, Peters EC, Bartholomew M, Landis R. Origins of cerebral palsy. Am J Dis Child 1989;143:1154–1161.
9. Curatolo P, Arpino C, Stazi MA, Medda E. Risk factors for the co-occurrence of partial epilepsy, cerebral palsy and mental retardation. Dev Med Child Neurol 1995;37:776–782.
10. Asku F. Nature and prognosis of seizures in patients with cerebral palsy. Dev Med Child Neurol 1990;32:661–668.
11. Ottman R, Annegers JF, Risch N, et al. Relations of genetic and environmental factors in the etiology of epilepsy. Ann Neurol 1996;39:442–449.
12. Badawi N, Watson L, Petterson B, et al. What constitutes cerebral palsy? Dev Med Child Neurol 1998;40:847–851.
13. Pharaoh PO, Cooke T, Cooke RW, Rosenbloom L. Birthweight specific trends in cerebral palsy. Arch Dis Child 1990;65:602–606.
14. Stanley FJ, Alberman E, Blair E. The cerebral palsies: epidemiology and causal pathways. Clin Dev Med 2000;151:208–211.
15. Hagberg B, Hagberg G, Olow I, von Wendt L. The changing panorama of cerebral palsy in Sweden: VII. Prevalence and origin in the birth year period 1987–90. Acta Paediatr 1996;85:954–960.
16. Topp M, Uldall P, Langhoff-Roos J. Trend in cerebral palsy birth prevalence in eastern Denmark: birth-year period 1970–89. Pediatr Perinatal Epidemiol 1997;11:451–460.
17. Pharaoh PO, Cooke T. Cerebral palsy and multiple births. Arch Dis Child Fetal Neonatal Ed 1996;75:F174–F177.
18. Petterson B, Nelson KB, Watson L, Stanley F. Twins, triplets and cerebral palsy in births in Western Australia in the 1980s. BMJ 1993;307:1239–1243.
19. Stanley FJ, Blair E, Hockey A, et al. Spastic quadriplegia in Western Australia. A genetic epidemiological study: 1. Case population and perinatal risk factors. Dev Med Child Neurol 1993;35:191–120.
20. Nelson KB, Ellenberg JH. Antecedents of cerebral palsy. Multivariate analysis of risk. N Engl J Med 1986;315:81–86.
21. Blair E, Stanley FJ. Intrauterine growth and spastic cerebral palsy: 1. Association with birth weight for gestational age. Am J Obstet Gynecol 1990;162:229–237.
22. Blair E, Stanley F. When can cerebral palsy be prevented? The generation of causal hypotheses by multivariate analysis of a case-control study. Paediatr Perinat Epidemiol 1993;7:272–301.
23. Kudrjveev T, Schoenberg B, Kurland L, Grouver H. Cerebral palsy: survival rates, associated handicaps, and distribution by clinical subtype. Neurology 1985;35:900–903.
24. Aicardi J. Epilepsy in brain-injured children. Dev Med Child Neurol 1990;32:191–202.
25. Hadjipanaysis A, Hadjichristodoulou C, Youroukos S. Epilepsy in patients with cerebral palsy. Dev Med Child Neurol 1997;39:659–663.
26. Kwong KL, Wong SN, Kwan TS. Epilepsy in children with cerebral palsy. Pediatr Neurol 1998;19:31–36.
27. Zafeiriou DI, Kontopoulos EE, Tsikoulas I. Characteristics and prognosis of epilepsy in children with cerebral palsy. J Child Neurol 1999;13:289–294.
28. Dooley JM, Gordon K, Camfield PR, et al. Discontinuation of anticonvulsant therapy in children free of seizures for 1 year. Neurology 1996;46:969–974.
29. Berg AT, Shinnar S. Relapse following discontinuation of antiepileptic drugs: a meta-analysis. Neurology 1994;44:601–608.
30. Camfield C, Camfield P, Smith B, et al. Biologic factors as predictors of social outcome of epilepsy in intellectually normal children: a population-based study. J Pediatr 1993;122:869–873.
31. Hollowach-Thurston J, Thurston DL, Hixon BB, Keller A. Prognosis of childhood epilepsy: additional follow-up of 148 children 5–23 years after withdrawal of anticonvulsant therapy. N Engl J Med 1982;306:831–836.

32. Peters ABC, Brouwer OF, Geerts AT, et al. Randomized prospective study of antiepileptic drugs in children with epilepsy. Neurology 1998;50:724–730.

33. Matricardi M, Brinciotti, M, Benedetti P. Outcome after discontinuation of antiepileptic drug therapy in children with epilepsy. Epilepsia 1989;30:582–589.

34. Roger J, Bureau M. Unilateral Seizures: Hemiconvulsions-Hemiplegia Syndrome and Hemiconvulsions-Hemiplegia Epilepsy. In F Broughton, H Gastaut (eds), The Neurosciences, Electroencephalography and Clinical Neurophysiology [Suppl 35]. Amsterdam: Elsevier, 1982;211–221.

35. Traverse L, Dravet C, Roger J, et al. Epilepsy in children with severe cerebral palsy: outcome and evolution. Dev Med Child Neurol 1994;36[Suppl 70]:32–33.

36. Sillanpaa M, Jalava M, Olli K, Shinnar A. Long-term prognosis of seizures with onset in childhood. N Engl J Med 1998;338:1715–1722.

37. Delgado MR, Riela AR, Mills J, et al. Discontinuation of antiepileptic drug treatment after two seizure-free years in children with cerebral palsy. Pediatrics 1996;97:192–197.

38. Camfield CS, Breau L, Camfield PR. Impact of pediatric epilepsy on the family: a new scale for clinical and research use. Epilepsia 2001;42:104–112.

Chapter 5

Sudden Unexpected Death in Epilepsy: An Update

Thaddeus Walczak

Tonic-clonic seizures are dramatic events, often including collapse, unresponsiveness, impaired respiration, and cyanosis. A first-time observer may well conclude that a person experiencing a tonic-clonic seizure is about to die. The dramatic character of tonic-clonic seizures has led to widespread fears that tonic-clonic seizures commonly result in death. In fact, such seizures are rarely responsible for death. Mortality in population-based studies of epilepsy is only mildly increased,[1] and much of this increase is attributable to the diseases responsible for the epilepsy rather than to the epileptic seizures themselves. Nonetheless, sudden, unexpected death has been reported in patients with epilepsy since the late 1800s.[2] For many years, this entity was considered a curiosity among forensic pathologists. More recent efforts have confirmed the existence of this entity, explored its incidence in various population studies, and begun to define its risk factors and investigate its pathophysiology. Sufficient information now is available to reassure most patients, identify high-risk patients, and suggest means to reduce risk. As one might expect, this topic continues to engender anxiety among patients and physicians. The increasingly available information is the best means by which to assuage such fears.

Definition

There is increasing consensus regarding a definition for sudden unexpected death in epilepsy (SUDEP), allowing comparison among various studies. Proposed definitions vary somewhat between investigators in the United Kingdom and North America because of higher autopsy rates in the former locale. U.K. investigators have proposed the following definition: "Sudden, unexpected, witnessed or unwitnessed, nontraumatic and nondrowning death in patients with epilepsy with or without evidence for a seizure and excluding documented status epilepticus, in which postmortem examination does not reveal a toxicologic or anatomic cause for death."[3] North American investigators have proposed that SUDEP subjects meet the following criteria: (1) The victim suffers from epilepsy (recurrent unprovoked seizures); (2) death occurs unexpectedly while the patient is in a reasonable state of health; (3) death occurs over minutes; (4) death occurs in benign circumstances while the patient is engaged in normal activities; and (5) no obvious cause of death, including status epilepticus, is present. SUDEP is further divided into four categories: definite (other causes excluded by sufficient description of circumstances of death and autopsy with toxicologic screening), probable (no obvious cause of death but no autopsy), possible (SUDEP possible but information regarding circumstances of death insufficient), and not SUDEP (SUDEP unlikely per circumstances of death or another cause of death established).[4] Because of low autopsy rates in the United States, a working definition of SUDEP includes both definite and probable SUDEP. Estab-

Table 5-1. Incidence of Sudden Unexplained Death in Epilepsy

Population Type	Location or Group Studied	Total Patient-Years	Incidence (per 1,000 patient-years)
Geographic population	Olmsted County (Ficker 1998)[6]	25,939	0.35
Large epilepsy cohort	Minnesota (Walczak 1998)[7]	17,376	1.0
	Stockholm (Nilsson 1999)[8]	40,508	1.3
	Saskatchewan (Tennis 1995)[9]	33,299	0.7–1.0
Drug or device development program	Gabapentin (PDR 1999)[10]		3.8
	Lamotrigine (Leestma 1997)[4]	5,745	3.5
	Vagal nerve stimulator (Annegers 1999)[11]	3,176	4.1
Epilepsy surgery program	Graduate hospital (Sperling 1999)[12]	1,502	4.0
	MINCEP (Walczak 1999)[13]	4,384	1.4

PDR = *Physicians' Desk Reference.*

lishing whether SUDEP exists in an individual situation, therefore, depends largely on the available information regarding circumstances of death, and this information may be incomplete. Because these judgments are somewhat subjective, contemporary studies require consensus by a panel of physicians familiar with SUDEP. Interobserver reliability of these individual observations is unknown.

Case History

A subject from the Cook County series[5] is presented to illustrate a typical SUDEP case.

M.J. was 46 years old at the time of his death. He experienced some seizures during childhood, followed by a relatively long seizure-free period. Seizures resumed at age 38 and occurred three to four times per year. Observer description suggested that these were complex partial seizures with secondary generalization. M.J. was last seen by his family physician in November 1983, when he was given a prescription for phenytoin, 300 mg. per day, and phenobarbital, 90 mg per day. He had abused alcohol in the past, but his medical history was otherwise unremarkable, and the family specifically denied head trauma. Family witnessed a tonic-clonic seizure on December 5 at 10:45 AM, after which M.J. got up to go to the bathroom. At this point, family heard a fall and found him in the midst of another tonic-clonic seizure. Tonic-clonic movements stopped after several minutes but he remained unresponsive, so an ambulance was

summoned. M.J. was taken to a nearby emergency room, where he was pronounced dead on arrival at 11:30 AM. General autopsy found no evidence of atherosclerotic heart disease, aspiration, or cause of death. Lungs weighed 1,426 g, approximately 2.2% of body weight. Gross examination revealed severe pulmonary edema. Toxicologic screening revealed no phenytoin, phenobarbital, or alcohol in bile or serum. A neuropathologic workup revealed encephalomalacia of the right temporal lobe together with right dorsal frontal and parietal contusions.

Incidence

The incidence of SUDEP appears to vary by the severity of epilepsy in the population studied (Table 5-1).[4,6–13] The only large population study found a relatively low incidence of 0.35 per 1,000 patient-years.[6] However, this rate was nearly 24 times the rate found in the general population without epilepsy. Selection bias probably is present in all other reasonably large cohort studies. The incidence of SUDEP in large epilepsy referral cohorts clusters around 1.0 per 1,000 patient-years. One would expect a range of seizure severity in these groups, although overall severity would likely be higher than in a population-based cohort.

The incidence in drug development programs and the vagal nerve stimulation development program is three to four times higher than in epilepsy referral cohorts and is similar to that found in epilepsy surgery cohorts (see Table 5-1). One would expect an increased severity of epilepsy in these groups. The increase in SUDEP incidence parallels an increase in epilepsy severity, arguing that severity of epilepsy is a risk factor for SUDEP. The relatively high incidence of SUDEP found in epilepsy drug and device development programs has raised concern that the medications and devices were responsible for sudden death. However, the presence of similar rates in virtually all populations of refractory epilepsy treated with new drugs has led to the conclusion that the severity of the epilepsy rather than the treatment is responsible for SUDEP.[4,14]

Circumstances of Death, Autopsy Studies, and Risk Factors in Uncontrolled Series

Initial speculations regarding risk factors for SUDEP came from medical examiner and autopsy case series. Circumstances at death are remarkably uniform. Of all SUDEP deaths examined, 33–63% of patients are found dead in bed,[5,15,16] being either asleep at the time of death or perhaps instinctively getting into bed after an epileptic seizure. Fifty to 75% die shortly after a witnessed seizure.[5,17,18] For those patients who were continuously observed, a seizure typically was followed by unresponsiveness, the patient was pulseless, and attempts to resuscitate the patient usually were unsuccessful.[5,15] However, some subjects have been observed to collapse and expire without a witnessed seizure.[19] When position of death is reported, 42–81% are noted to be in a prone position.[18,20,21] However, we encountered such cases infrequently in the Cook County series and so did not include them in the SUDEP group.

Autopsy studies have excluded other potentially fatal conditions by definition. Cardiovascular disease does not appear to be particularly prominent. Structural lesions, indicative of symptomatic epilepsy, appear more commonly than would be expected.[5,15,17] Pulmonary edema is almost invariably present, both by lung weight and histology.[5,17,21,22] Anticonvulsant drug levels assayed postmortem often are determined to be subtherapeutic,[5,15,16] suggesting that noncompliance is common in SUDEP cases. Nonfatal con-

centrations of alcohol were frequent in the Cook County series[5,15] but rare in the Norwegian series.[17]

Characteristics of the subjects in autopsy-based series also were reasonably uniform. Young men predominated. Seizures appeared to be more frequent and duration of the epilepsy disorder longer than would be expected in the general epilepsy population. Virtually all subjects had experienced tonic-clonic seizures at some time in the course of their epilepsy. Moreover, seizures witnessed prior to death were invariably of the tonic-clonic type. Developmental delay was more common and psychotropic medications were administered more frequently than was expected. However, these observations all were uncontrolled and therefore susceptible to selection bias. For example, the increased number of male subjects and the high prevalence of structural lesions found in these studies likely were due to referral bias.

Risk Factors for Sudden Unexpected Death in Epilepsy in Controlled Series

Three cohort-based case-control studies have begun to address concerns regarding selection bias (Table 5-2).[7–9] Even though substantial methodological differences were noted among the studies, the results are reasonably identical. Examination of the information revealed that an increased number of any seizures and of tonic-clonic seizures were associated with SUDEP. Longer duration of epilepsy also was associated with SUDEP. These findings, together with the observation that SUDEP follows witnessed tonic-clonic seizures, strongly support the notion that exposure to tonic-clonic seizures is a strong risk factor for SUDEP. A reasonable conclusion is that the number of anticonvulsant drugs is a surrogate for the severity of epilepsy.[9] However, Nilsson et al.[8] found that the number of anticonvulsant drugs and seizure frequency were independent risk factors for SUDEP, and further analysis of the Minnesota data set supports this finding (unpublished observation).

Whether SUDEP is more common in young male subjects remains unresolved, different trends being revealed in the various cohort-

Table 5-2. Risk Factors for Sudden Unexplained Death in Epilepsy in Cohort-Based Controlled Studies

	Saskatchewan (Tennis 1995)[9]	Stockholm (Nilsson 1999)[8]	Minnesota (Walczak 1998)[7]
Number of seizures	NE	+	+
Number of tonic-clonic seizures	NE	NE	+
Duration of epilepsy	NE	+	+
Number of anticonvulsant drugs	+	+	+
Psychotropic medications	+	+	−

NE = risk factor not examined; + indicates positive association between risk factor and SUDEP; − indicates negative association between risk factor and SUDEP.

based studies.[6–9] A population-based study[23] found that SUDEP was very rare in the pediatric age group, which supports the relative lack of pediatric cases in uncontrolled series. Structural lesions were not more common in SUDEP than in controls in the only assessment of this issue.[7]

Controlled studies have also questioned the notion that noncompliance with treatment regimens is more common in SUDEP. Walczak et al.[7] compared anticonvulsant drug levels at last antemortem visit in SUDEP subjects and controls and found no difference. All anticonvulsant drug levels were therapeutic in approximately 60% of both groups. At least some levels were therapeutic in more than 90% of both groups. One controlled study of postmortem anticonvulsant drug levels[24] found that subtherapeutic levels were significantly more common in SUDEP than in epilepsy patients dying of other causes, but another study[25] demonstrated no difference. Multiple factors can affect postmortem anticonvulsant drug levels, and whether postmortem levels adequately reflect antemortem compliance remains in question.

Only one controlled study asked whether developmental delay was more common in SUDEP than in control subjects.[7] Developmental delay was defined as an intelligence quotient of less than 70 or delay so severe that formal mental status examination was not possible. Intelligence quotient determinations had been performed in approximately 70% of both groups. Whereas 46% of SUDEP subjects had developmental delay, only 18% of the control group exhibited such delay ($p < .05$). Subsequent analysis has determined that developmental delay and seizure frequency were independent risk factors in this group (unpublished observation).

In summary, controlled studies uniformly indicate that the number of seizures in general and the number of tonic-clonic seizures are risk factors for SUDEP. The number of anticonvulsant drugs administered appears to be an independent risk factor, as does developmental delay. Information regarding age and gender is unclear, although SUDEP appears rare in the pediatric age group. In contrast to earlier reports, the presence of structural lesions and compliance with a prescribed medical regimen do not appear to be risk factors. However, this assessment remains tentative because the number of controlled assessments of risk factors still is relatively small.

Possible Mechanisms for Sudden Unexpected Death in Epilepsy

Initial reports suggested that fatal cardiac arrhythmia was responsible for SUDEP. The evidence supporting this theory has been reviewed.[26–28] Seizures are known to increase catecholamine levels, which, in turn, may increase ventricular ectopic activity. Cortical stimulation rarely induces ventricular ectopic activity, and seizures resulting in arrhythmia have been reported. Sleep induces both ventricular ectopic activity and epileptic seizures, which may explain the apparent increased rate of SUDEP during sleep. Some psychotropic medications may predispose to arrhythmia, which may explain the higher use of psychotropic medications in the SUDEP group. Finally, repeated surges of catecholamines induce subtle cardiac lesions, which may act as a nidus for a cortically or hormonally induced ventricular arrhythmia. Animal models have confirmed that interictal and ictal discharge increase the tendency to cardiac arrhythmia.[29]

The hypothesis that cardiac arrhythmia is responsible for SUDEP has been challenged by subsequent findings. Long-term monitoring of ictal electroencephalograms and electrocardiograms reveals that ictal arrhythmia is rare. This hypothesis does not account for the almost uniform finding of pulmonary edema in autopsy studies of SUDEP. Finally, animal models of SUDEP do not demonstrate cardiac arrhythmia prior to death.[30,31]

The presence of pulmonary edema in SUDEP led to the suggestion that neurogenic pulmonary edema is responsible for SUDEP. Neurogenic pulmonary edema has been reported as a consequence of a variety of neurologic conditions, including epilepsy. The mechanism is thought to be increased preload and pulmonary capillary permeability. The latter may be attributable to hydrostatic mechanisms or directly to an abnormal cortical discharge. This hypothesis is consistent with autopsy findings and with reports that death may occur an hour or more after the witnessed seizure. A sheep model of death after bicuculline-induced status epilepticus found that pulmonary edema was, in fact, more extensive in animals that died than in animals that survived.[30] The pulmonary edema was associated with increased left atrial and pulmonary artery pressures.

However, the degree of pulmonary edema was not sufficient to explain the degree of ventilatory failure observed in the animal model of SUDEP.[30] Further studies of eight animals found that central apnea was at least partially responsible for two deaths and that cardiac failure related to massive subendocardial necrosis was responsible for a third death.[31] These findings, together with the time course of the ventilatory failure, led to the conclusion that profound central apnea related to the seizure was more often responsible for death than pulmonary edema, at least in this model.[31] A skeptic would point out that this is a model of status epilepticus. Nonetheless, no evidence indicates that the seizures responsible for SUDEP are more severe than the patient's characteristic seizures.

Some degree of apnea is common during and after epileptic seizures in humans.[32,33] The apnea appears to be central in type, but its duration is not particularly long nor is the degree of oxygen desaturation profound. Two case reports of video electroencephalographic monitoring during SUDEP have demonstrated continuing regular heart rhythms more than 1 minute after seizure termination.[34,35] An apparent respiratory arrest in one case was seen to respond to brief cardiopulmonary resuscitation.[35] In both cases, intense postictal electroencephalographic suppression was noted, more profound than had been seen in other seizures in this patient.

A SUDEP case series suggested that SUDEP was far more common in an outpatient setting than in a group home setting where staff had received vigorous training in first aid treatment of tonic-clonic seizures.[18] The researchers of this series have suggested that attention to positioning, aggressive treatment of seizures, stimulation after seizures, and respiratory support when necessary may help to prevent SUDEP.

We believe that the mechanism of SUDEP remains speculative and that different mechanisms may be operational in different patients. A more complete understanding of the mechanism is necessary before sound recommendations for prevention are possible. Although the controlled series and circumstances at death argue strongly that tonic-clonic seizures cause SUDEP, most patients tolerate well even very lengthy and severe tonic-clonic seizures. Indeed, virtually all patients succumbing to SUDEP had experienced unwitnessed tonic-clonic seizures previously, and several in our case series had survived status epilepticus. We do not know how the tonic-clonic seizure responsible for death differs from all other such seizures that the patient has survived.

Approach to the Individual Epilepsy Patient

The diagnosis of epilepsy and the ensuing changes are traumatic for many patients. Distressing topics such as driving privileges, informing of employers, and pregnancy must be addressed. In the multiply impaired patient, SUDEP may appear to be yet another intractable problem in a long list. Patients and their caregivers already are anxious and raise difficult questions to which the practitioner may not have easy answers. Not surprisingly, many physicians shy away from discussing SUDEP, although it now is clear that SUDEP is a genuine phenomenon. Information regarding risk factors is fairly consistent, and it appears that developmental delay is an independent risk factor. Therefore, we consider it reasonable to address the issue of SUDEP directly in appropriate situations.

We tend to discuss SUDEP with patients experiencing established, relatively severe epilepsy that includes tonic-clonic seizures. We start with a general discussion of mortality in epilepsy—for example, stating that mortality in epilepsy is increased two to three times over that of the general population—and then add that 20–30% of the time, the death in epileptics may be sudden and unexpected. Sufficient information now is available to support a more quantitative discussion of risk based on epilepsy severity (see Table 5-1), assuming the patient is in a position to understand such information. We use the general discussion of SUDEP to emphasize other relevant issues such as compliance with anticonvulsant treatment regimens and medical appointments and avoidance of alcohol. Obviously, the potentially distressing topic of SUDEP must be discussed in a sensitive and balanced way, taking into account the patient's and family's individual circumstances. Emphasis on the fact that the great majority of patients tolerate the great majority of tonic-clonic seizures without much difficulty is critical.

No scientific proof exists that any specific intervention can prevent SUDEP; consequently, no firm recommendations for prevention are possible. Currently, the best way to treat SUDEP is to treat the patient's epilepsy aggressively and to ensure that caregivers receive proper education in the acute management of tonic-clonic seizures. Certainly, every effort should be made to control seizures, especially tonic-clonic seizures, with the fewest anticonvulsants possible. SUDEP should be discussed when consideration is being given to epilepsy surgery, because evidence now shows that successful epilepsy surgery decreases mortality.[12] Drug compliance and avoidance of alcohol should be emphasized, even though it is not clear that these are strong risk factors. Patients should be encouraged to sleep in the supine rather than prone position, because so many SUDEP subjects are found prone at the time of death.

Instructing caregivers in the delivery of appropriate first aid during and after tonic-clonic seizures is useful. Conditions for summoning emergency medical assistance should be clear. Ideally, caregivers should be able to distinguish between the ictal and postictal states and to evaluate the patient's respirations in the postictal period. Also ideally, caregivers should be instructed in how to position the patient and keep the airway open postictally and about how much apnea is tolerable. As some believe that vigorous stimulation may shorten the duration of the usual postictal central apnea, vigorous stimulation of the patient after a tonic-clonic seizure is reasonable, to ensure responsiveness.

As with many other aspects of epilepsy, the possibility of SUDEP is at first terrifying to patient, physician, and family. Research, education, and the engagement of patient and family in care is critical. This approach minimizes risk, increases understanding, alleviates anxiety, and helps patients with epilepsy to live the fullest lives possible.

References

1. Nilsson L, Tomson T, Farahmand BY, et al. Cause-specific mortality in epilepsy: a cohort study of more than 9,000 patients once hospitalized for epilepsy. Epilepsia 1997;38(10):1062–1068.
2. Bacon GM. On the modes of death in epilepsy. Lancet 1868;1:555–556.
3. Nashef L. Sudden unexpected death in epilepsy: terminology and definitions. Epilepsia 1997;38[Suppl 11]:S6–S8.
4. Leestma JE, Annegers JF, Brodie MJ, et al. Sudden unexplained death in epilepsy: observations from a large clinical development program Epilepsia 1997;38:47–55.
5. Leestma JE, Walczak TS, Hughes JR, et al. A prospective study on sudden unexpected death in epilepsy. Ann Neurol 1989;26:195–203.
6. Ficker DM, So EL, Shen WE, et al. Population-based study of incidence of sudden unexplained death in epilepsy. Neurology 1998;51:1270–1274.
7. Walczak TS, Hauser WA, Leppik IE, et al. Incidence and risk factors for sudden unexpected death in epilepsy: a prospective cohort study. Neurology 1998;50[Suppl 4]:A443–A444.
8. Nilsson L, Farahmand B, Persson PG, et al. Risk factors for sudden unexpected death in epilepsy: a case control study. Lancet 1999;353:888–893.
9. Tennis P, Cole T, Annegers J, et al. Cohort study of incidence of sudden unexplained death in persons with

seizure disorder treated with antiepileptic drugs in Saskatchewan, Canada. Epilepsia 1995;36(1):29–36.

10. Physicians' Desk Reference (PDR). Montvale, NJ: Medical Economics, 1999.

11. Annegers JF, Coan SP, Hauser WA, Leestma J. Epilepsy, vagal nerve stimulation by the NCP system, all-cause mortality, and sudden unexpected, unexplained death. Epilepsia 1999;40[Suppl 7]:165.

12. Sperling MR, Feldman H, Kinman J, et al. Seizure control and mortality in epilepsy. Ann Neurol 1999; 46:45–50.

13. Walczak TS, Radick JO, Hauser WA, et al. Mortality after epilepsy surgery. Neurology 1999;52[Suppl 2]:A108.

14. Annegers JF, Coan SP, Hauser WA, et al. Epilepsy, vagal nerve stimulation by the NCP system, all-cause mortality, and sudden, unexpected, unexplained death. Epilepsia 2000;41(5):549–553.

15. Leestma JE, Kalelkar MB, Teas SS, et al. Sudden unexpected death associated with seizures: analysis of 66 cases. Epilepsia 1984;25:84–88.

16. Terrence CF, Wisotzkey HM, Perper JA. Unexpected, unexplained death in epileptic patients. Neurology 1975;25:594–598.

17. Kloster R, Engelskjon T. Sudden unexpected death in epilepsy (SUDEP): a clinical perspective and a search for risk factors. J Neurol Neurosurg Psychiatry 1999; 67:439–444.

18. Nashef L, Garner S, Fish D. Circumstances of death in sudden death in epilepsy: interviews of bereaved relatives. J Neurol Neurosurg Psychiatry 1998;64:349–352.

19. Hirsch CS, Martin DL. Unexpected death in young epileptics. Neurology 1971;21:682–690.

20. Coyle HP, Baker-Brian N, Brown SW. Coroners' autopsy reporting of sudden unexplained death in epilepsy (SUDEP) in the UK. Seizure 1994;3:247–254.

21. Earnest MP, Thomas GE, Eden RA, Hossak FF. The sudden unexplained death syndrome in epilepsy: demographic, clinical and pathological features. Epilepsia 1992;33(2):310–316.

22. Terrence CF, Rao GR, Perper JA. Neurogenic pulmonary edema in unexpected, unexplained death of epileptic patients. Ann Neurol 1981;9:458–464.

23. Camfield CS, Camfield PR. Good news—a population-based study indicates that SUDEP is very unusual in childhood onset epilepsy. Epilepsia 1999;40[Suppl 7]:159.

24. George JR, Davis GG. Comparison of AED levels in different cases of sudden death. J Forensic Sci 1998; 43:598–603.

25. Opeskin K, Burke MD, Cordner SM, Berkovic SF. Comparison of antiepileptic drug levels in sudden unexpected deaths in epilepsy with deaths from other causes. Epilepsia 1999;40:1795–1798.

26. Jay GW, Leestma JE. Sudden death in epilepsy. Acta Neurol Scand Suppl 1981;63:1–66.

27. Lathers CM, Schraeder PL (eds). Epilepsy and Sudden Death. New York: Marcel Dekker, 1990.

28. Lathers CM, Schraeder PL, Boggs J. Sudden Unexplained Death and Autonomic Dysfunction. In J Engel Jr, TA Pedley (eds), Epilepsy: A Comprehensive Textbook. Philadelphia: Lippincott–Raven, 1997;1943–1955.

29. Lathers CM, Schraeder PL, Weinder FL. Synchronization of cardiac autonomic neural discharge with epileptogenic activity: the lockstep phenomenon. Electroencephalogr Clin Neurophysiol 1987;67:247–259.

30. Johnston SC, Horn JK, Valnete J, Simon RP. The role of hypoventilation in a sheep model of epileptic sudden death. Ann Neurol 1995;37:531–537.

31. Johnston SC, Siedenberg R, Min J, et al. Central apnea and acute cardiac ischemia in a sheep model of epileptic sudden death. Ann Neurol 1997;42:588–594.

32. Nashef L, Walker F, Allen P, et al. Apnea and bradycardia during epileptic seizures: relation to sudden death in epilepsy. J Neurol Neurosurg Psychiatry 1996;60:297–300.

33. Walker F, Fish DR. Recording respiratory parameters in patients with epilepsy. Epilepsia 1997;38[Suppl 11]:41–42.

34. Bird JM, Dembny KAT, Sandeman D, Butler S. Sudden unexplained death in epilepsy: an intracranially monitored case. Epilepsia 1997;38[Suppl 11]:52–56.

35. So EL, Sam MC, Lagerlund TL. Postictal central apnea as a cause of SUDEP: evidence from a case of near-SUDEP. Epilepsia 1999;40[Suppl 7]:90–91.

Part II

Epilepsy Syndromes in the Developmental Disability Population

Chapter 6

Neonatal Seizures and Neonatal Epilepsy

Josiane LaJoie and Solomon L. Moshe

Neonatal seizures are undoubtedly one of the most common neurologic conditions in the neonatal period. Neonatal seizures occur in 1.5–3.5 live births per 1,000.[1] Neonatal seizures occur, by definition, within the first 28 days of life, and usually within the first 10 days.

A neonatal seizure is defined as an abnormal, paroxysmal, stereotypical clinical behavior. When the clinical events are associated with changes in the electroencephalogram (EEG), they are known as *epileptic seizures*. At times, clear EEG changes are noted in the absence of any accompanying clinical changes. These are referred to as *electrographic seizures*. Finally, when a clinical event is not associated with EEG changes, it then is regarded as a *nonepileptic seizure*. In this case, concluding whether the event truly represents epileptic seizure activity or another behavioral manifestation is difficult.

Neonatal seizures most often are provoked seizures, meaning that they occur acutely in relation to a specific insult (e.g., hypoxia or ischemia, birth trauma, or metabolic disturbances). They can be symptomatic in nature, occurring without any provocation but related to a specific brain lesion. Much research has been performed regarding the recognition, etiology, treatment, and prognosis of neonatal seizures. What have been emphasized less are the neonatal epilepsy syndromes, which represent a collection of signs and symptoms, the recognition of which implies future genetic risk and specific syndrome-dependent prognosis. In this

chapter, we review certain aspects of neonatal seizures, including the recognition, prognosis, and treatment of the neonatal epilepsy syndromes.

Recognition of Neonatal Seizures

The manifestations of neonatal seizures include a limited repertoire of behaviors consisting mostly of motor or autonomic phenomena. Other types of seizures encountered in older individuals cannot be diagnosed in the newborn period, because they require the maturation of the central nervous system and language. Neonatal seizures can be classified according to their motor and autonomic manifestations (Table 6-1). The four major types are clonic, tonic, myoclonic, and subtle, and each can be further subdivided. Mizrahi and Kellaway[2] devised a system that depends on whether there is consistent, inconsistent, or no correlation between the clinical behavior and the ictal EEG discharges. Some debate remains as to whether all the behaviors classified as neonatal seizures have a consistent relationship with electrographic discharges (Table 6-2).

Clonic seizures are characterized by rhythmic contractions and relaxations of single or multiple muscle groups. Focal clonic seizures are the most common type. Clonic seizures are most consistently associated with EEG seizure discharges, which may be either focal or multifocal in origin.[3] Focal discharges are caused by not only focal lesions (i.e., stroke) but by conditions

Table 6-1. Behavioral Characteristics of Neonatal Seizures

I. Clonic
  A. Focal
  B. Multifocal
II. Tonic
  A. Focal
  B. Generalized
III. Myoclonic
  A. Focal
  B. Multifocal
  C. Generalized
IV. Subtle
  A. Ocular
    1. Eye deviation
    2. Sustained eye opening
    3. Eye jerking
  B. Oral-buccal-lingual
    1. Chewing
    2. Other
  C. Limb movement: pedaling
  D. Autonomic
    1. Brady tachycardia
    2. Hypertension
  E. Apnea

Source: Modified from JJ Volpe. Neonatal Seizures. In JJ Volpe (ed), Neurology of the Newborn. Philadelphia: Saunders, 1995;172–207.

affecting the brain diffusely, such as metabolic derangements.

Tonic seizures are characterized by sustained contractions of muscle groups either in flexion or extension. Premature infants are more likely to exhibit this type of seizure. Tonic seizures may be focal or generalized, the latter being more common. When generalized, they tend to mimic decorticate or decerebrate posturing and most frequently are seen with diffuse cerebral dysfunction. EEG recordings at the time of tonic seizures rarely show electrographic seizure patterns. Approximately 30% of focal tonic seizures are associated with EEG seizure discharges.

Myoclonic seizures also involve the contraction of individual muscle groups but are more rapid than clonic seizures and are more likely to involve flexor muscles. They may be focal, multifocal, or generalized. In focal myoclonic seizures, an arm or leg muscle is flexed. In multifocal seizures, asynchronous twitching of different muscle groups occurs in different parts of the body. Generalized myoclonic seizures are found in bilateral muscle groups. Of all of the types of myoclonic seizures, generalized myoclonic seizures are most likely to be associated with electrographic seizure patterns.

The recognition of subtle seizures may be difficult. They tend to be expressed as stereotypical, behavioral, or motor automatisms, such as oral-buccal-lingual movements, ocular signs, pedaling, bicycling, stepping, rotary arm movements, or other purposeless movements such as thrashing or struggling.[4] Subtle seizures are more common in the premature population. Many of the clinical manifestations are not associated consistently with EEG seizure discharges but, at some point, all the clinical manifestations have been documented with electrographic seizure discharges. Mizrahi and Kellaway[2] found that tonic horizontal deviation of the eyes is the most common subtle seizure exhibiting consistent EEG seizure discharges.

Table 6-2. Types and Likelihood of Accompanying Electrographic Correlates of Neonatal Seizures

Type	Volpe	Mizrahi and Kellaway
Clonic-focal	Common	Common
Clonic-multifocal	Common	Common
Tonic-focal	Common	Common
Tonic-generalized	Uncommon	Inconsistent
Myoclonic-focal	Uncommon	Common
Myoclonic-multifocal	Uncommon	Inconsistent
Myoclonic-generalized	Common	Inconsistent
Ocular signs	Common[a]	Inconsistent
Oral-buccal-lingual movements	Common[b]	Inconsistent
Limb movements	Inconsistent	Inconsistent
Apnea	Common[a]	Common

[a]In term infants.
[b]In preterm infants.
Sources: Modified from JJ Volpe. Neonatal Seizures. In JJ Volpe (ed), Neurology of the Newborn. Philadelphia: Saunders, 1995;172–207; and EM Mizrahi, P Kellaway. Characterization and classification of neonatal seizures. Neurology 1987;37:1837–1844.

The occurrence of epileptic apnea is a controversial subject. Apnea alone is rarely, if ever, epileptic in nature. As a seizure manifestation, it usually is associated with other "subtle" signs with or without autonomic instability (i.e., tachycardia, hypertension). Apnea is more commonly seen in premature infants who are already being treated with anticonvulsant medications and who are at increased risk for other medical conditions.[2] When presented with the possibility of subtle seizures, the practitioner must remark whether any relation exists between stimulation of the infant and the movement, whether the movement can be suppressed by manual restraint, and whether other associated autonomic phenomena are present. Nonepileptic phenomena usually are stimulus-sensitive, can be suppressed, and are not associated with other autonomic changes. The EEG can be helpful in this determination. Most practitioners require electrographic confirmation to continue antiepileptic drug (AED) therapy and will usually discontinue treatment if no EEG correlates can be found. In this case, it is assumed that subtle seizures may be primitive brainstem and spinal motor patterns released from the tonic inhibition exerted by forebrain structures (i.e., release phenomena).[2]

However, the lack of electrographic seizures does not always argue against the epileptic nature of the altered, paroxysmal behavior. Some seizures are known to originate from deep cerebral structures, including the limbic system, and therefore may not be detected by scalp electrodes. Although a controversial issue in humans, brainstem seizures occur in animals, and these discharges do not spread in cortical regions.[5,6] In fact, Danner et al.[7] reported a case of seizures in an atelencephalic infant.

Etiology of Neonatal Seizures

Neonatal seizures are most commonly provoked seizures but can also occur as part of symptomatic epilepsy or part of a neonatal epileptic syndrome (Table 6-3). The etiology of provoked neonatal seizures depends on the gestational age of the infant (Table 6-4). Hypoxic-ischemic encephalopathy is a well-known entity in both full-term and preterm newborns and is the cause of 50–65% of

Table 6-3. Etiology of Neonatal Seizures

Provoked neonatal seizures
Birth asphyxia
Birth trauma
Drug withdrawal
Infection
Metabolic disturbances
Vascular events
Onset of symptomatic neonatal epilepsies
Posthypoxic
Posttraumatic
Secondary to cerebrovascular accident
Association with cerebral dysgenesis
Association with metabolic disorders
Association with tumor (rare)
Neonatal epilepsy syndromes
Benign
Catastrophic

neonatal seizures.[4] Its incidence is on the rise, probably secondary to the advances in neonatal resuscitation. Many of these newborns would not have survived in previous decades. Seizures usually begin on the first day of life, usually within 12–24 hours. The seizures tend to be most severe in the first 72 hours.

Infants born after intrauterine drug exposure can also present with seizures secondary to intoxication or withdrawal. A history of maternal drug use is present, most commonly involving cocaine, methadone, tricyclic antidepressants, or alcohol. Seizures can present as early as 3 days or as late as 34 days after birth.

Infants in whom infections are seeding the subarachnoid space are extremely vulnerable to seizures. Intracranial infections account for approximately 5–10% of neonatal seizures.[4] Newborns with meningoencephalitis or sepsis (or both) usually present with seizures within 24 hours but can present as late as 10 days after birth. The most common bacterial pathogens are group B beta-streptococci, *Escherichia coli*, and *Listeria* species. In cases of encephalitis, herpes simplex virus is a common cause, as are toxoplasmosis, Coxsackie B virus, rubella, and cytomegalovirus infection. Seizures in the context of toxoplasmosis and cytomegalovirus infection tend to occur within the first 3 days, whereas

Table 6-4. Common Etiologies of Provoked Neonatal Seizures in Relation to Age, Frequency, and Onset

Etiology	Full-Term	Preterm	% Frequency	Seizure Onset (hrs)
HIE	+	+	50–65	0–24
ICH			10	
SAH	+			48
IVH		+		0–72
Subdural	+	+		0–48
Drug withdrawal	+	+		72
Infection	+	+	5–10	0–72
Hypoglycemia	+	+	12	0–72
Hypocalcemia	+	+	12	48–72
Local anesthetic	+	+		0–6

HIE = hypoxic-ischemic encephalopathy; ICH = intracerebral hemorrhage; IVH = intraventricular hemorrhage; SAH = subarachnoid hemorrhage.
Source: Modified from JJ Volpe. Neonatal Seizures. In JJ Volpe (ed), Neurology of the Newborn. Philadelphia: Saunders, 1995;172–207.

those in herpes simplex virus infections tend to occur later.[4]

Of all possible metabolic disturbances associated with seizures, disturbances of glucose and calcium are the most frequent.[4] Hypoglycemia is most commonly found in small-for-gestational-age newborns and those babies born to diabetic mothers. Early onset hypoglycemia tends to be associated with maternal diabetes mellitus, asphyxia, and intracerebral hemorrhage. The incidence of hypocalcemic seizures has been decreasing over the previous decades. When found, hypocalcemia frequently is associated with, but usually is not the sole cause of, neonatal seizures. These seizures tend to begin within the first 3 days of life. Low calcium levels can be associated with low birth weight, asphyxia, maternal diabetes mellitus, neonatal hypoparathyroidism, maternal hyperparathyroidism, and DiGeorge's syndrome. Hypocalcemia can also present in the later neonatal period and usually is found in infants in whom cow's milk is administered, as this preparation contains a low ratio of phosphorus to calcium.

Other, rarer causes of neonatal seizures include pyridoxine dependency, which can be seen at or shortly after birth. Some authors have even reported intrauterine seizures in association with this dependency. At birth, these infants tend to be meconium-stained and flaccid. Seizures have been reported to occur in those newborns who were mistakenly administered the local anesthetics (procaine substances) given to the mother.

This condition is underdiagnosed secondary to a lack of suspicion. Affected infants are confused with asphyxiated infants, tending to be meconium-stained, flaccid, and apneic, with cardiac arrhythmias and brainstem abnormalities, and often having a laceration of the scalp.[4]

Vascular causes of seizures include cerebral hemorrhage and infarction. The incidence of intracerebral hemorrhage, which can be subarachnoid, subdural, intraventricular, or intraparenchymal, is increasing. Volpe[4] reports that in his experience, intracerebral hemorrhages may account for approximately 10% of neonatal seizures. Intraventricular hemorrhages usually occur in premature patients and commonly are perceived to be due to lack of cerebral blood flow autoregulation. The seizures tend to begin at between 24 and 72 hours of life. Subarachnoid hemorrhage tends to occur in full-term infants. Seizures secondary to subdural hemorrhage are usually focal and occur within 48 hours of life.[4]

Neonatal seizures can present as the first episode of seizure in the onset of symptomatic neonatal epilepsies. Inborn errors of metabolism exhibit various constellations of signs and symptoms (Table 6-5). However, newborns with such metabolic errors commonly present with seizures, which occur as early as the third day of life because, when fed, the neonates are unable to tolerate the metabolic byproducts. Some will present as part of a catastrophic epilepsy syndrome (e.g., nonketotic hyperglycinemia). Neonatal adrenoleukodystrophy is a progressive neurodegenerative disorder that can present with clonic or myoclonic seizures within days of birth. Affected infants tend to be hypotonic, and their seizures are intractable to conventional therapies.

Pathophysiologic Features of Neonatal Seizures

Ongoing basic scientific research has shown that the immature brain is highly susceptible to seizures.[8–12] The increased susceptibility of the immature brain may be due to precocious development of excitatory synapses in certain brain regions, whereas in other brain areas, there may be delayed development of inhibition. Receptor heterogeneity is present at the molecular level. At a very young age, γ-aminobutyric acid, the main neurotransmitter involved in inhibition, may mediate excitatory effects.[13–15] The ionic microenvironment is different early in life, owing to its spatial features and the immaturity of glia. Thus, the immature brain is able to accumulate extracellular potassium to a much greater extent than is the mature brain secondary to altered clearance and slow ion pump systems. This ability to accumulate extracellular potassium contributes to and creates a hyperexcitable state.[12] The lack of organization of the newborn cerebral cortex and weak surround inhibition may make a less effective barrier for seizure spread and generalization.[12] Also, the maturation of circuits involved in the control of seizures is delayed. One such system is based on the connections of the substantia nigra pars reticulata and is under the control of gender hormones.[16]

Whether neonatal seizures affect brain development is a subject of ongoing research and much debate. Most studies have been performed in normal rodents. To date, information reveals that severe recurrent seizures in the neonatal rat can lead to depletion of high-energy phosphates, with a concomitant decrease in high energy and inhibition of DNA synthesis, leading to impaired synaptogenesis, myelination, and brain growth. However, some of these changes may be transient, depending on the total seizure load that the animal experiences.[17] Nonetheless, although it has increased susceptibility to seizures, the neonatal brain appears to be

Table 6-5. Symptoms and Signs of Selected Metabolic Diseases

Metabolic Disease	Symptoms and Signs
Maple syrup urine disease	Vomiting, hypertonia, seizures
Urea cycle defects	Vomiting (after protein-initiated lethargy), hypotonia, bulging fontanelle, seizures
Nonketotic hyperglycinemias	Hypotonia, lethargy, myoclonic seizures, coma between spells
Ketotic hyperglycinemias	Vomiting, dehydration, coma, seizures, acidosis, ketosis, thrombocytopenia
Isovaleric acidemia	Vomiting, acidosis, ketosis, seizures, body odor

more resistant to seizure-induced hippocampal injury of the type seen in adults.[18]

Neonatal Epilepsy Syndromes

Recently, work has led to the identification of neonatal epilepsy syndromes, consisting of a constellation of clinical signs and symptoms and a variable clinical course and EEG findings, which led researchers to identify these syndromes as their own entities. They have been classified as either benign or catastrophic encephalopathies (Table 6-6). Obviously, the nomenclature indicates the prognosis, with the catastrophic epileptic syndromes having an extremely poor outcome.

Benign Idiopathic Neonatal Convulsions

Benign idiopathic neonatal convulsions, also known as *fifth-day fits*, was first described by Dehan in 1977.[19] The current prevalence is between 2% and 7% of neonates.[20] Male infants are affected more than female infants (62%). The onset of seizures is between the fourth and sixth days of life (range, 1–7 days). The seizures are mostly partial clonic and frequently are associated with apnea. Tonic seizures do not occur. The clonic seizures tend to be lateralized and alternate sides. Generalized seizures are rare. Each seizure bout lasts 1–3 minutes but can recur for 24 to 48 hours

Table 6-6. Benign and Catastrophic Neonatal Epilepsy Syndromes

Benign
    Benign idiopathic neonatal convulsions
    Benign familial neonatal convulsions
    Benign neonatal sleep myoclonus
Catastrophic
    Neonatal myoclonic encephalopathy
    Early infantile epileptic encephalopathy

and can evolve into status epilepticus. In 60% of cases, a characteristic interictal EEG pattern, *theta pointu alternant*, is noted. *Theta pointu alternant* is characterized by a nonreactive pattern of dominant theta activity, which is discontinuous, with frequent alternating intrahemispheric activity intermixed with sharp waves. This pattern may persist even after the seizure stops, up to the second week of life. Thus, the diagnosis can be contemplated even if the EEG is performed later.

The differential diagnosis includes nonepileptic paroxysmal phenomena, tremulousness, provoked seizures of various etiologies, benign sleep myoclonus, and benign familial neonatal convulsions, as well as catastrophic epilepsies. Benign idiopathic neonatal convulsions is a diagnosis of exclusion and requires that the following criteria be met, as proposed by Plouin[20]:

1. Normal pregnancy and delivery
2. Full-term infant, normal birth weight
3. Apgar score greater than 7 at 1 minute
4. Normal interval between birth and onset of seizures
5. Normal neurologic state before and between seizures
6. Normal neuroimaging and metabolic examinations; no evidence of infection
7. No family history of either neonatal or later epilepsy

The etiology is unclear. Numerous attempts have been made to identify either metabolic or infectious causes. Herrmann et al.[21] reviewed 21 cases and found an association with rotavirus in stool in 95% of patients but no evidence of any infection in the cerebrospinal fluid. Goldberg and Sheehy[22] in 1982 proposed acute zinc deficiency in the cerebrospinal fluid of neonates as the cause,

but no further reports have substantiated this hypothesis.

The seizures tend to stop without therapy, yet the majority of clinicians believe that the seizures should be treated until the diagnosis is confirmed. Phenobarbital commonly is used. If treatment is initiated, then AEDs should be discontinued prior to the infant's discharge from the hospital.

Prognosis is excellent in that secondary epilepsy is found in only 0.5% of patients. Despite the identification of transient psychomotor delays, the prognosis for a normal developmental outcome is excellent.[19] Only one study identified various neurodevelopmental deficits in 50% of 33 infants followed up until their second birthday.[23] Plouin[20] implies that this percentage of abnormalities is excessively high and not concordant with her experience.

Benign Familial Neonatal Convulsions

Benign familial neonatal convulsions were first described by Rett and Teubel[24] in 1964. The incidence appears to be between 0.9% and 2% of neonates, making this a rare condition. No gender predilection has been identified. In this syndrome, seizures appear during the second or third day of life in 80% of cases, although they can appear from 1 day to 3 months after birth, the latter having been reported in two cases. The seizures are clonic at times, are associated with apnea, and occur repetitively during the first week. Tonic seizures can occur,[25,26] whereas myoclonus and spasms do not. Each seizure episode lasts for only a short period (1–3 minutes). The EEG findings are not specific, although on few occasions a *theta pointu alternant* pattern has been described. Benign familial neonatal convulsions is a diagnosis of exclusion, requiring that the following criteria be met:

1. Normal pregnancy and delivery
2. Full-term infant, normal birth weight
3. Apgar score greater than 7 at 1 minute
4. Normal neurologic state (although some authors have reported a mild transitory hypotonia)
5. Normal neuroimaging and metabolic examinations; no evidence of infection
6. A family history of either neonatal or later epilepsy is found

Family studies have revealed probable autosomal dominant inheritance with regular penetration but variable expression. Genetic studies have localized the gene to chromosome 20q13.2[27] or chromosome 8q24.[28] In 1991, Schiffman et al.[29] documented an autosomal recessive form; hence, this syndrome probably is multigenic. Molecular studies have identified abnormalities of the potassium channel and have found the two possible mutant genes responsible, known as *KCNQ2* and *KCNQ3*. These mutations may result in reduction of potassium currents, thus impairing membrane repolarization.[30,31] From long-term studies, we know that the future seizure frequency is low. If the abnormality in the potassium channel were persistent throughout life, one would expect that the percentage of patients with recurrent seizures would be greater than the 14% currently reported, unless an adaptive mechanism is engaged, the existence of which is as yet unknown.

Treatment usually consists of phenobarbital either acutely or for 2–6 months. Plouin[20] has documented successful treatment with valproate in some cases. Long-term treatment is unnecessary.

The prognosis in affected neonates is good. The seizures are easily controlled and usually disappear within days to weeks. All patients have a favorable outcome, and no cases of resultant severe epilepsy have been reported. Lombroso[32] reported a 14% incidence of later epilepsy, whereas Plouin[33] reported that 11% of her cases later developed epilepsy, with a 5% risk for febrile seizures.

Benign Neonatal Sleep Myoclonus

Benign neonatal sleep myoclonus involves episodes of myoclonus in normal full-term infants during all sleep states but most frequently during quiet sleep. Myoclonus does not occur during wakefulness. The onset can be as early as within the first week of life. The myoclonic jerks are rhythmic or sustained and usually are bilateral and synchronous. The arms, the legs, or both may be involved. The episodes may last a few minutes. No observable EEG changes occur with the myoclonus; the EEG appears normal. Myoclonus disappears spontaneously within days to weeks and almost always by 6 months of age. No treatment is necessary.

Neonatal Myoclonic Encephalopathy

Neonatal myoclonic encephalopathy (NME), which is also known as *early myoclonic encephalopathy*, was first described by Aicardi and Goutieres[34] in 1978, in an infant with myoclonic jerks and an EEG consistent with burst suppression for greater than 28 days. NME is a rare condition that shows no known gender predilection. Most cases are sporadic, although some familial cases have been reported, representing questionable autosomal recessive inheritance.[35]

The onset of seizures can occur within the first 3 months of life but usually is within the first month. This syndrome is composed of fragmentary or partial myoclonus, massive myoclonic jerks, simple partial seizures, and tonic infantile spasms. The myoclonic jerks may involve a part of or an entire limb. They are frequent, even continuous, usually in the awake state but may persist during sleep. Massive myoclonic jerks are not always present. The partial seizures follow the onset of myoclonus and generally are associated with respiratory arrest or oculomotor dysfunction. Spasms may be seen but, in most cases, they occur after 3–4 months of age and can evolve into an atypical West's syndrome. The clinical episodes in this syndrome tend to be brief at onset and then become more prolonged over time.[36]

Clinically, affected infants are severely hypotonic. In some cases, the neck and back muscles are hypotonic, and the infants exhibit bilateral pyramidal tract signs. Over time, these infants develop cortical blindness and moderate microcephaly and have poor mental development. In only two patients has peripheral nervous system involvement been documented. Brain computed tomography scans can appear normal at first, with subsequent evidence of cerebral or periventricular atrophy.[37]

The EEG reveals an abnormal background, with complex bursts of spikes, sharp waves, and slow waves and a burst suppression pattern. The EEG changes become more distinct in sleep. As the clinical picture progresses, the EEG tracing evolves into atypical hypsarrhythmia at 3–5 months of age. This is a transient event, as there is a return to the burst suppression pattern.[36]

Numerous etiologies have been proposed, including inborn errors of metabolism. Most work has been in the realm of the early glycine encephalopathies, such as nonketotic hyperglycinemia, propionic acidemia, and D-glycine acidemia. In 1990, Lombroso[38] reviewed 29 neonates whose clinical picture met criteria for NME. Of these, eight had inborn errors of metabolism (4 of whom had nonketotic hyperglycinemia), 5 had congenital brain malformations, 6 had a history of birth asphyxia, and 10 were cryptogenic.[38] Pathologically, NME is characterized by neuronal loss, astrocytic proliferation, and multiple areas of spongiosis in the white matter, with concentric, perivascular, and periodic acid–Schiff–positive bodies.[39]

The outcome in these infants is notably poor. More than 50% are expected to die within the first year of life. The majority of survivors have profound developmental impairments. Different courses of treatment consisting of adrenocorticotropic hormone, steroids, pyridoxine, and other AEDs are ineffective.

Early Infantile Epileptic Encephalopathy

Early infantile epileptic encephalopathy (EIEE), also known as *Ohtahara's syndrome*, was first described by Ohtahara in 1976.[40] Its onset is usually within 12 days to 3 months of birth. It is characterized mainly by tonic spasms, which can be flexor, extensor, unilateral, or bilateral in character. These spastic episodes occur in both the awake and asleep states. They often occur consecutively but can also be isolated events. In rare instances, partial clonic and very brief myoclonic jerks have been seen. Fragmentary myoclonus, a feature of NME, is not present in this syndrome. Neither a gender predilection nor familial cases have been reported.

The EEG reflects a burst suppression pattern in the awake and asleep states. It is characterized by high-voltage bursts lasting 1–3 seconds and alternating with a suppression phase of 3–4 seconds' duration. These EEG changes are present at onset

and disappear within 6 months. Later, the EEG picture evolves into atypical hypsarrhythmia. Imaging reveals progressive brain atrophy.[36]

The cause has been linked mostly to congenital malformations and cerebral dysgenesis, including atrophy, porencephaly, olivary dentate dysplasia, hemimegalencephaly, and Aicardi's syndrome—an X-linked dominant condition characterized by agenesis of the corpus callosum and chorioretinal lacunae in female individuals. No laboratory anomalies have been reported,[36] and no effective treatment is known. Therapy with adrenocorticotropic hormone at best results in a partial effect, although, in most cases, this agent is not at all effective.

Affected infants experience severe psychomotor retardation and continue to exhibit seizures that are usually intractable to AEDs. All affected infants have poor outcomes in that one-half evolve into West's or Lennox-Gastaut syndrome and the others succumb to an early death. All have abnormal brainstem auditory and visual evoked responses. Of 15 patients followed up by Ohtahara[41] in 1992, 8 survived but all with profound mental retardation. Of the 15 patients, 6 were quadriplegic and bedridden, 2 had persistent seizures, and 7 had persistent EEG abnormalities. Ohtahara showed that if the EEG evolved into a mostly focal EEG, the survival rate was higher.[41]

Kelly et al.[42] described a 5-month-old infant with a history of neonatal seizures. These investigators found that distinguishing EIEE from NME was difficult, not only in their case but in several others.[42] The cardinal differentiating point is the presence of myoclonus: NME is characterized by myoclonus, whereas EIEE neonates exhibit tonic spasms. NME has been shown to be familial and is associated with inborn errors of metabolism, whereas EIEE has been shown to be correlated with cerebral malformations. Though the burst suppression pattern is common to both syndromes, in EIEE it appears in the awake and asleep states, whereas in NME, the discontinuous EEG pattern may disappear in the awake state. In EIEE, the burst suppression pattern is apparent at onset and disappears within 6 months. It can then evolve into hypsarrhythmia and then to slow spike and waves. In contrast, the burst suppression pattern in NME appears at 1–5 months and persists for a longer period.[43] Finally, the onset of NME tends to be earlier than that of EIEE, and NME follows a rapid, progressive, degenerating course, whereas EIEE tends to be more static.

Treatment Issues

The major goals of treating any of the neonatal epilepsy syndromes are to eliminate all seizures and prevent recurrences. One must also balance the decision between the possible detrimental effects of neonatal seizures on the immature brain and the known side effects and complications of AEDs.

Many physiologic factors in the neonate affect the use of AEDs. The gastrointestinal system in the neonate is very immature, and gastric emptying is delayed up to 8 hours. Also, the gastric pH is initially high, with a rapid decrease in the first 24 hours and then a rapid increase for 10–20 days.[44] These conditions lead to decreased absorption of phenytoin, phenobarbital, valproate, and carbamazepine.[45]

Intramuscular administration of medication also poses difficulties. Neonates have higher muscular water content than do persons in other age groups. They also exhibit vasomotor instability with a strong tendency for vasoconstriction. Therefore, intramuscular absorption of most AEDs is erratic and unpredictable. Because their skeletal muscle mass is lower than that of other age groups, infants have a high potential for muscular necrosis and nerve paralysis.[45]

The water content in the neonate also affects AEDs. The newborn's total body water to total body weight ratio is high, with an even higher ratio of extracellular to intracellular water. Phenobarbital, carbamazepine, and phenytoin are distributed into total body water, whereas valproate tends to be restricted to extracellular water. Diazepam accumulates in adipose tissue.[46] The brain and liver volumes are higher in the newborn than in the mature organs. Furthermore, the neonatal brain has less myelin and the relative cerebral blood flow is higher as compared to the mature brain. Because the brain concentration of lipophilic drugs depends on blood flow, the brain of the neonate is exposed to higher amounts of diazepam and carbamazepine. This is not the case with phenytoin and valproate.[47]

The plasma protein binding of drugs is decreased in the newborn.[48] This is an important point, as phenytoin, carbamazepine, and valproate are highly bound (more than 70%) to plasma proteins. Albumin concentrations are decreased. Hence, an increased free fraction of the drug is seen in neonates, as is an increased volume of distribution, with more of the drug in specific tissues. It is important to note that some neonates with seizures are acutely sick with systemic conditions. Consequently, they may be receiving multiple medications, which also can interfere with or displace AEDs from protein-binding sites.

Hepatic metabolism in neonates differs from that in older persons. The rate of hepatic uptake of drugs in neonates is decreased because the activity of microsomal enzymatic systems is not yet fully developed. Phase I oxidation, which is needed for the metabolism of phenobarbital, phenytoin, diazepam, clonazepam, and valproate, is only approximately 50% efficient in the newborn. Phase II reactions also are significantly diminished. Valproate is oxidized by mitochondrial oxidation systems that process fatty acids. As the neonate matures, hepatic metabolic capacity increases, and so dosages must be monitored and adjusted closely.[46]

In addition, the renal system of neonates differs from that of even slightly older individuals. The glomerular filtration rate is decreased in the newborn. In the ensuing days after birth, increased cardiac output leads to decreased renal vascular resistance, which in turn increases renal blood flow and the glomerular filtration rate.[49] Therefore, initially there is decreased excretion and clearance of most AEDs. Because of all the complex interactions among the different systems in the neonate, the half-lives of most AEDs are increased. The concentration of "free drug" in the plasma and tissues also is increased, which can cause increased toxicity even with documented normal blood levels. For this reason, monitoring free drug levels can be helpful. It is noteworthy that these complications are even more exaggerated in the premature patient.

Finally, all AEDs may produce detrimental effects in the developing brain. These effects have been studied best in animals. Mikati et al.[50] provided data suggesting that phenobarbital may affect learning and memory in developing rats.

Brooks et al.,[51] in 1997, showed that N-methyl-D-aspartate agonists or antagonists given to immature rats caused a decrease in synaptic density in later life. Other reports claim that phenobarbital, phenytoin, and benzodiazepines can interfere with cortical neuronal proliferation in vitro.

Before pharmacologic therapy is initiated, simple metabolic disturbances such as hypoglycemia or hypocalcemia should be ruled out and addressed with replacement therapy. In practice, the most frequently used drug for neonatal seizures is phenobarbital, which is available in intravenous and oral forms. Its efficacy in treating seizures ranges from 32% to 85%. The recommended loading dose is 20 mg/kg, with a maintenance dose of 3–4 mg/kg per day. Doses as high as 30–40 mg/kg have been used to control seizures. Toxic effects include lethargy, apnea, and bradycardia.

Fosphenytoin is used as a second-line agent. The recommended loading dose is 20 mg/kg and a maintenance dose of 3–4 mg/kg in two divided doses, which are in phenytoin equivalents. Its metabolism is unpredictable and variable, and its half-life can be as much as 30 times normal. Its major toxicity includes cardiac arrhythmias.[52]

Of the benzodiazepines, diazepam, which is best administered intravenously, is the most commonly used. Usual doses begin at 0.1–0.3 mg/kg. In refractory cases, doses as high as 3–12 mg/kg daily or 0.7–2.8 mg per hour have been used. Toxic effects include hypotension, apnea, and lethargy.[53] Midazolam is best used in an infusion secondary to its short half-life and is gaining favor in the treatment of refractory seizures. It is given as a 0.1- to 0.3-mg/kg bolus followed by 0.05–0.40 mg/kg per hour. Lorazepam is given in a dose of 0.05–0.10 mg/kg, and clonazepam as 0.1 mg/kg intravenously. Lorazepam, which is less lipophilic than diazepam, has now gained favor secondary to its longer-acting effects. Of the other AEDs, lidocaine is used only in extreme refractory cases. At a dose of 4 mg/kg hourly, 80% of patients in one study responded over a period of 4 days.[54] Only eight patients were involved in this study, however, and so determining whether there were other confounding factors is difficult. Toxic side effects include seizures of different types, arrhythmias, hypotension, and bradycardia.[54] Valproate has been used primarily in Europe for the treatment of benign neonatal convulsions and has had only limited use

in neonates in the United States. If seizures are difficult to control, then 100 mg of pyridoxine should be administered with concurrent EEG monitoring to rule out pyridoxine dependency.[52]

As AEDs have their own effects on brain function, they should be used judiciously for the shortest period of time. Before treatment is initiated, the epileptic nature of the paroxysmal behavior should be documented with an EEG. The cessation of all clinical events and electrographic seizures is desirable, although some syndromes such as benign neonatal convulsions resolve spontaneously without any consequences attributable to seizures. Electrographic seizures may be resistant to initial doses of medications, and so toxic doses may be needed. Seizures may persist after phenobarbital, phenytoin, and benzodiazepines have been administered. No consensus has been reached on the use of other AEDs.

Before a patient's discharge from the hospital, AEDs should be discontinued if the patient is neurologically intact and the seizures are controlled. The length of time over which to taper the medication varies. The duration of treatment of a neurologically impaired infant is undetermined, as no consensus has been reached. To date, no studies have documented that continuous administration of AEDs prevents the development of epilepsy and avoids neurodevelopmental sequelae.

Prognosis

The prognosis of neonatal seizures and neonatal epilepsy syndromes depends on etiology, type, and duration of seizures and EEG patterns during the acute illness (Table 6-7). The practitioner who can recognize infants at risk for certain sequelae, such as epilepsy, mental retardation, cerebral palsy, and learning disabilities, can supply accurate information and ensure that rehabilitative services are rendered early.

Currently, the overall mortality for all neonatal seizures is approximately 15%.[55–57] Before 1969, the mortality rate approached 40%.[4] This substantial decrease represents marked advances in obstetric and neonatal care.

The risk of developing epilepsy is approximately 20%,[4] a percentage that is unchanged from the data supplied from the National Collaborative

Perinatal Study. Kuromori et al.[58] and Holden et al.[59] found that in those infants who developed epilepsy, the seizures returned either in the late neonatal period or, in most cases, by 6 months of age. Few patients may develop epilepsy many years later. The highest likelihood of subsequent epilepsy is in infants with cerebral dysgenesis or severe intracranial hemorrhage. Infants with mild to moderate hypoxic-ischemic encephalopathy have an approximate risk of subsequent epilepsy of 20%. Epilepsy does not occur in infants whose seizures were attributable to simple, transient metabolic disturbances.

At least 50% of newborns with neonatal seizures have normal global outcomes.[32] The incidence of neurodevelopmental sequelae in survivors has remained unchanged at 20–35% since the 1970s.[1,4] Neurodevelopmental sequelae constitute a broad spectrum of disabilities, including motor deficits, mental retardation, and other learning disabilities. The National Collaborative Perinatal Study found that 70% of infants with neonatal seizures were experiencing normal development at 7 years; only 13% fulfilled criteria for cerebral palsy.

Etiology of the seizures is the most important factor in determining prognosis. Patients whose seizures were secondary to hypoxic-ischemic encephalopathy, cerebral malformations, intraventricular hemorrhage, or unknown causes tend to have a worse prognosis than do infants with seizures secondary to hypocalcemia, subarachnoid hemorrhage, or drug withdrawal.[4,60] Infants with a history of hypoxic-ischemic encephalopathy or intraventricular hemorrhage are at a 20–53% risk of developing neurologic sequelae.[61,62]

Subtle, generalized tonic, and some myoclonic seizures have a worse prognosis than do focal clonic seizures.[2,3,63] Mizrahi and Kellaway[2] reported that infants with clonic seizures were more likely to be normal at the time of discharge from the nursery (approximately 71%) than were infants experiencing other seizure types. The National Collaborative Perinatal Study found that only tonic and myoclonic seizures were related to outcome. Tonic seizures occurred more often in children who later developed cerebral palsy, mental retardation, and epilepsy. Myoclonic seizures were related to the development of mental retardation. Myoclonic and tonic seizures occur either in premature infants with severe insults or in infants

Table 6-7. Neonatal Seizure Etiology and Neurodevelopmental Outcome

Seizure Etiology	Neonates with Normal Development (%)
Asphyxia	50
Primary subarachnoid hemorrhage	90
Intraventricular hemorrhage	<10
Hypoglycemia	50
Hypocalcemia (early)	50
Hypocalcemia (late)	80–100
Intracranial infection	20–65
Developmental defects	0
Drug withdrawal	100

Source: Modified from Hill A, Volpe JJ. Seizures, hypoxic-ischemic brain injury, and intraventricular hemorrhage in the newborn. Ann Neurol 1981;10:109–121.

with catastrophic epilepsies, and thus carry a worse prognosis.

Evidence indicates that seizures that persist beyond 3 days often are associated with neurologic impairments.[2,55,62,64] Because controlling these prolonged seizures is difficult, it is not surprising that when more than two drugs are required for the control of seizures, the affected neonates tend to have a poorer prognosis.[62]

The EEG patterns during the acute phase may provide important prognostic information.[62,65–68] Infants with a normal interictal EEG had an 86% chance of normal neurologic development; infants with focal EEG abnormalities had a 40–70% chance of normal development; and infants with flat, periodic, burst suppression or multifocal EEG abnormalities had only a 7–12% chance of normal neurologic outcome. Rowe et al.[67] noted that the presence of epileptiform activity was related to a poorer outcome but that the relationship was not as highly significant as abnormalities of background rhythms. Scher et al.[69,70] reported that infants whose seizures were accompanied by EEG seizure discharges had a higher mortality rate than did the general population (40–50%). Of those who survived, 65% had significant developmental abnormalities.[68] Although their presence often is associated with abnormal neurologic development, electrographic seizures should intensify the need to establish a diagnosis, as the cause of the seizures is the most important predictor of outcome.

Conclusion

Neonatal seizures are one of the most common neurologic conditions in the newborn period. They have multiple etiologies, each with its own clinical manifestations and prognosis. Neonatal seizures are extremely complex because newborns do not manifest the characteristic clinical signs seen in older patients, and EEG recordings do not always aid in characterizing an epileptic event. In addition, benign and catastrophic neonatal epilepsy syndromes are known. Their recognition is important in terms of treatment issues and prognosis. With new information that should be provided by future research, clinicians should be better able to identify, treat, and determine the outcome of neonatal seizures and syndromes.

Acknowledgments

This work was supported by National Institutes of Health (NS20253 SLM). Dr. Moshe is the recipient of a Martin A. and Emily L. Fisher Fellowship in Neurology and Pediatrics.

References

1. Lombroso CT. Prognosis in neonatal seizures. Adv Neurol 1983;34:101–113.
2. Mizrahi EM, Kellaway P. Characterization and classification of neonatal seizures. Neurology 1987;37:1837–1844.
3. Mizrahi EM. Neonatal seizures: problems in diagnosis and classification. Epilepsia 1987;28[Suppl 1]:S46–S55.
4. Volpe JJ. Neonatal Seizures. In JJ Volpe (ed), Neurology of the Newborn. Philadelphia: Saunders, 1995;172–207.
5. Tacke R, Tuomisto L, Danner R. Cortical spike wave discharges during audiogenic convulsions in rats. Exp Neurol 1984;85:233–238.
6. Ludvig N, Moshe SL. Cyclic AMP derivatives injected into the inferior colliculus induce audiogenic seizure-like phenomena in normal rats. Brain Res 1987;437:193–196.
7. Danner R, Shewmon DA, Sherman MP. Seizures in an atelencephalic infant. Is the cortex essential for neonatal seizures? Arch Neurol 1985;42:1014–1016.
8. Moshe SL, Albala BJ, Ackermann RF, Engel J Jr. Increased seizure susceptibility of the immature brain. Brain Res 1983;283:81–85.
9. Moshe SL. Epileptogenesis and the immature brain. Epilepsia 1987;28[Suppl 1]:S3–S15.
10. Moshe SL. Seizures in the developing brain. Neurology 1993;43:S3–S7.
11. Moshe SL, Sperber EF, Velisek L. Critical issues of developmental seizure disorders [editorial]. Physiol Res 1993;42:145–154.
12. Swann JW, Moshe SL. Developmental Issues in Animal Models. In JJ Engel, TA Pedley (eds), Epilepsy: A Comprehensive Textbook. New York: Raven Press, 1997;467–480.
13. Ben-Ari Y, Khazipov R, Leinekugel X, et al. GABAA, NMDA and AMPA receptors: a developmentally regulated "menage à trois." Trends Neurosci 1997;20:523–529.
14. Michelson HB, Wong RK. Excitatory synaptic responses mediated by $GABA_A$ receptors in the hippocampus. Science 1991;253:1420–1423.
15. Mueller AL, Chesnut RM, Schwartzkroin PA. Actions of GABA in developing rabbit hippocampus: an in vitro study. Neurosci Lett 1983;39:193–198.
16. Moshe SL. Sex and the substantia nigra: administration, teaching, patient care, and research. J Clin Neurophysiol 1997;14:484–494.
17. Wasterlain CG, Dwyer BE. Brain Metabolism During Prolonged Seizures in Neonates. In AV Delgado-Escueta, CG Wasterlain, DM Treiman, RJ Porter (eds), Advances in Neurology: Status Epilepticus—Mechanisms of Brain Damage and Treatment. New York: Raven Press, 1983;241–260.
18. Sperber EF, Moshe SL. The Effects of Seizures on the Hippocampus of the Immature Brain. In JJ Engel, DH Lowenstein, PA Schwartzkroin, SL Moshe (eds), Brain Plasticity and Epilepsy: A Tribute to Frank Morrell. San Diego: Academic Press, 2000.
19. Dehan M, Quillerou D, Navelet Y, et al. [Convulsions in the fifth day of life: a new syndrome?] Arch Fr Pediatr 1977;34:730–742.
20. Plouin P. Benign Familial Neonatal Convulsions and Benign Idiopathic Neonatal Convulsions. In JJ Engel, TA Pedley (eds), Epilepsy: A Comprehensive Textbook. Philadelphia: Lippincott–Raven, 1997;2247–2255.
21. Herrmann B, Lawrenz-Wolf B, Seewald C, et al. 5-Tages-Krampfe des Neugeborenen bei Rotavirusinfektionen. Monatsschr Kinderheilkd 1993;141:120–123.
22. Goldberg HJ, Sheehy EM. Fifth day fits: an acute zinc deficiency syndrome? Arch Dis Child 1982;57:633–635.
23. North KN, Storey GN, Henderson-Smart DJ. Fifth day fits in the newborn. Aust Paediatr J 1989;25:284–287.
24. Rett A, Teubel R. Neugeborenen Krampfe im Rahmen einer epileptisch belasten Familie. Wien Klin Wochenschr 1964;76:609–613.
25. Ronen GM, Rosales TO, Connolly M, et al. Seizure characteristics in chromosome 20 benign familial neonatal convulsions. Neurology 1993;43:1355–1360.

26. Hirsch E, Velez A, Sellal F, et al. Electroclinical signs of benign neonatal familial convulsions. Ann Neurol 1993;34:835–841.

27. Leppert M, Anderson VE, Quattlebaum T, et al. Benign familial neonatal convulsions linked to genetic markers on chromosome 20. Nature 1989;337:647–648.

28. Lewis TB, Leach RJ, Ward K, et al. Genetic heterogeneity in benign familial neonatal convulsions: identification of a new locus on chromosome 8q. Am J Hum Genet 1993;53:670–675.

29. Schiffmann R, Shapira Y, Ryan G. An autosomal recessive form of benign familial neonatal seizures. Clin Genet 1991;40:467–470.

30. Yang WP, Levesque PC, Little WA, et al. Functional expression of two KvLQT1-related potassium channels responsible for an inherited idiopathic epilepsy. J Biol Chem 1998;273:19419–19423.

31. Lerche H, Biervert C, Alekov AK, et al. A reduced K+ current due to a novel mutation in KCNQ2 causes neonatal convulsions. Ann Neurol 1999;46:305–312.

32. Lombroso CT. Neonatal seizures: a clinician's overview. Brain Dev 1996;18:1–28.

33. Plouin P. Benign Idiopathic Neonatal Convulsions. In J Roger, M Bureau, C Dravet, et al. (eds), Epileptic Syndromes in Infancy, Childhood, and Adolescence. London: John Libbey, 1992;3–11.

34. Aicardi J, Goutieres F. [Neonatal myoclonic encephalopathy (author's transl).] Rev Electroencephalogr Neurophysiol Clin 1978;8:99–101.

35. Aicardi J. Early Myoclonic Encephalopathy. In J Roger, M Bureau, C Dravet, et al. (eds), Epileptic Syndromes in Infancy, Childhood, and Adolescence. London: John Libbey, 1992;13–23.

36. Ohtahara S, Ohtsuka Y, Erba G. Early Epileptic Encephalopathy with Suppression Burst. In JJ Engel, TA Pedley (eds), Epilepsy: A Comprehensive Textbook. Philadelphia: Lippincott–Raven, 1997;2257–2261.

37. Murakami N, Ohtsuka Y, Ohtahara S. Early infantile epileptic syndromes with suppression-bursts: early myoclonic encephalopathy vs. Ohtahara syndrome. Jpn J Psychiatry Neurol 1993;47:197–200.

38. Lombroso CT. Early myoclonic encephalopathy, early infantile epileptic encephalopathy, and benign and severe infantile myoclonic epilepsies: a critical review and personal contributions. J Clin Neurophysiol 1990; 7:380–408.

39. Vigevano F, Cincinnati P, Bertini E, et al. [Neonatal myoclonic encephalopathy. Contribution of a case with suspected dysmetabolic etiology.] Rev Neurobiol 1981;27:458–466.

40. Ohtahara S, Ishida T, Oka E, et al. On the age-dependent epileptic syndrome: the early infantile epileptic encephalopathy with suppression-burst. No To Hattatsu 1976;8:270–280.

41. Ohtahara S, Ohtsuka Y, Yamatogi Y, et al. Early-Infantile Epileptic Encephalopathy with Suppression-Bursts. In J Roger, M Bureau, C Dravet, et al. (eds), Epileptic Syndromes in Infancy, Childhood, and Adolescence. London: John Libbey, 1992;25–34.

42. Kelley KR, Shinnar S, Moshe SL. A 5-month-old with intractable epilepsy. Semin Pediatr Neurol 1999;6:138–144; discussion 144–135.

43. Dalla BB, Dulac O, Fejerman N, et al. Early myoclonic epileptic encephalopathy. Eur J Pediatr 1983;140:248–252.

44. Heiman G. Enteral absorption and bioavailability in children in relation to age. Eur J Clin Pharmacol 1980;18:43–50.

45. Guillet P, Morselli PL. Pharmacokinetics of Anticonvulsants in the Neonate. In CG Wasterlain, P Vert (eds), Neonatal Seizures. New York: Raven Press, 1990;257–267.

46. Eadie MJ. Anticonvulsant drugs. An update. Drugs 1984;27:328–363.

47. Rowland M, Tozer TN. Clinical Pharmacokinetics: Concepts and Applications. Philadelphia: Lea & Febiger, 1980.

48. McElnay JC, D'Arcy PF. Protein binding displacement interactions and their clinical importance. Drugs 1983;25:495–513.

49. Morselli PL, Thiercelin JF. Human Neonatal Pharmacokinetics. In P Turner, DG Shand (eds), Recent Advances in Clinical Pharmacology. Edinburgh: Churchill Livingstone, 1983;21–43.

50. Mikati MA, Holmes GL, Chronopoulos A, et al. Phenobarbital modifies seizure-related brain injury in the developing brain. Ann Neurol 1994;36:425–433.

51. Brooks WJ, Weeks AC, Leboutillier JC, Petit TL. Altered NMDA sensitivity and learning following chronic developmental NMDA antagonism. Physiol Behav 1997;62:955–962.

52. LaJoie J, Moshe S. Treatment of Neonatal Seizures. In RT Johnson, JW Griffin, JC McArthur (eds), Current Therapy in Neurological Diseases. St. Louis: Mosby (in press).

53. Gamstorp I, Sedin G. Neonatal convulsions treated with continuous, intravenous infusion of diazepam. Ups J Med Sci 1982;87:143–149.

54. Norell E, Gamstorp I. Neonatal seizures; effect of lidocaine. Acta Paediatr Scand Suppl 1970;206:S297.

55. Andre M, Matisse N, Vert P, Debruille C. Neonatal seizures—recent aspects. Neuropediatrics 1988;19:201–207.

56. Torrence C. Neonatal seizures: II. Recognition, treatment, and prognosis. Neonatal Netw 1985;4:21–28.

57. Watkins A, Szymonowicz W, Jin X, Yu VV. Significance of seizures in very low-birthweight infants. Dev Med Child Neurol 1988;30:162–169.

58. Kuromori N, Arai H, Ohkubo O, et al. A prospective study of epilepsy following neonatal convulsions. Folia Psychiatr Neurol Jpn 1976;30:379–388.

59. Holden KR, Mellits ED, Freeman JM. Neonatal seizures: I. Correlation of prenatal and perinatal events with outcomes. Pediatrics 1982;70:165–176.

60. Doberczak TM, Shanzer S, Cutler R, et al. One-year follow-up of infants with abstinence-associated seizures. Arch Neurol 1988;45:649–653.

61. Minchom P, Niswander K, Chalmers I, et al. Antecedents and outcome of very early neonatal seizures in infants born at or after term. Br J Obstet Gynaecol 1987;94:431–439.

62. Bergman I, Painter MJ, Hirsch RP, et al. Outcome in neonates with convulsions treated in an intensive care unit. Ann Neurol 1983;14:642–647.

63. Scher MS, Painter MJ. Controversies concerning neonatal seizures. Pediatr Clin North Am 1989;36:281–310.

64. Lombroso CT. Neonatal seizures: historic note and present controversies. Epilepsia 1996;37[Suppl 3]:5–13.

65. Watanabe K, Miyazaki S, Hara K, Hakamada S. Behavioral state cycles, background EEGs and prognosis of newborns with perinatal hypoxia. Electroencephalogr Clin Neurophysiol 1980;49:618–625.

66. Rose AL, Lombroso CT. A study of clinical, pathological, and electroencephalographic features in 137 full-term babies with a long-term follow-up. Pediatrics 1970;45:404–425.

67. Rowe JC, Holmes GL, Hafford J, et al. Prognostic value of the electroencephalogram in term and preterm infants following neonatal seizures. Electroencephalogr Clin Neurophysiol 1985;60:183–196.

68. Scher MS, Painter MJ, Bergman I, et al. EEG diagnoses of neonatal seizures: clinical correlations and outcome. Pediatr Neurol 1989;5:17–24.

69. Scher MS, Aso K, Beggarly ME, et al. Electrographic seizures in preterm and full-term neonates: clinical correlates, associated brain lesions, and risk for neurologic sequelae [see comments]. Pediatrics 1993;91:128–134.

70. Scher MS, Hamid MY, Steppe DA, et al. Ictal and interictal electrographic seizure durations in preterm and term neonates. Epilepsia 1993;34:284–288.

Chapter 7

Lennox-Gastaut Syndrome

Tracy A. Glauser and Diego A. Morita

Epilepsy occurs more frequently in patients with developmental disabilities than in the general population.[1] A long-term study of 221 children with mental retardation (MR) found that 15% had epilepsy by 22 years of age,[2] in contrast to the approximately 1% of the general population that develops epilepsy. In this cohort, the cumulative risk of epilepsy for patients with only MR was 5% (at 22 years of age) but increased to 38% if MR was accompanied by cerebral palsy.[2]

A separate study, in a northern Swedish county, ascertained that 20.2% of patients with MR had active epilepsy.[3] Over time, mortality was significantly increased in patients in this cohort of patients with epilepsy and MR (regardless of the presence of cerebral palsy) as compared to the general population or to patients with only MR.[4] The highest mortality was noted in patients with generalized-onset seizures.[4]

The goals of epilepsy therapy in patients with developmental disabilities and epilepsy are the same as those in patients with only epilepsy: The best quality of life with the fewest seizures (none, if possible), the fewest treatment side effects, and the least number of medications. The obstacles to achieving these goals in this select population are numerous.[1] One of the most important factors in the proper management of patients with developmental disabilities and epilepsy is the recognition of epilepsy syndromes. Classifying patients according to epilepsy syndromes facilitates the identification of relatively homogeneous populations among this heterogeneous group. This, in turn, facilitates the selection of appropriate and optimal treatments, the provision of more accurate prognoses, and the delivery of better family education and counseling.

In patients with epilepsy and developmental disabilities, recognition of the epilepsy syndrome called *childhood epileptic encephalopathy with diffuse slow spike and waves* (the Lennox-Gastaut syndrome [LGS]) is important for three reasons. First, LGS is very common in children and institutionalized patients with MR (7% and 16.3%, respectively).[5,6] Second, patients with LGS have multiple disabilities and generalized-onset seizures, which increase their risk of death. Third, effective antiseizure treatments that can improve the patient's quality of life while reducing seizure frequency (and, in some cases, achieving seizure freedom) have recently become available.

History

The clinical manifestations of LGS have been recognized and described for more than two centuries.[7] Distinct from these clinical descriptions, in 1939 Gibbs et al.[8,9] identified an electroencephalographic (EEG) pattern similar to, yet slower than, the classic 3-Hz spike and wave discharge (petit mal pattern) and proposed to call it a *petit mal variant* to distinguish it. In 1945, Dr. William Lennox assembled the clinical and the

EEG manifestations into the first semblance of the electroclinical syndrome that we now call *childhood epileptic encephalopathy with diffuse slow spike and waves* or the *Lennox-Gastaut syndrome*.[10] Lennox's triad consisted of the slow spike and wave interictal EEG pattern, MR, and three types of seizures that were considered characteristic: myoclonic jerks, atypical absence, and drop attacks (also known as *akinetic seizures* or *astatic seizures*).[7,10-12]

Initially, this constellation of symptoms was not given a formal syndrome name. Renewed interest in this syndrome began in 1964 when Doose[13] and Sorel[14] each described approximately 20 cases. Three international meetings in Marseille (1964–1968) led by Henri Gastaut examined the syndrome in depth, confirmed its worldwide existence, and bestowed the name *Lennox-Gastaut*, reinforcing the significant contributions of both the U.S. and French groups to the understanding of the syndrome.[7]

The importance of recognizing patients with LGS increased in the early 1990s when this population was identified as a target group to participate in trials of investigational antiepileptic drugs (AEDs). The factors contributing to the targeting of this group for study with investigational AEDs include their high daily seizure frequency, the lack of highly effective therapy, and the desire to examine safety and efficacy issues for investigational AEDs in pediatric populations prior to general release of these agents.

Diagnostic Criteria

LGS, as defined by the International League Against Epilepsy classification,

> . . . manifests itself in children aged 1–8 years but appears mainly in preschool-age children. The most common seizure types are tonic-axial, atonic, and absence seizures, but other types such as myoclonic, generalized tonic clonic seizures (GTCS), or partial seizures frequently are associated with this syndrome. Seizure frequency is high, and status epilepticus is frequent (stuporous states with myoclonias, tonic and atonic seizures). The EEG usually has abnormal background activity, slow spike-waves <3 Hz and, often, multifocal abnormalities. During sleep, bursts of fast rhythms (10 Hz) appear. In general, there is MR. Seizures are difficult to control, and development is

unfavorable. In 60% of cases, the syndrome occurs in children suffering from a previous encephalopathy but is primary in other cases.[15]

A triad of basic elements usually is needed to make a diagnosis of LGS, based on the preceding definition coupled with clinical experience and research. This triad consists of

1. Multiple types of seizures including tonic, atypical absence, and atonic seizures
2. An EEG pattern consisting of interictal diffuse slow spike and wave discharges occurring at a 1.5- to 2.0-Hz frequency
3. Diffuse cognitive dysfunction or MR[7,15-20]

Among epileptologists, debate continues about the minimal necessary and sufficient criteria needed to diagnose LGS. Some investigators do not consider cognitive dysfunction or MR to be indispensable for diagnosis, especially at onset, if the seizures and EEG pattern are typical.[17,21-23] Other authors use a stricter EEG criterion, requiring that the diagnostic EEG pattern includes a burst of generalized fast spikes (10 Hz) during non–rapid eye movement (non-REM) sleep.[24]

Differential Diagnosis

Owing to the nonspecific nature of multiple seizure types and cognitive dysfunction, two other pediatric epilepsy syndromes may be confused with LGS. As compared with classic LGS, the myoclonic variant of LGS has less frequent and less severe MR, rarer tonic seizures, but an unusually marked myoclonic component and, frequently, faster (>2.5-Hz) spike and wave complexes on electroencephalography.[18,25]

Myoclonic-astatic epilepsy (Doose syndrome) and LGS have in common myoclonic, atonic, and atypical absence seizures. However, major differences exist: myoclonic-astatic epilepsy is predominantly idiopathic and genetically determined, usually has a favorable outcome, and does not follow West's syndrome, whereas LGS is mainly symptomatic and not genetically determined, usually has an unfavorable outcome, and can follow West's syndrome.[20,26]

Classification

LGS can be classified according to its suspected etiology as either idiopathic or symptomatic. Patients may be considered to have idiopathic LGS if normal psychomotor development is noted prior to the onset of symptoms, no underlying disorders or definite presumptive causes are known, and no neurologic or neuroradiologic abnormalities are seen.[21] In contrast, patients are considered to have symptomatic LGS if an identifiable factor is responsible for the syndrome. Population-based studies found that 22–30% of patients have idiopathic LGS, whereas 70–78% have symptomatic LGS.[21,22,27,28] Examples of underlying pathologic processes responsible for symptomatic LGS include encephalitis or meningitis, tuberous sclerosis, brain malformations (e.g., cortical dysplasias), birth injury, hypoxia-ischemia injury, frontal lobe lesions, and trauma.[20,21,25] Infantile spasms precede the development of LGS in 9–39% of cases.[16,23,25]

Some investigators consider cryptogenic LGS as a separate etiologic category, in which there is no identified cause when a cause is suspected and the epilepsy is presumed to be symptomatic. In an epidemiologic study in Atlanta, 44% of all LGS patients were classified in the cryptogenic group.[23]

Pathophysiology

Although a variety of possible pathophysiologic features have been proposed (including developmental, immunologic, and metabolic), the pathophysiology of LGS is not known.[16,20,29–32] No animal models have been identified.[20]

Epidemiology

LGS is common in children and institutionalized patients with MR (7.0% and 16.3%, respectively).[5,6] Overall, LGS accounts for 1–4% of all cases of childhood epilepsy, but it accounts for 10% of childhood epilepsy cases that begin in the first 5 years of life.[5,22,23,33–37] Boys are affected more often than girls,[23,28,38,39] but no racial differences in the occurrence of LGS are noted.[23] The mean age at epilepsy onset is 26–28 months (range, 1 day to 14 years).[22,39] The average age at diagnosis of LGS in a long-term outcome study in Japan was 6 years (range, 2–15 years).[22]

Electroclinical Features

Interictal Manifestations

Prior to syndrome onset, 20–30% of children with LGS are free from neurologic and neuropsychological deficits. These problems inevitably appear during the evolution of LGS. The frequency and severity of MR are increased in association with the following factors: symptomatic LGS, a history of West's syndrome, onset of symptoms before 12–24 months of age, and higher seizure frequency.[20,22,27,28,40] In young children, the psychiatric symptoms consist of mood instability and personality disturbances, whereas slowing or arrest of psychomotor development and educational progress characterize the neuropsychological symptoms. In older children, character problems predominate, and acute psychotic episodes or chronic forms of psychosis with aggressiveness, irritability, or social isolation may occur.[28] Prolonged reaction time and information processing are the most impaired of the cognitive functions.[20] Kaminska et al.[26] found that the main characteristics of mental deterioration were apathy, memory disorders, impaired visuomotor speed, and perseverance.

The interictal EEG is characterized by a slow background that can be constant or transient. Permanent slowing of the background is associated with poor cognitive prognosis.[28] The hallmark of the awake interictal EEG is the diffuse slow spike and wave. This pattern consists of bursts of irregular, generalized spikes or sharp waves followed by a sinusoidal 35- to 400-msec slow wave[20] with an amplitude ranging from 200 to 800 mV,[40] which can be symmetric or asymmetric. The amplitude very often is higher in the anterior region, in the frontal or frontocentral areas; however, in some cases, the activity may dominate in the posterior head regions.[40] The frequency of the slow spike and wave activity commonly is found between 1.5 and 2.5 Hz (Figure 7-1).[40]

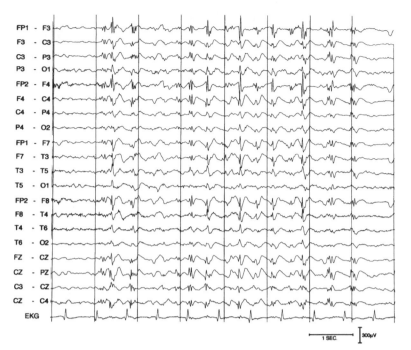

Figure 7-1. Slow spike and wave pattern in a 24-year-old awake man with Lennox-Gastaut syndrome. The slow posterior background rhythm displays frequent periods of 2.0- to 2.5-Hz discharges that are maximal in the bifrontocentral areas and occur in trains of up to 8 seconds without any associated clinical manifestations.

Slow spikes and waves are usually not activated by photic stimulation.[40] Likewise, hyperventilation rarely induces slow spike and waves.[20] During non-REM sleep, discharges are more generalized and more frequent and consist of polyspikes and slow waves. In REM sleep, spike and waves decrease.[20] During periods of frequent seizures, the total duration of REM sleep diminishes.[20]

Ictal Manifestations

Several types of seizures occur in LGS, including tonic, atonic, myoclonic, and atypical absence seizures, often associated with other less common types.

Tonic Seizures

Tonic seizures probably are the most characteristic type of seizures, and the reported frequency ranges from 17% to 95%.[18,25] Tonic seizures, which are more frequent during non-REM sleep, occur as one of three types: (1) axial tonic, involving the head and the trunk with head and neck flexion, contraction of masticatory muscles, and eventual vocalizations; (2) axorhizomelic tonic, in which there is tonic involvement of the proximal upper limbs with elevation of the shoulders and abduction of the arm; or (3) global tonic, with contraction of the distal part of the extremities, sometimes leading to a sudden fall and other times mimicking infantile spasms.[20,24,28] The EEG is characterized by a diffuse, rapid (10- to 13-Hz), low-amplitude activity, mainly in the anterior and vertex areas ("recruiting rhythm") that progressively decreases in frequency and increases in amplitude (Figure 7-2). A brief, generalized discharge of slow spike and waves or flattening of the recording may precede this pattern. Diffuse slow waves and slow spike and waves may follow it. These rapid discharges are common during non-REM sleep. Unlike tonic-clonic seizures, no postictal flattening occurs. Clinical manifestations appear 0.5–1.0 seconds after the onset of EEG manifestations and last several seconds longer than the discharge.[20,28]

Atonic Seizures, Massive Myoclonic Seizures, and Myoclonic-Atonic Seizures

Atonic, massive myoclonic, and myoclonic-atonic seizures can be difficult to differentiate by

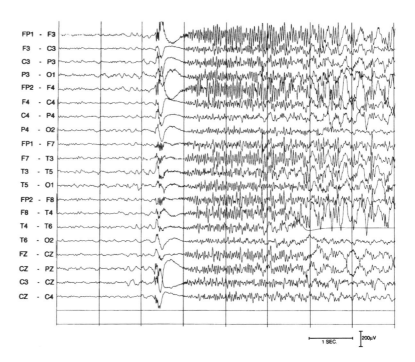

Figure 7-2. Tonic seizure with arm extension in a 24-year-old man with Lennox-Gastaut syndrome. Prior to the seizure, the patient was watching television; he then experienced a sudden body jerk and leaned forward, with his arms extended and fixed at shoulder level. The electroencephalogram shows a diffuse burst of high-voltage polyspike and slow wave activity followed by 1 second of relative attenuation and then paroxysmal rapid activity that is maximal in the bifrontocentral head regions.

clinical observation alone, and considerable discrepancies involve the application of these terms. The reported frequency ranges from 10% to 56%.[18,20,22,23,27,39] These types of seizures incite sudden falling, producing injuries (so-called drop attacks, *Sturzanfälle*); this falling sometimes is limited to the head, such that the head falls on the chest (head drop, head nod, *nictatio capitis*).[7,28,41] Ikeno et al.[41] found that pure atonic seizures are exceptional and that most involved a tonic or myoclonic component. The EEG is characterized by slow spike and waves, polyspike and waves, or diffuse rapid rhythms.[28] Simultaneous video EEG recording and polygraphy allows a more precise diagnosis. In 95% of patients, atonic, tonic, and myoclonic seizures coexist.[28]

Atypical Absence Seizures

The reported frequency of atypical absence seizures ranges from 17% to 100%.[18,24] In most studies, the frequency of the different types of seizures reported is based on parental counting of seizures or reviews of clinic charts or is not specifically stated. Unfortunately, parental ability to recognize and correctly identify atypical absence seizures is poor. In one study using video EEG monitoring in a cohort of children with LGS, parental recognition was 27% for atypical absence seizures, whereas the sensitivity was as high as 80% for myoclonic seizures and 100% for tonic, atonic, tonic-clonic, clonic, and complex partial seizures.[42]

Diagnosis of atypical absence seizures may be difficult because their onset may be gradual,[20,24,28] and loss of consciousness may be incomplete, thereby allowing the patient to continue activities to some degree. Automatisms may be observed.[20] The seizure end may be gradual in some cases but abrupt in others.[20,24,28] The EEG is characterized by diffuse, slow (2.0- to 2.5-Hz) and irregular spike and waves, which may be difficult to differentiate from interictal bursts.[20] Sometimes, discharges of rapid rhythms may be seen, preceded by flattening of the record for 1–2 seconds and followed by a progressive development of irregular fast rhythm in the anterior and central regions, ending with brief spike and waves.[24,28]

Other Types of Seizures

Generalized tonic-clonic seizures are reported in 15% of LGS patients, whereas complex partial seizures occur in 5%.[20] Status epilepticus of different types (absence status epilepticus, tonic status epilepticus, nonconvulsive status epilepticus) can occur[18,20] and often is prolonged and resistant to treatment. The EEG during absence status epilepticus reveals continuous spike and wave discharges, usually at a lower frequency than at baseline, and rapid rhythms during tonic status epilepticus.[28]

Prognosis

The long-term prognosis for LGS is variable but, overall, unfavorable. Four cohort studies have followed up children with LGS over time and found that a minority of patients eventually could work normally, but 47–76% still had typical characteristics (MR and treatment-resistant seizures) many years after onset and required significant help such as home care or institutionalization.[43–46] Patients with symptomatic LGS—particularly those with a history of West's syndrome,[27] early onset of seizures,[27] higher frequency of seizures,[20] or constant slow EEG background activity[28]—had a worse prognosis. In one report, tonic seizures became more difficult to control over time and persisted (97.8% of the patients), whereas myoclonic and atypical absence seizures

appeared easier to control, persisting in 22.5% and 39.3% of the patients respectively.[47] The characteristic diffuse slow spike and wave pattern of LGS gradually disappears with age and is replaced by focal epileptic discharges, especially multiple independent spikes.[27]

Mortality rates range from 3% (mean follow-up of 8.5 years) to 7% (mean follow-up of 9.7 years).[28]

Additional Considerations

The severity of the seizures, frequent injuries, developmental delays, and behavior problems take a large toll on even the strongest families. Attention must be paid to the psychosocial needs of the family (especially siblings). The proper educational setting is important to help the patient with LGS to reach his or her maximal potential.

Owing to the high rate of injuries associated with atonic and tonic seizures, some patients with LGS may need to wear a protective helmet. Helmets must have a face guard to maximize protection of the patient's forehead, nose, and teeth. Of course, some patients will not tolerate a helmet with face guards and, even if tolerated, helmets often are uncomfortable and rarely are cosmetically acceptable.[25]

Table 7-1. Treatments for Children with Lennox-Gastaut Syndrome

First-line treatments based on clinical experience or
    conventional wisdom
    Valproic acid
    Benzodiazepines
    Pyridoxine
Suspected effective treatments based on open-label,
    uncontrolled studies
    Adrenocorticotropic hormone–corticosteroids
    Intravenous immunoglobulin
    Vigabatrin
    Zonisamide
    Ketogenic diet
    Corpus callosotomy
    Vagus nerve stimulation
Effective treatments based on double-blind, placebo-
    controlled studies
    Felbamate
    Lamotrigine
    Topiramate

Treatment

Overview

The goals of treatment for patients with LGS, as for all epilepsy patients, are the best quality of life with the fewest seizures (none, if possible), the fewest treatment side effects, and the least number of medications. The various treatment options for patients with LGS can be divided into three major groups (as shown in Table 7-1): (1) first-line treatments based on clinical experience or conventional wisdom, (2) suspected effective treatments based on open-label, uncontrolled studies, and (3) effective treatments based on double-blind, placebo-controlled studies.

In the first and second groups, the efficacy and safety of individual treatment options have not been tested formally. Only options in the third group have been rigorously and scientifically evaluated and found to be effective and safe for specific seizure types in LGS patients. Because no single treatment in any of the three groups gives satisfactory relief for all or even a majority of patients with LGS, a combination of treatment modalities frequently is needed.[48]

First-Line Treatments Based on Clinical Experience or Conventional Wisdom

During the last two decades, valproic acid was considered as a first-line treatment option for children with LGS.[25,49,50] Valproic acid may be more effective in cryptogenic than symptomatic LGS.[51]

Benzodiazepines—specifically clonazepam, nitrazepam, and clobazam—are also first-line antiepileptic therapeutic options.[25,50,52] All are considered effective against seizures associated with LGS, but side effects and tolerance limit their usefulness over time.[25] Clonazepam's side effects include hyperactivity, sedation, drooling, and incoordination, which can significantly affect the quality of life for patients with LGS.[25] Nitrazepam's efficacy and tolerability profile is similar to that of clonazepam, but nitrazepam is not available in the United States.[25] Clobazam is considered the least sedating benzodiazepine and boasts the longest time to the development of tolerance but also is unavailable in the United States.[52] Some recommendations for slowing the development of tolerance include dosing on an every-other-day schedule or using two different benzodiazepines on an alternate-day basis.[53,54] However, not all benzodiazepines are beneficial: intravenous diazepam and lorazepam may induce tonic static epilepticus in some patients.[55,56]

Carbamazepine, phenobarbital, phenytoin, and ethosuximide are not considered first-line therapy for LGS. Carbamazepine may exacerbate atypical absence seizures, whereas phenytoin and ethosuximide are effective against some, but not all, of the seizures associated with LGS. Phenobarbital can exacerbate hyperactivity and aggressiveness or produce sedation and drowsiness (which may exacerbate tonic seizures).[25,48,51,57–59]

Because patients with pyridoxine (vitamin B_6) dependency may experience seizures and demonstrate a slow spike and wave pattern on EEG, some clinician-investigators have suggested trials of vitamin B_6 in all children younger than 5 years who have treatment-resistant epilepsy.[50] In one study of the efficacy of high-dose vitamin B_6 in five patients with LGS, three patients had no response, whereas the others exhibited a more noticeable response.[60] It is reasonable and appropriate to conduct a vitamin B_6 trial early in the treatment of a child with LGS, given the lack of serious side effects and the ease of performing such a therapeutic trial.[61] Doses and duration of vitamin B_6 therapy vary widely. In the aforementioned clinical trial, 50–100 mg vitamin B_6 was given intramuscularly each day for the first 5 days, followed by 200–300 mg per day orally.[60] Some clinicians (mainly in Japan) will administer high doses of pyridoxal phosphate (30–40 mg/kg per day).[50] Wheless and Constantinou[50] prescribe 100 mg of vitamin B_6 three times daily for 2 weeks, stopping if there is no response to therapy after 2 weeks.

At this time, the ketogenic diet, corpus callosotomy, and vagus nerve stimulation are not considered first-line therapeutic measures for the seizures associated with LGS.

Suspected Effective Treatments Based on Open-Label, Uncontrolled Studies

Medications suspected to have some effectiveness against seizures associated with LGS based on open-label, uncontrolled trials include (in alphabetic order) adrenocorticotropic hormone (ACTH),[62,63] corticosteroids,[28,50,64] intravenous immunoglobulin (IVIG),[65,66] vigabatrin,[67] and zonisamide.[68] Roger et al.[28] propose that prolonged corticosteroid therapy initiated at the onset of cryptogenic LGS can yield excellent results. Despite this effectiveness, Corticosteroid therapy and ACTH carry the risk of multiple potentially significant side effects, and relapse frequently occurs when the drugs are withdrawn.[25,50,61–64]

The efficacy of adjunctive high-dose IVIG in patients with LGS has been investigated in at least seven open-label trials,[65,66,69–71] the results of which were very encouraging. In one review, 30–92% of LGS patients receiving IVIG experienced at least a 50% seizure reduction during treatment.[65] Dosing schedules varied between studies. Subsequent well-controlled trials (detailed later) have not yet confirmed IVIG's effectiveness against seizures associated with LGS.[72,73]

Six studies involving 78 patients treated with vigabatrin showed that 15% of these patients became completely seizure-free, and 44% experienced at least a 50% reduction in their seizure frequency.[67,74–78] Vigabatrin's most common adverse effects are generally central nervous system–related and include hyperactivity, agitation, weight gain, drowsiness, insomnia, facial edema, ataxia, stupor, and somnolence.[76,79–81] Further, vigabatrin is not available in the United States, may exacerbate myoclonic seizures (and even absence seizures in some patients), and can cause visual field constriction in children.[75,76,79,82,83]

The effectiveness of zonisamide in LGS has been investigated in three small studies. Between 26% and 50% of patients with LGS treated with zonisamide experienced at least a 50% reduction in seizure frequency (Dianippon Pharmaceutical, Japan, data on file).[68,84]

No formal, published, open-label studies have investigated the effectiveness and safety of gabapentin, tiagabine, levetiracetam or oxcarbazepine in the treatment of seizures associated with LGS. Single reports have suggested that L-tryptophan (transient improvement), amantadine, and DN-1417 (a thyrotropin-releasing hormone analog) may reduce seizure frequency in patients with LGS.[85–87]

A number of studies have shown the ketogenic diet to be useful for patients with LGS.[61,62,88,89] Response to the diet usually is evident within 1 month of its initiation.[50] In a recent study, the atonic or myoclonic seizures in 17 consecutively treated patients with LGS at the Johns Hopkins Hospital decreased "by more than 50% immediately."[90] The benefits of the diet can include fewer seizures, less drowsiness, better behavior, and fewer concomitant AEDs.[50]

Surgical procedures that have been reported to be beneficial for patients with LGS include corpus callosotomy, vagus nerve stimulation (VNS), and, rarely, focal resection.[50] Corpus callosotomy is effective in reducing drop attacks but typically does not appear to be helpful for other seizure types.[25,91–93] In general, callosotomy is considered palliative rather than curative, and seizure freedom after this treatment is rare but can occur.[51,94]

In six studies (three published reports and three abstracts), VNS appears to be effective for patients with LGS.[95–100] The three published studies, for which follow-up was as long as 5 years, reported that a total of 13 of 18 (72%) patients with LGS experienced at least a 50% reduction in seizure frequency.[95–97] In the largest cohort of LGS patients treated with VNS (n = 46), Frost et al.[98] reported in abstract form that the mean reduction in seizure frequency at 1 (n = 46), 3 (n = 29), and 6 (n = 15) months was 38%, 41%, and 71%, respectively. Two other studies (reported in abstract form) also concluded that VNS is effective as adjunctive therapy for patients with LGS.[99,100]

Effective Treatments Based on Double-Blind, Placebo-Controlled Studies

The gold standard for evaluating the safety and efficacy of an AED is the randomized, double-blind, placebo-controlled clinical trial. Five drugs—cinromide, IVIG, felbamate, lamotrigine, and topiramate—have undergone this rigorous testing to determine their safety and efficacy in patients with LGS. The latter three AEDs successfully demonstrated efficacy against seizures in patients with LGS, whereas the first two did not. Despite the lack of proven efficacy for cinromide and IVIG in double-blind studies, both therapeutic options had undergone open-label trials that suggested their efficacy in patients with LGS. This discrepancy reinforces the need for randomized, double-blind, controlled trials to definitively establish the efficacy of any proposed therapy.

Cinromide

In 1980, cinromide, in an open-label, uncontrolled trial, was reported to be effective for seizures associated with LGS.[101] These results prompted a subsequent double-blind, placebo-controlled, adjunctive therapeutic trial of cinromide in patients with LGS that found no difference between cinromide adjunctive therapy and placebo adjunctive therapy in terms of seizure reduction or global evaluations.[102] The development of cinromide was halted in 1981.[102]

Immunoglobulins

Two blinded, placebo-controlled studies have been published examining the efficacy of IVIG in children with LGS.[72,73] The first study enrolled 10 children,

Table 7-2. Responder Rates (≥50% Reduction in Seizure Frequency) for Three Antiepileptic Medications Tested in Double-Blind, Placebo-Controlled Trials in Lennox-Gastaut Syndrome

Seizpure Type	Felbamate vs. Placebo[103]	Lamotrigine vs. Placebo[115]	Topiramate vs. Placebo[119]
Total seizures	50% vs. 11%*		
All major seizures (drop attacks plus tonic-clonic)		33% vs. 16%*	33% vs. 8%*
Drop attack or atonic seizures	57% vs. 9%*	37%* vs. 22%*	28% vs. 14%
Tonic-clonic seizures	60% vs. 23%*	43% vs. 20%*	

*p <.05.

ages 4–14 years, in an add-on, placebo-controlled, single-blind study design. Only two children showed a response to IVIG (42% and 100% decrease in seizure frequency), whereas the remaining eight children reportedly were unaffected.[72] The second study involved 61 patients with various forms of refractory epilepsy (including LGS and West's syndrome), who participated in a randomized, double-blind, placebo-controlled, dose-ranging (three different doses) trial of IVIG. Despite the fact that 52.5% of the IVIG group experienced a greater than 50% reduction in seizure frequency, as compared to the 27.8% in the placebo group, this difference did not reach statistical significance.[73]

Felbamate

Felbamate was found to be safe and effective in patients with LGS in a randomized, double-blind, placebo-controlled adjunctive therapeutic trial.[103] Seventy-three patients with LGS, ages 4–36 years, were enrolled. The felbamate dose in the double-blind portion was 45 mg/kg per day (maximum, 3,600 mg per day). The felbamate treatment group experienced a 34% reduction in atonic seizures, as compared with 9% in the placebo group (p = .01). Total seizure frequency dropped 19% in the felbamate group, as compared with a 4% increase in the placebo group (p = .002). The percentage of patients experiencing at least a 50% reduction in atonic seizures and total seizure frequency was significantly higher for the felbamate group than for the placebo group (p <.001) (Table 7-2). In addition, felbamate was significantly better than placebo in improving global evaluation scores.[103] During a 12-month follow-up period in patients who completed the con-

trolled part of the study, long-term efficacy was confirmed.[104]

Despite its apparent efficacy, felbamate is associated with idiosyncratic reactions involving the formed elements of the blood and liver. The most common severe felbamate-associated idiosyncratic reaction is aplastic anemia,[105] the incidence of which is approximately 127 cases per million treated with felbamate (approximately 1 in 4,000–8,000 treated patients), as compared with 2.0–2.5 cases per million persons in the general population.[80,105,106] Another report estimates the risk of aplastic anemia in patients receiving felbamate to be 1 in 3,000, with a death rate of 1 in 10,000 felbamate-treated patients.[80,107] This estimated risk is roughly up to 20 times greater than that for carbamazepine-associated aplastic anemia.[105] Risk factors for felbamate-associated aplastic anemia are being white, adult, and female and having a history of an autoimmune disorder, AED toxicity or allergy, cytopenia, and treatment with felbamate for less than 1 year.[105,108]

The second most common severe felbamate-associated idiosyncratic reaction is hepatotoxicity. Its estimated incidence is between 64 and 164 cases per million (approximately 1 in 18,500–25,000 felbamate-treated patients).[105] This suggests that the frequency of felbamate-associated and valproic acid–associated hepatotoxicity is roughly the same.[105] A suggested management strategy is to employ careful clinical monitoring and routine laboratory testing and to discontinue felbamate use if no substantial clinical benefit is observed after 3–6 months of therapy.

Despite felbamate's efficacy, the significant risks associated with felbamate use cause this agent to be regarded as a good third-line or fourth-line drug for LGS.

Lamotrigine

Lamotrigine's efficacy against seizures associated with LGS was examined in multiple open-label studies and two controlled trials. In five open-label trials of lamotrigine in patients with LGS, 58% (31 of 53) experienced at least a 50% reduction in seizure frequency.[109–113] A double-blind, placebo-controlled, crossover study of lamotrigine as adjunctive therapy in 30 patients with treatment-resistant generalized epilepsy (20 of whom had LGS) was reported in 1998. Seven of the twenty children with LGS responded to lamotrigine therapy with a greater than 50% reduction in seizure frequency, and two became seizure-free.[114]

Lamotrigine proved to be safe and effective in patients with LGS in a randomized, double-blind, placebo-controlled, adjunctive therapeutic trial in which 169 patients enrolled and were randomized to either lamotrigine (n = 79) or placebo (n = 90) adjunctive therapy.[115] Patients on the lamotrigine treatment arm had a greater median percentage reduction from baseline in weekly seizure counts (for drop attacks, tonic-clonic seizures, and all major seizures [defined as drop attacks plus tonic-clonic seizures]) as compared with patients on the placebo treatment arm. The responder rate (percentage of patients experiencing at least a 50% reduction in seizures) for major seizures (drop attacks and tonic-clonic seizures) was greater in the lamotrigine group than in the placebo group (see Table 7-2).[115]

Despite its efficacy, lamotrigine can be associated with idiosyncratic reactions predominantly involving the skin. The most common skin manifestation is a rash affecting 10–12% of lamotrigine-treated patients.[80,116,117] After lamotrigine withdrawal, the rash rapidly resolves; sometimes the rash may even resolve without changing the lamotrigine dosage.[118] However, this dermatologic reaction can progress in some patients to erythema multiforme, Stevens-Johnson syndrome, or even toxic epidermal necrolysis.[80,116,118] Stevens-Johnson syndrome and toxic epidermal necrolysis are considered to be related severe mucocutaneous disorders with mortality rates of less than 5% and 30%, respectively.[116] The risk of a potentially life-threatening rash (based on clinical trials and postmarketing reports) is 0.3% in adults and approximately 1% in children 16 years of age and younger.[118] Risk factors for lamotrigine-associated severe dermatologic reactions include younger age (children more than adults), comedication with valproic acid, a rapid rate of lamotrigine titration, and a high lamotrigine starting dose.[80,116,118]

Despite the risk of idiosyncratic reactions, lamotrigine is a very valuable medication for patients with LGS and should be considered for use as soon as the diagnosis of LGS is made. Proper attention to concomitant medications, a low starting dose, and a very slow titration rate can minimize the risk of dermatologic idiosyncratic reactions. The prompt evaluation of any rash is prudent.

Topiramate

Topiramate was found to be safe and effective as adjunctive therapy for patients with LGS in a multicenter, double-blind, placebo-controlled trial.[119] Ninety-eight patients with LGS (ages 1+ to 30 years) were randomized to either topiramate adjunctive therapy (target dose, 6 mg/kg per day) or placebo adjunctive therapy. The median percentage reduction from baseline in average monthly seizure rate for drop attacks was 14.8% for the topiramate group and –5.1% (an increase) for the placebo group (p = .04). Using parental global evaluations, topiramate-treated patients demonstrated greater improvement in seizure severity than did placebo-treated patients (p = .04). The responder rate for major seizures (drop attacks and tonic-clonic seizures) was greater in the topiramate group (15 of 46, or 33%) than in the control group (4 of 50, or 8%; p = .002). The responder rate for drop attacks in the topiramate group was higher than in the placebo group (28% vs. 14%) but did not reach statistical significance (see Table 7-2).[119]

In the long-term, open-label extension portion of the preceding trial, 97 patients were followed up, and their topiramate dose was adjusted as clinically indicated.[120] The mean topiramate dosage in those patients who had completed 6 months of open-label therapy was 10 mg/kg per day. For those patients who had completed 6 months of open-label topiramate therapy, drop attacks were reduced by at least 50% in 55% of patients (as compared to 28% during the double-blind portion of the trial), and 15% of patients were free of drop attacks for at least 6 months at the last visit. In this open-label extension phase, the median percentage reduction in drop attacks was 56% (as compared to 14.8% during the double-blind portion of the trial). The median percentage reduction in overall seizure frequency was 44%, with 45% of the patients having at least a 50% reduction in all seizure types and 2% being seizure-free for the previous 6 months. The most common adverse events were somnolence, injury, and anorexia. Only 5% of the patients reported behavioral problems during the last 6 months of topiramate long-term therapy. Therefore, topiramate was well tolerated during long-term therapy and was effective in controlling drop attacks and seizures associated with LGS.[120]

Comparison among Felbamate, Lamotrigine, and Topiramate

As the felbamate, lamotrigine, and topiramate double-blind, placebo-controlled adjunctive therapeutic trials for patients with LGS show efficacy and safety of each of these agents, attention turns to the issue of which medication is better. Because no comparative trial of AEDs has been performed in patients with LGS, the best method of resolving the issue is a meta-analysis of these three trials.

A clinically useful measure of treatment effect of a study medication is the number needed to treat (NNT).[121] This calculated number represents the number of patients that a clinician must treat with a study medication in order to find one with the desired outcome. The NNT is calculated as $1/(A - P)$, where *A* is the percentage of responders in the active treatment arm and *P* is the percentage of responders in the placebo treatment arm. This represents the inverse of the absolute risk reduction.[121] In clinical trials of AEDs involving patients with treatment-resistant epilepsy, the desired outcome is usually at least a 50% reduction in seizure frequency. A patient who achieves this reduction is called a *responder*. The 95% confidence interval (CI) can then be calculated (G. Pledger, personal communication, 1998).

To date, only trials involving adults with treatment-resistant partial seizures have been considered in other meta-analyses of AEDs.[122] The NNT can be calculated using the felbamate, lamotrigine, and topiramate double-blind placebo-controlled adjunctive therapy trials described earlier. In each study, drop attacks (atonic and tonic seizures) were used as the seizure outcome variable, because they are the most debilitating seizure type. The NNT for felbamate was 2.1 (95% CI, 1.4–3.8); for lamotrigine, 6.4 (95% CI, 3.4–54.8); and for topiramate, 7.2 (95% CI, 33–1,000). Although felbamate had a lower NNT than

did the other two agents, the confidence intervals overlap. Therefore, it is not possible to conclude that there will be an observable clinical difference among these three AEDs in terms of efficacy against drop attacks.

The efficacy of the ketogenic diet for patients with LGS currently is being examined in an ongoing double-blind, controlled trial (J. Freeman, personal communication, 2000). No double-blind trials either have been completed to date or are under way to examine the efficacy of surgical intervention in patients with LGS.

References

1. Alvarez N, Besag F, Iivanainen M. Use of antiepileptic drugs in the treatment of epilepsy in people with intellectual disability. J Intellect Disabil Res 1998;42:1–15.
2. Goulden KJ, Shinnar S, Koller H, et al. Epilepsy in children with mental retardation: a cohort study. Epilepsia 1991;32:690–697.
3. Forsgren L, Edvinsson SO, Blomquist HK, et al. Epilepsy in a population of mentally retarded children and adults. Epilepsy Res 1990;6:234–248.
4. Forsgren L, Edvinsson SO, Nystrom L, Blomquist HK. Influence of epilepsy on mortality in mental retardation: an epidemiologic study. Epilepsia 1996;37:956–963.
5. Steffenburg U, Hedstrom A, Lindroth A, et al. Intractable epilepsy in a population-based series of mentally retarded children. Epilepsia 1998;39:767–775.
6. Mariani E, Ferini-Strambi L, Sala M, et al. Epilepsy in institutionalized patients with encephalopathy: clinical aspects and nosological considerations. Am J Ment Retard 1993;98[Suppl]:27–33.
7. Gastaut H. The Lennox-Gastaut syndrome: comments on the syndrome's terminology and nosological position amongst the secondary generalized epilepsies of childhood. Electroencephalogr Clin Neurophysiol Suppl 1982;35:71–84.
8. Gibbs F, Gibbs E, Lennox W. Influence of blood sugar level on wave and spike formation in petit mal epilepsy. Arch Neurol Psychiatry 1939;41:1111–1114.
9. Gibbs F, Davis H, Lennox W. Electroencephalogram in epilepsy and in conditions of impaired consciousness. Arch Neurol Psychiatry 1935;34:1133–1148.
10. Lennox W. The petit mal epilepsies: their treatment with tridione. JAMA 1945;129:1069–1074.
11. Lennox WG, Davis JP. Clinical correlates of the fast and the slow spike-wave electroencephalogram. Pediatrics 1950;5:626–644.
12. Lennox W. Epilepsy and Related Disorders, vol 1. Boston: Little, Brown, 1960.
13. Doose H. Das akinetische Petit Mal. Arch Psychiatr Nervenkr 1964;205:625–654.

14. Sorel L. L'epilepsie myokinetique grave de la premiere enfance avec pointe-onde lente (petit mal variant) et son traitement. Rev Neurol 1964;110:215–233.

15. Commission on Classification and Terminology of the International League Against Epilepsy. Proposal for revised classification of epilepsies and epileptic syndromes. Epilepsia 1989;30:389–399.

16. Beaumanoir A, Dravet C. The Lennox-Gastaut Syndrome. In J Roger, M Bureau, C Dravet, et al. (eds), Epileptic Syndromes in Infancy, Childhood and Adolescence. London: John Libbey, 1992;115–132.

17. Farrell K. Classifying epileptic syndromes: problems and a neurobiologic solution. Neurology 1993;43:S8–S11.

18. Aicardi J. Epileptic syndromes in childhood. Epilepsia 1988;29:S1–S5.

19. Livingston JH. The Lennox-Gastaut syndrome. Dev Med Child Neurol 1988;30:536–540.

20. Dulac O, N'Guyen T. The Lennox-Gastaut syndrome. Epilepsia 1993;34:S7–S17.

21. Ohtahara S. Lennox-Gastaut syndrome. Considerations in its concept and categorization. Jpn J Psychiatry Neurol 1988;42:535–542.

22. Oguni H, Hayashi K, Osawa M. Long-term prognosis of Lennox-Gastaut syndrome. Epilepsia 1996;37[Suppl 3]:44–47.

23. Trevathan E, Murphy CC, Yeargin-Allsopp M. Prevalence and descriptive epidemiology of Lennox-Gastaut syndrome among Atlanta children. Epilepsia 1997;38:1283–1288.

24. Yaqub BA. Electroclinical seizures in Lennox-Gastaut syndrome. Epilepsia 1993;34:120–127.

25. Aicardi J. Epilepsy in Children. In PG Procopis, I Rapin (eds), The International Review of Child Neurology. New York: Raven Press, 1994.

26. Kaminska A, Ickowicz A, Plouin P, et al. Delineation of cryptogenic Lennox-Gastaut syndrome and myoclonic astatic epilepsy using multiple correspondence analysis. Epilepsy Res 1999;36:15–29.

27. Ohtsuka Y, Amano R, Mizukawa M, Ohtahara S. Long-term prognosis of the Lennox-Gastaut syndrome. Jpn J Psychiatry Neurol 1990;44:257–264.

28. Roger J, Dravet C, Bureau M. The Lennox-Gastaut syndrome. Cleve Clin J Med 1989;56:S172–S180.

29. Smeraldi E, Scorza Smeraldi R, Cazzullo CL, et al. Immunogenetics of the Lennox-Gastaut syndrome: frequency of HL-A antigens and haplotypes in patients and first-degree relatives. Epilepsia 1975;16:699–703.

30. van Engelen BG, de Waal LP, Weemaes CM, Renier WO. Serologic HLA typing in cryptogenic Lennox-Gastaut syndrome. Epilepsy Res 1994;17:43–47.

31. Theodore WH, Rose D, Patronas N, et al. Cerebral glucose metabolism in the Lennox-Gastaut syndrome. Ann Neurol 1987;21:14–21.

32. Chugani HT, Mazziotta JC, Engel J Jr, Phelps ME. The Lennox-Gastaut syndrome: metabolic subtypes determined by 2-deoxy- 2[18F]fluoro-D-glucose positron emission tomography. Ann Neurol 1987;21:4–13.

33. Hauser WA. The prevalence and incidence of convulsive disorders in children. Epilepsia 1994;35[Suppl 2]:S1–S6.

34. Kramer U, Nevo Y, Neufeld MY, et al. Epidemiology of epilepsy in childhood: a cohort of 440 consecutive patients. Pediatr Neurol 1998;18:46–50.

35. Prats JM, Garaizar C. Etiology of epilepsy in adolescents. Rev Neurol 1999;28:32–35.

36. Beilmann A, Talvik T. Is the International League Against Epilepsy classification of epileptic syndromes applicable to children in Estonia? Eur J Paediatr Neurol 1999;3:265–272.

37. Cavazzuti GB. Epidemiology of different types of epilepsy in school age children of Modena, Italy. Epilepsia 1980;21:57–62.

38. Heiskala H. Community-based study of Lennox-Gastaut syndrome. Epilepsia 1997;38:526–531.

39. Chevrie JJ, Aicardi J. Childhood epileptic encephalopathy with slow spike-wave. A statistical study of 80 cases. Epilepsia 1972;13:259–271.

40. Markand ON. Slow spike-wave activity in EEG and associated clinical features: often called "Lennox" or "Lennox-Gastaut" syndrome. Neurology 1977;27:746–757.

41. Ikeno T, Shigematsu H, Miyakoshi M, et al. An analytic study of epileptic falls. Epilepsia 1985;26:612–621.

42. Bare MA, Glauser TA, Strawsburg RH. Need for electroencephalogram video confirmation of atypical absence seizures in children with Lennox-Gastaut syndrome. J Child Neurol 1998;13:498–500.

43. Beaumanoir A. The Lennox-Gastaut syndrome: a personal study. Electroencephalogr Clin Neurophysiol Suppl 1982;35:85–99.

44. Roger J, Remy C, Bureau M, et al. [Lennox-Gastaut syndrome in the adult.] Rev Neurol 1987;143:401–405.

45. Ohtahara S, Ohtsuka Y, Kobayashi K. Lennox-Gastaut syndrome: a new vista. Psychiatry Clin Neurosci 1995;49:S179–S183.

46. Yagi K. Evolution of Lennox-Gastaut syndrome: a long-term longitudinal study. Epilepsia 1996;37:48–51.

47. Ohtsuka Y, Ohmori I, Oka E. Long-term follow-up of childhood epilepsy associated with tuberous sclerosis. Epilepsia 1998;39:1158–1163.

48. Mattson RH. Efficacy and adverse effects of established and new antiepileptic drugs. Epilepsia 1995;36:S13–S26.

49. Jeavons P, Clark J, Maheshwari M. Treatment of generalized epilepsies of childhood and adolescence with sodium valproate ("Epilim"). Dev Med Child Neurol 1977;19:9–25.

50. Wheless JW, Constantinou JEC. Lennox-Gastaut syndrome. Pediatr Neurol 1997;17:203–211.

51. Farrell K. Secondary Generalized Epilepsy and Lennox-Gastaut Syndrome. In: E Wyllie (ed), The Treatment of

Epilepsy: Principles and Practice. Philadelphia: Lea & Febiger, 1993;604–613.

52. Gastaut H, Lowe M. Antiepileptic properties of cloba-zam, a 1.5 benzodiazepine, in man. Epilepsia 1979; 20:437–446.

53. Snead OC, Saito M. Encephalopathic Epilepsy After Infancy. In: WE Dodson, JM Pellock (eds), Pediatric Epilepsy: Diagnosis and Therapy. New York: Demos Publications, 1993;147–156.

54. Sher P. Alternate day clonazepam treatment of intractable seizures. Arch Neurol 1985;42:787–788.

55. Bittencourt PR, Richens A. Anticonvulsant-induced status epilepticus in Lennox-Gastaut syndrome. Epilepsia 1981;22:129–134.

56. DiMario FJ Jr, Clancy RR. Paradoxical precipitation of tonic seizures by lorazepam in a child with atypical absence seizures. Pediatr Neurol 1988;4:249–251.

57. Snead O. Exacerbation of seizures in children by carbam-azepine. N Engl J Med 1985;323:916–921.

58. Horn CS, Ater SB, Hurst DL. Carbamazepine-exacer-bated epilepsy in children and adolescents. Pediatr Neurol 1986;2:340–345.

59. Erba G, Browne T. Atypical Absence, Myoclonic, Atonic and Tonic Seizures and the Lennox-Gastaut syndrome. In T Browne, R Feldman (eds), Epilepsy, Diagnosis and Management. Boston: Little, Brown, 1983;75–94.

60. Zouhar A, Slapal R. Administration of high doses of B_6 in age-related epileptic encephalopathies. Cesk Neurol Neurochir 1989;52:28–31.

61. Bourgeois BFD. Antiepileptic drugs in pediatric practice. Epilepsia 1995;36:S34–S45.

62. Brett E. The Lennox-Gastaut Syndrome: Therapeutic Aspects. In E Niedermeyer, R Degen (eds), The Lennox-Gastaut Syndrome. New York: Alan Liss, 1988;317–339.

63. Yamatogi Y, Ohtsuka Y, Ishida T, et al. Treatment of the Lennox syndrome with ACTH: a clinical and electroen-cephalographic study. Brain Dev 1979;1:267–276.

64. Snead O, Benton J, Myers C. ACTH and prednisone in childhood seizure disorders. Neurology 1983;33:966–970.

65. Duse M, Notarangelo LD, Tiberti S, et al. Intravenous immune globulin in the treatment of intractable child-hood epilepsy. Clin Exp Immunol 1996;104[Suppl 1]:71–76.

66. van Engelen BG, Renier WO, Weemaes CM, et al. High-dose intravenous immunoglobulin treatment in cryptogenic West and Lennox-Gastaut syndrome; an add-on study. Eur J Pediatr 1994;153:762–769.

67. Feucht M, Brantner-Inthaler S. Gamma-vinyl-GABA (vigabatrin) in the therapy of Lennox-Gastaut syndrome: an open study. Epilepsia 1994;35:993–998.

68. Sakamoto K, Kurokawa T, Tomita S, et al. Effects of zonisamide on children with epilepsy. Curr Ther Res 1988;43(3):378–383.

69. van Rijckevorsel-Harmant K, Delire M, Rucquoy-Ponsar M. Treatment of idiopathic West and Lennox-Gastaut syndromes by intravenous administration of human poly-valent immunoglobulins. Eur Arch Psychiatry Neurol Sci 1986;236:119–122.

70. Gross-Tsur V, Shalev RS, Kazir E, et al. Intravenous high-dose gammaglobulins for intractable childhood epilepsy. Acta Neurol Scand 1993;88:204–209.

71. Ariizumi M, Baba K, Shiihara H. High dose gammaglob-ulin for intractable childhood epilepsy. Lancet 1983;2:162–163.

72. Illum N, Taudorf K, Heilmann C, et al. Intravenous immunoglobulin: a single-blind trial in children with Lennox-Gastaut syndrome. Neuropediatrics 1990;21:87–90.

73. van Rijckevorsel-Harmant K, Delire M, Schmitz-Moor-man W, Wieser HG. Treatment of refractory epilepsy with intravenous immunoglobulins. Results of the first double-blind/dose finding clinical study. Int J Clin Lab Res 1994;24:162–166.

74. Livingston J, Beaumont D, Arzimanoglou A. Vigabatrin in the treatment of epilepsy in children. Br J Clin Pharma-col 1989;27:S109–S112.

75. Gibbs J, Appleton R, Rosenbloom L. Vigabatrin in intrac-table childhood epilepsy: a retrospective study. Pediatr Neurol 1992;8:338–340.

76. Luna D, Dulac O, Pajot N. Vigabatrin in the treatment of childhood epilepsies. A single-blind placebo-controlled study. Epilepsia 1989;30:430–437.

77. Fois A, Buoni S, Bartolo RD. Vigabatrin treatment in children. Childs Nerv Syst 1994;10:244–248.

78. Maldonado C, Castello J, Fuentes E. Vigabatrin in the management of Lennox-Gastaut syndrome. Epilepsia 1995;36:S102.

79. Dulac O, Chiron C, Luna D, et al. Vigabatrin in child-hood epilepsy. J Child Neurol 1991;[Suppl 2]:S30–S37.

80. Pellock JM. New antiepileptic drugs in pediatric epilepsy syndromes. Pediatrics 1999;104:1106–1116.

81. Shields WD, Sankar R. Vigabatrin. Semin Pediatr Neurol 1997;4:43–50.

82. Appleton RE. Vigabatrin in the management of general-ized seizures in children. Seizure 1995;4:45–48.

83. Sankar R, Wasterlain CG. Is the devil we know the lesser of two evils? Vigabatrin and visual fields. Neurology 1999;52:1537–1538.

84. Yamatogi Y, Ohtahara S. Current topics of treatment. In S Ohtahara, J Roger (eds), Proceedings of the International Symposium, New Trends in Pediatric Epileptology. Okayama, Japan: Okayama University Medical School, 1991;136–148.

85. Prusinski A, Stepien-Barcikowska A. A trial of using tryptophan in the treatment of Lennox-Gastaut syndrome. Neurochir Polska 1984;18:287–289.

86. Slapal R, Zouhar A. Therapeutic effect of dopaminergic substances in drug-resistant Lennox-Gastaut syndrome. Cesk Neurol Neurochir 1989;52:32–35.

87. Inanaga K, Kumashiro H, Fukuyama Y, et al. Clinical study of oral administration of DN-1417, a TRH ana-log, in patients with intractable epilepsy. Epilepsia 1989;30:438–445.

88. Ros Perez P, Zamarron Cuesta I, Aparicio Meix M, Sastre Gallego A. Evaluation of the effectiveness of the ketogenic diet with medium-chain triglycerides, in the treatment of refractory epilepsy in children. Apropos of a series of cases. An Esp Pediatr 1989;30:155–158.

89. Wheless J. The ketogenic diet: fa(c)t or fiction. J Child Neurol 1995;10:419–423.

90. Freeman JM, Vining EP. Seizures decrease rapidly after fasting: preliminary studies of the ketogenic diet. Arch Pediatr Adolesc Med 1999;153:946–949.

91. Wheless J. Evaluation of children for epilepsy surgery. Pediatr Ann 1991;20:41–49.

92. Baumgartner J, Clifton G, Wheless J. Corpus callostomy. Tech Neurosurg 1995;1:45–51.

93. Chevrie J-J, Aicardi J. Lennox-Gastaut Syndrome. In H Luders (ed), Epilepsy Surgery. New York: Raven Press, 1991;197–202.

94. Kwan SY, Wong TT, Chang KP, et al. Seizure outcome after corpus callosotomy: the Taiwan experience. Childs Nerv Syst 2000;16:87–92.

95. Hornig GW, Murphy JV, Schallert G, Tilton C. Left vagus nerve stimulation in children with refractory epilepsy: an update. South Med J 1997;90:484–488.

96. Ben-Menachem E, Hellstrom K, Waldton C, Augustinsson LE. Evaluation of refractory epilepsy treated with vagus nerve stimulation for up to 5 years. Neurology 1999;52:1265–1267.

97. Lundgren J, Amark P, Blennow G, et al. Vagus nerve stimulation in 16 children with refractory epilepsy. Epilepsia 1998;39:809–813.

98. Frost M, Gates J, Conry J, et al. Vagus nerve stimulation (VNS) in Lennox-Gastaut syndrome (LGS). Epilepsia 1999;40[Suppl 7]:95.

99. Hosain S, Harden C, Nikolov B, et al. Vagus nerve stimulation in children with symptomatic generalized epilepsy. Epilepsia 1999;40[Suppl 7]:125.

100. Tatum W, Ferriera J, Benbadis S, Vale F. Vagus nerve stimulation and antiepileptic drug reduction. Epilepsia 1999;40[Suppl 7]:223.

101. Lockman L, Rothner A, Erenberg G, et al. Cinromide in the treatment of seizures in the Lennox-Gastaut syndrome. Epilepsia 1980;22:241.

102. Group for the Evaluation of Cinromide in the Lennox-Gastaut Syndrome. Double-blind, placebo-controlled evaluation of cinromide in patients with the Lennox-Gastaut syndrome. Epilepsia 1989;30:422–429.

103. Ritter FJ. Efficacy of felbamate in childhood epileptic encephalopathy (Lennox-Gastaut syndrome). N Engl J Med 1993;328:29–33.

104. Jensen PK. Felbamate in the treatment of Lennox-Gastaut syndrome. Epilepsia 1994;35[Suppl 5]:S54–S57.

105. Pellock JM. Felbamate. Epilepsia 1999;40:S57–S62.

106. Patton W, Duffull S. Idiosyncratic drug-induced haematological abnormalities. Incidence, pathogenesis, management and avoidance. Drug Saf 1994;11:445–462.

107. Bourgeois BF. Felbamate. Semin Pediatr Neurol 1997;4:3–8.

108. Pellock JM, Brodie MJ. Felbamate: 1997 update. Epilepsia 1997;38:1261–1264.

109. Donaldson JA, Glauser TA, Olberding LS. Lamotrigine adjunctive therapy in childhood epileptic encephalopathy (the Lennox Gastaut syndrome). Epilepsia 1997;38:68–73.

110. Timmings PL, Richens A. Lamotrigine as an add-on drug in the management of Lennox-Gastaut syndrome. Eur Neurol 1992;32:305–307.

111. Schlumberger E, Chavez F, Palacios L, et al. Lamotrigine in treatment of 120 children with epilepsy. Epilepsia 1994;35:359–367.

112. Uvebrant P, Bauziene R. Intractable epilepsy in children. The efficacy of lamotrigine treatment, including non-seizure related benefits. Neuropediatrics 1994;25:284–289.

113. Buchanan N. Lamotrigine: clinical experience in 93 patients with epilepsy. Acta Neurol Scand 1995;92:28–32.

114. Eriksson AS, Nergardh A, Hoppu K. The efficacy of lamotrigine in children and adolescents with refractory generalized epilepsy: a randomized, double-blind, crossover study. Epilepsia 1998;39:495–501.

115. Motte J, Trevathan E, Arvidsson JF, et al. Lamotrigine for generalized seizures associated with the Lennox-Gastaut syndrome. N Engl J Med 1997;337:1807–1812.

116. Pellock JM. Overview of lamotrigine and the new antiepileptic drugs: the challenge. J Child Neurol 1997;12:S48–S52.

117. Schlienger RG, Shapiro LE, Shear NH. Lamotrigine-induced severe cutaneous adverse reactions. Epilepsia 1998;39:S22–S26.

118. Matsuo F. Lamotrigine. Epilepsia 1999;40:S30–S36.

119. Sachdeo RC, Glauser TA, Ritter F, et al. A double-blind, randomized trial of topiramate in Lennox-Gastaut syndrome. Neurology 1999;52:1882–1887.

120. Glauser TA, Levisohn PM, Ritter F, Sachdeo RC. Topiramate in Lennox-Gastaut syndrome: open-label treatment of patients completing a randomized controlled trial. Topiramate YL Study Group. Epilepsia 2000;41:S86–S90.

121. Cook RJ, Sackett DL. The number needed to treat: a clinically useful measure of treatment effect. BMJ 1995;310:452–454.

122. Marson AG, Kadir ZA, Chadwick DW. New antiepileptic drugs: a systematic review of their efficacy and tolerability. BMJ 1996;313:1169–1174.

Chapter 8

Landau-Kleffner Syndrome and Its Variants

Ruth Nass and Anna Gross

The nosology of Landau-Kleffner syndrome (LKS) and its putative variants are a subject of current controversy.[1] Although the classic form of LKS has been well described, clinical and electroencephalographic similarities between LKS and other developmental and acquired cognitive and behavioral disorders associated with an epileptiform electroencephalogram (EEG) raise questions as to the boundaries of the LKS syndrome. It is unclear whether LKS is a distinct entity or a subtype of a broader syndrome that has a single etiology but multiple clinical phenotypes. The fact that a given child may exhibit features common to several different disorders (e.g., LKS, autism, disintegrative disorder [DD]), either simultaneously or at various times over the course of development, adds to the confusion. Given this uncertainty, attempts have been made to delineate homogeneous subgroups within the developmental language disorders, autistic spectrum disorders, and DDs on the basis of the presence or absence of language, behavioral, cognitive, or electroencephalographic abnormalities. Without a clear understanding of etiology or pathophysiology, however, the rationale for these demarcations remains controversial. The central, unresolved issue is whether the epileptiform discharges cause or contribute to language, behavioral, or cognitive regression in these disorders.[2–4]

Our aim in this chapter is to outline the boundaries of LKS and its putative variants, shedding light on where they both diverge and overlap. We first characterize the clinical findings that may distinguish LKS from its putative variants and then describe the electroencephalographic features that may distinguish them. We call special attention to the debate regarding the relationship between the presence and severity of epileptiform discharges and language and cognitive dysfunction. Finally, we summarize the results of treatment and the outcome.

Clinical Features of the Landau-Kleffner Syndrome

Landau and Kleffner[5] were the first to report an acquired aphasia occurring in childhood that was associated with a convulsive disorder.[6–11] Typically, language comprehension in a previously normal, usually male, child between the ages of 3 and 7 years deteriorates over days to weeks. Initially, parents often are concerned that their child is becoming deaf. The child, however, *is* able to hear, as proven by the facts that he or she is alert to environmental sounds and that the audiogram or brainstem auditory responses are normal. However, the child cannot process meaningful language (verbal auditory agnosia).[12–15] The language comprehension deficit generally is followed by the insidious loss of speech. Poorly articulated, dysprosodic speech is the rule. Mutism occurs occasionally. (This is believed to occur because expressive language is not yet automatized in the young child and therefore deteriorates without reinforcement.) Many children with classic LKS can access language in the visual modality; that is, they can gesture, learn sign language, read,

Table 8-1. Comparison of Landau-Kleffner Syndrome (LKS),
Autistic Epileptiform Regression, and Disintegrative Epileptiform Disorder

	Aphasia	Social	Cognitive	Abnormal EEG	Prior Normal Development
Acquired epileptiform aphasia (LKS)	Yes	No	No	Yes	Yes
Autistic regression	Yes	Yes	No	No	Yes or no
Autistic epileptiform regression	Yes	Yes	No	Yes	Yes or no
Disintegrative disorder	Yes	Yes	Yes	No	Yes until 2 yrs
Disintegrative epileptiform disorder	Yes	Yes	Yes	Yes	Yes until 2 yrs

EEG = electroencephalogram.

and write. Older children with this disorder often have greater expressive (including writing) than receptive language deficits.[16–19] Except for the language impairment, children with LKS are intellectually normal, as measured (for example) by nonverbal reasoning tests. Sometimes they have behavioral difficulties such as hyperactivity or attention deficit, presumably as a secondary response to their communication impairment. Rarely, psychosis has been described.

Clinical Features of Landau-Kleffner Syndrome Variants

Although classic LKS is rare, putative clinical variants are relatively common.[1,3,20,21] Tuchman[21] has proposed a schema that takes into account cognitive, language, social, and behavioral deficits, age of onset, and the EEG and epilepsy status. LKS is contrasted with autistic epileptiform regression (AER) and disintegrative epileptiform disorder (DED) (Table 8-1).

Autistic Epileptiform Regression

AER is the most common of the putative LKS variants. The clinical picture differs from LKS in several important respects. Unlike children with LKS, children with AER show impairments in social relatedness, both verbal and nonverbal communication skills, and symbolic play. They also demonstrate a restricted, ritualized pattern of interests and activities. Motor, vocal, or visual stereotypies may be observed. Other behavioral disturbances may include distractibility, hyperactivity, tantrums, and difficulty in making the transition from one activity to another. Cognitive impairment is relatively common in children with autistic spectrum disorders who regress.[22]

Autistic regression tends to occur between 12 and 36 months, generally earlier than LKS. At this age, the normality of prior development is difficult to ascertain. Approximately one-fourth of autistic children ultimately experience seizures. Epileptiform EEGs are even more common. In Tuchman and Rapin's[22] cohort of almost 600 children with autistic spectrum disorders, nearly one-third experienced a regression. Of those who regressed, one-third had epilepsy and one-half had epileptiform EEGs. Of those who regressed but did not have epilepsy, one-fifth had epileptiform EEGs. Epileptiform EEGs were thus more common in those who regressed and had epilepsy (60% with epilepsy, 15% without). An epileptiform EEG with or without concurrent epilepsy was more likely to be associated with regression (15% vs. 5%). Thus, almost one-third of this cohort had AER. A number of investigators have reported on individual patients with AER who have responded variably to treatment with antiepileptic drugs.[23–28] Some patients responding to surgical management (multiple subpial transections) have also been reported (see later).

Disintegrative Epileptiform Disorder

DD involves an even broader range of deficits than are seen in the autistic spectrum disorders. By definition, DD begins after age 2 years and before age 10 years in a previously normal child. Some DD children have seizures or epileptiform EEGs—hence the designation *DED*. Behavioral disturbances may include attention deficit, hyperactivity, impulsiveness, aggression, mood changes, disinhibition, and psychosis.[27] Cognitive deterioration tends to be more severe than in the autistic spectrum disorders. Comparing 18 DED children with 51 and 145 autistic children with and without speech loss, respectively, Kurita and Michiko[29] found that by age 7 years (approximately 4 years after regression), children with DED showed significantly more severe mental retardation than did those with autism. Autistic symptomatology among the groups was similar. Treatment responses in DED are reported on a case study basis.[27,30,31] Although not designated as such, patients with DED often are included in series of patients with continuous spikes and waves during slow sleep (CSWS).[32–34]

Other Clinical Variants

A single case study documents significant improvement during valproate treatment in a child with severe learning disabilities and an extremely epileptiform EEG without clinical seizures.[35] Another single case study documents a child with a prolonged isolated deficit of prosody in association with an epileptiform EEG.[36]

Diagnosis of Landau-Kleffner Syndrome and Its Variants

Features of Epilepsy

Approximately 75% of patients with classic LKS experience seizures, which can predate or postdate the onset of aphasia; the rest, by definition, have an epileptiform EEG. Virtually all seizure types have been reported in association with LKS. Generally, seizures are easily controlled, although seizures may be intractable in rare cases and require surgery.[37–39] No specific differences have been reported for the variants.

Electroencephalographic Features

Other than the electroencephalographic variants described later, the abnormalities seen on the EEG in LKS and its putative clinical variants are, for the most part, nonspecific and consist of a variety of generalized or focal (approximately 10%) epileptiform discharge patterns. Centrotemporal spikes (considered apart from the possible Rolandic variant) probably are the most common morphologic pattern found in LKS. Centrotemporal spikes also are seen commonly in children with autistic spectrum disorders and AER.[22] Electroencephalographic abnormalities generally increase during sleep. (The relationship between LKS and CSWS is discussed later.) Overnight EEG recording definitely picks up more abnormalities than does a routine sleep recording. Prolonged recording (over several nights) may be necessary to document epileptiform discharge, including CSWS.[40–42] Amitriptyline activation may increase the likelihood of observing these discharges in some cases.[43]

Recent studies suggest that magnetoencephalography (MEG) may represent yet another level of sensitivity for diagnosis. MEG identified epileptiform activity in 41 of 50 (82%) patients with AER, whereas only 34 of 50 (68%) had epileptiform activity as revealed on the EEG.[44] Contrasting LKS patients with AER patients, Lewine et al.[44] documented during stage III sleep primary epileptiform activity only in the perisylvian region in the LKS patients (bilaterally in five of six). By contrast, in addition to the intrasylvian cortex, 75% of the AER patients showed extrasylvian zones of independent epileptiform activity. MEG has also been used in classic LKS patients to localize the primary epileptogenic region to intrasylvian cortex prior to multiple subpial transection (MST) surgery.[45]

In addition to the clinically defined variants already discussed, a number of electroencephalographic variants exist in the LKS spectrum.

Ictal Aphasia

LKS must be distinguished from prolonged ictal aphasia and prolonged postictal aphasia secondary to frequent seizures, each with associated ictal aphasia. For example, the patient of Jambaque et al.[46] who had had a history of transient ictal aphasia developed a prolonged (6-month) postictal transcortical motor aphasia when he began to experience several seizures per night.

Seizure control (with antiepileptic medications) resulted in recovery from the aphasia as well as virtual normalization of regional cerebral blood flow, which had exhibited diffusely depressed left hemisphere metabolism during the period of aphasia.

Patients with Rolandic status epilepticus and associated oromotor symptoms have been reported.[47–51] A few patients with documented structural pathology, intractable epilepsy, and severe focal epileptiform activity have shown clear improvement in language that correlated with improved seizure control and decreased epileptiform activity after hemispherectomy.[38,39]

Continuous Spikes and Waves during Slow Sleep

In most patients with LKS, epileptiform abnormalities increase during sleep. CSWS is relatively frequent. For example, in a series of 17 LKS patients reported by da Silva et al.,[52] 7 patients had CSWS, as did almost half of the patients with LKS or one of its variants seen by Veggiotti et al.[34] Not all patients with CSWS, however, have LKS[53]: The electroencephalographic pattern of CSWS is associated with different clinical phenotypes.[34,54,55] CSWS was first described by Patry et al.[56] and was called *electrical status epilepticus during sleep.* This term has been supplanted by CSWS because patients with electrical status epilepticus during sleep do not necessarily have epilepsy and because the presence of clinical status epilepticus cannot be demonstrated during sleep.

Some investigators consider CSWS to be a syndrome in its own right, one that lies along the same spectrum as LKS and shares a similar pathophysiology.[57,58] Hence, Bureau[59] has reviewed and mapped its natural history. In terms of early electroclinical features, the first seizure generally occurs between ages 1 and 10 years, with a peak at 4–5 years. In approximately half the patients, this is a hemiclonic seizure that frequently is prolonged. Other seizure types are seen and occur mostly during sleep. The initial EEG reveals a multifocal spike and slow wave pattern or a diffuse spike and wave pattern. The EEG abnormalities worsen during sleep. In nearly two-thirds of patients, development is normal. The other one-third experience delays predominantly in language.

In nearly one-third, brain abnormalities can be demonstrated neuroradiologically. During the CSWS period, seizure characteristics change; atypical absence seizures (including status epilepticus) and atonic seizures occur. A diffuse spike and wave pattern appears on the awake EEG; CSWS appears during non–rapid eye movement sleep (present for >85% of the time) and may continue for months to years. The exact age of onset and duration of CSWS can be difficult to determine clinically, as knowledge of these features depends on the timing of electroencephalography. The average age for diagnosis is 8 years. Atypical absence seizures (including status epilepticus) and atonic seizures predominate, and epilepsy generally is severe. Tonic seizures have never been reported. Previously normal children deteriorate (leading to a diagnosis of LKS, AER, or DED, depending on the clinical features), and previously delayed children regress. In the third phase of CSWS syndrome, epilepsy remits and CSWS disappears. However, at least half of the patients remain significantly impaired. The duration of CSWS on the EEG appears to affect prognosis.

In a comprehensive literature review of 209 patients with CSWS on EEG, Rousselle and Revol[53] differentiated three main clinical groups based on neuropsychological profile during the period when CSWS was present. This profile correlated directly with the duration of CSWS and the site of the main epileptogenic focus. The largest group of children with CSWS experienced global neuropsychological deterioration rather than language deterioration alone; the main epileptiform focus was frontal. A second group included children with language deterioration (primarily LKS) and CSWS; epileptiform activity was found primarily in the temporal region. A third group showed no neuropsychological deterioration; CSWS was found to be of shorter duration, and the main focus on EEG had a Rolandic topography.

Centrotemporal (Rolandic) Spikes

Centrotemporal spikes probably are the most common specific epileptiform abnormalities found in classic LKS and in children with autistic spectrum disorders with and without regression.[22] Extreme cases of Rolandic epilepsy (which usually is a benign, age-dependent form of epilepsy) with prolonged deficits including drooling, oromotor dyspraxia, dysphagia, isolated deterioration of speech, and a complete anterior opercular syndrome have been described.[47,49,51,60–63] Deonna et al.[48] have suggested that an oromotor deficit may be the initial symptom in Rolandic epilepsy, preceding the appearance of overt seizures and paralleling the appearance of verbal auditory agnosia in classic LKS prior to the onset of seizures. Deonna speculates that the variations in clinical symptoms are related to the main site, local extension, and bilaterality of the epileptic foci, rather than to a basic difference in pathophysiology (between classical LKS and its variants). The patients reported with centrotemporal spikes and classic LKS do not appear to have greater expressive deficits, however. Deonna[48] hypothesizes that oromotor difficulties interfere either with simple voluntary oromotor functions or with complex movements including speech production, depending on the location and spread of the epileptic focus around the perisylvian region. Thus, nonlinguistic deficits such as intermittent drooling, oromotor apraxia, or dysfluency, as well as linguistic deficits involving phonologic production, all can occur. The most severe deficit produced in this context is a complete anterior operculum syndrome. The reported rapidity of onset, duration, progression, and recovery of the deficit varies widely. Such differences could reflect the degree of epileptic activity. Like LKS, rapid improvement with antiepileptic medication occurs in some cases, and the paroxysmal EEG activity (which usually is bilateral) and the clinical deficit sometimes run in parallel.

Occipital Spikes or Spikes and Waves

Occipital spikes or spikes and waves generally present as an age-dependent, EEG-defined benign focal epilepsy[64] manifesting in the younger child as autonomic symptoms followed by brief or prolonged partial motor seizures and, in the older child, as visual symptoms and headache. Occipital spikes are not always benign, however. Nass et al.[65] reported 7 (5 from a consecutive series of 42) young children presenting clinically with autism or autistic regression and possible or definite seizures who had solely or predominantly occipital spikes

or spikes and waves on the EEG. These children all exhibited severe language and behavior deficits. Tenembaum et al.[66] reported two teenagers who had carried the diagnosis of benign occipital epilepsy but who deteriorated cognitively and behaviorally when they developed CSWS and persistent occipital paroxysms that extended anteriorly. Beaumanoir[67] suggests that the semiology of seizures with occipital spikes or spikes and waves depends on the child's age, the maturation of the occipital cortex, and the cortex's connection with other structures. Occipital maximal spikes can have fields extending to posterior temporal and parietal regions, both of which are involved in language acquisition and cognitive development. This effect could be most prominent in the young child, who is in the process of acquiring language.

Relationship between Epilepsy and Epileptiform Electroencephalographic Abnormalities and Language and Cognitive Disorders

The relationship between epilepsy and epileptiform EEG abnormalities and language and cognitive deficits in classic LKS continues to be debated. Some investigators consider the epileptiform abnormalities an epiphenomenon reflecting underlying brain pathology rather than the direct cause of the language, cognitive, or behavioral disorder.[4,68,69] They cite the lack of clear correlation between the status of the epilepsy and EEG abnormalities and the status of the language, cognitive, or behavioral disorder as well as the lack of consistent response to medication (see later). Although structural lesions are uncommon,[70] metabolic abnormalities consistent with primary dysfunctional cortex are described more frequently as technology advances (see later).

Other researchers believe that the language, cognitive, or behavioral disorder is a direct consequence of the epileptiform activity.[3,20,71–73] In essence, LKS and its variants are a form of epileptic encephalopathy. Studies documenting transient cognitive impairment during epileptiform discharge lend support to this position.[24,74–78] By way of contrast, however, electrical status epilepticus can occur without cognitive correlates.[79] The anatomic specificity between the particular clinical deficit and the focus of epileptiform abnormalities also supports this position: That is, LKS and its variants each seem to reflect different areas of maximal epileptiform activity. The intrasylvian cortex appears to be the pacemaker of epileptiform discharges in classic LKS.[44,45] By contrast, AER has both sylvian and extrasylvian pacemakers.[44] Occipital spike fields extend to posterior temporal and parietal areas. Centrotemporal spikes interfere with simple oromotor functions or complex movements including speech production.

Consistent with the argument that the epileptiform activity per se has a specific, negative effect on language processing, Seri et al.[80] found that left hemisphere spike–triggered auditory evoked responses are associated with a greater reduction in amplitude and an increase in latency of responses than are right-triggered auditory evoked responses. Morrell's group[81] demonstrated that intracarotid amobarbital (Amytal) injection into the hemisphere having the primary epileptiform focus causes the disappearance of discharges over both hemispheres, whereas contralateral Amytal injection suppresses spikes on only the injected side. Patients with significant focal seizure diathesis have shown dramatic improvement of language and cognitive function when hemispherectomy eliminates seizures.[38,39]

Theoretically, epileptiform activity could disrupt the development of language and cognitive function during a critical period.[71] Neurons and axons affected by abnormal electrical discharge may not develop or perform normally.[8] Epileptiform activity could interfere with the establishment of normal cortical circuitry.[7,11,67,71,82–85] Synaptic contacts that should have degenerated by apoptosis could instead be strengthened.[2] From a clinical perspective, the time of onset of epileptiform discharges may further obscure the boundaries of LKS and its variants. For example, LKS might start early in the course of language development, making difficult the distinction between it and a developmental language disorder.[86] Verbal auditory agnosia is a well-described developmental language disorder subtype.[87] Epileptiform activity is relatively frequent in developmental language disorder cohorts.[88–91]

Parallel between the Presence and Severity of Epilepsy and Electroencephalographic Abnormalities and the Aphasic Disorder

Controversy also exists as to the extent of the parallel between the presence and severity of the epilepsy and EEG abnormalities and the aphasic disorder. Such a parallel must be distinguished from ictal aphasia (see earlier). Many investigators have demonstrated a parallel between the status of the aphasia and the EEG.[37] Several investigators have noted that children who received early treatment with anticonvulsants demonstrated a remarkable clinical improvement paralleled by normalization of their EEG.[92–94] De Volder et al.[95] published a report of a patient with an arachnoid cyst whose language and EEG improved after the cyst was shunted. The status of CSWS correlates with aphasia in some cases. Because the disappearance of CSWS may harbinger an improvement in aphasia (although not coinciding with it), some investigators suggest that long-term expectant treatment with anticonvulsants or corticosteroids (or both) is worthwhile if the EEG is improved significantly by this treatment.[96] By contrast, most long-term prospective case studies generally fail to demonstrate a parallel between the EEG and clinical status.[97–104]

Etiology

LKS probably is not a single entity. In most instances, the cause is unknown. The relative rarity of a focal etiology may explain why the outcome of this disorder generally is much poorer than that of other acquired aphasias of childhood (see van Hout[105] for a recent review). Some cases of LKS may be a form of chronic focal encephalitis in the tradition of Rasmussen's encephalitis. However, only one of the few pathologic specimens is consistent with encephalitis, and the case itself had atypical features.[106] A few patients with documented structural lesions, including tumors and cysts, have been reported.[37,73,95,107–110] Treatment of these lesions has been associated with temporally related improvement of the aphasia. For example, placement of a temporal lobe arachnoid cyst peritoneal shunt resulted in significant metabolic improvement (as evidenced by single-photon emission computed tomography [SPECT]) in all cortical regions, especially the inferior frontal gyrus and the perisylvian area, but with residual deficit in the left superior temporal gyrus. The patient showed a pronounced increase in word fluency and some progress in verbal auditory comprehension.[95] Tumor and cyst removal also has coincided with improved language function. In one patient with a unilateral intrasylvian pacemaker, a small transection of a sylvian pacemaker resulted in cessation of all epileptogenic activity. Her auditory agnosia improved, although her speech did not.[45]

Increasingly sophisticated electrophysiologic data suggest a focal origin for the epileptiform activity in some patients. MEG documents that the intrasylvian cortex is the pacemaker of the epileptiform discharge in LKS.[44,45] In some patients with a unilateral pacemaker, spread to the contralateral hemisphere is rapid.

Metabolic imaging studies (see more details later) support a focal origin in a number of cases, even when the EEG abnormalities appear generalized. For example, Park et al.[111] reported on an 11-year-old boy with partial seizures and cognitive and behavioral regression whose sleep EEG showed CSWS and whose EEG during wakefulness showed epileptiform discharges over the right parietal region, suggesting that the CSWS were a manifestation of secondary bilateral synchrony. Bilateral suppression of the spike and wave activity was observed after right-sided intracarotid Amytal injection, and fluorodeoxyglucose–positron emission tomographic (FDG-PET) imaging revealed hypermetabolism in the right superior temporoparietal region.

Relationship between Epileptiform Abnormalities and Metabolic Abnormalities

Generally, the location of metabolic abnormalities and epileptiform abnormalities in LKS and its variants are correlated. Abnormalities appear predominantly in the temporal lobes.[30,95,112–115] Chez et al.[116] found that the temporal lobe EEG abnormalities corresponded with the side of the SPECT abnormalities. In the cohort of da Silva et al.,[52] the area of hypometabolism, although more extensive, corresponded with the location of epileptiform discharges in 11 of 17 children. A patient of Cole et al.[37] who had intractable epilepsy was seen to have temporal hypometabolism or hypermetabolism, depending on his seizure status at imaging. de Volder et al.[95] found focal hypometabolism in the area of a left temporal lobe arachnoid cyst, which decreased after shunting. In the largest series to date, 2 of 17 patients had focal hypermetabolism in

the left temporal cortex, one of whom also showed right temporal cortex hypometabolism (FDG-PET). The remaining 15 patients showed bilateral temporal (middle temporal gyrus) hypometabolism.[52] MEG reveals left perisylvian epileptiform abnormalities in classic LKS and left perisylvian as well as additional nonsylvian zones of independent epileptiform activity in AER.[44] In another series, brain SPECT imaging demonstrated abnormal perfusion in the left temporal lobe in all five patients aged 3 and 9 years.[112]

The metabolic abnormalities in LKS children with CSWS tend to be more extensive than in those without CSWS. Metabolic abnormalities tend to increase in sleep. During metabolic imaging (FDG-PET), patients with CSWS had bitemporal and bifrontal hypometabolism.[52] Two patients with CSWS were discussed by Rintahaka et al.[117] In the first patient, the awake interictal PET study revealed moderate hypometabolism in the thalamus and frontal and temporal cortex and mild hypometabolism in the parietal and anterior cingulate cortex bilaterally. The occipital cortex was severely hypometabolic bilaterally. In a repeat PET study performed during sleep in which CSWS was present, the only difference noted (as compared with the awake study) was a marked bilateral increase in temporal cortex metabolism. The awake interictal PET in the second child was normal, except for mildly increased relative glucose metabolism in the left inferior temporal cortex. The sleep PET study with CSWS in this child showed hypermetabolism in both temporal lobes, although the finding was more pronounced and had a wider distribution in the left temporal cortex. In normal subjects, PET studies performed during awake and sleep states have not revealed such differences. Whether the temporal lobes are involved in the generation of CSWS remains to be confirmed in a larger group of patients.

Maquet et al.[30] culled four basic metabolic characteristics of LKS via FDG-PET studies:

1. The metabolism of the cortical mantle was higher than in the subcortical structures, especially in the thalamic nuclei. This metabolic pattern is characteristic of an immature brain.
2. The metabolic abnormalities involved focal or regional areas of the cortex. This finding agrees well with recent neurophysiologic data

suggesting a focal origin of the spike and wave discharges.

3. The metabolic disturbances predominantly involved associative cortices. The pattern of neuropsychological deterioration agrees well with the topography of the disturbances of cortical glucose metabolism.

4. The thalamic nuclei remained symmetric despite significant cortical asymmetries, suggesting either that corticothalamic neurons do not participate in the generation of spike and wave discharges or that they are inhibited by pathologic mechanisms.

Maquet et al.[30] hypothesized that the acquired deterioration of cognitive function with CSWS is caused by an alteration of the maturation of one or several associative cortices, primarily involving local interneurons and corticocortical associative neurons. An adrenocorticotropic hormone (ACTH) responder with LKS variant had bitemporal and left frontal pathology on SPECT scan and steady-state auditory evoked potentials.[118]

Treatment

Treatment for both LKS and AER, when instituted, has generally consisted of traditional antiepileptic drugs and steroids or ACTH, immunoglobulins,[119,120] and calcium channel blockers. ACTH probably has the greatest efficacy, although detailed prospective outcome studies are lacking.[28,94,112] Some have suggested that AER and infantile spasms lie on the same spectrum, given their phenotypic overlap. If this is true, the neuroendocrine underpinnings of infantile spasms[121] provide the backdrop for anticipating the efficacy of ACTH and, possibly, steroids. Several investigators suggest that early treatment is extremely important.[92,94]

Surgical treatment has also been tried recently. MEG provides useful presurgical information about the cortical spike dynamics in LKS patients.[45] Morrell et al.[81] first used MSTs in 14 children with aphasia, seizures, and markedly abnormal EEGs. Of the 14 patients, 7 recovered age-appropriate speech, are in regular classes in school, and no longer require speech therapy. Four of the 14 showed marked improvement, are

speaking and understanding verbal instruction, but still are receiving speech therapy. Thus, three-fourths of the patients, none of whom had used language to communicate for at least 2 years, improved significantly after MSTs.

Sawhney et al.[122] reported on the efficacy of MSTs in 18 patients with medically intractable epilepsy, 3 of whom had LKS. Their ages ranged from 6 to 47 years (mean, 15 years), and the duration of epilepsy ranged from 0.33 to 42.00 years (mean, 8.60 years). Preoperative magnetic resonance imaging showed focal abnormalities in eight cases. In addition, MSTs were performed in 12 patients, none of whom had LKS. MSTs were carried out mainly in the precentral and postcentral regions. Eighteen patients have been followed up for 1 – 5 years, and three have been followed up for 10 months. The three patients with LKS were mute before their operations and have exhibited substantial recovery of speech. Among the other 18 patients, 11 showed a worthwhile decrease in seizure frequency.

Gillberg et al.[123] also reported positive responses to surgery in two preadolescent autistic boys with tuberous sclerosis. One had a corticectomy in addition to the MSTs. Neville et al.[124] reported two preschoolers with autistic regression and intractable epilepsy. One improved after left temporal lobectomy and the other after MSTs.

In the series by Grote et al.,[125] 11 of 14 children demonstrated significant postoperative improvement on measures of receptive or expressive vocabulary. Results indicate that early diagnosis and treatment optimize outcome and that gains in language function are most likely to be seen years, rather than months, postoperatively. The best predictor of postoperative improvements in language function was the length of time since surgery.[125]

In one of the patients of Rintahaka et al.,[117] CSWS disappeared and language function improved after MST surgery. Nass et al.[126] reported 7 patients (derived from a cohort of 36 children who had been referred originally for video EEG monitoring) with refractory epilepsy and AER who responded to varying degrees to MSTs after medical management had failed. Surgical treatment variously involved MSTs of the left neocortex in temporal, parietal, and frontal regions, often including regions within the classic perisylvian language areas. One patient also had a left temporal lobectomy. In all seven patients, seizure control or electroencephalographic features (or both) improved after MSTs. Language, social, and overall behavior improved to a moderate degree, although most improvements were temporary.

In another cohort, 12 of 18 AER patients showed improved behavior or language ability postoperatively, despite the multifocal nature of the epileptiform activity on MEG.[44]

Outcome

Outcome in LKS is generally poor. Fewer than one-third of the original LKS patients ultimately had normal language ability, one-third had mild to moderately impaired language ability, and one-third had severely impaired language ability.[127] Dugas et al.[40] recently reviewed the literature on the follow-up of 55 LKS patients (at least 14 years of age at the time of follow-up and followed for at least 7 years) with and without CSWS and found a similar distribution, with perhaps a slightly smaller percentage of patients experiencing a good outcome. Another follow-up study conducted on a group of 12 patients (75% of whom had exhibited some language disturbance prior to acquired epileptic aphasia) followed for 2–15 years (mean, 8 years) found that only 3 achieved normal language ability, even though the EEG normalized in 9 patients.[102] During very long-term follow-up (20–30 years), all four patients studied showed marked recovery in language without any intellectual handicap but with some disability in spoken language, auditory verbal perception, and a discrepancy between Wechsler Verbal and Performance IQ scores.[13]

Case studies provide important information about particular linguistic features and linguistic recovery patterns. The features of verbal auditory agnosia have been examined in some detail, particularly in longitudinal studies. For example, a case study describes a 27-year-old woman with chronic auditory agnosia after LKS was diagnosed at age 4.5 years. Manually coded (signed) English allowed for good communication. Comprehension and production of spoken language remain severely compromised. Disruptions in auditory processing were observed in tests of pitch and duration, suggesting that her disorder is not specific to language. Linguistic analysis of signed, spoken, and written English indicated that her language system is intact but compromised because of impoverished input during the critical period for acquisition of spoken phonology. Specifically, although her sign language phonology is intact, her spoken language phonology is markedly impaired. Deprivation of auditory input during a period critical for the development of a phonological grammar and auditory-verbal short-term memory may limit lexical and syntactic development.[97]

Another patient followed from age 6 to 15 years had a fluctuating clinical course with improvement and worsening of aphasia and epilepsy. At the end of the follow-up period, the boy was seizure-free and had moderately disturbed language production and comprehension. The results of linguistic evaluation suggest that the aphasic disturbance was related to a deficiency in phonologic decoding, which leads to phonologic, morphosyntactic, and lexical disturbances. A temporal relationship between the electroclinical picture and the aphasia was observed; persisting improvement in linguistic performances took place only after disappearance of the seizures and the epileptiform abnormalities during sleep.[104] In addition, intraoperative evoked potential recording (during MST) documented the ability to distinguish between different consonant-vowel syllables (despite verbal-auditory agnosia).[12]

Clinical or EEG features may affect outcome. Younger patients fare less well than do older patients,[128] and those with CSWS on electroencephalography may have a poorer outcome. In only 2 (18.2%) of 11 patients with CSWS (mean follow-up, 9 years) was language recovery complete; 7 (63.6%) of these patients were mentally retarded.[100] Those with good language outcome show evidence of "crowding"[87,127,129]: recovery of language at the expense of ordinarily right hemisphere–mediated functions. This pattern suggests that reorganization with transfer of language to the right hemisphere underlies recovery. This subgroup with seemingly focal pathology may be distinguishable from other patients with LKS and its variants.

Conclusion

In sum, LKS is an uncommon and as yet incompletely understood disorder. Its putative variants, particularly AER, are considerably more common. Whether LKS exists along a spectrum of language-behavior encephalopathies that share a common etiology or represents a biologically distinct syndrome remains unclear. In either case, multiple factors likely interact to produce the range of language, behavioral, and cognitive deficits seen. Among the most important may be the location of the underlying brain abnormalities, epileptic focus or foci, the precise language disturbance, and the timing of the regression. The notion that LKS and its variants reflect different areas of maximal epileptiform activity merits further investigation. Future electrophysiologic and metabolic studies will improve our understanding of the etiology of these disorders.

References

1. Landau W. Landau-Kleffner syndrome: an eponymic badge of ignorance. Arch Neurol 1992;49:353.
2. Brown S. Epileptic Dementia: Intellectual Deterioration as a Consequence of Epileptic Seizures. In M Sillanpaa (ed), Epilepsy and Mental Retardation. Philadelphia: Wrightson Biomedical Publishing, 1999; 120–131.
3. Deonna T. Cognitive and behavioral manifestations of epilepsy in children. Semin Neurol 1995;2:254–260.
4. Rapin I. Autistic regression and disintegrative disorder: how important the role of epilepsy? Semin Pediatr Neurol 1995;2(4):278–285.
5. Landau WM, Kleffner FR. Syndrome of acquired aphasia with convulsive disorder in children. Neurology 1957;7(8):523–530.
6. Appleton RE. The Landau-Kleffner syndrome. Arch Dis Child 1995;72(5):386–387.
7. Gascon G, Victor D, Lombroso CT. Language disorders, convulsive disorder, and electroencephalographic abnormalities. Acquired syndrome in children. Arch Neurol 1973;28(3):156–162.
8. Gordon N. The Landau-Kleffner syndrome: increased understanding. Brain Dev 1997;19(5):311–316.
9. Mouridsen SE. The Landau-Kleffner syndrome: a review. Eur Child Adolesc Psychiatry 1995;4(4):223–228.
10. Paquier P, van Dongen H, Loonen C. The LKS or "acquired aphasia with convulsive disorder." Arch Neurol 1992;49:354–359.
11. Shoumaker RD, Bennett DR, Bray PF, Curliss R. Clinical and EEG manifestations of an unusual aphasic syndrome in children. Neurology 1974;24:10–16.
12. Boyd S, Rivera-Gaxiola M, Towell A, et al. Discrimination of speech sounds in LKS. Neuropediatrics 1996;27:1–5.
13. Kaga M. Language disorders in Landau-Kleffner syndrome. J Child Neurol 1999;14(2):118–122.
14. Korkman M, Granstrom M, Appelqvist K, Liukkonen E. Neuropsychological characteristics of five children with the Landau-Kleffner syndrome: dissociation of auditory and phonological discrimination. J Int Neuropsychol Soc 1998;4(6):566–575.
15. Rapin I, Mattis S, Rowan A, Golden G. Verbal auditory agnosia. Dev Med Child Neurol 1977;19(2):197–207.
16. Deonna T, Davidoff V, Roulet E. Isolated disturbance of written language acquisition as an initial symptom of epileptic aphasia in a 7-year-old child: a 3-year follow-up study. Aphasiology 1993;7(5):441–448.
17. Gerard CL, Dugas M, Valdois S, et al. Landau-Kleffner syndrome diagnosed after age nine: another Landau-Kleffner syndrome. Aphasiology 1993;7(5):463–473.
18. Marien P, Saerens J, Verslegers W, et al. Some controversies about type and nature of aphasic symptomatology in Landau-Kleffner's syndrome: a case study. Acta Neurol Belg 1993;93:183–203.
19. Papagno C, Basso A. Impairment of written language and mathematical skills in a case of Landau-Kleffner syndrome: acquired childhood aphasia. Aphasiology [Special Issue] 1993;7(5):451–461.
20. Deonna TW. Acquired epileptiform aphasia in children (Landau-Kleffner syndrome). J Clin Neurophysiol 1991;8:288–298.
21. Tuchman RF. Acquired epileptiform aphasia. Semin Pediatr Neurol 1997;4(2):93–101.
22. Tuchman R, Rapin I. Regression in pervasive developmental disorders: seizures and epileptiform electroencephalogram correlates. Pediatrics 1997;99:560–566.
23. Deonna T, Ziegler AL, Moura-Serra J, Innocenti G. Autistic regression in relation to limbic pathology and epilepsy: report of two cases. Dev Med Child Neurol 1993;35:166–175.
24. Deonna T, Ziegler A, Maeder M, et al. Reversible behavioural autistic-like regression: a manifestation of a special (new?) epileptic syndrome in a 28-month-old child. A 2-year longitudinal study. Neurocase 1995; 1:91–99.
25. Gillberg C, Schaumann H. Epilepsy presenting as infantile autism. Neuropediatrics 1983;14:406–412.
26. Nass R, Petrucha D. Epileptic aphasia: a pervasive developmental disorder variant. J Child Neurol 1990; 5:327–328.
27. Roulet Perez E, Davidoff V, Despland PA, Deonna T. Mental and behavioural deterioration of children with

epilepsy and CSWS: acquired epileptic frontal syndrome. Dev Med Child Neurol 1993;35(8):661–674.

28. Stefanatos GA. Case study: corticosteroid treatment of language regression in pervasive developmental disorder. J Am Acad Child Adolesc Psychiatry 1996;35(4): 404–405.

29. Kurita H, Michiko K. A comparative study of development and symptoms among disintegrative psychosis and infantile autism with and without speech loss. J Autism Dev Disord 1992;22(2):175–188.

30. Maquet P, Hirsch E, Metz-Lutz MN. Regional cerebral glucose utilization in children with deterioration of one or more cognitive functions and CSWS. Brain 1995;118:1497–1520.

31. Roulet E, Deonna T, Gaillard F, et al. Acquired aphasia, dementia, and behavior disorder with epilepsy and continuous spike and waves during sleep in a child. Epilepsia 1991;32(4):495–503.

32. Beaumanoir A, Bureau M, Deonna T, et al (eds). Continuous Spikes and Waves During Slow Sleep. London: John Libbey Eurotext, 1995.

33. Perez E. Syndromes of acquired epileptic aphasia and epilepsy with continuous spike and wave during sleep: models for prolonged cognitive impairment of epileptic origin. Semin Neurol 1995;2:261–268.

34. Veggiotti P, Beccaria F, Guerrini R, et al. Continuous spike and wave activity during slow wave sleep: syndrome or EEG pattern? Epilepsia 1999;40:1593–1601.

35. Gordon K, Bawden H, Camfield P, et al. Valproate treatment of LD and severely epileptiform EEG without clinical seizures. J Child Neurol 1996;11:41–43.

36. Deonna T, Chevrie C, Hornung E. Childhood epileptic speech disorder: prolonged isolated deficit of prosody features. Dev Med Child Neurol 1987;29:100–105.

37. Cole AJ, Andermann F, Taylor A, et al. The Landau-Kleffner syndrome of acquired epileptic aphasia: unusual clinical outcome, surgical experience and absence of encephalitis. Neurology 1988;38:31–38.

38. Rosenblatt B, Vernet O, Montes J, Andermann F. Continuous unilateral epileptiform activity and language delay: effect of functional hemispherectomy on language acquisition. Epilepsia 1998;39:787–792.

39. Vargha-Khadem F, Carr LJ, Isaacs E, et al. Onset of speech after left hemispherectomy in a nine-year-old boy. Brain 1997;120[Pt 1]:159–182.

40. Dugas M, Franc S, Gerard CL, Lecendreux M. Evolution of Acquired Epileptic Aphasia With or Without CSWS. In A Beaumanoir, M Bureau, T Deonna, et al (eds), Continuous Spikes and Waves During Slow Sleep. London: John Libbey Eurotext, 1995;47–55.

41. Nass R, Gross A, Devinsky O. Patterns of electroencephalographic abnormalities in autistic spectrum disorders: correlation with clinical status and outcome. Ann Neurol 1998;44(3):578–579.

42. Tuchman R, Jayakar P, Yaylali I, Villalobos R. Seizures and EEG findings in children with autistic spectrum disorder. CNS Spectrums 1998;3:61–65.

43. Kollros PR, Stefanatos G, Rabinovich H, Streletz LJ. Sleep and amitriptyline enhance the sensitivity of electroencephalograms in children with a pervasive developmental disorder and language regression. Ann Neurol 1996;40(2):303–304.

44. Lewine JD, Andrews R, Chez M, et al. Magnetoencephalographic patterns of epileptiform activity in children with regressive autistic spectrum disorders. Pediatrics 1999;104(3):405–418.

45. Paetau R, Granstrom ML, Blomstedt G, et al. Magnetoencephalography in presurgical evaluation of children with the Landau-Kleffner syndrome. Epilepsia 1999;40(3):326–335.

46. Jambaque I, Chiron C, Kaminska A, et al. Transient motor aphasia and recurrent partial seizures in a child: language recovery upon seizure control. J Child Neurol 1998;13(6):296–300.

47. Colamaria V, Sgro V, Caraballo R, et al. Status epilepticus in BRE manifesting as an anterior opercular syndrome. Epilepsia 1991;32:329–334.

48. Deonna TW, Roulet E, Fontan D, Marcoz JP. Speech and oro-motor deficits of epileptic origin in benign partial epilepsy of childhood with Rolandic spikes (BPERS). Relationship to the acquired aphasia–epilepsy syndrome. Neuropediatrics 1993;24(2):83–87.

49. Fejerman N, Di Blasi AM. Status epilepticus of benign partial epilepsies in children: report of 2 cases. Epilepsia 1987;28:351–355.

50. Fusco L, Vigevano F. Reversible operculum syndrome caused by progressive epilepsia partialis continua in a child with left hemimegalencephaly. J Neurol Neurosurg Psychiatry 1991;54:556–558.

51. Shafrir Y, Prensky AL. Acquired epileptiform opercular syndrome: a second case report, review of the literature, and comparison to the Landau-Kleffner syndrome. Epilepsia 1995;36(10):1050–1057.

52. da Silva EA, Chugani DC, Muzik O, Chugani HT. Landau-Kleffner syndrome: metabolic abnormalities in temporal lobe are a common feature. J Child Neurol 1997;12(8):489–495.

53. Rousselle C, Revol M. Relations Between Cognitive Functions and Continuous Spikes and Waves During Slow Sleep. In A Beaumanoir, M Bureau, T Deonna, et al. (eds), Continuous Spikes and Waves During Slow Sleep. London: John Libbey Eurotext, 1995; 123–133.

54. Benton P, Guerrini R. What differentiates Landau-Kleffner syndrome from the syndrome of continuous spikes and waves during slow sleep? Arch Neurol 1993;50:1008–1009.

55. Benton P, Maton B, Ogihara M, et al. Continuous focal spikes during REM sleep in a case of acquired aphasia (Landau-Kleffner syndrome). Sleep 1992;15(5):454–460.

56. Patry G, Lyagoubi S, Tassinari C. Subclinical status epilepticus induced by sleep in children. Arch Neurol 1971;24:242–252.

57. Hirsch E, Marescaux C, Maquet P. Landau-Kleffner syndrome: a clinical case and EEG study of five cases. Epilepsia 1990;31:756–767.

58. Marescaux C, Kiesmann M, Hirsch E. Are the LKS and CSWS one and the same? Epilepsia 1989;30:693–696.

59. Bureau M. CSWS: Definition of the Syndrome. In A Beaumanoir, M Bureau, T Deonna, et al. (eds), Continuous Spikes and Waves During Slow Sleep. London: John Libbey Eurotext, 1995;17–26.

60. Boulloche J, Husson B, Le Luyer B, Le Roux P. Dysphagia, speech disorders and centrotemporal spikes. Arch French Pediatr 1990;47:115–117.

61. Nass R, Devinsky O. Autistic regression with Rolandic spikes. Neuropsychiatr Neuropsychol Behav Neurol 1999;12(3):193–197.

62. Roulet E, Deonna T, Despland PA. Prolonged intermittent drooling and oro-motor dyspraxia in benign childhood epilepsy with centrotemporal spikes. Epilepsia 1989;30(5):564–568.

63. Scheffer IE, Jones L, Pozzebon M, et al. Autosomal dominant Rolandic epilepsy and speech dyspraxia: a new syndrome with anticipation. Ann Neurol 1995; 38(4):633–642.

64. Andermann F, Beaumanoir A, Mira L, et al. (eds). Occipital Seizures and Epilepsies in Children. London: John Libbey, 1993.

65. Nass R, Gross A, Devinsky O. Autism and autistic epileptiform regression with occipital spikes. Dev Med Child Neurol 1998;40(7):453–458.

66. Tenembaum S, Deonna T, Fejerman N, et al. Continuous spike-waves and dementia in childhood epilepsy with occipital paroxysms. J Epilepsy 1997;10:139–145.

67. Beaumanoir A. Semiology of Occipital Seizures in Infants and Children. In F Andermann, A Beaumanoir, L Mira, et al. (eds), Occipital Seizures and Epilepsies in Children. London: John Libbey, 1993;71–86.

68. Eslava-Cobos J, Mejia L. Landau-Kleffner syndrome: much more than aphasia and epilepsy. Brain Lang 1997;57(2):215–224.

69. Holmes H, McKeever M, Saunders Z. Epileptiform activity in aphasia of childhood: an epiphenomenon? Epilepsia 1981;22:631–639.

70. Nass R, Heier L, Walker R. Acquired aphasia with convulsive disorder due to tumor responding to surgery. Pediatr Neurol 1993;9:303–308.

71. Morrell F. Electrophysiology of CSWS in Landau-Kleffner Syndrome. In A Beaumanoir, M Bureau, T Deonna, et al. (eds), Continuous Spikes and Waves During Slow Sleep. London: John Libbey Eurotext, 1995;77–90.

72. Paetau R, Kajola M, Korkman M. LKS: epileptic activity in auditory cortex. Neuroreport 2 1991;201–204.

73. Solomon G, Carson D, Pavlakis S, et al. Intracranial EEG monitoring in LKS associated with left temporal lobe astrocytoma. Epilepsia 1993;34:557–560.

74. Aarts JHP, Binnie CD, Smit A, Wilkins AJ. Selective cognitive impairment during focal and generalized epileptiform EEG activity. Brain 1984;107:293–308.

75. Aldenkamp A. Effect of seizures and epileptiform discharge on cognitive function. Epilepsia 1997;38[Suppl 1]:S52–S55.

76. Binnie C, Marston D. Cognitive correlates of interictal discharge. Epilepsia 1992;33[Suppl]:S11–S17.

77. Kasteleijn-Nolst Trenite D, Smit A, Velis D, et al. On line detection of transient neurological disturbances during EEG discharges in children with epilepsy. Dev Med Child Neurol 1990;32:46–50.

78. Rugland A. Subclinical Epileptogenic Activity. In M Sillanpaa (ed), Pediatric Epilepsy. Norway: Wrightson Biomedical Publishing, 1990;212–220.

79. Gokyigit A, Caliskan A. Diffuse spike-wave status of 9-year duration without behavioral change or intellectual decline. Epilepsia 1995;36(2):210–213.

80. Seri S, Cerquiglini A, Pisani F. Spike-induced interference in auditory sensory processing in Landau-Kleffner syndrome. Electroencephalogr Clin Neurophysiol 1998;108(5):506–510.

81. Morrell F, Whisler WW, Smith MC, et al. Landau-Kleffner syndrome: treatment with subpial intracortical transection. Brain 1995;118[Pt 6]:1529–1546.

82. Ansynk BJJ, Sarphatie H, von Dongen HR. The LKS. Neuropediatrics 1989;20:170–172.

83. De Negri M. The maturational development of the child: developmental disorders and epilepsy. In A Beaumanoir, M Bureau, T Deonna, et al. (eds), Continuous Spikes and Waves During Slow Sleep. London: John Libbey Eurotext, 1995;3–8.

84. Gordon N. Acquired aphasia in childhood. Dev Med Child Neurol 1990;32:270–274.

85. Kellerman K. Recurrent aphasia and subclinical status epilepticus during sleep. Eur J Pediatr 1978;128:207–212.

86. Deonna T, Roulet E. AEA: definition of the syndrome and current problems. In A Beaumanoir, M Bureau, T Deonna, et al. (eds), Continuous Spikes and Waves During Slow Sleep. London: John Libbey Eurotext, 1995;37–46.

87. Nass R. Developmental Language Disorders. In B Berg (ed); Principles of Child Neurology. New York: McGraw-Hill, 1996;140–144.

88. Duvelleroy-Hommet C, Billard C, Lucas B, et al. Sleep EEG and developmental dysphasia: lack of a consistent relationship with paroxysmal EEG activity during sleep. Neuropediatrics 1995;26(1):14–18.

89. Echenne B, Cheminal R, Rivier F, et al. Epileptic EEG abnormalities and developmental dysphasia. Brain Dev 1992;14:216–220.

90. Klein S, Tuchman R, Rapin I. Relationship of language impairment and seizures in children with verbal auditory agnosia. Ann Neurol 1989;26:482.

91. Maccario M, Hefferen SJ, Keblusek SJ, Lipinsky KA. Developmental dysphasia and electroencephalo-

graphic abnormalities. Dev Med Child Neurol 1982; 24:141–155.

92. Deuel RK, Lenn N. Treatment of acquired epileptic aphasia. J Pediatr 1977;90:959–961.

93. Lanzi G, Veggiotti P, Conte S, et al. A correlated fluctuation of language and EEG abnormalities in a case of the Landau-Kleffner syndrome. Brain Dev 1994;16(4):329–334.

94. Lerman P, Lerman-Sagie T, Kivity S. Effect of early corticosteroid therapy for Landau-Kleffner syndrome. Dev Med Child Neurol 1991;33:257–260.

95. De Volder A, Michel C, Thauvoy C, et al. Brain glucose utilization in acquired childhood aphasia associated with a sylvian arachnoid cyst: recovery after shunting as demonstrated by PET. J Neurol Neurosurg Psychiatry 1994;57(3):296–302.

96. Li M, Hao XY, Qing J, Wu XR. Correlation between CSWS and aphasia in Landau-Kleffner syndrome: a study of three cases. Brain Dev 1996;18(3):197–200.

97. Baynes K, Kegl JA, Brentari D, et al. Chronic auditory agnosia following Landau-Kleffner syndrome: a 23-year outcome study. Brain Lang 1998;63(3):381–425.

98. Deonna T, Peter C, Ziegler AL. Adult follow-up of the acquired aphasia-epilepsy syndrome in childhood. Report of 7 cases. Neuropediatrics 1989;20(3):132–138.

99. Lou H, Brandt S, Bruhn P. Progressive Aphasia and Epilepsy with a Self-Limited Course. In JK Penny (ed), Epilepsy: The Eighth International Symposium. New York: Raven Press, 1977;85–94.

100. Rossi PG, Parmeggiani A, Posar A, et al. Landau-Kleffner syndrome (LKS): long-term follow-up and links with electrical status epilepticus during sleep (ESES). Brain Dev 1999;21(2):90–98.

101. Sandt-Koenderman W, Smit I, Dongen H, Hest JBC. A case of acquired aphasia and convulsive disorder: some linguistic aspects of recovery and breakdown. Brain Lang 1984;21:174–188.

102. Soprano AM, Garcia EF, Caraballo R, Fejerman N. Acquired epileptic aphasia: neuropsychologic follow-up of 12 patients. Pediatr Neurol 1994;11(3):230–235.

103. van Dongen H, Meulstee J, Blaw-van Mourik M. LKS: a case study with a fourteen year followup. Eur Neurol 1989;29:109–114.

104. Zardini G, Molteni B, Nardocci N, et al. Linguistic development in a patient with Landau-Kleffner syndrome: a nine-year follow-up. Neuropediatrics 1995;26(1):19–25.

105. van Hout A. Acquired aphasia in children. Semin Pediatr Neurol 1997;4(2):102–108.

106. Lou C, Brandt S, Bruhn P. Aphasia and epilepsy in childhood. Acta Neurol Scand 1977;56:46–54.

107. Bhatia MS, Shome S, Chadda RK, Saurabh S. Landau-Kleffner syndrome in cerebral cysticercosis. Ind Pediatr 1994;31(5):584–587.

108. McKinney W, McGreal DA. An aphasic syndrome in children. Can Med Assoc J 1974;110:637–639.

109. Nass RD, Peterson H, Koch D. Differential effects of early left versus right brain injury on intelligence. Brain Cogn 1989;9:258–266.

110. Otero E, Cordova S, Diaz F. Acquired epileptic aphasia (the Landau-Kleffner syndrome) due to neurocysticercosis. Epilepsia 1989;30:569–572.

111. Park YD, Hoffman JM, Radtke RA, DeLong GR. Focal cerebral metabolic abnormality in a patient with continuous spike waves during slow-wave sleep. J Child Neurol 1994;9(2):139–143.

112. Guerreiro MM, Camargo EE, Kato M, et al. Brain single photon emission computed tomography imaging in Landau-Kleffner syndrome. Epilepsia 1996;37(1):60–67.

113. Maquet P, Hirsch E, Dive D, et al. Cerebral glucose utilization during sleep in the LKS: a PET study. Epilepsia 1990;31:778–783.

114. O'Tuama L. Functional imaging in neuropsychiatric disorders. J Child Neurol 1999;14:207–222.

115. Treves S, O'Tuama A, Urion D. Cerebral perfusion abnormalities in Landau-Kleffner syndrome. Neurology 1991;41:267.

116. Chez M, Major S, Smith M. SPECT evaluation of cerebral perfusion in LKS. Epilepsia 1992;33[Suppl 3]:52.

117. Rintahaka PI, Chugani HT, Sankar R. Landau-Kleffner syndrome with continuous spikes and waves during slow-wave sleep. J Child Neurol 1995;10(2):127–133.

118. Stefanatos GA, Grover W, Geller E. Case study: corticosteroid treatment of language regression in pervasive developmental disorder. J Am Acad Child Adolesc Psychiatry 1995;34(8):1107–1111.

119. Fayad MN, Choueiri R, Mikati M. Landau-Kleffner syndrome: consistent response to repeated intravenous gamma-globulin doses: a case report. Epilepsia 1997;38(4):489–494.

120. Lagae LG, Silberstein J, Gillis PL, Casaer PJ. Successful use of intravenous immunoglobulins in Landau-Kleffner syndrome. Pediatr Neurol 1998;18(2):165–168.

121. Baram TZ. Pathophysiology of massive infantile spasms (MIS): perspective on the role of the brain adrenal axis. Ann Neurol 1993;33:231–237.

122. Sawhney IM, Robertson IJ, Polkey CE, et al. Multiple subpial transections: a review of 21 cases. J Neurol Neurosurg Psychiatry 1995;58(3):344–349.

123. Gillberg C, Uvebrant P, Carlsson G, et al. Autism and epilepsy (and tuberous sclerosis?) in two pre-adolescent boys: neuropsychiatric aspects before and after epilepsy surgery. J Intellect Disabil Res 1996;40:75–81.

124. Neville BG, Harkness WF, Cross JH, et al. Surgical treatment of severe autistic regression in childhood epilepsy. Pediatr Neurol 1997;16(2):137–140.

125. Grote C, van Slyke P, Hoeppner J. Language outcome following multiple subpial transection for Landau-Kleffner syndrome. Brain 1999;122(3):561–566.

126. Nass R, Gross A, Wisoff J, Devinsky O. Outcome of multiple subpial transections for autistic epileptiform regression. Pediatr Neurol 1999;21(1):464–470.

127. Mantovani JF, Landau W. Acquired aphasia with convulsive disorder: course and prognosis. Neurology 1980;30:524–529.

128. Bishop DV. Age of onset and outcome in "acquired aphasia with convulsive disorder" (Landau-Kleffner syndrome). Dev Med Child Neurol 1985;27(6):705–712.

129. Teuber H. Why Two Brains? In F Schmitt, F Worden (eds), The Neurosciences: Third Study Program. Cambridge, MA: MIT Press, 1974;782–787.

Chapter 9

Status Epilepticus

John M. Pellock and David J. Leszczyszyn

Status epilepticus (SE) represents a true neurologic emergency.[1–4] Its incidence is greatest at the extremes of age, with the highest occurrence in young children and the elderly, and at these ages there is greater morbidity and mortality.[1–6] The disorder is more common than previously noted. Hospital-based studies suggest that SE is underrecognized and is the cause of coma in a significant number of patients who demonstrate no overt seizure activity or in outpatients who seem confused and disoriented.[7–9] Prompt recognition and management may significantly reduce morbidity and mortality by decreasing the prolonged duration of seizures and halting the biochemical cascade that accompanies SE both in brain and systemically.[10]

The significant morbidity and mortality that can accompany SE supports an operational definition of SE as seizures lasting longer than 5–10 minutes, so that acute therapies may begin prior to seizures becoming more refractory.[11] The population with multiple handicaps is at increased risk not only for SE but for clusters of seizures that may become prolonged as a consequence of the refractory epilepsy and, thus, may meet the definition of SE. Several recent advances in treatment have allowed more prompt therapy, both in and out of hospital, with the potential benefit of significantly decreasing the duration of SE.[1,2]

Definition and Classification

Any type of seizure, when prolonged, may be classified as being SE. The International League against Epilepsy and the World Health Organization suggested that SE be defined as "condition characterized by an epileptic seizure that is so frequently repeated or so prolonged as to create a fixed and lasting condition."[12] The traditional universal definition of SE is a seizure lasting 30 minutes but, as noted earlier, clinical care requires intervention for seizures lasting longer than 5 minutes.[11] DeLorenzo et al.[13] found a nearly 10-fold greater mortality in seizures lasting 30 minutes or more as compared with those lasting 10–29 minutes.

Although medical and paramedical personnel think of SE as being composed of seizures that are tonic-clonic (grand mal) in nature, all types of seizures may become prolonged or recur without recovery for 30 minutes. Either primary generalized or secondarily generalized seizures can evolve to SE, and these may occur at any age. SE may also be composed of several nonconvulsive entities including complex partial, simple partial, and absence seizures. Table 9-1 summarizes a proposed classification of SE.

Complex partial SE usually is characterized by an epileptic twilight state in which there is cyclic variation between periods of partial responsiveness and episodes of motionless staring and complete unresponsiveness accompanied, at times, by automatic behavior.[7,14,15] Simple partial SE is characterized by focal seizures that may persist or be repetitive for at least 30 minutes without impairment of consciousness. When this condition lasts for hours or days, it is termed *epilepsia partialis continua*. Absence status (petit mal status or spike and wave stupor) is a type of

Table 9-1. Proposed Classification of Status Epilepticus

Partial		
Convulsive		
Tonic	Hemiclonic status epilepticus, hemiconvulsion-hemiplegia-epilepsy, hemi–grand mal	
Clonic	Status epilepticus, grand mal	
Nonconvulsive		
Simple	Focal motor status, focal sensory, epilepsia partialis continuans, adversive status epilepticus	
Complex partial	Epileptic fugue state, prolonged epileptic stupor, prolonged epileptic confusional state, temporal lobe status epilepticus, psychomotor status epilepticus, continuous epileptic twilight state	
Generalized		
Convulsive		
Tonic-clonic	Grand mal, epilepticus convulsivus	
Tonic		
Clonic		
Myoclonic	Myoclonic status epilepticus	
Nonconvulsive		
Absence	Spike and wave stupor, spike and slow wave or 3-sec spike and wave status epilepticus, petit mal epileptic fugue, epilepsia minora continua, epileptic twilight state, minor status epilepticus	
Undetermined		
Subtle	Epileptic coma	
Neonatal	Erratic status epilepticus	

Source: From DJ Leszczyszyn, JM Pellock. Status Epilepticus. In JM Pellock, WE Dodson, B Bourgeois (eds), Pediatric Epilepsy, Diagnosis and Treatment. New York: Demos, 2000; and H Gastaut, Classification of Status Epilepticus. In AV Delgado-Escueta, RJ Porter, CG Wasterlain (eds), Status Epilepticus: Mechanisms of Brain Damage and Treatment. New York: Raven Press, 1982.

nonconvulsive SE that may be extremely difficult to differentiate from complex partial SE without electroencephalography. Classically, in absence status, a continuous alteration of consciousness occurs without the cyclic variations seen in complex partial SE. The electroencephalographic (EEG) recording exhibits prolonged, sometimes continuous, generalized synchronous 1.5- to 4.0-Hz spike and slow wave complexes rather than focal ictal discharges, which characterize partial SE.[7,16] The patient presenting with a prolonged confused state, with a fluctuating level of consciousness, or with prolonged uncon-sciousness requires both clinical and EEG evaluations in addition to other studies.

Myoclonic, generalized clonic, and generalized tonic SE are seen primarily in children. These children usually have encephalopathic epilepsies,[5,7,17] and their consciousness seems to be preserved throughout the attacks. The EEG pattern is bilaterally symmetric with polyspike discharges coinciding with the myoclonic jerks. The term *myoclonic SE* should not be used when children with severe encephalopathy exhibit repetitive myoclonic jerks not accompanied by ictal discharges on the EEG recording. These patients have subtle, generalized, convulsive SE, as defined by Treiman.[7] Approximately one-half of the cases of generalized clonic SE occur in otherwise healthy children and are associated with prolonged febrile seizures; the other half are distributed among those with acute and chronic encephalopathies.[18] Generalized tonic SE appears most frequently in children, particularly those with the Lennox-Gastaut syndrome. Prolonged generalized tonic convulsions may be precipitated by benzodiazepine administration.

Epidemiology

SE usually is a manifestation of symptomatic epilepsy with preexisting neurologic dysfunction or a manifestation of acute disease primarily or secondarily affecting the central nervous system (CNS). In patients of all ages, SE rarely occurs in the unstressed patient with idiopathic epilepsy. Those with prolonged resistant seizures should receive a full diagnostic evaluation for all etiologies of seizures, along with a search for those precipitating events noted in Table 9-2.

Interestingly, evidence exists for a genetic predisposition for SE.[19] The major causes vary with age, such as febrile SE in children 1–2 years of age and remote symptomatic etiologies in the 5- to 10-year range.[18,20] Acute symptomatic etiologies most commonly lead to prolonged SE lasting longer than 1 hour.[1,6,18] Similarly, recurrent SE is more frequent in children with remote symptomatic etiologies or progressive degenerative disease.[20–23] This population with remote symptomatic SE best characterizes the population with mental retardation and multiple handicaps.

A recent, prospective, population-based study of SE revealed the incidence of SE to be 41 patients per year per 100,000 population, resulting in a total of 50 episodes of SE per year per 100,000. It is projected that between 102,000 and 152,000 events occur in the United States annually, an incidence two to two and a half times greater than that previously proposed.[4,14] Approximately one-third of the cases present as the initial seizure of epilepsy, one-third occur in patients with previously established epilepsy, and one-third occur as the result of an acute isolated brain insult. Among those individuals in whom epilepsy was previously diagnosed, estimates of SE occurrence range from 0.5% to 6.6%. Within 5 years of the initial diagnosis of epilepsy, 20% of all patients will experience an episode of SE. A greater incidence of SE is reported from cohorts of patients with childhood-onset epilepsy.[24] One-third of the patients experienced SE over a 30-year period, 50% of such instances presenting as the first seizure and an additional 22% occurring within 12 months of onset of epilepsy. In this group, SE occurred in 44% of those with remote symptomatic epilepsy and 20% of those with idiopathic or cryptogenic epilepsy.

Although adults in whom SE occurs as their first unprovoked seizure often develop subsequent epilepsy,[25] a prospective study of children with SE found that only 30% of those initially presenting with SE later develop epilepsy.[20] Hesdorffer et al.[25] has presented more recent data indicating a greater likelihood of epilepsy after SE in a group of 95 people, one-third of whom were children. Over the ensuing 10-year period after symptomatic SE, a 41% risk of an unprovoked seizure was noted.[25]

Among children, SE is most common in infants and young toddlers, with more than 50% of cases of SE occurring in children younger than 3 years.[26] In the study from Richmond, Virginia, total SE events and incidence per 100,000 individuals per year showed a bimodal distribution, with the highest values during the first year of life and after 60 years of age.[14,27,28] Infants younger than 1 year represent a subgroup of children with the highest incidence of SE, whether events, total incidents, or recurrence is counted. The recurrence rate of SE in the Richmond study was 10.8%,[1,22] but 38% of patients

Table 9-2. Status Epilepticus Precipitating Events

Antiepileptic drug alterations
  Withdrawal
  Noncompliance
  Interactions
  Toxicity
Infections
  Central nervous system
  Systemic
Toxins
  Alcohol
  Drugs
  Poisons
  Convulsive agents
Structural
  Trauma
  Ischemic stroke
  Hemorrhagic stroke
  Acute hydrocephalus
Hormonal change
Electrolyte imbalance
Diagnostic procedures and medications
Emotional stress
Progressive-degenerative disease
Sleep deprivation
Primary apnea
Cardiac arrhythmias
Fever

Source: From DJ Leszczyszyn, JM Pellock. Status Epilepticus. In JM Pellock, WE Dodson, B Bourgeois (eds), Pediatric Epilepsy, Diagnosis and Treatment. New York: Demos, 2000.

ings supported by the Finnish study.[24] In another cohort of pediatric epilepsy patients followed up for 5 years by Berg et al.,[29] only 4.3% had experienced their first episode of SE, whereas 19.6% of those who presented with SE had experienced one or more episodes.

In persons with mental retardation and multiple handicaps, most have SE of a remote symptomatic etiology. Their epilepsy frequently is refractory to therapy and is chronic. In a population of 221 children, Goulden et al.[30] reported that 15% had developed epilepsy by age 22 years. Further, the cumulative risk increases substantially in mentally retarded persons when other disabilities, such as cerebral palsy, are evident.[31] Epilepsy in this population frequently is characterized by its refractory nature, the use of polypharmacy, multiple seizure types, lifelong antiepileptic drug (AED) treatment, and frequent

SE.[32] Patients who experience many seizures before therapy is initiated or who have an inadequate response to the initial treatment are most likely to have refractory epilepsy. A population-based series of mentally retarded children revealed that 45% had intractable seizures.[32] In this series, predictive factors for frequent seizures were the number of seizure types, severe mental retardation, SE, and tonic seizures. In another series, four risk factors for SE were identified in children with symptomatic epilepsy: focal background EEG abnormalities, partial seizures secondarily generalized, first seizure being SE, and generalized abnormalities on neuroimaging.[33] In an ongoing prospective study of SE in Richmond, Virginia, we estimate that nearly 20% of all cases of SE in children are in those with mental retardation, nearly 30% of this group experiencing recurrent episodes.

Extrapolating these figures worldwide, more than 1 million cases of SE occur throughout the world annually. Furthermore, the population with mental retardation and epilepsy is at an increased risk for SE. Because SE is a neurologic emergency that requires immediate, effective treatment to prevent residual neurologic complications or death, SE poses a substantial health risk. Mortality rates as high as 30% and as low as 10% have been reported in overall studies. Children have a far lower mortality rate than do adults, with the exception of those in the first year of life.[20,28,29] Age, etiology, and duration directly correlate with mortality.[1,6,13,28] Multiple studies confirm the lower mortality rate in most children after adequate emergency treatment.[1,4,20,21,34,35]

Pathophysiology

The mechanisms by which chronic seizures evolve to SE remain unclear.[1] An apparent loss of inhibitory mechanisms occurs, and neuronal metabolism is unable to keep up with the demand of continuing ictal activity. The pathophysiologic changes that accompany SE can be divided into neuronal (cerebral) and systemic effects. Continuing seizures lead to both biochemical changes within the brain and systemic

derangements that further complicate these cerebral changes.

Prolonged convulsive seizures can lead to excitotoxic brain injury. Glutamate, the primary excitatory amino acid neurotransmitter, binds to several neuronal receptors, including the N-methyl-D-aspartate (NMDA) receptor, which is activated by depolarization. The resulting calcium influx causes further depolarization and perpetuates seizures. Glutamate also activates receptors that open channels that conduct sodium and calcium into the cell. Through this excessive excitatory neurotransmission, further neuronal damage results. Although γ-aminobutyric acid (GABA) is the most prevalent inhibitory neurotransmitter in the brain, excessive GABA may, in fact, increase activity on both GABA(A) and GABA(B) receptors. Activation of the presynaptic GABA(B) receptors can provide feedback inhibition of GABA(A) receptors and, paradoxically, exacerbate seizures. Other neurotransmitters that may help to initiate and maintain SE include acetylcholine, adenosine, and nitric oxide.[29]

Neuronal injury and cell death from SE are most prominent in areas rich in NMDA glutamate receptors, including the limbic region. The increase in intracellular calcium concentration is critical to cell death. Calcium activates proteases and lipases that degrade intracellular elements, leading to mitochondrial dysfunction and cellular necrosis. Laminar necrosis and neuronal damage after prolonged seizures are similar to that following cerebral hypoxia. Although young animals appear to develop brain damage from SE,[36] studies using alternative models demonstrate hippocampal cellular injury even in immature rodents.[37] The glutamate-initiated calcium-dependent cascade appears similar to the mechanism of NMDA receptor–mediated cell death during cerebral ischemia. Absence SE associated with excessive inhibitory influences generated by GABA(B)-mediated hyperpolarization and activation of folinic T-type calcium channels, however, does not cause cerebral injury.[29] Further, acute and long-term changes in gene expression may occur after prolonged seizures and may contribute directly to hyperexcitability.[38]

Systemic metabolic abnormalities increase the rim of brain damage in convulsive SE. These

Table 9-3. Prognosis of Childhood Status Epilepticus

	Aicardi[41]	Dunn[34]	Maytal[20]	MCV[5]
Patients	239	97	193	29
Status epilepticus duration	60	30	30	30
Symptomatic (%)	75	72	77	73
Morbidity (%)	>50	23	9.1	11–15
Mortality (%)	11	8	3.6	3

MCV = Medical College of Virginia.

include alterations of blood pressure, heart rate, respiratory function, and body temperature, acidosis, hypoxia, leukocytosis, rhabdomyolysis, and heightened demands on cerebral oxygen and glucose use.[10] Circulating catecholamine concentrations increase during the initial 30 minutes of SE, resulting in a hypersympathetic state. Tachycardia sometimes associated with severe cardiac dysrhythmias occurs and may rarely be fatal.[39] Furthermore, cardiac output diminishes and total peripheral resistance increases along with mean arterial blood pressure, perhaps because of the sympathetic overload. Hyperpyrexia may become significant during the course of SE, even without prior febrile illness, in both children and adults and may contribute to neuronal injury.[40]

Hypoventilation leads to hypoxia and respiratory acidosis. In addition, serum pH and glucose levels frequently are abnormal, as lactic acidosis develops after increased anaerobic metabolism. A leukemoid reaction of peripheral blood frequently occurs in the absence of infection. Rhabdomyolysis, not uncommonly seen, may compromise renal function. Recovery from this complicated derangement of metabolism is time-dependent. More prolonged seizures produce further neuronal injury and death.[10]

Prognosis

The morbidity and mortality of SE are direct consequences of its basic pathophysiology and the efficiency of treatment. Previously, overall mortality figures for SE were quoted as 10–30%.[41,42] The mortality rate for the Richmond, Virginia, population was 22% overall. On the basis of this study, which includes all age groups, approximately 126,000–195,000 SE events associated with 22,000–42,000 deaths per year occur within the United States. However, the mortality rate in children was only 3%, and most of the pediatric deaths occurred between the ages of 1 and 4 years (Table 9-3). The pediatric as well as the elderly population experienced more recurrences of SE after a single episode. These children, in general, had chronic neurologic disabilities but rarely died.[22] Among those patients who died, death rarely occurred during the acute episode of SE. Rather, most succumbed 15–30 days later.[6] Children with chronic epilepsy and low AED levels have the lowest mortality rate overall but, with advancing age, mortality increases.

The morbidity of SE in children was examined in the same database from Virginia. Before their SE event, 81% of children with no history of seizures were neurologically normal, in contrast to only 31% of children with seizure histories. Of the neurologically normal children with no prior seizures, more than 25% deteriorated after their first SE event, in comparison with fewer than 15% of neurologically normal children with a seizure history. Children who were neurologically abnormal without prior seizures deteriorated further in 6.7% of cases, as compared with 11.3% of the neurologically abnormal children who had a seizure history. Morbidity was determined at the time of hospital discharge and, in some children, the abnormalities may not persist. Minor degrees of ataxia, incoordination, or motor deficits, for example, may be attributed to the acute therapies or clinical changes after prolonged seizures and may improve over time. Determining whether language deficits and school performance difficulties were transient or more permanent was more difficult.[1] In a prospective study, 11–15% of affected children had significant morbidity after an episode of SE (see Table 9-3). These findings suggest a neurologic morbidity substantially lower than the "greater than 50%" rate previously reported in children having SE,[41] but the morbidity and mortality of very sick infants is higher than in older children.[28]

Hesdorffer et al.[25] in Rochester, Minnesota, found that the 10-year risk of having an unprovoked seizure after an acute seizure of SE was 41%. This 95-person cohort included 17 individuals younger than 1 year and 17 persons aged 1–19 years. This risk was increased 18.8-fold for SE due to anoxic encephalopathy, 7.1-fold for structural causes, and 3.6-fold for metabolic causes, as compared with patients who experienced a less prolonged acute symptomatic seizure.[25]

Electrographic and biochemical markers for increased morbidity and mortality in SE exist. The duration of the individual seizure, especially if it evolves to nonconvulsive SE (NCSE), has been directly correlated with death or poor outcome as defined by one's inability to return to a prehospitalization level of function.[43] Serum and cerebrospinal fluid (CSF) levels of neuron-specific enolase rise above normal after both brief and prolonged seizures. Serum levels after SE are significantly higher and are at their highest in patients after NCSE, in whom levels exceeding 37 ng/ml correlate with poor outcome.[44] The CSF lactate level also is elevated after SE, and levels three times greater than the accepted normal are associated with poor outcome, whereas those whose levels are elevated twofold or less have better outcomes. CSF lactate dehydrogenase and creatinine kinase levels do not indicate prognosis in SE.[45] In addition, CSF pleocytosis is not a valid indicator of prognosis in SE. In all age groups, prognosis typically is related to the acute illness or injury precipitating the seizure. More than 6 white blood cells per cubic millimeter or the presence of any polymorphonuclear cells in an adult, or more than eight white blood cells or more than four polymorphonuclear cells per cubic millimeter in a child, should prompt a search for an etiology other than the seizure itself.[46,47]

Radiographic findings after SE, typically reversible focal T2-weighted magnetic resonance imaging abnormalities, are benign for years.[48] Case reports, however, suggest that brain injury occurs despite radiographic normalization, as evidenced by persistent EEG abnormalities and proton magnetic resonance spectroscopy abnormalities.[49,50] This injury may be more prevalent in those with prior focal injury and subsequent prolonged seizures.[51,52] Strong evidence also exists to suggest that structural brain injury in the form of ischemic stroke has a synergistic effect with SE, leading to increased mortality.[53]

Therapeutic Considerations

SE requires mobilization of personal and medical resources and is a substantial public health concern. With mortality rates as high as 30% reported in all-age inclusive studies, immediate and effective treatment is needed to prevent residual neurologic complications or death. Age, etiology, and duration of the SE episode directly correlate with mortality.[1,4,6] The highest mortality is seen in the elderly, and children have a far lower mortality rate than do adults.[1,6,14,20,21,24,34,35] Some of this improved prognosis in children is likely a result of fewer coexisting medical conditions.[5,18,20]

Because SE frequently occurs out of hospital, appropriate first aid recommendations will be discussed for completeness. The Epilepsy Foundation of America[54] recommends that the person attending follow these guidelines: (1) Look for medical identification; (2) protect the person from nearby hazards; (3) loosen ties or shirt collars; (4) protect the head from injury; (5) turn the person on her or his side to keep the airway clear; (6) reassure when consciousness returns; (7) if a single seizure has lasted more than 5 minutes, ask whether hospital evaluation is desired; (8) if multiple seizures occur, or if one seizure lasts longer than 5 minutes, call an ambulance; (9) if the person is pregnant, injured, or diabetic, call aid at once. The EF also recommends that the attending person adhere to the following restrictions: (1) Do not put any hard implement in the patient's mouth; (2) do not try to hold the tongue so that it cannot be swallowed; (3) do not try to give liquids during or just after the seizure; (4) do not use artificial respiration unless breathing is absent after muscle jerks subside or unless water has been inhaled; and (5) do not restrain the person. The patient should be transferred to a medical center as soon as possible if the seizure continues beyond 5 minutes or if, after ceasing, it begins again.

The neurologic emergency of SE requires maintenance of respiration, general medical support, and specific treatment of seizures while the etiology is sought.[2] Every medical setting must develop a protocol for the treatment of SE. Time wasted while deciding on which therapeutic regimen to use and when and how to administer it delays optimal care. A typical and frequent mistake made in the treatment of SE is that inadequate doses of drugs are given initially, and then physicians wait for more seizures to occur before administering the necessary total dose.[1,2,5]

The ideal AED for the treatment of SE should have the following properties: rapid onset of action; broad spectrum of activity; ease of administration, including intravenous and intramuscular preparations; minimal redistribution from the CNS; and a wide therapeutic safety margin. Because of these desired properties and particularly because it is longer-acting, lorazepam as the initial agent is more popular than diazepam in many centers. Recent studies in both children and adults also support the use of rectal diazepam or midazolam. Rapid absorption of benzodiazepine agents from varied sites of administration and rapid onset of anticonvulsant activity make this a very attractive agent for use in multiple settings. If, however, SE continues after the initial dosing of a benzodiazepine and persists after a primary AED such as phenytoin (as fosphenytoin) or phenobarbital is given, a second dose of the same AED should be administered before switching to alternative medications. SE that is refractory to these established agents carries a more grave prognosis.[55] Numerous studies suggest that additional bolus administration and then titrated intravenous infusions of diazepam, midazolam, pentobarbital, or the anesthetic agents lidocaine or propofol may break these seizures. The role of intravenous valproic acid in the treatment of SE currently is being studied. Our experience to date suggests additional benefit in hemodynamically unstable patients and those resistant to prior therapies.[56]

The first goal of treatment is to stop the convulsive discharges in the brain. Table 9-4 lists the steps in the emergency management of SE.[1,4,57] Cardiorespiratory function must be assessed immediately by vital sign determination, auscultation, airway inspection, arterial blood gas determination, and suction, when necessary. Although spontaneously breathing on presentation, the patient can develop hypoxia with respi-

Table 9-4. Status Epilepticus Emergency Management

Ensure adequate brain oxygenation and cardiorespiratory function.
Terminate clinical and electrical seizure activity as rapidly as possible.
Prevent seizure recurrence.
Identify precipitating factors such as hypoglycemia, electrolyte imbalance, lowered drug levels, infection, and fever.
Correct metabolic imbalance.
Prevent systemic complications.
Further evaluate and treat the etiology of status epilepticus.

Source: From DJ Leszczyszyn, JM Pellock. Status Epilepticus. In JM Pellock, WE Dodson, B Bourgeois (eds), Pediatric Epilepsy, Diagnosis and Treatment. New York: Demos, 2000.

ratory or metabolic acidosis from apnea, aspiration, or central respiratory depression.[1] The need for ventilator support depends not only on respiratory status at the time of presentation but also on the conditions prior to arrival at a hospital and the ability to maintain adequate oxygenation throughout ongoing seizures and during the intravenous administration of drugs, all of which cause some amount of respiratory depression. In the neurologically depressed patient, elective intubation and respiratory support are urged. In most patients, placement of an oral airway or nasal cannula oxygen is insufficient, as respiratory drive is depressed. Significant hypoxia is a principal factor determining morbidity and mortality.[6] Rapid assessment of vital signs and general neurologic examination give clues to the etiology of SE. Blood drawn to determine blood gases, levels of glucose, calcium, and electrolytes, complete blood count, AED levels, culture, and virologic and toxicologic studies helps with the overall determination of etiology. Similarly, urine should be collected for drug and metabolic screens. The roles of CSF neuron-specific enolase and lactate, as well as serum neuron-specific enolase, in prognostication of outcomes in SE were discussed earlier.

Intravenous fluids should be administered judiciously, with appropriate corrections for fever, suction, and chemical abnormality. Fluid restriction rarely is necessary. Immediately after placement of the intravenous line, 25% glucose (2–4 ml/kg) should be given by bolus. In a case in which intravenous access cannot be established, rectal administration of diazepam or use of the intraosseous route is efficient for both fluid and medication administration.[58] Because of the high incidence of febrile SE resulting from CNS infection in infants, a lumbar puncture should be performed early in the course of management but not necessarily during the initial phase of stabilization. Rarely is waiting for imaging studies necessary in this group. If lumbar puncture is deferred for any reason, appropriate antimicrobial coverage for possible meningitis or encephalitis should be considered. Electrocardiographic (ECG) and EEG monitoring is desirable when available. EEG monitoring is extremely useful in both the initial and subsequent management of SE.[57,59–61] The classification of SE, clues to its etiology, and the prognosis may be suggested from the EEG recording and the patient's response to therapy as indicated by EEG monitoring. Patients with conversion attacks and those presenting with overdose of drugs or focal pathologic processes are among those in whom electroencephalography may reveal such important information. Definition of seizures as being mainly partial versus primarily or secondarily generalized is easily recognized; in nonconvulsive cases, the EEG recording easily establishes the diagnosis as complex partial or absence seizures. The use of electroencephalography is mandatory in the presence of neuromuscular blockade or whenever recurrence of seizures cannot be documented on a clinical basis.[1,2,7,57]

An electroclinical dissociation may exist after large doses of AEDs have been given, so that the clinical manifestations are absent while electrographic seizures continue. The recognition of such EEG patterns as paroxysmal lateralized epileptiform discharges, periodic epileptiform discharges, and evidence of continued post-SE ictal discharges without clinical correlation while the patient remains in a coma that requires ongoing therapy may help to establish the etiologic diagnosis and prognosis.[7] One recent study of 50 patients with SE reported poor outcomes, including death or persistent vegetative states, in 44% of those whose records demonstrated periodic epileptiform discharges, as compared with 19% of those without periodic epileptiform discharges.[62] ECG changes seen in adults during and after SE range from evidence of ischemia to tachyarrhythmias.[63] These must be promptly and appropriately treated.[39,63] These findings suggest that both EEG and ECG

monitoring be more aggressively used in the evaluation and treatment of SE. Practical limitations, however, must be realized, as many treatment sites do not have EEG equipment readily available. Urgent use of this monitoring must be considered, nevertheless, when patients do not regain consciousness or when seizures are continuous or recur.

Drug Therapy for Status Epilepticus

Multiple regimens are available for treating SE successfully. Benzodiazepines and fosphenytoin (FOS; phenytoin prodrug equivalent) as initial therapy are preferred for most patients by our group at the Medical College of Virginia of Virginia Commonwealth University, but alternative agents are used if the patient is on maintenance therapy, has already received smaller doses of phenytoin (PHT) or phenobarbital, or has shown resistance to these agents in the past.[1,56,64,65] Lorazepam, diazepam, PHT, FOS, and phenobarbital are accepted agents for initial and continued therapy of SE. The large SE treatment study undertaken in adults and sponsored by the U.S. Veterans Administration suggests that, for initial management of generalized convulsive SE when results were measured at 20 minutes, no significant difference is found among three intravenous drug regimens: (1) diazepam, 0.15 mg/kg, and PHT, 18 mg/kg; (2) lorazepam, 0.1 mg/kg; and (3) phenobarbital, 15 mg/kg.[55] Each was superior to PHT (18 mg/kg) used alone. Importantly, the rate of PHT administration probably biased the study. The much more rapid speed at which FOS can be administered may significantly alter these results. The choice of an initial agent may depend on individual patient characteristics, prior AED therapy, and physician preference. Recommended doses of commonly used drugs for the treatment of convulsive SE are listed in Table 9-5. Protocols presently used by our group for the management of SE in children, adolescents, and adults are given in Tables 9-6 and 9-7.[1,2]

Benzodiazepines

Benzodiazepines are the most potent and efficacious drugs in the treatment of SE.[66] Lasting con-

Table 9-5. Recommended Initial Intravenous Drug Doses for Status Epilepticus

Patient Age	Lorazepam (0.1 mg/kg)	Diazepam (0.3 mg/kg)	Midazolam (0.15–0.30 mg/kg)	Fosphenytoin (Phenytoin Equivalents) (20 mg/kg)	Phenobarbital (20 mg/kg)
<6 mos	0.3–1.0	1–2	0.5–2.0	60–200	60–200
6–12 mos	0.5–1.2	2–4	1.0–4.0	100–250	100–250
1–5 yrs	0.8–2.5	3–10	1.5–10.0	160–250	160–250
5–12 yrs	1.5–6.0	5–15	2.5–15.0	300–1,200	300–1,200
13+ yrs	3.0–6.0	10–20	5.0–20.0	500–1,500+	500–1,500+

Source: From DJ Leszczyszyn, JM Pellock. Status Epilepticus. In JM Pellock, WE Dodson, B Bourgeois (eds), Pediatric Epilepsy, Diagnosis and Treatment. New York: Demos, 2000.

trol of SE is achieved in approximately 80% of patients treated with lorazepam, diazepam, or clonazepam.[66] As the intravenous preparation of clonazepam is not available in the United States, lorazepam and diazepam are used most frequently. A recent prospective, randomized study determined that intramuscular midazolam is as effective as diazepam in stopping seizures and is faster than diazepam because it avoids the requirement of starting an intravenous line.[67] Nasal and buccal administration of benzodiazepines has demonstrated efficacy in aborting acute seizures, but no prospective studies support these routes in treating SE.[68,69] Significant sedation is a disadvantage of benzodiazepines when continued observation of level of consciousness is necessary.

Lorazepam

Lorazepam is a potent benzodiazepine with rapid onset and more prolonged duration of anticonvulsant action as compared to diazepam. With a half-life of approximately 10–15 hours in adults and children, lorazepam continues to have an effective brain level for 8–24 hours. A favorable lipid partition coefficient allows lorazepam to remain in the brain longer than diazepam, which redistributes more rapidly. The recommended intravenous bolus lorazepam dose is 0.1 mg/kg up to a total of 5–8 mg/kg. Tachyphylaxis develops, making repeated doses less effective.[70,71] Lorazepam is also less useful in patients receiving chronic benzodiazepine therapy.

The efficacy of lorazepam equals diazepam in neonates, children, and adults.[70–77] Adverse effects include hypoventilation, ataxia, vomiting, amnesia, lethargy, respiratory depression, and hypotension. These symptoms are exacerbated when barbiturates, paraldehyde, or other depressant drugs are administered prior to lorazepam. After rectal administration, lorazepam has a more delayed onset of action than does diazepam.[76] Sedation that follows intravenous administration of lorazepam is longer-lasting than that after diazepam.

Diazepam

Diazepam enters the brain within seconds after intravenous administration and successfully stops convulsive and nonconvulsive seizures in the majority of adults and children.[66] Its primary disadvantages are similar to those of lorazepam. In addition, because of rapid redistribution, seizures frequently recur after 15–20 minutes following intravenous administration, requiring that a second longer-acting drug be given or a second dose of diazepam be administered. The active desmethyl metabolite of diazepam has a physiologic half-life of 46–78 hours. Respiratory support should be available when this drug is used to treat SE. Recommended dose estimates by age are given in Table 9-5 and are based on 10.0–15.0 mg/m^2, or 0.3 mg/kg. An initial estimate of dose may be made by taking the patient's age and giving 1 mg per year plus 1 mg.[1] Diazepam may be given by intraosseous or rectal route or by a continuous intravenous infusion.[78] Respiratory depression and laryngospasm may develop during the administration of diazepam.

As lorazepam is supplanting diazepam in many hospital emergency situations, diazepam has taken on another important role: prehospital treatment by

Table 9-6. Medical College of Virginia Hospitals Status Epilepticus Protocol for Children

Step	Time from Start of Intervention	Procedure
1	0–5 mins	Determine whether status epilepticus is present and of what type. As soon as the diagnosis is made, institute monitoring of temperature, blood pressure, pulse, respirations, ECG, and EEG. Insert oral airway and administer O_2 if necessary. Insert an IV catheter and draw venous blood levels of anticonvulsants, glucose, electrolytes, calcium, BUN, and CBC. Draw arterial blood for antipyretics (acetaminophen). Perform frequent suctioning.
2	6–9 mins	Place an IV line with normal saline. Administer a bolus of 2 ml/kg 50% glucose.
3	10–30 mins	Initial treatment consists of an infusion by IV lorazepam given at a rate of 1–2 mg/min (0.1 mg/kg) to a maximal dose of 8 mg. This is followed by IV FOS infused at 150 mg/min (or PHT infused at a rate not to exceed 1 mg/kg per min or 50 mg/min). Monitor ECG and blood pressure. May repeat FOS (PHT) 10 mg/kg before proceeding to next step.
4	31–59 mins	If seizures persist, administer a bolus infusion of phenobarbital at a rate not to exceed 50 mg/min until seizures stop or to a loading dose of 20 mg/kg.
5	60 mins	If control is not achieved, other options include the following:
		Dilute diazepam (50 mg) in a solution of 250 ml 0.9% NaCl or D5W and run as a continuous infusion at 1 ml/kg per hr (2 mg/kg per hr) to achieve blood levels of 0.2–8.0 mg/ml. Change the IV solution every 6 hrs, as advised by certain authors, and use short-length tubing.
		Administer pentobarbital with an initial IV loading dose of 5 mg/kg, with additional amounts given to produce a burst suppression pattern on EEG. Maintain pentobarbital anesthesia for approximately 4 hrs by an infusion of 1–3 mg/kg per hr. Then check the patient for the reappearance of seizure activity by decreasing the infusion rate. If clinical seizures or generalized discharges persist on EEG, repeat the procedure; if not, taper the pentobarbital over 12–24 hrs.
		Administer valproate with an initial IV loading dose of 25 mg/kg given at a rate of 6 mg/kg per min. As necessary, administer additional doses of 10–20 mg/kg can be administered. This preparation is particularly useful in patients with primary generalized epilepsy or when cardiovascular complaints such as arrhythmia or hypotension are present.
6	61–80 mins	If seizures still are not controlled, call anesthesia department to begin general anesthesia with halothane and neuromuscular blockade.

BUN = blood urea nitrogen; CBC = complete blood cell count; D5W = 5% dextrose in water; ECG = electrocardiogram; EEG = electroencephalogram; FOS = fosphenytoin; PHT = phenytoin.

Note: Continuous monitoring of EEG is recommended in an obtunded patient to ensure that status epilepticus has not recurred. In the management of intractable status epilepticus, a neurologist who has expertise with this condition should be consulted, and advice from a regional epilepsy center should be sought. Lumbar puncture should be performed as soon as possible, especially in a febrile child or infant younger than 1 year. For infants with a history of neonatal seizures, infantile spasms, or early-onset seizures, pyridoxine (100 mg IV) should be administered while EEG monitoring is ongoing to diagnose and treat the rare patient with seizures and a vitamin B_6 deficiency.

family or other caregivers for prolonged or acute repetitive seizures. A new viscous solution of 5 mg/ml diazepam was developed specifically for rectal administration. Its safety and efficacy have been established in two U.S. trials. Considerably fewer of the diazepam gel–treated patients required subsequent emergency medical attention for continued seizures after the treatment of their episode.[65,79–81] This leads to a reduced cost of care and, in the future, may decrease the prolongation of some seizures to SE.[81]

Midazolam

Midazolam has been used successfully as a first-line treatment for convulsive SE and for refractory convulsive SE. Clinical evidence supports that intramuscular midazolam is more effective than intramuscular diazepam and as effective as intravenous diazepam in abolishing interictal spikes on EEG recordings. At doses from 0.15 to 0.30 mg/kg, intramuscular midazolam terminated convulsive seizures.[82] Many causes of SE were treated successfully with midazolam,

Table 9-7. Medical College of Virginia Hospitals Status Epilepticus Protocol for Adults

Step	Time from Start of Intervention	Procedure
1	0–5 mins	Determine whether status epilepticus is present and of what type. As soon as the diagnosis is made, institute monitoring of temperature, blood pressure, pulse, respirations, ECG, and EEG. Insert oral airway and administer O_2 if necessary. Insert an IV catheter and draw venous blood levels of anticonvulsants, glucose, electrolytes, Ca, Mg, BUN, and CBC. Draw arterial blood for ABG analysis. If necessary, perform nasotracheal suctioning.
2	6 9 mins	Place an IV line with normal saline containing vitamin B complex. Administer a bolus of 50 ml 50% glucose.
3	10–30 mins	Infuse IV lorazepam given at a rate of 2 mg/min (0.1 mg/kg) to a maximal dose of 8 mg or, alternatively, administer IV diazepam given at a rate not to exceed 2 mg/min until seizures stop or to a total of 20 mg. This is followed by IV fosphenytoin phenytoin, 20 mg/kg, at a rate no faster than 50 mg/min. Monitor ECG and blood pressure.
4	31–59 mins	If seizures persist, perform elective endotracheal intubation before starting a bolus infusion of phenobarbital at a rate not to exceed 100 mg/min until seizures stop or to a loading dose of 20 mg/kg.
5	60 mins	If control is not achieved, other options include the following: Administer pentobarbital at an initial IV loading dose of 5–10 mg/kg, with additional amounts given to produce a burst suppression pattern on EEG. Maintain pentobarbital anesthesia for approximately 4 hrs by an infusion of 1–3 mg/kg per hr. Then check the patient for the reappearance of seizure activity by decreasing the infusion rate. If clinical seizures or generalized discharges persist on EEG, repeat the procedure; if not, taper the pentobarbital over 12–24 hrs. Dilute diazepam (50–100 mg) in a solution of 500 ml 0.9% NaCl or D5W and run as a continuous infusion to achieve blood levels of 0.2–8.0 mg/ml. Change the IV solution every 6 hrs, as advised by certain authors, and use short-length tubing. Administer valproate at an initial IV loading dose of 25 mg/kg given at a rate of 6 mg/kg per min. Administer additional doses of 10–20 mg/kg as necessary. This preparation is particularly useful in patients with primary generalized epilepsy or when cardiovascular complaints such as arrhythmia or hypotension are present.
6	61–80 mins	If seizures still are not controlled, call anesthesia department to begin general anesthesia and neuromuscular blockade.

ABG = arterial blood gas; BUN = blood urea nitrogen; CBC = complete blood cell count; D5W = 5% dextrose in water; ECG = electrocardiogram; EEG = electroencephalogram.
Note: Continuous monitoring of EEG is recommended in an obtunded patient to ensure that status epilepticus has not recurred. In the management of intractable status epilepticus, a neurologist who has expertise with this condition should be consulted, and advice from a regional epilepsy center should be sought.

without drug-related cardiac side effects or urgent intubation for ventilatory support.[83,84] The dosing of midazolam for SE in children is not established, although suggested values are found in Table 9-5.

Although lorazepam, diazepam, and now midazolam usually are considered as the initial drugs of choice, they sometimes are useful as the second or third agents when seizures continue. Respiratory support should be available when any of the benzodiazepines are used, because of the cumulative blunting of the respiratory drive centers. Additional intensive monitoring should also be performed to guard against hypotension.

Midazolam undergoes rapid hepatic breakdown, leaving no active metabolites. The elimination half-life of midazolam in children ages 6 months to 10 years ranges from 1.17 to 4.00 hours, in contrast to longer values in adults (1.8–6.4 hours) and elderly men (5–6 hours).[85] When midazolam is administered as a continuous intravenous drip, dosing must be adjusted upward to achieve continued anticonvulsant or sedative action because of marked tachyphylaxis.

Phenobarbital

Phenobarbital remains the initial drug of choice in some institutions for the treatment of childhood SE.[17,86] Its time to onset of action is longer than that of lorazepam and diazepam, with peak brain levels being reached in 20–60 minutes. Slow intravenous bolus infusion of 20–25 mg/kg is suggested initially. Repeated 10–20-mg/kg doses may be necessary to be successful.[1,2,87] Principal side effects are hypotension and respiratory and sensorial depression. Phenobarbital should be administered by intravenous push at a rate no faster than 100 mg/min. In the Veterans Administration cooperative study, phenobarbital was just as efficacious in treating SE as was lorazepam and lorazepam plus PHT and was a better first drug (regimen) than PHT alone.[55]

Fosphenytoin

FOS has replaced injectable PHT at many institutions because of its safety advantages. This prodrug is nearly 100% bioavailable and, unlike its product, PHT, is freely soluble in aqueous solutions.[88] Given intravenously, FOS is rapidly converted to PHT by phosphatases in the bloodstream. PHT then enters the brain, reaching peak brain levels at 15 minutes.[89,90] FOS is an excellent agent for the treatment of convulsive SE, both partial and generalized, but it is ineffective in the treatment of absence status.[1,2] A marked advantage is that it does not depress respiration as do other drugs in this situation.[1,65]

The dose is prescribed as milligrams of PHT equivalents (PE). In young children, the initial intravenous FOS dose should be 15–25 mg PE/kg.[65] In adolescents and adults, a PHT dose of 18 mg PE/kg provides initial serum PHT levels greater than 25 µg/ml and is effective in maintaining serum levels of 10 µg/ml for 24 hours.[91] Cardiac conduction disturbances have not been seen with FOS, and hypotension is rare with infusion rates up to 150 mg PE/minute.[92] According to data from animal and human studies, most systemic adverse effects are due to the derived PHT, and so the most common CNS effects include nystagmus, headache, ataxia, and somnolence. Intramuscular administration of FOS at doses from 10–20 mg PE/kg may allow for treatment in the field or when no intravenous access is present, potentially allowing for more rapid seizure control.

Therapeutic blood levels can be attained in 20–30 minutes intramuscular injection of FOS but not PHT.[93,94]

Although it has many advantages over PHT (intramuscular route, safe when the intravenous site infiltrates, faster rates of administration, and lack of solvent, cardiosuppressive effects), FOS is not available in all facilities. Where it is available, it should be substituted for PHT for the treatment of SE.

Phenytoin

PHT is an excellent agent for treating convulsive SE, both partial and generalized, but it is not indicated in the treatment of absence status.[1,2] After intravenous administration, PHT reaches peak brain levels at 15 minutes.[89,90] A marked advantage of PHT is lack of respiratory depression.[1,2] As demonstrated by the Veterans Administration study, PHT is best administered in combination with a benzodiazepine, to assure a rapid anticonvulsant effect, followed by the long-lasting efficacy of PHT.[55] Because of hypotension and cardiac conduction disturbances, primarily in adults or children with preexisting cardiac disease, ECG monitoring should be conducted during the drug's administration.[1,2,65] The rate of infusion should be less than 50 mg per minute in adults or 25 mg per minute in children and the elderly. Intravenous injection should be directly into the vein or intravenous line close to venous access, because precipitation is likely to occur in most intravenous solutions. Intramuscular administration of PHT is discouraged because of crystallization, muscle destruction, and unpredictable absorption.[94]

Pentobarbital

Pentobarbital is used at many institutions for refractory SE. After administration of a loading dose of 20 mg/kg, 1–2 mg/kg per hour is given intravenously to maintain the serum level at 20–40 µg/ml to produce electrographic suppression or a burst suppression pattern. Pentobarbital's half-life is approximately 20 hours. Most authorities stop pentobarbital coma at 24–48 hours to determine whether SE subsides.[95] At levels exceeding 40 µg/

ml, cardiac output and blood pressure are compromised. Refractory SE requiring coma induction with pentobarbital or other anesthetic agents to produce EEG suppression is associated with a higher rate of morbidity and mortality.[96]

Other Agents

In cases of SE that are resistant to benzodiazepines, phenobarbital, and PHT, paraldehyde previously was used.[2] Paraldehyde intravenous solution no longer is commercially available in the United States, but a rectal solution sometimes still is used. For rectal administration, a 2 to 1 paraldehyde oil (vegetable or peanut) mixture is administered at 0.3 ml/kg per dose, with doses repeated every 2–4 hours.[97] Intravenous lidocaine may alternatively be used for the treatment of SE. No large, double-blind, placebo-controlled studies of lidocaine's efficacy are available; however, numerous case reports and case series suggest an initial bolus of 1–3 mg/kg followed by slow infusion of 4–10 mg/kg per hour.[98] The principal side effect is cardiovascular dysfunction. As levels of lidocaine elevate, paradoxical convulsions may occur.

In addition to lidocaine, other anesthetic agents have been used for seizure and EEG suppression.[1,2] The foremost is propofol, and its use in the treatment of refractory SE has recently been reviewed.[99] Propofol seems no more efficacious than other second-line agents for ultimate control of prolonged seizures but, as compared with high-dose barbiturate therapy, seizure control is attained more rapidly.[100] This promising property of propofol is offset in children, however, by two drawbacks: The metabolism of this drug is exceedingly rapid, and escalating doses are required to maintain adequate blood levels, without which breakthrough seizures and SE are common. In addition, severe metabolic acidosis and rhabdomyolysis may occur.[101]

Intravenous valproic acid may be given to patients with epilepsy when it is not possible to maintain concentrations of this agent by the oral route. Although no multicenter, controlled trials of intravenous valproate in SE are known, two small studies have reported improvement in patients with diazepam-resistant SE.[56,102] Another small open study demonstrated control of seizures

within 20 minutes in more than 80% of patients.[103] Doses in these studies of seizures and SE usually were an IV bolus of 15 mg/kg, followed by continuous or intermittent infusions at rates of 0.5–1.0 mg/kg per hour. We recommend doses of 20–30 mg/kg, administering the available valproic acid for intravenous use diluted 1 to 1 at a rate of 6 mg/kg per minute for rapid replacement or in cases in which seizures are refractory to other therapies.[56,65,104] Steady-state concentrations exceeding 50 mg/liter have been reported after administration of intravenous valproic acid, 15 mg/kg, followed 1–3 hours later by either intravenous valproic acid or sustained-release oral divalproex sodium, 7 mg/kg every 8 hours or 4 mg/kg every 6 hours. When valproic acid concentrations must be maintained above 100 mg/liter, the drug may have to be infused every 4 hours.[56] When oral valproic acid is to follow intravenous loading, it must be given soon after the intravenous dose is administered.[105] Experience with the use of intravenous valproic acid is growing because of the lack of association with cardiovascular compromise, which is frequently a limiting factor when barbiturates, PHT, or other sedative drugs are used.

Discussions concerning the optimal or first-choice drug therapy of SE examine morbidity, mortality, and the practical issues of drug administration and adverse effects. As Holmes[64] recently concluded, no one drug of choice may be acceptable to all clinicians. Lorazepam, diazepam, midazolam, PHT, and phenobarbital are all useful agents for both the initial and continued treatment of SE.[87,106,107] Thus, one's choice of the initial and subsequent medications for the treatment of SE may depend on individual patient characteristics, prior AED therapy, and physician preference. Most important, a protocol should be established so that prompt and appropriate emergency treatment can be given in an efficient manner.[4] The use of intravenous valproic acid in SE is currently being better defined, as are the roles for alternate forms of administering benzodiazepines.

Medical Complications of Status Epilepticus

The treatment of SE requires close monitoring of physiologic variables and excellent nursing to

Table 9-8. Medical Complications of Status Epilepticus

Tachycardia
Bradycardia
Cardiac arrhythmia
Cardiac arrest
Conduction disturbance
Congestive heart failure
Hypertension
Hypotension
Altered respiratory pattern
Pulmonary edema
Pneumonia
Oliguria
Uremia
Renal tubular necrosis
Lower nephron nephrosis
Rhabdomyolysis
Increased creatine phosphokinase
Myoglobinuria
Apnea
Anoxia
Hypoxia
CO_2 narcosis
Intravascular coagulation
Metabolic and respiratory acidosis
Cerebral edema
Excessive perspiration
Dehydration
Endocrine failure
Altered pituitary function
Elevated prolactin
Elevated vasopressin
Hyperglycemia
Hypoglycemia
Increased plasma cortisol
Autonomic dysfunction
Fever

Source: From DJ Leszczyszyn, JM Pellock. Status Epilepticus. In JM Pellock, WE Dodson, B Bourgeois (eds), Pediatric Epilepsy, Diagnosis and Treatment. New York: Demos, 2000.

prevent secondary complications.[1,2,7,59] Besides the underlying or precipitating disease states associated with SE, subsequent medical complications are common. Pulmonary care, proper positioning, and careful observation of seizures, noting the possible changes in seizure pattern, are mandatory. Frequent surveillance and normalization of glucose and electrolyte levels, particularly in neonates and small infants, is mandatory. Optimal oxygenation and expectant observation and treatment for hyperthermia and other medical complications can reduce morbidity and mortality. Cardiovascular, respiratory, and renal effects may be severe. Medical complications of SE are listed in Table 9-8.

When hyperthermia is resistant to rectally administered antipyretics and cooling blankets, muscular blockade may be necessary. EEG monitoring is a necessity when such blockade is performed. A rise in blood pressure consistently accompanies seizures but rarely requires antihypertensive medication unless the child is at risk for malignant hypertension. Treatment may result in hypotension and reduce cerebral perfusion pressure. Cerebral edema or increased intracranial pressure rarely becomes problematic during most cases of SE not associated with an intracranial mass. Therefore, the use of osmotic diuretics and steroids rarely is indicated in the routine treatment of SE.

Nonconvulsive Status Epilepticus

Convulsive generalized tonic-clonic SE may evolve into NCSE or subtle SE either without treatment as part of its natural history or due to partially successful drug treatment. The incidence of post-treatment subtle SE has been placed as high as 48% in patients requiring intensive care unit management.[1,8,9] The mortality in such cases has been difficult to isolate from the associated acute medical illnesses but ranges from 33% to 52%, rising well above that for the SE population as a whole. Similarly, cases of NCSE may present as coma or stupor in the emergency department or in the intensive care setting.[9] Multifactorial analysis does suggest, however, that the morbidity and mortality in this group is most closely correlated with the delay in time to diagnosis (duration of seizure) and also with serum levels of neuron-specific enolase.[43,44] Treatment of subtle SE is identical to that of refractory SE, and the central theme to improving outcome is early recognition and intensive EEG monitoring.

In addition to postconvulsive subtle seizures, NCSE also presents as prolonged complex partial, absence, myoclonic, or atonic seizures. These confusional or fugue states are a separate entity from the previously described subtle SE and may be more common in the elderly. Childhood conditions with periods of frequently occurring seizures that meet the definition of SE include the syndromes of West (infantile spasms or hypsarrhythmia), Lennox-Gastaut, Landau-Kleffner, childhood absence (pyknolepsy), continuous spike and wave during sleep, and continuous occipital spike and wave during sleep.[2] Further, neonatal seizures with their various subtle and sometimes variable symptomatology sometimes may represent SE. Specific etiologies should always be considered in these cases.

EEG monitoring reveals continuous or noncontinuous, generalized, symmetric, or diffuse and irregular 1.5- to 4.0-Hz multispike and wave complexes in absence status, as opposed to the partial discharges seen in SE due to complex partial seizures.[1,7] Clinically, a child in absence status usually demonstrates partial responsiveness with confusion, disorientation, speech arrest, amnesia, and, sometimes, automatisms.[108] Total unresponsiveness with stereotyped automatisms usually is lacking in absence status. Complex partial SE is more likely to be fluctuating, sometimes with nearly cyclic impairment of consciousness, including total unresponsiveness and more complex stereotyped automatisms, with wandering eye movements or eye deviations.[109,110]

The therapy for complex partial SE is similar to that noted earlier for convulsive SE. For absence status, intravenous lorazepam or diazepam is excellent. This medication should then be followed quickly by intravenous valproic acid or oral, nasogastric, or rectal doses of ethosuximide or clonazepam. Rarely, combined administration of valproic acid and clonazepam may produce absence status. Some children with the Lennox-Gastaut syndrome have seizures that are exacerbated by benzodiazepines.[87] Case reports demonstrate the response of refractory partial SE to clobazam[111] and the response of refractory absence SE to propofol or intravenous valproic acid.[112,113] Respiratory support is less problematic in NCSE than in convulsive forms; however, some patients have difficulties handling secretions in their "twilight state" or spike and wave stupor.

Conclusion

Similar to other seizure types, SE represents a symptom of CNS dysfunction. However, it signifies

severe malfunction. The etiology of SE must be sought because the highest percentage of SE is symptomatic, particularly in young children and the elderly. Furthermore, SE is more common in those with mental retardation, multiple handicaps, and refractory epilepsy. Judicious use of routine laboratory tests coupled with neuroradiologic studies and lumbar puncture should be employed in most patients. Those patients who remain in prolonged coma may harbor a disease such as intracranial hemorrhage, meningitis, or encephalitis, or may be continuing in SE although the symptoms seem subtle. In general, such patients have a poorer prognosis as do all those with prolonged or uncontrollable SE. Recent studies dispute the prior morbidity and mortality figures for SE at approximately two-thirds, but mortality rates at 20–30% for adults continue, and morbidity is significant. A better prognosis seems possible if seizures are controlled rapidly while optimal support is given. Prompt recognition of medical complications and treatment of concomitant diseases further improve outcome in all patients with SE. A plan should be developed to provide a standard approach and algorithms at each institution and in each setting to allow optimal and prompt care.

References

1. Pellock JM, DeLorenzo RJ. Status Epilepticus. In RJ Porter, D Chadwick (eds), The Epilepsies, vol 2. Boston: Butterworth–Heinemann, 1997;267.
2. Leszczyszyn DJ, Pellock JM. Status Epilepticus. In JM Pellock, WE Dodson, B Bourgeois (eds), Pediatric Epilepsy, Diagnosis and Treatment. New York: Demos, 2000.
3. Treiman DM. Generalized Convulsive Status Epilepticus. In J Engel, TA Pedley (eds), Epilepsy: A Comprehensive Textbook. Philadelphia: Lippincott–Raven, 1997;669–680.
4. Dodson WE, DeLorenzo RJ, Pedley TA, et al. For the Epilepsy Foundation of America's Working Group on Status Epilepticus. Treatment of convulsive status epilepticus. JAMA 1993;270:854.
5. Pellock JM. Status epilepticus: update and review. J Child Neurol 1994;9[Suppl 2]:S27–S35.
6. Towne AR, Pellock JM, Ko D, et al. Determinants of mortality in status epilepticus. Epilepsia 1994;35:27.
7. Treiman DM. Status Epilepticus. In J Laidlaw, A Richems, D Chadwick (eds), A Textbook of Epilepsy. Edinburgh: Churchill Livingstone, 1993;205.
8. DeLorenzo RJ, Waterhouse EJ, Towne AR, et al. Persistent nonconvulsive status epilepticus after the con-

trol of convulsive status epilepticus. Epilepsia 1998;39:833–840.

9. Towne AR, Waterhouse EJ, Boggs JG, et al. Prevalence of nonconvulsive status epilepticus in comatose patients. Neurology 2000;54(2):340–345.

10. Simon RP, Pellock JM, DeLorenzo RJ. Acute Morbidity and Mortality of Status Epilepticus. In J Engel, TA Pedley (eds), Epilepsy: A Comprehensive Textbook. Philadelphia: Lippincott–Raven, 1997;741–753.

11. Lowenstein DH, Bleck T, Macdonald RL. It's time to revise the definition of status epilepticus. Epilepsia 1999;40:120–122.

12. Gastaut H. Classification of Status Epilepticus. In AV Delgado-Escueta, RJ Porter, CG Wasterlain (eds), Status Epilepticus: Mechanisms of Brain Damage and Treatment. New York: Raven Press, 1982.

13. DeLorenzo RJ, Garnett L, Towne AR, et al. Comparison of status epilepticus with prolonged seizure episodes lasting from 10 to 29 minutes. Epilepsia 1999;40:164–169.

14. DeLorenzo RJ, Towne AR, Pellock JM, et al. Status epilepticus in children, adults, and the elderly. Epilepsia 1992;33[Suppl 4]:S15.

15. Delgado-Escueta AV, Treiman DM. Focal Status Epilepticus: Modern Concepts. In H Luders, RP Lesser (eds), Epilepsy Electroclinical Syndromes. London: Springer, 1987;347.

16. Porter RH, Penry JK. Petit Mal Status. In AV Delgado-Escueta, CG Wasterlain, et al. (eds), Status Epilepticus: Mechanisms of Brain Damage and Treatment. New York: Raven Press, 1983;61.

17. Lockman LA. Treatment of status epilepticus in children. Neurology 1990;40:43–46.

18. Shinnar S, Pellock JM, Moshé SL, et al. In whom does status epilepticus occur? Epilepsia 1997;38:907–914.

19. Corey LA, Pellock JM, Boggs JG, et al. Evidence for a genetic predisposition for status epilepticus. Neurology 1998;50:558–560.

20. Maytal J, Shinnar S, Moshé SL, Alvarez LA. Low-morbidity and mortality of status epilepticus in children. Pediatrics 1989;83:323–331.

21. Driscoll SM, Jack RE, Teasley JE, et al. Mortality in childhood status epilepticus. Ann Neurol 1988;24: 318.

22. Driscoll SM, Pellock JM, Towne A, et al. Recurrent status epilepticus in children. Neurology 1990;40:14[Suppl 1]:297.

23. Hauser WA, Rich SS, Annegars JF, et al. Seizure recurrence after a first unprovoked seizure: an extended follow-up. Neurology 1990;40:1163.

24. Sillanpaa M, Jalava M, Shinnar S. Status epilepticus in a population-based cohort with childhood-onset epilepsy in Finland. Epilepsia 1998:39[Suppl 6]:219–220.

25. Hesdorffer D, Logroscino G, Cascino G, et al. Risk of unprovoked seizure after acute symptomatic seizure: effect of status epilepticus. Ann Neurol 1998:44;908–912.

26. Shinnar S, Pellock JM, Berg AT, et al. An inception cohort of children with febrile status epilepticus:

cohort characteristics and early outcomes [abstract]. Epilepsia 1995;36[Suppl 4]:31.

27. DeLorenzo RJ, Pellock JM, Towne AR, et al. Pathophysiology of status epilepticus. J Clin Neurol 1995;12:316.

28. Morton LD, Watemberg NM, Driscoll-Bannister S, et al. Long-term outcome of status epilepticus in the first year of life [abstract]. Epilepsia 1998;39[Suppl 6]:220.

29. Berg AT, Shinnar S, Levy SR, et al. Status epilepticus in children with newly diagnosed epilepsy. Ann Neurol 1999;45:618–623.

30. Goulden KJ, Shinnar S, Koller H, et al. Epilepsy in children with mental retardation: a cohort study. Epilepsia 1991;32:690–697.

31. Pellock JM, Hunt PA. A decade of modern epilepsy therapy in institutionalized mentally retarded patients. Epilepsy Res 1996;25:263–268.

32. Steffenbeurg U, Hedstrom A, Lindroth A, et al. Intractable epilepsy in a population-based series of mentally retarded children. Epilepsia 1998;39(7):767–775.

33. Kwan P, Brodie MJ. Early identification of refractory epilepsy. N Engl J Med 2000;342(5):314–319.

34. Dunn W. Status epilepticus in children: etiology, clinical features, and outcome. J Child Neurol 1988;3:167.

35. Phillips SA, Shanahan RJ. Etiology and mortality of status epilepticus in children. Arch Neurol 1989;46:74–76.

36. Moshé SL. Brain injury with prolonged seizures in children and adults. J Child Neurol 1998;13[Suppl 1]:S3–S6.

37. Thompson K, Wasterlain C. The model of status epilepticus that produces neuronal necrosis in the immature brain. Neurology 1994;44:A272.

38. Rice AC, DeLorenzo RJ. Kindling Induces Long-Term Changes in Gene Expression. In M Cocoran, SL Moshé (eds), Kindling, vol 5. New York: Plenum, 1998;267–284.

39. Boggs JG, Painter JA, DeLorenzo RJ. Analysis of electrocardiographic changes in status epilepticus. Epilepsy Res 1993;14:87–94.

40. Liu Z, Gatt A, Mikati M, et al. Effect of temperature on kainic acid-induced seizures. Brain Res 1993;631:51–58.

41. Aicardi JF, Chevrie JJ. Convulsive status epilepticus in infants and children: a study of 239 cases. Epilepsia 1987;11:187.

42. Whitty CWM. Status Epilepticus. In JH Tryer (ed), The Treatment of Epilepsy. Philadelphia: Lippincott, 1980.

43. Young GB, Jordan KG, Dolg GS. An assessment of nonconvulsive seizures in the intensive care unit using continuous EEG monitoring: an investigation of variables associated with mortality. Neurology 1996;47:83–89.

44. DeGiorgio CM, Heck CN, Rabinowicz AL, et al. Serum neuron-specific enolase in the major subtypes of status epilepticus. Neurology 1999;52:746–749.

45. Calabrese VP, Gruemer HD, James K, et al. Cerebrospinal fluid lactate levels and prognosis in status epilepticus. Epilepsia 1991;32:816–821.

46. Barry E, Hauser WA. Pleocytosis after status epilepticus. Arch Neurol 1994;51:190–193.

47. Rider LG, Thapa PB, Del Beccaro MA, et al. Cerebrospinal fluid analysis in children with seizures. Pediatr Emerg Care 1995;11:226–229.

48. Chan S, Chin SS, Kartha K, et al. Reversible signal abnormalities in the hippocampus and neocortex after prolonged seizures. Am J Neuroradiol 1996;17:1725–1731.

49. Juhasz C, Scheidl E, Szirmai I. Reversible focal MRI abnormalities due to status epilepticus. An EEG, single photon emission computed tomography, transcranial Doppler follow-up study. Electroencephalogr Clin Neurophysiol 1998;107:402–407.

50. Fazekas F, Kapeller P, Schmidt R, et al. Magnetic resonance imaging and spectroscopy findings after focal status epilepticus. Epilepsia 1995;36:946–949.

51. van Landingham KE, Heinz ER, Cavazos, JE, Lewis DV. Magnetic resonance imaging evidence of hippocampal injury after prolonged focal febrile convulsions. Ann Neurol 1998;43(4):413–426.

52. Shinnar S. Prolonged febrile seizures and mesial temporal sclerosis. Ann Neurol 1998;43(4):411–412.

53. Waterhouse EJ, Vaughan JK, Barnes TY, et al. Synergistic effect of status epilepticus and ischemic brain injury on mortality. Epilepsy Res 1998;29:175–183.

54. Epilepsy Foundation of America. Seizure Recognition and First Aid. Landover, MD: Epilepsy Foundation of America, 1989.

55. Treiman DM, Meyers PD, Walton NY, et al. A comparison of our treatments for generalized convulsive status epilepticus. Veterans Affairs Status Epilepticus Cooperative Study Group. N Engl J Med 1998; 339:792–798.

56. Morton LD, Towne AR, Garnett LK, et al. Safety and efficacy of intravenous valproate in status epilepticus. Epilepsia 2000;41[Suppl 7]:252.

57. Pellock JM, Myer EC, eds. Neurologic emergencies in infancy and childhood (2nd ed). New York: Butterworth, 1993.

58. Orlowski JP, Porembha DT, Gallagher BB, et al. Comparison study of intraosseous, central intravenous and peripheral intravenous infusions of emergency drugs. Am J Dis Child 1990;144:112–117.

59. Leppik WA. Status epilepticus: the next decade. Neurology 1990;40[Suppl]:4–9.

60. Jaitly R, Sgro JA, Towne AR, et al. Prognostic value of EEG monitoring after status epilepticus: a prospective adult study. J Clin Neurophysiol 1997;14:326–334.

61. Alehan FK, Morton LD, Pellock JM. Electroencephalogram in the pediatric emergency department: is it useful [abstract]? J Child Neurol 2001;16(in press). AAN Annual Conference Supplement.

62. Nei M, Lee JM, Shanker VL, et al. The EEG and prognosis in status epilepticus. Epilepsia 1999;40:157–163.

63. Boggs JG, Marmarou A, Agnew JP, et al. Hemodynamic monitoring prior to and at the time of death in status epilepticus. Epilepsy Res 1998;31:199–209.

64. Holmes GL. Drug of choice for status epilepticus. I Epilepsy 1990;3:1.

65. Morton LD, Pellock JM. Treatment Options for Acute Seizure Care. In G Mallarkey, KJ Palmer (eds), Issues in Epilepsy. Auckland, NZ: Adis International, 1999;29–41.

66. Treiman DM. The role of benzodiazepines in the management of status epilepticus. Neurology 1990;40 [Suppl]:32–42.

67. Chamberlain J, Alterieri M, Futterman C, et al. A prospective, randomized study comparing intramuscular midazolam with intravenous diazepam for treatment of seizures in children. Pediatr Emerg Care 1997;13:92–94.

68. Wallace S. Nasal benzodiazepines for management of acute childhood seizures? Lancet 1997;25:222.

69. Scott RC, Besag FMC, Neville BGR. Buccal midazolam and rectal diazepam for treatment of prolonged seizures in childhood and adolescence: a randomized trial. Lancet 1999;353:623–626.

70. Homan RW, Unwin DH. Benzodiazepines: Lorazepam. In RH Levy, FE Dreifuss, RH Mattson, et al. (eds), Antiepileptic Drugs (3rd ed). New York: Raven Press, 1989;849–854.

71. Crawford TO, Mitchell WG, Snodgrass SR. Lorazepam in childhood status epilepticus and serial seizures: effectiveness and tachyphylaxis. Neurology 1987;37:190–195.

72. Deshnukh A, Wittert W, Schnitzler E, Margutten HH. Lorazepam in the treatment of refractory neonatal seizures. Am J Dis Child 1986;140:1042–1044.

73. Graing DW, McBride MC. Lorazepam versus diazepam for the treatment of status epilepticus. Pediatr Neurol 1988;4:358–361.

74. Lacey DJ, Singer WD, Horwitz SJ, Gilmore H. Lorazepam therapy of status epilepticus in children and adolescents. J Pediatr 1986;198:771–774.

75. Levy RJ, Krall RL. Treatment of status epilepticus with lorazepam. Arch Neurol 1984;41:605–611.

76. Relling MV, Mulhern RK, Dodge RK, et al. Lorazepam pharmacodynamics and pharmacokinetics in children. J Pediatr 1989;114:641–646.

77. Graves NM, Kriel RL. Rectal administration of antiepileptic drugs in children. Pediatr Neurol 1987;3:321–326.

78. Enrile-Bacsal F, Delgado-Escueta AV. IV Diazepam Drip in Tonic-Clonic Status Epilepticus. In AV Delgado-Escueta, RJ Porter, CG Wasterlain (eds), Status Epilepticus: Mechanisms of Brain Damage and Treatment. New York: Raven Press, 1982.

79. Dreifuss F, Rosman N, Cloyd J, et al. A comparison of rectal diazepam gel and placebo for acute repetitive seizures. N Engl J Med 1998;338:1869–1875.

80. Cereghino JJ, Mitchell W, Murphy J, et al. Treating repetitive seizures with a rectal diazepam formulation: a randomized study. The North American Diastat Study Group. Neurology 1998;51:1274–1282.

81. Pellock JM. Management of acute seizure episodes. Epilepsia 1998;39[Suppl 1]:S28–S35.
82. Egli M, Albani C. Relief of status epilepticus after IM administration of the new short-acting benzodiazepine midazolam (Dormicum) (abstract 137). In Program and Abstracts of the Twelfth World Congress of Neurology. Princeton: Excerpta Medica, 1981;44.
83. Bebin M, Bleck TP. New anticonvulsant drugs. Focus on flunarizine, fosphenytoin, midazolam, and stiripentol. Drugs 1994;48:153–171.
84. Pellock JM. Use of midazolam for refractory status epilepticus in pediatric patients. J Child Neurol 1998;13:581–587.
85. Greenblatt D, Abernathy D, Locniskar A, et al. Effect of age, gender, and obesity on midazolam kinetics. Anesthesiology 1984;61:27–35.
86. Lombroso CT. The treatment of status epilepticus. Pediatrics 1974;53:536–542.
87. Shaner DM, McCurdy SA, Herring MO, Gabor AJ. Treatment of status epilepticus: a prospective comparison of diazepam and phenytoin versus phenobarbital and optional phenytoin. Neurology 1988;38:202–207.
88. Quon C, Stampfi, H. In-vitro hydrolysis of ACC-9653 (phosphate ester prodrug of phenytoin) by human, dog, rat blood and tissues (abstract). Pharmacol Res 1987;3[Suppl]:1349.
89. Wilder BJ, Ramsay RE, Hillmore U, et al. Efficacy of intravenous phenytoin in the treatment of status epilepticus: kinetics of central nervous system penetration. Ann Neurol 1977;1:511–518.
90. Ramsey RE, Hammond EJ, Perchalski RJ, et al. Brain uptake of phenytoin, phenobarbital and clonazepam. Arch Neurol 1979;36:535–539.
91. Cranford RE, Leppick IE, Patrick B, et al. Intravenous phenytoin: clinical and pharmacokinetic aspects. Neurology 1979;29:1474–1479.
92. Eldon M, Loewen G, Voightman R, et al. Pharmacokinetics and tolerance of fosphenytoin and phenytoin administration intravenously to healthy subjects. Can J Neurol Sci 1993;20:5180.
93. Knapp LE, Kugler AR. Clinical experience with fosphenytoin in adults: pharmacokinetics, safety, and efficacy. J Child Neurol 1998;13[Suppl 1]:S15–S18.
94. Wilensky AJ, Lowden JA. Inadequate serum levels after intramuscular administration of diphenylhydantoin. Neurology 1973;23:318–321.
95. Raskin MC, Younger C, Penowish P. Pentobarbital treatment of refractory status epilepticus. Neurology 1987;37:500–503.
96. van Ness PC. Pentobarbital and EEG burst suppression in treatment of status epilepticus refractory to benzodiazepines and phenytoin. Epilepsia 1990;31:61–67.
97. Shields WD. Status epilepticus. Pediatr Clin North Am 1989;36:383–393.
98. Walker I, Slovis C. Lidocaine in the treatment of status epilepticus. Acad Emerg Med 1997;4:918–922.
99. Brown LA, Levin GM. Role of propofol in refractory status epilepticus. Ann Pharmacother 1998;32:1053–1059.
100. Stecker MM, Kramer TH, Raps EC, et al. Treatment of refractory status epilepticus with propofol: clinical and pharmacokinetic findings. Epilepsia 1998;39:18–26.
101. Hanna JP, Ramundo ML. Rhabdomyolysis and hypoxia associated with prolonged propofol infusion in children. Neurology 1998;50:301–303.
102. Price DJ. Intravenous valproate: experience in neurosurgery. R Soc Med Int Cong Symp Ser 1989;152:197–203.
103. Marlow N, Cooke RWI. Intravenous sodium valproate in the neonatal intensive care unit. R Soc Med Int Cong Symp Ser 1989;152:208–210.
104. Wheless J, Venkataraman V. Safety of high intravenous valproate doses in epilepsy patients. J Epilepsy 1999;11:319–324.
105. Cavanaugh JH, Hussein Z, Lamm J, et al. Effect of multiple oral dose divalproex sodium after intravenous loading dose administration in healthy volunteers. Drug Invest 1994;7:1–7.
106. Gabor AJ. Lorazepam versus phenobarbital: candidates for drug of choice for treatment of status epilepticus. J Epilepsy 1990;3:3–6.
107. Mitchell WG, Crawford TO. Lorazepam is the treatment of choice for status epilepticus. J Epilepsy 1990;3:7–10.
108. Porter RJ, Penry JK. Petit mal status. Adv Neurol 1987;34:61–67.
109. McBride MC, Dooling EC, Oppenheimer IN. Complex partial status epilepticus in young children. Ann Neurol 1981;9:526–530.
110. Treiman DM, Delgado-Escueta AV. Complex partial status epilepticus. Adv Neurol 1987;34:69–68.
111. Corman C, Guberman A, Benavente O. Clobazam in partial status epilepticus. Seizure 1998;7:243–247.
112. Crouteau D, Shevell M, Rosenblatt B, et al. Treatment of absence status in the Lennox-Gastaut syndrome with propofol. Neurology 1998;51:315–316.
113. Alehan FK, Morton LD, Pellock JM. Treatment of absence status with intravenous valproate. Neurology 1999;52:889–890.

Part III

Associated Disorders and Their Treatment

Chapter 10

Developmental Speech, Language, and Communication Problems among Children with Epilepsy

Renée Toueg

Communication disorders affect a significant proportion of our population. In the last year before the beginning of the new millennium, the American Speech-Language-Hearing Association[1] reported that 17% of the people in the United States have some kind of communication disorder. Specifically, it has been approximated that 11% have a hearing loss and 6% have a speech, voice, or language disorder. Of children who are preschoolers or who are first developing speech and language, 8–12% exhibit language disorders. In 1986, the vast majority of individuals with traumatic brain injury were reported to exhibit dysarthria (a weakness, incoordination, or paralysis of the speech mechanism that interferes along a continuum with the intelligibility of speech) that may impair communication.[2]

Communication is the use of verbal (speech, reading, writing, listening) and nonverbal language (gestures, facial expression, pictures, and signs). Communication is a basic and vital part of life, allowing us to (1) maintain contact with others, (2) gain information, (3) give information, and (4) accomplish goals. When an impairment exists in the ability to receive, send, process, or comprehend verbal, nonverbal, or graphic symbols,[3] then a *communication disorder* is said to exist. A *language disorder* is more specifically defined as an impairment in the comprehension or use of spoken, written, or other symbol systems.[4] It may involve a combination of the form of the language (e.g., the phonology and the syntax of the utterance), the content or semantics of language, and

the use of language (how we use language to interact with others in a social context). Communication with oral language involves the use of speech.

Speech can be defined as a verbal means of communicating or conveying meaning via the sounds of language. A *speech disorder* is defined as a disruption in any of the elements that add meaning to the sound system, such as sound combinations, voice quality, intonation, rhythm, and rate.

Epilepsy is not necessarily associated with speech, language, and communication disorders. Many children who experience seizures do not experience disruptions in their communicative growth. Their language function may be disrupted only during the seizure or the ictal state or in the immediate postictal period. The speech-language pathologist is concerned with the evaluation and treatment of only interictal (between seizures) language difficulties or deficits.[5]

Interictal language and communication difficulties seen in children with epilepsy may be affected by a variety of factors including the following:

1. *The frequency of the seizures*: The time between the interictal periods is important in relation to the learning of speech and language and the opportunities for communication to occur. When seizures occur frequently, less environmental and internal stimulation occur and, as a result, learning can be delayed or suppressed.

Table 10-1. Antiepileptic Drugs and Their Effects on Speech, Language, and Communication

General effects
  Cognitive and linguistic difficulties
  Difficulty in retaining and recalling information and
    symbols
  Difficulty with problem solving
  Concreteness in thinking: not being able to generalize
    symbols and information into other contexts
  Word retrieval difficulties: not being able to retrieve, at a
    given moment, a word from the mental lexicon
  Producing paraphasic errors (i.e., a problem with the
    selection of words or sounds)
    Literal paraphasia: substitution of a word that basically
      has the same sound elements (e.g., "I have roubles/
      troubles")
    Semantic paraphasia: substitution of a word that is
      generally within the same category as the desig-
      nated word (e.g., *yes* for *no*, and vice versa)
Speech difficulties
  Slurred speech or imprecision of the articulators
  Decreased rate of speech due to impreciseness of articu-
    lators and amount of time needed for the articulators to
    move from one target area to another
  Disfluencies and reformulations: discoordination of the
    articulators and difficulty with linguistic organization
    and formulation
Nonverbal behaviors contributing to speech and language
    delay
  Drooling, due to poor mobility of the lips to effect clo-
    sure; possibly due also to decreased sensory feedback
    and monitoring of the tongue movements and pooling
    of saliva
  Hyperactivity leading to poor attending abilities for con-
    sistent speech and language development
  Drowsiness
  Depression or the lack of motivation to engage in inter-
    acting with linguistic and physical environment
  Irritability
  Dizziness

Source: Adapted from O Devinsky, A Guide to Understanding and Living with Epilepsy. Philadelphia: FA Davis, 1994.

2. *The presence of structural lesions*: Abnormalities in language functioning may be more common when the seizures originate in the dominant side of the brain for speech and language. The temporal lobes are the most common sites of epileptogenicity and therefore are more subject to difficulties with learning and retention of speech and language in young children.[4] Approximately 95% of people who are right-handed have left-sided language localization, whereas 70% of left-handers are left hemisphere–dominant for speech and language.[5] However, in very young children who have sustained left brain injury, language function can be displaced to the nondominant hemisphere or to other parts of the brain.[5]

3. *The presence of subclinical epileptiform discharges*: Electrical discharges may occur even though seizures do not and may disrupt cognitive processes related to speech and language.

4. *Side effects of antiepileptic medications*: The dosage and the type of drug being administered can affect the mental and speech abilities of a child, delaying or disrupting speech and language development. Table 10-1 describes the cognitive and linguistic, speech, and nonverbal behaviors that may be modified as a result of medications.[6]

5. *Psychosocial factors*: Limited opportunities may exist for communication experiences and independence. Owing to the physical or emotional limitations on the part of both the child and the parent or caregiver, the developing child may not be given opportunities to experience and manipulate his or her environment. For the child whose needs are anticipated, sensorimotor experiences will be limited, thereby limiting the accompanying verbal and nonverbal languages that are part of language stimulation.

Medical Syndromes Associated with Both Epilepsy and Speech, Language, and Communication Disorders

Certain medical syndromes in which both epilepsy and speech, language, and communication disorders are predominantly featured have been identified and include Angelman's syndrome, Landau-Kleffner syndrome, Rett syndrome, Rasmussen's syndrome, Lennox-Gastaut syndrome, cerebral palsy, temporal lobe epilepsy, and frontal lobe epilepsy. Specific characteristics of the speech, language, and communication difficulties associated with each of these syndromes are addressed next.

Angelman's Syndrome

Angelman's syndrome, a nonprogressive neurologic disorder, was first reported by Dr. Harry Angelman in 1965. It is characterized by seizures, developmental delays, severe cognitive impairment, oral motor dysfunction, short attention span, and hyperactivity. The level of mental retardation may be related to the severity of the expressive language disorder; many affected children are nonverbal. The characteristically wide mouth (macrostomia), irregularly spaced teeth, tongue thrust, prominent jaw, mouthing, biting, and drooling may specifically contribute to a phonologic and articulatory disorder. In addition, impaired imitative skills may exist that further inhibit verbal and nonverbal language. The short attention span and hyperactivity may additionally confound the speech and language disorder. Children with Angelman's syndrome are typically happy, affectionate, and sociable, and so their communication may not be as impaired as their cognitive, receptive, and expressive language skills. They may engage in behaviors that regulate and express their wants and needs, but they will infrequently initiate social interaction. Augmentative communication would be appropriate for these children who cannot express themselves verbally. However, their unusual motor movement patterns—such as hand flapping, fine tremors, and jerky movements—may impair their ability to learn and imitate fine motor movements for cued speech, finger spelling, and certain gestures and signs.[7]

Landau-Kleffner Syndrome

The Landau-Kleffner syndrome is associated with epilepsy and a progressive loss of the understanding of verbal language over days, weeks, and months. Affected children develop speech and language normally for the first 3–7 years, after which time an abrupt interruption occurs in their communication skills. They initially lose their ability to recognize and assign meaning to the auditory signal, even though their auditory acuity is within normal limits.[8] This disruption in auditory coding and processing is known as *word deafness, acquired epileptic aphasia,* or *auditory agnosia.*[9] Because the children no longer experience an auditory-kinesthetic link in their internal and external monitoring of speech and language, expressive language then regresses from complex sentence structures to telegraphic speech, jargon, and difficulties with resonation and articulation. These articulatory and phonologic problems may take the form of simplification processes, such as deletion of final consonants (*ca* for *cat*) and juxtaposition of phonemes (*psghetti* for *spaghetti*). These phonologic processes eventually may regress to mutism. Because language and communication were developing normally prior to the epileptic seizures, the children become confused, frightened, and frustrated about their inability to comprehend and produce language and, as a result, hyperactivity, social isolation, aggressiveness, and poor attending behaviors are noted. Aphasia does not affect cognition but only the understanding and expression of the symbols of verbal language. Nonverbal language may be a viable substitute for continued language development. In older children, the beginning metalinguistic skills of reading and writing may be relatively spared and so these can be avenues for increased language learning and monitoring of the linguistic system.

Rett Syndrome

Rett syndrome, which exclusively affects female youngsters, was first described by Dr. Andreas Rett in 1966 and is characterized by normal development during the first 9–12 months of life. The predominant features of this syndrome are seizures, mental retardation, apraxia of speech, and the inability to program, initiate, and sequence motor movements. In addition, voluntary hand movements are lost.[10] Prior to the neurologic regression, the infants might have engaged in cooing and vocal play behaviors and, possibly, babbling. Thereafter, cognitive speech and language development deteriorate and, after a certain point, abnormal breathing patterns emerge (e.g., hyperventilation, breath holding). These abnormal respiratory patterns interfere further with the production and modulation of the breath stream to drive the energy for speech and expressive language production.

During the beginning stages of the syndrome, fine and gross motor movements deteriorate also, and atrophy of the muscles is common as the child matures. This motor muscle regression impairs the child's ability to swallow adequately, leading to feeding problems or dysphagia and an inability to feed oneself owing to loss of purposeful use of the fingers.[10] This loss of gross and fine motor skills can lead to problems in learning augmentative communication, such as signing of nonverbal language and the use of communication boards and computers. As a result, highly visible pictures and objects may be the most viable medium for language development. Mental retardation reduces the child's ability to think, reason, and comprehend abstract sentence structures and concepts. Therefore, language comprehension is better for functional, concrete vocabulary and for both comprehending and producing simple sentence constructions.[10]

Rasmussen's Syndrome

Rasmussen's syndrome is associated with a slow deterioration of cognitive, language, and speech abilities, especially if the neurologic site is on the dominant side of the brain for language functioning. This syndrome may begin in children between the ages of 14 months and 14 years. A mild hemiparesis may begin as an initial symptom 1–3 years after the onset of epileptic seizures.[11] Because the brain injury may occur any time after linguistic development, aphasia or a disturbance in the understanding or expression of speech and language may occur in the developing child, causing a regression of previously attained language. If children also experience a loss of the tactile and visual areas of sensation, language and speech will be further compromised, as these areas are important in internal and external monitoring and feedback.

Lennox-Gastaut Syndrome

The Lennox-Gastaut syndrome is characterized by mental retardation that ranges from mild to severe and is accompanied by seizures that are difficult to control. These seizures can begin in children between the ages of 1 and 6 years and, in some cases, even later. Important in determining the speech, language, and behavioral development is the amount of control of the seizures, the effect of drugs on the linguistic system, the site of the neurologic injury, and the amount of intellectual impairment involved.[11]

Cerebral Palsy

At least half of the children with cerebral palsy have some difficulty in speaking. The speech may vary on a continuum of oromotor involvement from feeding difficulties and drooling to dysarthria, which involves weakness, incoordination, or paralysis of any of the muscles of articulation, phonation, respiration, and fluency. Prosodics, which involves stress, rate, fluency, volume, and pitch, commonly are affected, as are the sounds of the language. Children with cerebral palsy may be apraxic and display difficulty in programming motor movements for initiating and sequencing of phonemes and syllabic units. Other factors such as intellectual, auditory, visual, and language impairments may complicate the communication disorder.

Approximately 25–35% of children with cerebral palsy also have epilepsy.[12] Mental retardation, ranging from educable to profoundly impaired, can occur among children with cerebral palsy approximately 33% of the time (as opposed to 2% of the time in the general population), resulting in diminished expression and understanding of language as well as the inability to think and reason symbolically. Antiepileptic drugs may further complicate attentional and learning abilities, decreasing consistent speech and language development.

Children who have spasticity have increased muscle tone, perhaps decreased strength of the muscles involved in the speech mechanism, and limited range and direction of motion of the tongue. Therefore, their speech lacks precision and control. After linguistic development begins, those children who have acquired spastic hemiplegia involving their dominant hemisphere for language (after age 18 months to 2 years) may have more significant communication and language difficulties than those children who are prelinguistic in development when the motor difficulties present.[13] Goulden and Hoge[13] write that children at this early age develop language in the opposite hemisphere and do not have major oromotor problems.

Children with athetoid cerebral palsy have problems of consistent voluntary motor movement and experience difficulties with oromotor control. Their speech is characterized by excessive jaw movement, limited tongue mobility, and velopharyngeal insufficiency resulting in impreciseness of phoneme production and nasality. Hearing and auditory discrimination may also be affected, resulting in poor reception and interpretation of the verbal symbol as well as poor internal monitoring of their own speech and lack of generalization. Affected children's rate of speech is decreased, and they stress each syllable equally rather than linking syllables together by generally stressing the first syllable in English. Volume may be low due to decreased subglottal air pressure; hence, voiced phonemes may be devoiced, especially at the end of phrases. Little variety in pitch is noted and, as such, a monotone of the voice is perceived; also, affected children may employ a falsetto pitch, using the upper limit of their vocal range.

Because breath control often depends on proper positioning and good energy levels, fatigue and poor posture may interfere with the resonance and phonation of the sound production. When such children are placed in a supine position, the oral musculature appears to be more relaxed, as it is when humming, singing, and rhyming and, therefore, better breath control may be facilitated.

Children with ataxic cerebral palsy may exhibit defective kinesthetic and tactile feedback of articulatory movements, imprecise production of phonemes, and a decreased rate of speech. Augmentative communication using communication form boards with pictures or writing and low- and high-tech computer devices may be the venue for language and communication development. The pacing board also can aid in development of phonologic and syllabic structures, thus increasing intelligibility of speech. Table 10-2 illustrates the various parameters of speech that are affected when incoordination, paresis, or paralysis occurs within the speech mechanism.

Temporal Lobe Epilepsy

In infants who have incurred an early left hemisphere cerebral injury or a left temporal seizure focus, language function may transfer from the left to the right hemisphere. The presence of dominant temporal lobe seizure foci in the infant during language development usually is associated with a widespread or diverse distribution of the temporal language areas into other areas of the brain.[5] When a chronic temporal seizure focus is present from early childhood, language function may then be displaced from the temporal lobe into the parietal lobe in the dominant left hemisphere or to the right hemisphere. However, interictal language functioning, especially in the area of memory, word retrieval, and emotional responses, may be compromised in some children with chronic temporal lobe seizures.[11]

Table 10-2. Checklist of Dysarthric Speech

Intelligibility				
Intelligible	Fairly intelligible	Unintelligible		
Articulation				
Few sound errors	Some sound errors	Many sound errors		
Segmentation of syllables				
Correct linking of syllables	Omission of syllables	Addition of syllables		
Rate of speech				
Normal	Somewhat slow	Very slow	Fast	
Voice quality				
Within normal limits	Breathy	Hoarse	Harsh	Strained
Pitch				
Normal pitch levels	High pitch	Low pitch	Pitch breaks	Monopitch
Volume				
Normal volume	Loud	Decreased	No variation in volume	
Resonation				
Within normal limits	Nasal	Intermittent nasality	Denasality	
Rhythm				
Normal fluency	Repetitions	Reformulations	Difficulty initiating speech	Equal stress for all syllables

Frontal Lobe Epilepsy

When the motor areas of the frontal lobe are involved with epilepsy, paresis of the muscles of articulation, resonance, and phonation may ensue, resulting in reduced intelligibility of speech and decreased mobility of the speech mechanism.[11] Therefore, comprehension of the verbal symbol may not be impaired—only the expression of oral language, including intelligibility of speech.

Interventions

A plethora of interventions can be applied in the treatment of speech, language, and communication problems. Many of these interventions can be taught to caregivers and applied during daily interactions to enhance language and speech development. The following list reflects a few examples within each domain of communication.

Enhancing Development of Language Comprehension

1. Vocabulary that is functional for the child should be introduced. Talk should center around those objects, people, or places that are meaningful and that exist in the child's environment. The child should be familiar with the labels, actions, and events that are within the immediate domain so that the thoughts that he or she acquires can be conveyed into the medium of language.

2. Gestures and sign language used should supplement verbal input, especially for those children who are not able to use the auditory avenue in an efficient and effective manner. It is imperative that children develop a language system for meaningful communication, and the medium of nonverbal language is a viable accompaniment to or, if need be, a substitute for helping children gain knowledge about their world.

3. The physical and linguistic environment should be structured so as to reduce hyperactivity and increase attention span for consistent learning of the linguistic system. The reduction of extraneous stimuli and ambient noise can be most helpful for those children who are easily distracted and have difficulty focusing on a desired object, subject, or

linguistic utterance. Children need consistency and repetition for language and speech development.

4. Time pressures should be alleviated so as to reduce frustration, aggressiveness, and isolation. When given sufficient time to process information, children are more at ease and receptive to language stimulation.[5] Establishing routines or rote language lends a certain amount of automaticity, thus freeing attentional capacity for processing the content, form, and use of language.[14]

5. Simplified language should be used by the child's conversational partner, and one should pause frequently to decrease processing and memory limitations. Some children experience difficulty in processing auditory, visual, or other sensory stimuli, and so a decreased rate of speech with meaningful pauses will allow time for a message to be relayed to the child's brain for meaningful comprehension. Snow[14] wrote that mothers generally increase pause intervals at sentence and phrase boundaries and use a slower rate of speech when speaking to younger as opposed to older children.

6. Multisensory stimulation should be used to heighten the desired lexical items or concepts. Many children with speech, language, and communication disorders do not have efficient sensory receptors, and so a collection of sensory avenues needs to be applied to heighten and reinforce language. Touching, seeing, hearing, and smelling may be effective means of fostering generalization.

7. Use synonyms, antonyms, descriptions, associations ("grass is green"), or alphabet letters to develop the child's vocabulary.

Enhancing Development of Expressive Language

1. The child's utterances should be expanded so as to impart new vocabulary into the situation of the moment. If the child says, "Mommy ball," the mother could respond with "Mommy throws the ball." This will bring the child's attention to the cohesiveness of language (i.e., the use of other parts of speech). These words may be repeated within various contexts and situations so that the child can generalize the action and develop an awareness that language can represent objects as well as events and relationships.

2. One should speak slowly and clearly so that the child has time to process the language and the

speech sounds. This will also serve as a good model for the child to emulate. This habit is particularly important if the child has a hearing impairment. It affords the youngster an opportunity to see the facial area more distinctly and to attend to the stimuli at hand. This kind of speech has been known in the literature as *Motherese*[14] and functions as a learning tool, even for children who speak to younger children.

3. Emphasis should be placed on designated lexical items by the use of increased duration, volume, or pausing. In overlapping speech, attending to unstressed words such as prepositions, articles, and conjunctions is difficult. In addition, the content words, such as nouns, verbs, and adjectives, may not be heard if there are distractions in the linguistic and physical environment. These suprasegmental parameters of language add extra meaning to the sounds of the language.

4. If a child cannot learn to produce verbal language, gestures, sign language, and pictures can be used to develop vocabulary and linguistic concepts.

5. All verbal and nonverbal attempts and approximations of language production by the child should be reinforced so as to develop and foster greater self-confidence and self-esteem about the child's ability to communicate. Successful communication breeds greater experiences with communication and the motivation to want to interact with one's animate environment.

Enhancing Development of Speech

1. The important phonemes should be emphasized when speaking, such as ends of words, unstressed syllable endings (play*ing*, ba*by's*, eat*s*), and the segmentation of syllables in multisyllabic words (*ra-di-o*). Many children with speech, language, and communication disorders have difficulty attending to the auditory and verbal signal and, if unstressed or low-intensity sounds are part of the speech signal, they will not comprehend or focus on the entire message. By singling out those parts of the auditory signal, the speaker can help to heighten such children's attention, thereby facilitating their imitation of such signals. For those children who cannot imitate very well through one particular sensory avenue (i.e., auditory), other

avenues of stimulation might be tried (e.g., visual, tactile, kinesthetic) and a great deal of repetitiveness employed.

2. One's speech should be clear and include normal inflections. With children who are experiencing difficulty comprehending the auditory signal, eye contact is important, so that the visible parts of speech will be apparent. Vowels and the front sounds, such as /p/, /b/, /f/, /v/, /th/, /w/, /s/, /m/ are most visible and can be more easily imitated than the back sounds, such as /k/, /g/, /y/, /ch/, and /sh/. When the visual and auditory avenues are impaired, feeling vibrations on the neck and nasal areas can aid in differentiating the voiceless and voiced phonemes (e.g., /p/ vs. /b/).

3. Oral motor strengthening and awareness exercises should be paired with some form of speech sound so that the process is more meaningful. When working on tongue strengthening, the child should be asked to produce the tongue tip sounds followed by the universal vowel /ah/ (e.g., /la/, /ta/, /da/, /na/). When attempting to foster greater lip mobility, ask the child to use spread and pucker sounds such as /e/ and /o/. Use of a mirror is beneficial, as is having the child feel his or her lips to obtain a greater sense of proprioception and kinesthetic stimulation.

Enhancing Development of Pragmatic Language

1. Increased eye contact between the speaker and the listener will ensure that the message is transmitted more efficiently and in a cooperative manner. Facial expression and head movements can be very important sources of nonverbal language communication. This will also aid in supplementing the verbal message.[10]

2. Turn-taking skills should be fostered so that the child can experience the communicative act and become an active participant. This discourse act also develops a sense of awareness about communication and encourages positive self-esteem and confidence in the interactive process.

3. Joint attention and joint action skills should be encouraged[10]: for example, "You look at what I do and try to do it." This will aid in the development of imitative skills that are important for motor development and communication.

4. The use of speech acts such as questioning, negating, requesting, and commenting should be

plentiful so as to give the child experience with different ways of communicating his or her thoughts and ideas. Nonverbal language, such as the use of gestures and facial expression, can also express these speech acts.

Summary

Communication is a very important part of life. It permits one to express feelings, thoughts, and needs to another human being. It is an act of sharing on an intellectual, emotional, or motor level. The process of communicating can be accomplished through the use of verbal or nonverbal language. However, the mental, motor, and emotional system must be fairly intact for communication to be efficient and self-satisfying. The environmental surroundings must also be conducive to reinforcing communication.

All the syndromes (or groups of behaviors that differentiate a number of individuals from other individuals)[4] that were discussed in this chapter share the disorder of epilepsy. In all these clinical categories of developmental language disorders, epilepsy affects a child's communication and language development. However, epileptic seizures need not necessarily affect a child's overall communication system: Language and communication may be affected only during the ictal and postictal stage and may not have any other repercussions. However, antiepileptic drugs that are prescribed may have a negative effect on a child's speech mechanism, cognition, and nonverbal behaviors.

The speech and language pathologist can help to plan and implement a program that will help to remedy some of the child's behaviors and can counsel members of the child's environment to aid them in providing a stimulating and satisfying language and communicative space in which the child can grow and reach full potential.

References

1. Castrogiovanni A. Incidence and Prevalence of Speech, Voice and Language Disorders in the United States. Communication Facts. Rockville, MD: American Speech-Language-Hearing Association, 1999.
2. Sarno MT, Buonaguro A, Levita E. Characteristics of verbal impairment in closed head injury. Arch Phys Med Rehab 1986;67:403.
3. Owens RE, Metz DE, Haas A. Introduction to Communication Disorders. Needham Heights, MA: Allyn & Bacon, 2000;14.
4. Lahey M. Language Disorders and Language Development. New York: Macmillan, 1988;5,48.
5. Johnson AF, Jacobson BH. Language and Its Management in the Surgical Epilepsy Patient. In AF Johnson, BH Jacobson (eds), Medical Speech-Language Pathology: A Practitioner's Guide. New York: Thieme Medical, 1998.
6. Devinsky O. Antiepileptic Drug Therapy. In O Devinsky, A Guide to Understanding and Living with Epilepsy. Philadelphia: FA Davis, 1994.
7. Richard GJ, Hoge DR. Angelman Syndrome. In GJ Richard, DR Hoge, The Source for Syndromes. East Moline, IL: Linguisystems, 1999;9–16.
8. Richard GJ, Hoge DR. Landau-Kleffner Syndrome. In GJ Richard, DR Hoge, The Source for Syndromes. East Moline, IL: Linguisystems, 1999;80–88.
9. Nelson N. Childhood Language Disorders in Context: Infancy Through Adolescence (2nd ed). Needham Heights, MA: Allyn & Bacon, 1998;124.
10. Richard GH, Hoge DR. Rett's Syndrome. In GJ Richard, DR Hoge, The Source for Syndromes. East Moline, IL: Linguisystems, 1999;98–106.
11. Devinsky O. Classification of Epileptic Syndromes. In O Devinsky, A Guide to Understanding and Living with Epilepsy. Philadelphia: FA Davis Company, 1994.
12. Devinsky O. Epilepsy, Mental Retardation and Cerebral Palsy. In O Devinsky, A Guide to Understanding and Living with Epilepsy. Philadelphia: FA Davis Company, 1994;220.
13. Goulden KJ, Hoge M. Neurogenic Communication Disorders of Childhood. In AF Johnson, BH Jacobson (eds), Medical Speech-Language Pathology: A Practitioner's Guide. New York: Thieme Medical, 1998;409–419
14. Snow C. Mother's speech to children learning language. Child Dev 1972;43:549–565.

Chapter 11

Augmentative and Alternative Communication Technologies: A Review

Nancy Lenhart Jones, Christine Baudin,
and Charles A. Kincaid

This chapter is designed to give readers an overview of the field of augmentative and alternative communication (AAC) technologies and assessment techniques. The complexity and range of AAC technology has grown considerably over the last 5 years. The authors present current state-of-the art information on AAC. A description and history of AAC, current developments in AAC, and detailed descriptions of devices and assessment techniques are covered.

Definition of Augmentative and Alternative Communication

Beukelman et al.[1] defined AAC as "any approach designed to support, enhance, or augment the communication of individuals who are not independent verbal communicators in all situations" (p. 3). According to the American Speech-Language-Hearing Association,[2] an AAC system is "an integrated group of components, including the symbols, aids, strategies, and techniques used by individuals to enhance communication" (p. 10).

The definition of AAC can be divided into its component parts: *Augmentative* means "to add to, help with, or assist something." *Alternative* means "to be available in place of something." *Communication* is "making known, conveying,

transmitting, exchanging, and/or passing news or information to and from people." In effect, AAC is anything that is used to communicate in place of intelligible speech.

Users of Augmentative and Alternative Communication

Individuals with various types of disabilities and disorders use AAC in their daily lives. Among these are persons with such congenital or developmental conditions as cerebral palsy, mental retardation, epilepsy, severe profound hearing impairment, deafness or blindness, autism, developmental apraxia, developmental aphasia, and Rett syndrome. Individuals with acquired disabilities also use AAC. Among this group are persons who are affected by traumatic brain injury, cerebrovascular accident, spinal cord injury, laryngectomy; glossectomy, and locked-in syndrome. Persons with such progressive neurological diseases such as multiple sclerosis, muscular dystrophy, amyotrophic lateral sclerosis (Lou Gehrig's disease), Parkinson's disease, Huntington's chorea, and the acquired immunodeficiency syndrome also use AAC in their daily lives. Temporary conditions that might necessitate the use of AAC in a person include intubation, tracheotomy, shock, trauma, and the Guillain-Barré syndrome. Any of these conditions may cause dysarthria, anarthria, or an inability to produce vocal output that results in poor speech intelligibility and difficulty in communicating.

History of Augmentative and Alternative Communication

More than 50 million Americans live with disabilities. According to the American Speech-Language-Hearing Association,[2] approximately 2 million Americans are unable to speak sufficiently to meet their communication needs.

A number of AAC techniques are available that range from simple to complex. In fact, many AAC techniques are used by most people everyday, including gesture, body language, vocalizations, facial expressions, handwriting, typing, and, with the computer age, e-mail. When these techniques are insufficient for communicating an intended message, AAC devices may be enlisted to assist a person in conveying a message to others.

Types of Devices

A wide variety of AAC devices—attention-getting devices, communication boards, manual systems, and electronic systems—may be used by individuals with speech impairments to communicate their thoughts and needs to others. An attention-getting device is anything used by a person to gain another person's attention, such as noise, vocalizations, movement, or lights. Some individuals may attempt the use of inappropriate techniques to gain attention (e.g., head banging), but appropriate devices are available to substitute for these techniques (e.g., a beeper or a voice output device).

Communication boards can be found to match an individual's abilities. For example, communication boards may be constructed with concrete objects, pictures, symbols, or the alphabet and certain words. A board can easily be personalized for an individual's unique communication needs or may be activity-specific. The size of a communication board can be reduced or expanded based on a user's communication environment and physical abilities. Communication books may also be used and are highly portable.

Sign language is a manual system of communicating. The higher range of AAC devices includes electronic communication devices, among which are electronic indicators, voice output devices, and speech processors. Electronic indicators present the user with a limited number of word or message choices that are designated by either a flashing light near the selection or a clock-like level pointing to the choice. These devices typically are battery-operated and do not have voice output. Voice output devices use either digitized or synthesized speech to convey messages. *Digitized speech* refers to the recorded voice of another person (in any language) that is converted into a digital format and played back when the device user activates it by either pressing a button directly or flipping a switch connected to the device. Synthesized speech is electronically reproduced speech created through spelling.

Speech processors enhance a person's own speech. Speech processors are used by individuals who are unable to produce a consistent, intelligible volume of speech due to injury or disease. The device clarifies and amplifies a user's voice.

Device Features

Electronic communication devices can be further categorized based on their features, which are numerous. A device's output may be vocal (synthesized or digitized) or visual (message window, liquid crystal display). Printed (visual) output is either incorporated directly within the device or is accessed by attaching a printer.

Message selection techniques vary also. Direct selection may be accomplished by way of a pointer (finger pointing, hand pointer, mouth stick, and head pointer); indicators (electronic selection methods such as a laser-light pointer, an optical indicator, and infrared); or a directional (inverse) device, which is operated by a joystick or switch. With a directional device, a cursor begins to move when a user activates the joystick or switch and, as long as the joystick or switch is activated, the cursor moves through a preset scanning pattern. Selection is made when the user releases the joystick or switch. Another direct selection option is an emulated mouse; using such devices as a Head Mouse (Origin Instruments, Grand Prairie, Texas), Tracker (Madentec, Edmonton, Alberta, Canada), or Head Master (Prentke Romich Company, Wooster, Ohio), an operator can use his or her head movements to control the movement and operation of the mouse cursor. Finally, direct selection may involve *modifications* and *selections*, terms that refer to changes on an electronic device such as keystroke acceptance time, activation and hold-down time, touch-enter, touch-exit, and audio touch.

Choice scanning takes many forms also. If linear, the cursor moves across each item. In circular selection, the cursor moves across each item and repeats for a predetermined number of times until a selection is made. Row and column scanning involves highlighting of first each row and then each item within the column. In quadrant scanning, the entire display is highlighted in four quadrants, then each row, and, finally, each item is highlighted. Group scanning is similar, in that the entire display is highlighted in two, three, or four groups, then each row, and, finally, each item is highlighted. In auto scanning, movement of the cursor is automatic and continuous according to a preset pattern; a user activates a switch to interrupt the cursor to make a selection. Step scanning moves the cursor through a preset selection pattern one step at a time for each activation of a switch; to select an item, the user stops activating the switch for an extended period or activates a second switch that indicates selection of an item displayed. Auditory scanning provides auditory feedback with each communication option (i.e., letters of the alphabet, communication symbols). Items are announced one at a time. Morse code, a dot-dash system of representing the letters of the alphabet, also may be used.

Number and size of the message areas, a fixed versus adjustable choice grid (a fixed device consisting of a set grid and predetermined picture size), and levels of messages available to the user (i.e., grid of 8 messages with 4 levels equals 32 total messages from which to choose) are distinctive features of AAC devices. Levels are incorporated into such devices through the use of overlays

and changeable grids. Different message levels add flexibility to communication devices.

The symbol system used by the device will vary. Open systems allow for additional choices or types of symbols (picture, symbol sets, concrete object), whereas closed systems use a fixed symbol set whose symbols can be combined to produce unique utterances.

Approaches to vocabulary organization are methods for expanding language and increasing the rate of speech output. As previously mentioned, the use of a number of overlays of symbols and text allows the creation of several levels; as overlays are changed, new communication options are created. Sequential coding or abbreviation expansion allows the user to produce several words or a phrase with a few keystrokes. Dynamic display uses page linking, which is similar to a folder system: When a user selects one button or item, it opens up to a new page. Page linking is similar to a menu bar on a software program. Linguistic prediction or semantic compaction capitalizes on the fact that 85% of language needs may be satisfied using only 250 words of core vocabulary. The user of semantic compaction systems is presented with logical word choices based on his or her initial selection.

Table 11-1 delineates the characteristics of the full range of AAC devices. In addition, Table 11-1 lists the skills that are needed to use each of the described devices successfully. This table can be used as a resource to identify the appropriate AAC tools for meeting the communication needs of individuals with speech impairments. AAC devices are placed into four categories in the table, on the basis of device characteristics. They include high-tech AAC devices with vocabulary expansion, low-tech and mid-tech AAC devices, text-to-speech AAC devices, and nondedicated or computer-based AAC devices.

Device Determination

The process of evaluating an individual for an AAC device requires the gathering of information about the person's abilities, experiences, skills, communication needs, and goals. Selection of an AAC device is made after a comprehensive AAC assess-

Table 11-1. Description of Augmentative and Alternative Communication (AAC) Devices and Skills Needed to Use Them*

Name of Device	Characteristics of Device	Skills Needed to Use Device
High-tech AAC devices with vocabulary expansion		
DeltaTalker, Prentke Romich Co., 1022 Heyl Rd., Wooster, OH 44691; (800) 262-1933; e-mail: info@prentrom.com	Synthesized speech; computer compatibility; Minspeak and UNITY; lightweight, portable; multiaccess	Symbol level: Minspeak; ability to construct novel utterances; good visual and memory skills; sequencing skills; varied motor skills; abstract thinking
DynaMyte, Dynavox Systems, Inc., a division of Sunrise Medical, 2100 Wharton St., Pittsburgh, PA 15203; (888) 697-7332	Synthesized speech; digitized speech also available; touch screen; multiaccess; auditory scan; page linking; lightweight, portable; English–Spanish capability; switch port, infrared capability; computer compatibility	Symbol level: varied visual, motor, and cognitive skills; vocabulary expansion needs; category knowledge; page-linking capability
Dynamo, Dynavox Systems, Inc., a division of Sunrise Medical, 2100 Wharton St., Pittsburgh, PA 15203; (888) 697-7332	Digitized speech; lightweight, portable (small black and white screen); durable case; quick communication; dynamic screen, page linking; switch port, infrared capability; multiple selection methods (direct and scanning); language capability; easily programmable; built-in remote control; touch screen; multiaccess; auditory scan; page linking	Symbol level: phrase- or single word–based; good visual skills; varied motor skills; knowledge of categories; page-linking capability; advanced communication capability not needed; limited communication needs; ideal for ambulatory population
DynaVox 3100, Dynavox Systems, Inc., a division of Sunrise Medical, 2100 Wharton St., Pittsburgh, PA 15203; (888) 697-7332	Synthesized speech; digitized speech also available; large color screen; durable case; touch screen; multiaccess; visual and auditory scanning; dynamic screen-page linking; bilingual (Spanish) capability; switch port, infrared capability; environmental controls	Symbol level: phrase- or single word–based; varied visual and motor skills; category knowledge; vocabulary expansion; page-linking capabilities; varied communication needs
Liberator II, Prentke Romich Co., 1022 Heyl Rd., Wooster, OH 44691; (800) 262-1933; e-mail: info@prentrom.com	Synthesized speech; Minspeak and UNITY; multiaccess; visual display; print output; icon prediction; word prediction; carrying case; lightweight; new model scans; uses familiar symbols; flexible symbol set; computer capability	Symbol level: Minspeak; good visual skills; varied motor skills; abstract thinking skills; good memory skills; sequenced selection; grammatical knowledge; vocabulary expansion; varied communication needs; need to construct novel utterances
Palm Top, Portable Impact, Enkidu Research, Inc., 247 Pine Hill Rd., Spencer Port, NY 14559; (716) 352-0507; www.enkidu.net	Symbol-based; touch access only; expansion cards increase recording time; lightweight, portable; unlimited communication boards capability; digitized speech; runs on AA batteries; black-and-white LCD; dynamically linked	Symbol level: good motor and visual skills; basic page-linking capability; limited vocabulary skills; good for ambulatory patients; category skills
Pathfinder, Prentke Romich Co., 1022 Heyl Rd., Wooster, OH 44691; (800) 262-1990; e-mail: info@prentrom.com	UNITY included; word prediction; predictive selection scanning; icon prediction; multiaccess; display backlighting; prestored activities; digitized speech: 15 minutes; synthesized speech: 6 users; language capability	Symbol level: Minspeak; good visual skills (small); varied motor skills; good memory skills; sequenced selection; abstract thinking skills; grammatical knowledge; varied communication needs; ideal for ambulatory population; need to construct novel utterances
Vanguard, Prentke Romich Co., 1022 Heyl Rd., Wooster, OH 44691; (800) 262-1933; e-mail: info@prentrom.com	Synthesized speech; symbol-based: Minspeak icons, UNITY; multiaccess, touch screen; scan, infrared head pointing; word prediction supplement; 12-minute digitized speech; dynamic screen; switch-activated; word prediction supplement; fringe vocabulary; auditory scanning; selection flexibility; optional keyguard	Symbol level: varied visual skills; good memory skills; varied motor skills; abstract thinking skills; need to construct novel utterances; sequenced selection; grammatical knowledge

Table 11-1. *continued*

Name of Device	Characteristics of Device	Skills Needed to Use Device
Low-tech/mid-tech AAC devices		
Action Voice, Ability Research, Inc., P.O. Box 1721, MN 55345-0721; (952) 939-0121; email: ability@skypoint.com	Digitized speech: 120 seconds of speech; single-switch scanning; external switches; lightweight, portable; easily programmable; uses any symbol set; prompted auditory scanning; records in any language; inexpensive; multi-level (2)	Photograph-symbol level: concrete skills; good visual skills; varied motor skills; limited communication needs; limited vocabulary available
Action Voice 2A, Ability Research, Inc., P.O. Box 1721, MN 55345-0721; (952) 939-0121; email: ability@skypoint.com	Digitized speech: 120 seconds of speech; single-switch scanning; external switches; lightweight, portable; uses any symbol set; prompted auditory scanning; multilevel; inexpensive; records in any language	Photograph-symbol level: concrete skills; good visual skills; limited communication needs; limited vocabulary available; ideal for ambulatory population
Alpha Talker, Prentke Romich Co., 1022 Heyl Rd., Wooster, OH 44691; (800) 262-1990; (800) 262-1933; e-mail: info@prentrom.com	Digitized speech: 3–5 minutes; recorded speech can be increased to 14 and 25 minutes; theme keys; memory modules; multiaccess; lightweight; records in any language	Photograph-symbol level: phrase- or single word–based; varied visual and motor skills; simple sequencing skills; concrete skills; limited communication needs; limited vocabulary expansion (can be expanded by changing levels)
Bedside Communicator, Enabling Devices, 385 Warburton Ave., Hastings-on-Hudson, NY 10706; (800) 832-8697	Scanning device; easily programmable; digitized speech; single level; 8 locations; inexpensive; records in any language	Concrete skills: limited communication needs; limited motor skills and needs; switches
Big Mac, Ablenet, 1081 Tenth Ave. SE, Minneapolis, MN 55414; (800) 322-0956	Digitized speech; low-level, single message; requires battery; easily programmable; 20 seconds of recording time; records in any language; can also be used as switch	Photograph-symbol level: phrase level; cause-and-effect relationships; concrete skills; limited vocabulary skills
Black Hawk, AdamLab, 33500 Van Born Rd., Wayne, MI 48184; (734) 334-1610	Digitized speech: 3.75 seconds per selection area; records in any language; 4 levels of 16 selections; switch accessible; lightweight, portable	Symbol level: varied motor skills; good visual skills; limited vocabulary needs, limited communication skills
Chatbox, Saltillo Corp., 2143 TR 112, Millersburg, OH 44654; (330) 674-6722; email: aac@saltillo.com	Low level; digitized speech; lightweight, portable; Minspeak: icon prediction; multiple levels; limited 4 level; scanning capability; inexpensive; records in any language	Photograph-symbol level: phrase level; good visual and fine motor skills; direct selection; limited vocabulary and communication needs; ideal for ambulatory patients
Cheap Talk, Enabling Devices, 385 Warburton Ave., Hastings-on-Hudson, NY 10706; (800) 832-8697	Inexpensive; digitized speech; jacks into which external switches corresponding to each plate can be plugged; scan-and-touch model; Cheap Talk 4: 4 locations; Cheap Talk 8: 8 locations; multilevel; scan model; records in any language	Photograph-symbol level: good visual skills; concrete skills; varied motor skills; limited communication needs; good for topic-based overlays
Dec-Aid, Adaptivation, Inc., 2225 West 50th Street, Suite 100, Sioux Falls, SD 57105; (800) 723-2783	Digitized speech: 10 messages; use of external switch; lightweight; switch capabilities; records in any language	Object-photo-symbol level: phrase level; cause-and-effect; choice making; limited vocabulary and communication needs
Double-Message Chatter Switch, Partner Two, ERI, 31 Watermill Lane, Great Neck, NY 11021; (516) 501-0235	Digitized speech; easily programmable; two external jacks; records in any language	Object-photo-symbol level: concrete skills; any symbol set; limited vocabulary needs; choice making; varied motor skills

Table 11-1. *continued*

Name of Device	Characteristics of Device	Skills Needed to Use Device
Dynamic Deluxe Talk Back 24, Crestwood Company, 6625 N. Sidney Place, Milwaukee, WI 53209; (414) 352-5678	Digitized speech; lightweight, portable; 6–24 locations; single-level; easy to program; switch selection; records in any language	Object-photo-symbol level: good motor and visual skills; limited vocabulary and communication needs
Easy Talk, ACCI, The Great Talking Box, Co., 2245A Fortune Drive, San Jose, CA 95131; (408) 456-0133; www.greattalkingbox.com	Digitized speech; easily programmable; records in any language; small, lightweight; inexpensive; multilevel (4); adjustable keyboard layout; direct selection or scan	Photograph-symbol level: good visual and fine motor skills; direct selection; limited communication needs
Four Compartments Speech and Lights, Enabling Devices, 385 Warburton Ave., Hastings-on-Hudson, NY 10706; (800) 832-8697	Beginning device; digitized speech; records in any language; 20-second record time; voice output; pairs objects with symbols; teaches language skills; permits individual and group activities	Concrete skills: object discrimination; object-to-picture transition; choice making; limited communication skills
Grooved Platform Communicator, Enabling Devices, 385 Warburton Ave., Hastings-on-Hudson, NY 10706; (800) 832-8697	Direct select; low level; digitized speech; records in any language	Object discrimination: object-to-picture transition; choice making; concrete skills; limited communication needs
Hawk II & III Communication Device, AdamLab, 33500 Van Born Rd., Wayne, MI 48184; (734) 334-1610	Digitized speech; switch accessibility; 2 levels of 8 selection areas; records in any language; includes keyguard; 7.5 seconds of digitized speech per selection area	Photo-symbol-based: phrase-based; good motor skills; direct selection; limited vocabulary needs
Hawk, AdamLab, 33500 Van Born Rd., Wayne, MI 48184; (734) 334-1610	Digitized speech: 6.5 seconds of per selection area; records in any language; lightweight, portable	Symbol-photograph level: limited vocabulary on each level; good fine motor skills; limited vocabulary needs; good for ambulatory patients
Hip Talk, Enabling Devices, 385 Warburton Ave., Hastings-on-Hudson, NY 10706; (800) 832-8697	Digitized speech; low level; simple–easy to program; varied message capabilities; records in any language; lightweight, portable; carrying case	Symbol level: good visual and motor skills; limited communication needs; ideal for ambulatory population
Holly.Com, Communication Devices, Inc., 4830 Industrial Way, West Coeur d'Alene, ID 83815; (800) 604-6559	Digitized speech; built-in disk drive; tilt-up adjustable keyboard, 8 or 32 key; unlimited speech capacity; multiaccess, direct or scan; unlimited disc and overlay sets; records in any language	Photograph-symbol level: good visual skills; varied motor skills; limited communication needs; limited vocabulary for each page
Lighthawk, AdamLab, 33500 Van Born Rd., Wayne, MI 48184; (734) 334-1610	Digitized speech; scanning; 2.4 seconds per selection area; switch accessible; 7 jacks; records in any language; total 24 messages	Symbol-photograph level: varied motor and visual skills; scanning ability; limited vocabulary needs
Macaw, ZYGO Industries, Inc., P.O. Box 1008, Portland, OR 97207-1008; (800) 234-6006	Digitized speech; multiaccess: direct or scan, auditory scan available; lightweight, portable; multilevel; records in any language; linking capability; keyguard; adaptable overlay 2/4/8/32	Photograph-symbol level: phrase- or single word–based; varied visual, motor, and cognitive skills; limited vocabulary on each level; good for patients needing auditory prompts
Message Mates, Words +, 1220 West Ave. J, Lancaster, CA 93534; (800) 869-8521	Multilevel Message Mate 40; 10 minutes' total recording time; multiaccess mode; digitized speech; lightweight, portable; durable carrying case; easily programmed; records in any language; optional keyguard; mem-keyboard	Photograph-symbol level: phrase-based; good visual skills; varied motor skills; ideal for ambulatory population; limited vocabulary needs; vocabulary expansion possible by changing levels

Table 11-1. *continued*

Name of Device	Characteristics of Device	Skills Needed to Use Device
Message Mate 40/20, Words +, 1220 West Ave. J, Lancaster, CA 93534; (800) 869-8521	Single level; 150 seconds' total recording time; multiaccess mode; digitized speech; durable, lightweight; carrying case; optional keyguard; mem-keyboard; records in any language	Photograph-symbol level: good visual skills; varied motor skills; limited communication and vocabulary needs; ideal for ambulatory population
Mini Message Mate, Words +, 1220 West Ave. J, Lancaster, CA 93534; (800) 869-8521	Eight large keys; 60-second recording time; digitized speech; lightweight, durable; direct selection; good for group activities; records in any language	Photograph-symbol level: fair to good visual skills; good motor skills; limited vocabulary needs; ideal for ambulatory population
One-Step Communicator, Ablenet, 1081 Tenth Ave. SE, Minneapolis, MN 55414; (800) 322-0956	Digitized speech: 20 seconds per single message; easily programmable; records in any language; inexpensive	Concrete skills: object-photo-symbol level; phrase level; no precursor; cause-and-effect relationships; limited communication needs
Personal Talker, Innocomp, 26210 Emory Rd., Warrensville Heights, OR 44128; (800) 382-8622	Digitized speech: 10 seconds per single message; direct selection; inexpensive; records in any language	Phrase level: limited communication needs; good fine motor skills to access; no precursor; cause and effect
Rocking Plate Talker/Twin Talker, Enabling Devices, 385 Warburton Ave., Hastings-on-Hudson, NY 10706; (800) 832-8697	Digitized speech; photographs, symbols or objects can be attached; inexpensive; easily programmed; choice making; records in any language	Concrete skills: object-photo-symbol level; good motor skills for direct selection; beginning communication; choice making; limited communication needs
Say It Simply Plus, Innocomp, 26210 Emory Rd., Warrensville Heights, OR 44128; (800) 382-8622	Synthesized speech; large display area; lightweight; multilevel; durable construction; keyguard available; direct selection; records in any language	Good for person with fisted points: photograph-symbol level; phrase level; good to fair motor skills; able to change overlays
Scan-It-All, Innocomp, 26210 Emory Rd., Warrensville Heights, OR 44128; (800) 382-8622	Lightweight; synthesized speech; visual display; multiaccess: scan, laser pointer; multilevel; adaptable overlay size; inexpensive; records in any language	Photograph-symbol level: single word–based; motor difficulties; good head control or switch use
Shadow Talker, Enabling Devices, 385 Warburton Ave., Hastings-on-Hudson, NY 10706; (800) 832-8697	2-in. display; activated by body movement that creates shadow on box; digitized speech; inexpensive; easily programmed; records in any language	Low level: object-photo-symbol level; choice making; varied motor skills; limited communication needs
Side Kick, Prentke Romich Co., 1022 Heyl Rd., Wooster, OH 44691; (800) 262-1933; www.prentrom.com	Digitized speech; 24 location keyguard; sequence selections; 4 user areas; small, lightweight; carrying case; multiaccess; records in any language	Photograph-symbol level: good visual and memory skills; varied motor skills; limited communication needs; sequenced selections
Single-Message Chatter Switch, Partner Two, ERI, 31 Watermill Lane, Great Neck, NY 11021; (516) 501-0235	Digitized speech; easily programmable; external jacks; battery-run; inexpensive; records in any language	Photograph-symbol level: limited vocabulary needs; cause and effect; no precursor
Speak Easy, Ablenet, 1081 Tenth Ave. SE, Minneapolis, MN 55414; (800) 322-0956	Digitized speech; multiaccess; keyguard; portable, lightweight; carrying case; external jacks; records in any language; conducive to group activities using external jacks	Photograph-symbol level: good visual skills; good fine motor skills for direct selection; limited communication and vocabulary needs

Table 11-1. *continued*

Name of Device	Characteristics of Device	Skills Needed to Use Device
Step-by-Step Communication with Levels, Ablenet, 1081 Tenth Ave. SE, Minneapolis, MN 55414; (800) 322-0956	Sequenced message capability: 75 seconds; easily programmable; digitized speech; level capability; records in any language	Object-photo-symbol level: phrase level; no precursor; cause and effect
Step-by-Step Communicator, Ablenet, 1081 Tenth Ave. SE, Minneapolis, MN 55414; (800) 322-0956	Digitized speech: 75 seconds; easily programmable; multimessage capability; records in any language	Object-photo-symbol level: concrete skills; no precursor; cause and effect
Super Hawk, AdamLab, 33500 Van Born Rd., Wayne, MI 48184; (734) 334-1610	Digitized speech; single-switch auditory scanning; 4 switch inputs; 72 programmable cells; records in any language	Symbol- and photograph-based; phrase- or word based–level: varied motor, visual, and cognitive skills; need auditory prompts
Super Hawk Plus, AdamLab, 33500 Van Born Rd., Wayne, MI 48184; (734) 334-1610	Digitized speech: 72 minutes; single- and multiple-switch auditory scanning; 72 programmable cells; 4 switch inputs; unlimited message length	Photograph-symbol level: word- or phrase-level capability; varied motor, visual, and cognitive skills; ability to construct sentences; auditory scanning
Talking Buddy, Innocomp, 26210 Emory Rd., Warrensville Heights, OR 44128; (800) 382-8622	Digitized speech; single message; easily programmable; battery-run; records in any language	Object-photo-symbol level: phrase level; concrete skills; no precursor; cause and effect
Talking Switch Plate, Enabling Devices, 385 Warburton Ave., Hastings-on-Hudson, NY 10706; (800) 832-8697	Digitized speech; inexpensive; easily programmable; records in any language	Object-photo-symbol level: concrete skills; cause and effect; limited communication needs
Tech/Four, AMDI, 31 Watermill Lane, Great Neck, NY 11021; (516) 466-2288	Digitized speech; lightweight, portable; durable; easily programmable; records in any language	Photo- and symbol-based: direct selection or concrete phrase level; choice making in any language; limited vocabulary needs
Tech/Scan, AMDI, 31 Watermill Lane, Great Neck, NY 11021; (516) 466-2288	Digitized speech: multilevel 2/4/6; 32 locations; direct selection; scan: linear, row or column, step; relatively inexpensive; lightweight, portable; durable	Phrase level: photograph- and symbol-based; expand vocabulary by changing levels; good visual skills; varied motor ability; limited communication needs
Tech/Speak, AMDI, 31 Watermill Lane, Great Neck, NY 11021; (516) 466-2288	Low-tech and simple; digitized speech; inexpensive; new model scans; lightweight; durable; multilevel: 32 locations; interchangeable overlays; easily programmable; flexible symbol set; direct selection; records in any language; uses familiar symbols	Photograph-symbol level: topic-based exchanges; good visual and fine motor skills; good for ambulatory or nonambulatory users; limited communication needs; limited vocational needs; expand vocabulary by changing overlays
Tech Talk, AMDI, 31 Watermill Lane, Great Neck, NY 11021; (516) 466-2288	Digitized speech: multilevel 6/8/12; 8 locations; easily programmable; lightweight; durable; water-resistant; direct selection; records in any language; limited vocabulary per page	Object-photo-symbol level: phrase-based; good motor skills; limited communication needs; expand vocabulary by changing pages; direct selection
Talking Box Voice In Box, Enabling Devices, 385 Warburton Ave., Hastings-on-Hudson, NY 10706; (800) 832-8697	Digitized device; records up to 4–8 messages; plugs into one's own switches to activate messages; multiple switch capability for one child or group activities; varied models; records in any language	Object-based system (objects could be placed on switches): limited communication needs
Ultimate, TASH, Unit 1, 91 Station St., Ajax, Ontario, Canada L1S 3H2; (800) 463-5685	Digitized speech; direct selection; 4 messages; small, lightweight; durable; records in any language	Photograph-symbol level: good motor skills; good visual skills; choice making; limited vocabulary needs

Table 11-1. *continued*

Name of Device	Characteristics of Device	Skills Needed to Use Device
Ultimate 8, Tash, Unit 1, 91 Station St., Ajax, Ontario, Canada L1S 3H2; (800) 463-5685	Digitized speech: 32 seconds; small, light-weight, portable; direct selection; 8 locations	Photograph-symbol level: good visual skills and motor skills; limited communication needs
Vocal Assistant 90S, GMR Labs; www.gmrlabs.com	Digitized speech: 90 seconds; multiaccess; auditory scan; 6 regular 9-volt batteries; small, lightweight; keyguard available; 15 active keys; records in any language	Good visual skills: varied motor skills; limited communication needs; limited vocabulary; ideal for ambulatory population
Voice Mate, TASH, Unit 1, 91 Station St., Ajax, Ontario, Canada L1S 3H2; (800) 463-5685	Low-tech; digitized speech; direct scan models; 4–8 messages; portable/light-weight; records in any language	Good visual skills: varied motor skills; limited vocabulary needs; good for ambulatory population
VoicePal, Innocomp, 26210 Emory Rd., Warrensville Heights, OR 44128; (800) 382-8622	Digitized speech; 20-second recording time; can create vocal output when objects or switches are touched; connections for up to 5 switches or 5 taction pads; records in any language; direct selection	Object level: limited communication needs; discrimination skills teaching of pictures or symbols; phrase level
VoicePal Plus, Innocomp, 26210 Emory Rd., Warrensville Heights, OR 44128; (800) 382-8622	Digitized speech: 60 seconds; 10 one-inch symbols or 2 two-inch symbols; scanning: auditory or visual (or both); flexible change overlay configuration; connections for up to 10 external switches or taction pads; records in any language	Object-symbol level: direct selection; limited communication needs; good visual and motor skills if using keyboard; choice making

Nondedicated, computer-based AAC devices

Name of Device	Characteristics of Device	Skills Needed to Use Device
Access 1600, Prentke Romich Co., 1022 Heyl Rd., Wooster, OH 44691; (800) 262-1990; (800) 262-1933; e-mail: info@prentrom.com	Computer-based; Windows Operating System; synthesized speech; multiaccess; Unity; limited battery time	Symbol level: varied motor skills; single-word level: abstract skills; sequenced selections; good memory skills; computer knowledge; academic potential; page-linking capability; intact high-level cognition; vocabulary expansion needs; varied communication needs
Freedom 2000, Words +, 1220 West Ave. J, Lancaster, CA 93534; (800) 869-8521	Computer-based; Windows Operating System; durable; EZ keys and talking screen; multiaccess modes	Symbol- or word-based: intact high-level cognition; academic potential; computer knowledge; page-linking capability; vocabulary expansion needs; large vocabulary set
Freestyle, Assistive Technology, 7 Wells Ave., Newton, MA 02459; (800) 793-9227; www. assistivetech.com	Computer-based; MAC platform; holds MAC software: Speaking Dynamically, DynaVox, Mayer Johnson; CD-ROM/disk; synthesized speech; multiaccess; symbol- or letter-based; portable	Symbol-letter level: intact high-level cognition; vocabulary expansion needs; page-linking capabilities; varied motor skills; academic potential; computer knowledge
Synergy Mac, Synergy, 412 High Plain St., Ste. 19, Walpole, MA 02081; (508) 668-7424	Computer-based; MAC platform; portable; multiaccess; CD-ROM/disk; synthesized speech; symbol or letter based	Symbol-letter level: academic potential; page-linking capability; computer knowledge; intact high-level cognition; vocabulary expansion needs
The Communication Station, Innocomp, 26210 Emory Rd., Warrensville Heights, OR 44128; (800) 382-8622	Computer-based; Windows Operating System; touch screen; dynamic display; external keyboard; CD-ROM/disk; battery life up to 5 hours; includes AAC software; synthesized speech; multiaccess; portable	Symbol-letter level: vocabulary expansion needs; page-linking capability; academically based; computer knowledge; high-level cognition; academic potential

Table 11-1. *continued*

Name of Device	Characteristics of Device	Skills Needed to Use Device
Text-to-speech AAC devices		
Cannon Communicator, Crestwood Company, 6625 N. Sidney Place, Milwaukee, WI 53209; (414) 352-5678	Text-to-speech scanning capability; print output; prints frequently used phrases; enlarges print; digitized speech; message memory; records up to 240 seconds of speech in any language; calculator function	Spelling skills; need for print output; limited speech capability; good fine motor skills; good visual skills; varied communication needs
Crespeaker, Crestwood Company, 6625 N. Sidney Place, Milwaukee, WI 53209; (414) 352-5678	Synthesized speech; text-to-speech capability; inexpensive; easy to operate; not a dedicated device: Spanish-English dictionary; small, lightweight; direct selection	Good for ambulatory population; spelling skills; good visual and motor skills (for small keys); varied communication needs
Dubby, TASH Unit 1, 91 Station St., Ajax, Ontario, Canada L1S 3H2; (800) 463-5685	Synthesized speech; multiple voice options; text-to-speech capability; direct selection; split LCD display; lightweight, portable; membrane keyboard features computer capability; ABC or QWERTY layout; word prediction; storing storage; keyguard	Spelling skills; good fine motor and visual skills; grammatical skills; varied communication needs; keyboard use; rate enhancement techniques
Light Writer, Zygo, ZYGO Industries, Inc., P.O. Box 1008, Portland, OR 97207-1008; (800) 234-6006	Synthesized speech; text-to-speech capability; large, clear visual display; print capability light-touch keyboard; keyguard; small, lightweight; durable; acceleration techniques; scanning capability; user memory	Spelling skills; grammatical skills; good fine motor skills; keyboard use; good visual skills; high cognitive skills; varied communication needs; rate enhancement technique
Link, Assistive Technology, 7 Wells Ave., Newton, MA 02459; (800) 793-9227; www. assistivetech.com	Keyboard; text-to-speech capability; DecTalk: 8 voices; lightweight; computer compatibility; visual display; storing labels; abbreviation expansion; instant phrases	Higher level; spelling skills; keyboard use; good fine motor skills; rate enhancement techniques; good visual skills
Speaking Speller, Crestwood Company, 6625 N. Sidney Place, Milwaukee, WI 53209; (414) 352-5678	Voice output (with spell checker); synthesized speech; one-line screen display; lightweight; not dedicated	Grammatical skills; good visual and fine motor skills; spelling skills; keyboard use

LCD = liquid crystal display; MAC = Macintosh.
*Communication devices as of March 2000.

ment, for which typically one will obtain information about a user in the following areas:

- Background information
- Motor abilities
- Visual and visual motor status
- Auditory skills
- Cognitive skills
- Physical access needs
- Behavioral status
- Speech and language skills

General Skills Assessment

Background information is gathered to help personalize the choice of ACC interventions. The evaluator determines what the person's communication experience has been, the nature of his or her speech impairment, current and future communication environments, and goals.

Motor abilities are a central concern in choosing an AAC device. The user's ability to ambulate, upper-extremity function, and head control are analyzed during the assessment process. Ambulation affects the determination of portability of AAC devices recommended. Individuals using wheelchairs may benefit from mounting of AAC devices on the wheelchair. In addition, the positioning needs of an individual, especially the wheelchair user, are paramount to successful use of an AAC device. Even ambulatory individuals with low tone may need positioning support to keep their feet flat on the floor, forearms on the table, and proper table height. The optimal goal of positioning assessment is that proximal stability leads to distal mobility. Other issues that are examined in positioning are head control, seating needs, lateral support, tilt and recline needs, and lap-tray design. Mobility status affects the need for a portable AAC device.

Visual status includes such factors as visual motor integration, visual attention, visual deficits, and visual perception (e.g., field cuts, figure-ground orientation, eye gaze). An AAC device user's vision affects the speech-language pathologist's recommendation for size of symbols and symbol set. Photographs may be easier to discriminate than abstract symbols. In addition, contrasting colors (e.g., black letters on a yellow background) may accommodate for certain vision deficits.

Determinations of hearing status, auditory localization, and auditory identification are used to assess auditory skills. Individuals using AAC devices must be able to hear their own speech output or to use an augmentative communication device with a visual display of their message to determine its accuracy.

Cognitive skills are assessed by determining an individual's ability to follow simple (i.e., one- or two-step) to complex commands and to comprehend concrete to abstract concepts, as well as the capability of that person's short- and long-term memory. The complexity of the symbol set recommended for an individual with speech impairment will be based primarily on cognitive skills.

Within an AAC assessment, *physical access needs* encompass a person's ability to indicate directly or to select (e.g., by pointing, eye gaze, optical indicators, joystick, emulated mouse) a communication choice from a selection set. Physical access evaluation includes such factors as reflexes, tone, gross and fine motor skills, strength, range of motion, endurance, and coordination. For individuals who are unable to select a communication choice directly, access to AAC devices may be accomplished through

use of indirect selection. Indirect selection incorporates scanning of the selection set, whereby the user may choose an item by activating a switch. Presentation of items may be visual, auditory, or tactile.

Often, switch assessment is an integral part of an AAC assessment. This part of the evaluation is concerned with determining voluntary reproducible movement, strength and endurance, accuracy and control of movements, and activation and release of a switch. Switch sites can range from head to knee to eye. Presence of any consistent reproducible movement can be matched with a switch.

Behavioral status must be determined because such behaviors as defensiveness, perseveration, short attention span, distractibility, and delayed response may interfere with a person's ability to use an AAC device. Therapeutic interventions may be recommended by a speech-language pathologist to help a person overcome his or her behavioral difficulties so that he or she might better use an AAC device.

No AAC assessment is complete without examination of a user's language skills. Speech and language skills are assessed via an oral peripheral examination and by determining speech intelligibility, receptive and expressive language aptitude, and communication needs. Language skills assessment also entails a much more detailed workup, as discussed in the next section.

Language Assessment

A language assessment will help to determine the type of symbol set that a user will be able to access. Symbol sets range from concrete to abstract. The hierarchy of symbols includes (1) concrete object identification (actual objects, miniatures); (2) photographs; (3) symbols (colored, black and white, line drawings); and (4) written words.

The type of vocabulary output (phrase- or word-based) and additional features (e.g., page linking, word prediction) will be selected on the basis of language assessment. This assessment examines such cognitive and language skills as cause and effect, object permanence, matching skills, sorting, categorization, vocabulary knowledge, ability to follow simple and complex directions, sequencing skills, and semantic representation of symbols. With phrase- or sentence-based vocabulary output systems, a complete phrase or sentence is stored in each location of a voice output communication device. This approach is beneficial for individuals at the cause-and-effect level, cognitively low-functioning individuals, and individuals using scanning techniques. In contrast, word-based systems contain a single word or carrier phrase at each location that is represented by a symbol or written word, and these words are combined to create an utterance. This type of system is beneficial for the cognitively young individual as well as for those individuals who have cognitive levels within functional limits.[3]

In some cases, AAC device users may benefit also from vocabulary expansion techniques. *Vocabulary expansion* is the term applied to approaches that allow the user access to a vocabulary larger than the one provided instantly by the selection set. The specific techniques include page linking and semantic compaction. *Page linking* involves a main board consisting of category symbols linked to other boards consisting of items related to each category. This technique may be beneficial for the cognitively young individual and those within functional cognitive levels. To use this technique, a person would need to be able to identify multiple symbols, follow two-step directions, and exhibit good categorization skills. *Semantic compaction* uses one set of multiple-meaning icons in sequences to represent a variety of ideas. The skills needed to use semantic compaction include multiple symbol identification (i.e., *apple* = apple, fruit, eat, hungry, food) and ability to follow complex directions, follow sequences, and understand a semantic representation of symbols.[4,5]

Some users benefit from rate enhancement or acceleration techniques that cause the number of characters generated to be greater than the number of selections made by the individual. *Linguistic–word prediction* describes computer software that presents a list of the most likely next word or phrase choices after one or more letters have been input, whereas *word completion* provides a user with a list of possible words containing the initial letters provided. *Abbreviation expansion* is a tool that permits two to three letters to represent a longer, prestored phrase. When the letters are input, the whole phrase is printed or spoken out (i.e., *wp* = Where is my paycheck?).

Only after completion of a comprehensive augmentative communication evaluation can an individual's needs be matched to the device features of a specific AAC system.

References

1. Beukelman D, Yorkston K, Dowden P. Communication Augmentation: A Casebook of Clinical Management. San Diego: College Hill Press, 1985.
2. American Speech-Language-Hearing Association. Report: Augmentative and alternative communication. ASHA 1991;33[Suppl 5]:9–12.
3. Goosens C, Sapp Crain S, Elder P. Engineering the Preschool Environment for Interactive Symbolic Communication. Birmingham: Southeast Augmentative Communication Conference Publication, 1995.
4. Prentke Romich Company. What Is Minspeak? Wooster, OH: Prentke Romich Company, 1993.
5. Prentke Romich Company. Exploring UNITY/128: Language for Life. Wooster, OH: Prentke Romich Company, 1995.

Chapter 12

Progressive Cognitive and Behavioral Changes in Epilepsy

Orrin Devinsky and Andrew Tarulli

Cognitive impairment and behavioral problems were recognized in patients with epilepsy in ancient times[1] and documented in nineteenth century neurologic literature.[2,3] Gowers[4] found that although most patients demonstrated a normal intellect and pattern of behavior, interictal abnormalities occurred in some. He recognized that the etiology of this change was multifactorial but hypothesized that epilepsy was the most important cause. Lennox[5] expanded on Gowers' work, identifying five potential factors in the cognitive and behavioral decline associated with epilepsy: heredity, brain injury prior to seizure onset, medication, psychological handicaps, and epilepsy itself. The insights of Gowers and Lennox remain valid; the study of mental deterioration in epilepsy focuses on their observations and their suggested mechanisms.

Understanding the frequency, nature, and cause of mental deterioration in epilepsy poses several methodological issues. Were the cognitive and behavioral data valid? Were the testing procedures appropriate for the constructs that they were designed to measure? Two main strategies were employed to document progressive changes. First, longitudinal studies were used to track the progression of patients with epilepsy over time. Second, factors that have time as a variable were studied. Earlier age of onset, longer duration, and higher frequency of seizures should be associated with poorer cognitive function if the changes in cognitive function are indeed progressive. Etiol-ogy of epilepsy must be considered so that the effects of seizures on intellectual function can be separated from underlying neurologic damage, especially progressive neurologic disorders (e.g., brain tumors, metabolic disorders). The type, frequency, severity, and laterality of seizures are potentially important variables that may correlate with subsequent behavioral and cognitive change. The continuous[6] and transitory[7] neuronal dysfunctions associated with epilepsy may be critical factors contributing to cognitive and behavioral problems in epilepsy patients, but measuring these factors is extremely difficult. Behavioral changes associated with epilepsy, such as depression, psychosis, and impaired social function, can all be important but difficult to quantify. The anatomic substrates of cognitive and behavioral change can best be studied via radiology and pathology. Physiologic substrata of cognitive and behavioral changes may be partly defined by blood flow, metabolic, or other functional studies. Other factors such as antiepileptic drugs (AEDs) and psychosocial function can contribute to these problems and must be addressed.

Measurement of Cognitive Function

The ideal test of cognitive function in epilepsy would be both sensitive and specific for deficits produced by the disorder, reproducible, easily and quickly administered, and accepted as the standard by epilepsy researchers. Unfortunately, none of these criteria is met by the tests that are used most often. The tests and batteries designed to evaluate cognitive decline in epilepsy have limitations, and their use varies. Often, familiar tests or tests that are tailored to prove certain hypotheses are selected, thus complicating the literature with inconsistency and inaccuracy.

The Wechsler Adult Intelligence Scale–Revised (WAIS-R) is the most commonly used assessment of intelligence in epilepsy.[8] This test evaluates 11 different abilities, 6 verbal and 5 performance: information, comprehension, similarities, arithmetic, vocabulary, picture assembly, picture completion, block design, object assembly, digit span, and digit symbol.[9] The verbal scale measures previously acquired verbal information, whereas the performance scale measures visuospatial ability and visuomotor speed. The average range of the WAIS-R intelligence quotient (IQ) is 90–110, with mental retardation being defined as an IQ of less than 70.

Neuropsychological testing often is used to evaluate cognitive and behavioral deficits, and, although it often includes the WAIS-R, neuropsychological testing lacks a standard such as the WAIS-R. The problems created by this lack of standardization are illustrated by a literature search to determine the number of neuropsychological tests that were used in randomized controlled trials of AEDs.[10] In the 43 papers found, 87 different tests were administered, the most commonly used being applied only 13 times. Administration of tests and methods of reporting results were not uniform, further compounding this inconsistency. However, neuropsychological evaluation is currently the standard for assessing cognitive function in epilepsy patients. No equivalent exists with regard to careful and comprehensive evaluation of behavioral functions. Although mood and thought disorder can be assessed with standardized inventories, other behavioral functions, such as ability to comprehend emotional signals and ability to function successfully in social settings, are not readily tested.

Test batteries such as the Halstead-Reitan and Luria-Nebraska are commonly used as comprehensive measurements of neuropsychological functioning.[11,12] However, neither of these batteries was designed to assess the function of patients

with epilepsy, and their use for this purpose can be misleading. For example, the Halstead-Reitan battery was designed for head-injured patients and those who have undergone lobectomy.[10] In addition, neither of these batteries is truly comprehensive, and each one often fails to provide a detailed evaluation of specific deficits.[13]

The first attempt to create a test specific for the cognitive deficits of epilepsy was the Continuous Performance Test.[14] In 1978, Dodrill[15] designed the Neuropsychological Battery for Epilepsy.[15] He selected 16 tests on the basis of their ability to discriminate between normal subjects and patients with epilepsy and then performed an independent cross-validation assessment. In Dodrill's battery, factors such as verbal and nonverbal memory, sustained attention, and verbal problem solving receive a more thorough treatment than they do in the Halstead-Reitan battery. The Neuropsychological Battery for Epilepsy also attempted to standardize component tests, gender differences, and selection of an appropriate control population. Adoption of assessment protocols specific for epilepsy has been far from unanimous. In a review of 43 AED trials, only 2 used the Neuropsychological Battery for Epilepsy, and these both were conducted by Dodrill and associates.[10]

FePsy, a computerized assessment of neuropsychological functioning in patients with epilepsy, was developed by Alpherts and Aldenkamp.[16] This system includes tests of simple reaction time, binary choice reaction time, tapping speed, visual searching, and recognition. The advantage to this system is that performance in patients can be tracked over time via a database, but the system is not comprehensive or widely used.

Longitudinal Studies

Studies that track cognitive change in patients with epilepsy over time are among the most important data documenting or refuting mental deterioration. Most longitudinal studies of this type provided proof that intellectual decline is indeed progressive.[17–19] However, some such studies showed no deterioration, or even improvement, possibly related to AED therapy.[20,21] Among longitudinal studies, those with prospective designs that provide cognitive and neuropsychological data before the onset of

Table 12-1. Changes in Intelligence Quotient (IQ) over Time in Patients with Epilepsy

IQ Pattern over Time	No. of Patients (%) (n = 72)	IQ at First Testing (mean ± SD)	IQ at Last Testing (mean ± SD)
Decrease	8 (11.1)	108.1 ± 19.5	88.0 ± 19.5*
Increase	12 (16.7)	93.7 ± 24.2	108.8 ± 23.5*
Fluctuation	29 (40.3)	99.3 ± 19.0	100.8 ± 19.3
No change	23 (31.9)	100.3 ± 19.8	101.6 ± 19.8

Notes: The mean time between first and last testing was 4 years. Definition of groups: decrease = consistent decrease in IQ of 10 or more points over time; increase = consistent increase in IQ of 10 or more points over time; fluctuation = difference of 10 or more points between the highest and lowest scores, but no permanent increase or decrease; no change = less than a 10-point difference between the highest and lowest score.
*Significantly different from IQ on first testing ($p < .0001$).
Source: From BFD Bourgeois, AL Prensky, HS Palkes, et al. Intelligence in epilepsy: a prospective study in children. Ann Neurol 1983;14:438–444.

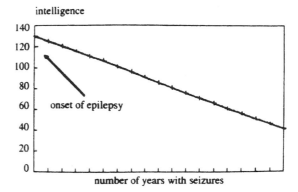

Figure 12-1. Deterioration as a continuous process. (Reprinted with permission from H Meinardi, AP Aldenkamp, B Nunes. Mental deterioration at epilepsy onset: a hypothesis. Acta Neurochirurg 1992;55:68–71.)

epilepsy are the most useful. They are, however, also uncommon. Furthermore, studies that report percentages of patients undergoing decline rather than simple patient test score means are infrequent.

A prospective study of 35 adults with epilepsy was performed to determine the nature of changes in cognitive or neuropsychological performance over a 10-year period.[22] Although some changes in subtests were noted, no overall changes in the WAIS-R or the Neuropsychological Battery for Epilepsy were observed over the 10 years of the trial. However, the mean duration of epilepsy before the initial evaluation was 20 years, an interval in which substantial, unobserved cognitive decline was possible.

Bourgeois et al.[23] evaluated children with epilepsy within 2 weeks of seizure onset and then over a period of 4 years. Unaffected siblings were used as controls. The mean IQ of the affected children did not change appreciably over time, but 8 of the 72 patients demonstrated persistent decreases of 10 points or more (Table 12-1). These patients were more likely to have toxic drug levels, epilepsy that was difficult to control, and earlier onset of seizures. Of these three factors, drug toxicity and early age of onset were the best predictors of poor prognosis. These results suggest that progressive

cognitive deterioration may take place in a percentage of children with epilepsy and that complete seizure control should not be sought at the expense of overall cognitive outcome.

Other studies have attempted to demonstrate that most cognitive change takes place early in the course of epilepsy. Meinardi et al.[24] described the cascadic model of deterioration, in which irreversible decline occurs shortly after the onset of seizures. In subsequent years, intellectual function plateaus, and no changes may be noted on cognitive testing (Figures 12-1, 12-2). This model could

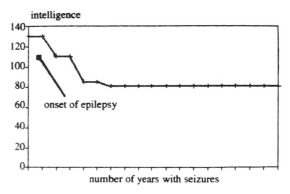

Figure 12-2. Deterioration as a step-like process. (Reprinted with permission from H Meinardi, AP Aldenkamp, B Nunes. Mental deterioration at epilepsy onset: a hypothesis. Acta Neurochirurg 1992;55:68–71.)

Table 12-2. Duration of Epilepsy in Relation to Intelligence Quotient (IQ) Scores in Longitudinal Studies

| Study | First Assessment | | Second Assessment | |
	Mean Duration of Epilepsy (yrs)	Mean IQ Score	Mean Period of Follow-Up (yrs)	Mean IQ Score
Aldenkamp et al.[25]	6.8	84.7	4.2	81.9
Bourgeois et al.[23]	ND	99.7	4.2	101.0
Rodin et al.[26]	3.7	91.6	9.6	90.2
Seidenberg et al.[27]	12.3	87.2	1.8	91.2

ND = no data.

Source: From LGJ Neyens, AP Aldenkamp, HM Meinardi. Prospective follow-up of intellectual development in children with a recent onset of epilepsy. Epilepsy Res 1999;34:85–90.

explain previous longitudinal studies in which epilepsy is associated with a baseline of impaired intellectual function but no further deterioration (Table 12-2).[23,25–27] To detect and control for the early cognitive decline that they hypothesized, Neyens et al.[28] chose patients with a maximum 3-year duration of epilepsy as subjects for a longitudinal study. These patients were matched to controls and underwent cognitive assessment every 6 months for 1.5 years. At the onset of the study, children with epilepsy demonstrated a lower level of intelligence as compared to the control group. Follow-up testing revealed that most subjects experienced a gain in IQ score; this gain was greatest for normal controls. The children with the longest duration of epilepsy (who had presumably already undergone their greatest period of cognitive decline) had smaller gains in IQ scores. Those who had epilepsy for 2 years or fewer showed an even more modest gain in IQ. The group of children with the most recent onset of epilepsy showed a relative decline in performance. These results were consistent with an early deterioration followed by relatively little change later in the course.

Seidenberg et al.[27] conducted a longitudinal study in which they administered the WAIS to patients with epilepsy on two occasions 18 months apart. The patients were divided into two groups: In one group, seizure frequency had decreased during the test-retest interval, whereas in the other group, seizure frequency was unimproved. Although both groups showed higher WAIS scores on the second test administration, the increase in the group with unimproved seizures was smaller and was present in fewer tests. These findings support some intellectual deterioration in the more severely affected group. The *practice effect*, a phenomenon that describes improved scores on subsequent test administration resulting from familiarity, may also explain improvement of IQ scores in patients with uncontrolled epilepsy.

A prospective trial by Ellenberg et al.[29] tested children at ages 4 and 7 years. Those who experienced seizure onset between these two ages did not show significant decreases in mean IQ scores as compared to normal controls. This finding challenges the notion of intellectual deterioration in epilepsy. However, IQ was measured using two different scales: the Stanford-Binet Intelligence Scale at age 4 and the Wechsler Intelligence Scale for Children at age 7. Also, children with epilepsy were compared to their unaffected siblings. The IQ was slightly (but not significantly) higher in the unaffected group. However, a higher prevalence of mental retardation and a greater degree of variation in the IQ of the children with seizures was noted. The authors did not believe that these findings indicated intellectual deterioration, because mental retardation was present in the group with epilepsy before the onset of seizures and probably reflects preexisting neurologic damage and not changes caused by seizures.

Age of Onset, Frequency, and Duration

Most studies indicate that early age of onset of seizures is an important correlate of poor cognitive function in epilepsy.[30–36] Several studies emphasize that age of onset is, in fact, the most important predictor of cognitive outcome in patients with epilepsy.[37,38] In a series of 1,141 patients, Strauss et al.[38] demonstrated a linear decline in IQ, from age of onset before 1 year (mean IQ, 84.4) to adult onset (mean IQ, 93.4). A similar study measured the WAIS Full-Scale IQ (FSIQ) scores of 410 patients with various seizure types.[32] The scores were 90.6 with onset between 0 and 5 years; 94.9 with onset between 6 and 12 years; 96.7 with onset between 13 and 18 years; and 100.8 with onset between 19 and 28 years. The average percentages of scores below normal limits in the Neuropsychological Battery for Epilepsy were 62.5 (onset before 5 years), 56.4 (onset ages 6–12), 51.1 (onset ages 13–18), and 49.9 (onset ages 19–28).

Several studies found that seizure frequency was negatively correlated with cognitive outcome.[19,39–41] Other researchers found that this was not the case.[23,42] In monozygotic twins with the same form of epilepsy but different seizure frequency, the twin with the more frequent seizures showed greater cognitive impairment.[43] Another twin study involved two sets of twins with tuberous sclerosis. One twin from each set experienced frequent generalized seizures, whereas the second twin had infrequent or short-lived seizures; the more severely affected twins were more likely to be mentally retarded.[34] Another group found that significant cognitive impairment was best correlated with the number and severity of seizures.[44] However, the number of seizures around the time of testing was not correlated with IQ changes, consistent with a slowly progressive and sustained effect of seizures.

Long duration of epilepsy is another factor associated with cognitive decline.[23,40,45] Jokeit and Ebner[46] separated patients with epilepsy into groups on the basis of seizure duration. They found that patients with epilepsy of more than 30 years' duration had statistically significantly lower FSIQ scores than patients with epilepsy of 15–30 years' duration or fewer than 15 years of epilepsy. A statistic derived from duration of seizures is "years with seizures."[40] This number is obtained by subtracting from the seizure duration the number of 12-month periods in which no seizures occurred. Years with seizures showed a stronger negative correlation to intelligence than did simple duration of seizures.[40] Other researchers found that years with seizures may be the best way to relate time to neuropsychological functioning in epilepsy, because it combines measurement of frequency of attacks with the length of time over which they occurred.[47]

Although most evidence indicates that earlier age of onset, more frequent seizures, and longer duration correlate with the severity of cognitive impairment, the question about whether younger patients are at greater risk for cognitive change as adults remains unanswered. Patients who had an earlier age of onset had a smaller gain in FSIQ score during 1.5 years of follow-up than did children with later-onset seizures.[28] Poor prognosis may result from disruption of intellectual development at an earlier age.[28] Children with later-onset seizures may have a greater opportunity for intellectual growth before being affected by seizures. Support for this theory is provided by Gomez's study of the prevalence of mental retardation in children with tuberous sclerosis.[34] Mental retardation was observed in 72 of 79 children with seizure onset before age 1 year, whereas only 6 of 25 children with seizures after age 4 exhibited mental retardation.

Education also may contribute to the effects of epilepsy duration and cognitive outcome. Jokeit and Ebner[46] found that patients with higher educational levels had stable FSIQs for longer periods. This suggests that education level as an indicator of higher brain reserve may contribute to cognitive preservation, a theory that has been similarly advanced for other neurologic disorders.[48–52]

Holmes[53] explored the role of age at seizure onset in the cognitive outcome of rodents. He induced status epilepticus (SE) with kainic acid in prepubescent and mature rats and then compared their mental development. The mature group showed greater cognitive impairment, suggesting a role for neuronal plasticity in adapting to the adverse consequences of severe seizures. A similar protective effect during early human development may exist, but studies have not yet demonstrated this protection. It is possible that this effect is indeed found in humans but that underlying structural damage causes irreversible cognitive dysfunction that masks any independent effect of seizures.

Etiology

Etiology of epilepsy is a factor in determining cognitive function and intellectual changes over time. The main distinction is between symptomatic (i.e., identified cause such as stroke or cortical dysplasia) and idiopathic (i.e., no identified cause other than genetic factors) epilepsy. Lennox[5] recognized that cognitive function was twice as likely to deteriorate in the presence of a known cause of epilepsy even if the idiopathic group had more frequent seizures. In another study, children with idiopathic epilepsy were more likely to conform to the expected normal distribution of intellectual ability for their age.[54] A third study demonstrated that patients with symptomatic epilepsy had a mean 6-point drop in IQ during follow-up periods between 1 and 9 years, as compared to a drop of 0.7 points in a normal control group.[17]

More recent work has confirmed the poorer prognosis in patients with symptomatic epilepsy. In a longitudinal study of a group of 72 patients with epilepsy, those with the symptomatic form had a significantly lower IQ than those with idiopathic epilepsy (89.1 vs. 102.5 on initial evaluation).[23] At their last evaluation, the symptomatic group again had lower test scores: 88.9 as compared to 104.1 for the idiopathic group.

Type and Severity

The potential of SE to cause permanent neurologic sequelae has long been recognized. One study indicated that SE was the most important predictor of poor performance on the WAIS and the Neuropsychological Battery for Epilepsy.[55] Several studies from the early 1970s estimated the rate of cognitive impairment from SE to be as much as 25%.[56–58] Among the risk factors for the development of cognitive and behavioral decline after an episode of SE are early age of onset,[56] longer duration of SE,[58,59] failure to treat with AEDs,[56,60,61] and symptomatic etiology.[58,61]

In a retrospective study of 98 patients with SE, Aminoff and Simon[59] found that only 10 patients had permanent cognitive decline. Of these 10 patients, 6 had damage clearly related to SE, and 5 of the 6 had SE lasting 2 hours or longer. In

Table 12-3. Intelligence Quotient (IQ) Scores before and after Status Epilepticus

Test Variable	Control Group		Status Group	
	Mean	SD	Mean	SD
Beginning of 5-year period				
WAIS Verbal IQ	100.00	10.69	90.44	22.16
WAIS Performance IQ	99.89	17.02	81.11	20.55
WAIS Full-Scale IQ	99.78	12.77	85.56	22.32
End of 5-year period				
WAIS Verbal IQ	103.30	19.63	85.89	23.90
WAIS Performance IQ*	107.80	15.53	84.89	21.77
WAIS Full-Scale IQ*	105.60	17.40	84.67	23.57

WAIS = Wechsler Adult Intelligence Scale.
*$p <.05$, indicating a significant decrease in performance and full-scale IQ scores for the status group as compared to the control group.
Source: From CB Dodrill, AJ Wilensky. Intellectual impairment as an outcome of status epilepticus. Neurology 1990;40[Suppl 2]:23–27.

another study, 10 of 193 children with SE showed cognitive impairment after a follow-up of 1–2 years.[61] Of these children, though, 8 had other possible causes of cognitive decline such as symptomatic epilepsy or progressive encephalopathy. Dodrill and Wilensky[62] found cognitive and neuropsychological impairment on initial testing of patients with SE and evidence of deterioration in these patients (Table 12-3).

Nonconvulsive status epilepticus (NCSE) also was evaluated as a potential cause of cognitive decline. The impact of NCSE on cognitive function was traditionally considered minimal because it does not produce such adverse systemic consequences of convulsive SE as hyperthermia, acidosis, hyperkalemia, pulmonary compromise, or cardiovascular collapse.[63] A review of the literature found no evidence of long-term cognitive changes induced by NCSE.[64] In 20 consecutive patients, Cockerell et al.[65] found no intellectual sequelae with complex partial SE in the absence of acute neurologic precipitants. Stores et al.[66] found that 28 of 50 patients with NCSE demonstrated intellectual deterioration, but the likelihood that NCSE was the primary pathologic factor remains unknown, as the etiology of the epilepsy was not reported in each case. Thus, the likelihood that NCSE was the primary pathogenic factor remains unknown. Krumholz et al.[67] found nine patients with NCSE with persistent or permanent cognitive dysfunction or memory loss. However, the patients in this study were enrolled over a 10-year period from two academic medical centers, and so the overall prevalence of poor cognitive outcomes from NCSE was actually low.

Dodrill[55] found that adults who experienced more than 100 episodes of generalized tonic-clonic seizures were more likely to show poorer intellectual, neuropsychological, psychosocial, and emotional function than those who had experienced fewer episodes. Patients who had experienced SE, however, showed the poorest overall function, independent of the number of generalized tonic-clonic seizures.

The association of absence seizures with cognitive decline is not clear. In a study of 118 patients with epilepsy, Farwell et al.[40] found that patients with all seizure types except those with classic absence seizures demonstrated subnormal intelligence. Bourgeois et al.[23] found that the IQ of patients with absence seizures was higher than the mean of all patients with epilepsy. Dam[68] recognized that despite the observation that patients with absence seizures showed normal intelligence, they demonstrated impaired attention and poor social adaptation. Loiseau et al.[69] found that one-third of patients with absence seizures had a social maladjustment.

Wirrell et al.[70] compared a consecutive, population-based series of children, some of whom had absence epilepsy and others of whom had juvenile rheumatoid arthritis (JRA), diseases that share a similar incidence, high remission rate, and outpatient manageability. Five categories of outcome were measured: academic-personal, behavioral, employment-financial, family relations, and social-personal relations. At follow-up after 10 or more years, those with absence epilepsy had significantly greater difficulties than their JRA peers in the academic-personal and behavioral categories. JRA controlled, in large

part, for stigma and the effects of chronic medication and illness. These findings suggest that many of the academic and social problems among patients with absence seizures result from the biological effects of their epilepsy (the underlying pathophysiology and interictal epileptiform activity) and, possibly, its treatment.

Comparison of partial and generalized seizures reveals more specific deficits associated with partial epilepsy.[71] Although early onset of generalized seizures is associated with poorer outcome than is early onset of partial seizures, in one study, overall no significant difference between the neuropsychological functioning of these two groups was observed.[35] Memory deficits are more frequent and severe with partial seizures than with primary generalized epilepsies.[72,73] The cognitive effects of partial epilepsy differ based on lateralization and localization of the seizure focus, with left temporal, right temporal, and frontal lobe epilepsy each producing different phenomena.

Classically, left temporal lobe epilepsy (left TLE) causes verbal memory deficits, whereas right TLE causes visuospatial impairment.[26,38,74,75] Hermann et al.,[76] though, found that the overall effects of the laterality of TLE on hemisphere-dependent cognitive functions were the exception rather than the rule. Mesial TLE is associated with generalized cognitive impairment: impaired intelligence, academic achievement, language, and visuospatial function.[76] It is not, however, associated with deficits in tests of attention, concentration, or executive function.

Extratemporal foci cause a different set of long-term cognitive changes from those caused by temporal foci. Brier et al. found that extratemporal lobe epilepsy patients performed better than right TLE patients on nonverbal memory measures and better than left TLE patients on measures of verbal memory. Long-term cognitive change resulting from frontal lobe epilepsy (FLE) involves impairment of executive behavior: attention, movement programming, spontaneity, conceptualization, and planning.[77] Wieser[78] found that psychopathology was more common in FLE than in TLE. Helmstaedter et al.[77] compared 35 patients with TLE to 23 patients with FLE with respect to attention, speed, motor coordination, verbal and nonverbal fluency, concept formation, response inhibition, anticipatory behavior, and memory span. FLE was associated with significantly poorer results on almost all tests, fluency being the exception. No group differences were found with regard to the lateralization of the epileptic focus or the presence of cerebral lesions. Smith and Milner[79] found that patients with right-sided FLE had a higher incidence of cognitive estimation error than did patients with left-sided FLE or TLE. Further, a correlation between error score in cognitive estimation and lesion size for the left FLE group was found.

Psychosis and Epilepsy

A possible association between epilepsy and psychosis was first recognized in antiquity but gained attention in the middle of the nineteenth century with the writings of Benedict Morel[80] and Jules Falret.[81] Hill,[82] in 1953, made the first modern report of a schizophrenia-like syndrome in patients with TLE. Psychosis in epilepsy can occur during interictal and postictal periods.

The prevalence of interictal psychosis (IIP) in epilepsy ranges from 0% to 16%, with a mean of 7–8%.[83,84] Compared to schizophrenia, IIP may be associated with a greater incidence of empathic persecutory delusions, auditory hallucinations, appropriate affect, a lack of autistic traits, and suicidality.[85,86] As compared to patients with only epilepsy, those with IIP have a later age of onset of epilepsy and more complex partial seizures, are more likely to experience auras, and are less likely to have generalized epilepsy.[86] Seizure onset is typically 18–21 years before the onset of psychosis,[87,88] but other evidence suggests that both sets of symptoms begin at the same time.[89] Some studies show that dominant TLE is positively correlated with IIP,[90,91] whereas other studies demonstrate a positive correlation with bitemporal foci[85] or no correlation with laterality.[92]

Postictal psychosis (PIP) is characterized by fluctuating combinations of delirium; persecutory and other delusions; auditory, visual, and other hallucinations; and affective changes.[89,93] It is distinguished from postictal confusion by a lucid interval that lasts from 2 to 72 hours; confusion is typically maximal immediately or shortly after a single seizure or cluster of seizures.[93] Bilateral seizure foci and clustering of seizures are significantly associated with episodes of PIP.[84,93] Generalized seizures[93] and complex partial seizures,[89,94] however, were associated with PIP in other studies.

Drug withdrawal can be temporally associated with PIP and IIP, probably by increasing seizure frequency in most cases.[86,93,94] An important question is whether recurrent PIP lasting hours, days, or weeks can evolve into chronic IIP. Logsdail and Toone[89] found minimal evidence of progression from PIP to IIP in their patients. Tarulli and colleagues, though, found that approximately 15% of patients with PIP went on to develop an interictal psychosis.[95]

Pathologic and Radiologic Findings

The earliest microscopic examinations of autopsy and surgically resected temporal lobes demonstrated mesial temporal sclerosis (MTS) as the characteristic finding of intractable TLE.[96,97] Subsequent studies have verified the correlation of MTS with TLE.[98–100] Hippocampal pathologic findings are associated with long-term cognitive deficits. In one study, 59 patients with TLE underwent neuropsychological testing before surgical resection of mesial temporal lobe structures was performed.[101] After resection, volumetric cell densities for hippocampal subfields cornu ammonis 1 (CA1), cornu ammonis 2 (CA2), cornu ammonis 3 (CA3), the hilar area, and the granule cell layer of area dentata were determined. Significant correlation between verbal memory impairment and hippocampal neuronal loss in CA3 and the hilar area for patients with left temporal seizure foci was demonstrated. Verbal intellectual ability and language skills, however, were not correlated with pathologic change.

The role of an initial precipitating injury (IPI) in producing anatomic changes was studied by examining hippocampi in resected temporal lobes (Figure 12-3).[102] The precipitating injuries were divided into four groups: IPI without seizures; IPI with prolonged seizures; IPI with repetitive, nonprolonged seizures; and no IPI. Patients with an IPI had MTS, whereas those with idiopathic TLE demonstrated less promi-

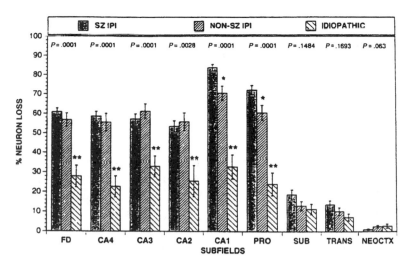

Figure 12-3. Comparison of mean neuronal loss in mesial temporal lobe epilepsy patients with initial precipitating injuries (IPIs) that involved seizures (SZ IPI), IPI events without seizures (NON-SZ IPI), and patients with idiopathic epilepsy (IDIOPATHIC). In cornu ammonis 1 (CA1) and prosubiculum (PRO), small differences in neuronal loss were noted between the two categories of IPI patients. These differences resulted from the longer duration of seizures in patients with IPIs that involved an initial severe seizure. (Subfields: FD = fascia dentata; CA4 = cornu ammonis 4; CA3 = cornu ammonis 3; CA2 = cornu ammonis 2; SUB = subiculum; TRANS = transitional cortex; NEOCTX = parahippocampal neocortex.) (Reprinted with permission from GW Mathern, TL Babb, JP Leite, et al. The pathogenetic and progressive features of chronic human hippocampal epilepsy. Epilepsy Res 1996;26:151–161. Copyright 1996, with permission from Elsevier Science.)

nent neuronal loss. Patients in whom the IPI was not associated with seizure were older at age of injury, had a longer latent period between injury and seizures, and showed more modest neuronal loss in Ammon's horn, CA1, and the presubiculum than did patients whose IPI initially produced seizures. An IPI that produced repetitive, nonprolonged seizures showed the shortest latent period, earliest age of TLE onset, and less CA2 damage than did other categories of IPI. CA1 and presubiculum neuronal losses were greater in patients with TLE of longer duration. An IPI after the age of 4 years was associated with shorter latent periods than an IPI occurring before the age of 4.

Correlation of pathologic findings and cognitive impairment has several methodological limitations. Emphasis has been placed almost exclusively on the temporal lobe, whereas extratemporal sites have largely been ignored. Patients requiring epilepsy surgery provide the vast majority of samples for microscopical evaluation; there are no surgical data on patients with less severe epilepsy. Similarly, control specimens from the contralateral hemispheres of surgically resected brains are not available. The issue of whether pathologic changes predate cognitive decline remains unknown. Complex and interwoven mechanisms related to preexisting neuropathologic lesions, seizure frequency and severity, and other factors likely contribute to cognitive and behavioral changes. Further, the role of different factors probably varies among different patients.

Lencz et al.[103] compared quantitative magnetic resonance imaging (MRI) in patients with refractory TLE and normal controls. They found that the left and right hippocampi were symmetric in the controls but, in patients with seizures, the hippocampus was smaller on the side of the focus. Additionally, the affected temporal lobe was smaller in patients with seizures as compared to that in normal controls. Neuronal densities were proportional to the ipsilateral-contralateral MRI volume ratio for every hippocampal subfield except CA2. Cognitive testing showed significant correlation between MRI measurement of the left hippocampus and logical memory retention scores and between the left temporal lobe volume and verbal memory testing.

The progressive nature of intellectual disability is also supported by MRI studies. In a case report of a 28-year-old patient with complex partial and secondary generalized seizures, a progressive decrease in the left hippocampal volume on MRI scans obtained 4 years apart was associated with moderate decline in verbal learning and memory functions and mild decline in visuospatial memory functions.[104] Patients with SE have demonstrated MRI abnormalities including cytotoxic and vasogenic edema, hyperperfusion of the epileptic region, and alteration of the leptomeningeal blood-brain barrier.[105] The changes were reversed on subsequent MRI, but these follow-up studies also showed subtle signs of atrophy, evidence of irreversible change. Other evidence indicating that recurrent seizures cause ongoing hippocampal damage include the observation that prolongation of ipsilateral T2 relaxation time in the body of the hippocampus correlated with the total number of both partial and generalized seizures and with the duration of TLE symptoms.[106]

MRI studies also demonstrated that repeated seizures correlate with progressive neuronal loss. This additional loss is small, usually occurs over long time intervals, and is found in limited subfields including granule cells, CA1, and the presubiculum.[107] This radiologic evidence is consistent with the cascadic model of deterioration, in which most cognitive change occurs early in the course of the disorder, followed by later stabilization of function.[24] Autopsies of patients who had seizures of 30 years' duration or patients with frequent generalized seizures showed greater neuronal losses than were seen in patients with fewer years of seizures.[108]

To evaluate the progressive neuronal losses that take place in TLE, Tasch et al.[109] evaluated patients using the neuron marker N-acetyl aspartate and MRI measurement of hippocampal volume. These researchers found that duration of epilepsy was negatively correlated with N-acetyl aspartate concentration bilaterally and hippocampal volume ipsilateral to the seizure focus. The number of complex partial seizures was not correlated with any radiologic measurement, but the number of generalized tonic-clonic seizures,

like seizure duration, was negatively correlated with N-acetyl aspartate measurements bilaterally and hippocampal volume ipsilaterally. These findings suggest that early fixed injuries can cause temporal lobe damage and that progressive neuronal losses also can result from multiple generalized seizures.

van Paesschen et al.[110] studied the hippocampus within 1 year of new onset of partial seizures, to identify possible change. Of 36 patients, 4 had MTS at onset and 32 had no changes on MRI. Twenty-three experienced seizures between the time that the baseline and follow-up MRI scans were obtained. Of the four patients with MTS, one had increased T2 relaxation time, suggesting progressive hippocampal damage. None of the 32 patients with negative MRI progressed to MTS, but two had significant hippocampal changes. The authors hypothesize that these hippocampal changes were the result of inflammatory swelling or edema after seizures were controlled.

Several MRI studies found evidence that SE can cause neuronal loss in the hippocampus. A 32-month-old child with an episode of SE was a subject for study of the progression of MTS.[111] Initial MRI demonstrated an increased T2 signal of the right hippocampus but no atrophy. Serial MRI performed at 2 months and then 13 months later demonstrated progressive hippocampal atrophy with resolution of the increased T2 signal. This study demonstrates the progressive changes induced by epilepsy. In an adult patient with generalized tonic-clonic SE, MRI scans showed bilateral hippocampal atrophy on initial evaluation.[112] Progressive hippocampal atrophy was detected in follow-up studies by hippocampal atrophy and coregistration of scans.

Using quantitative MRI, Baxendale et al.[113] found a significant association between global memory impairment and an abnormal proportion of gray to white matter. Patients with this structural abnormality did not have a WAIS-R score that differed significantly from that of normal patients. Extrahippocampal structural abnormalities were associated with further disruptions of memory in patients with MTS. Fluorodeoxyglucose–positron emission tomography measurement showed that prefrontal glucose hypometabolism is associated with lower verbal and performance intelligence scores.[114,115]

Drug Effects

The separation of AED toxicity from seizure effects is one of the most important obstacles in defining the progressive cognitive and behavioral decline of epilepsy. Studies that demonstrate stable or improving cognitive function over time may actually reflect benefits gained from seizure control. The AED that provides better seizure control for an individual may be more likely to provide a cognitive or behavioral benefit than the AED that has a statistically better cognitive-behavioral profile in controlled clinical studies.[116]

The cognitive benefits of treating epilepsy are supported by several studies. Seidenberg et al.[27] showed increased Wechsler verbal, performance, and full scale IQ measurements in patients with improved seizure control but no change in patients with poor seizure control. In another study, neuropsychological testing showed that unmedicated epilepsy patients performed poorly on fine motor, attention, and cognitive tasks as compared to normal controls.[117] Bourgeois et al.,[23] though, found that toxic drug levels and early age of onset were the factors most closely correlated with poor cognitive performance. Seizure control, therefore, should not be achieved at the price of repeated episodes of drug toxicity. Another study showed that treatment with AEDs, especially phenobarbital, caused decreased Wechsler Intelligence Scale for Children–Revised scores.[118]

Debate concerning the precise cognitive and behavioral effects of different AEDs is far from resolved. In the Holmfrid study, 100 children with epilepsy were seizure-free for 1 year on monotherapy with carbamazepine, phenytoin, or valproic acid.[119] The AEDs were withdrawn over a 3-month period, and the children were reevaluated 3–4 months later. Significant improvement attributable to drug withdrawal was noted on only the psychomotor speed test, suggesting a limited role for AEDs on cognitive function. This study showed, however, that phenytoin patients experienced greater cognitive impairment on tests of motor and mental speed than did carbamazepine patients.

Another drug withdrawal study involved children on monotherapy with carbamazepine, valproate, or phenytoin.[120] Withdrawal of the AED produced improvement in binary choice and visual search tasks, but similar improvements were noted in the normal control group. The performance of the children taking carbamazepine was similar to that of the children in the control group both before and after drug withdrawal. Children taking phenytoin, however, performed poorly both before and after drug discontinuation. A similar impairment, but to a lesser degree, was noted with the valproate group. The authors noted, however, that these differences among drugs might reflect differences among the children taking them rather than in the drugs themselves—a finding that may apply to other drug studies.

After 12 months of treatment, subjects taking valproic acid had higher cognitive scores than those taking carbamazepine or ethosuximide.[121] In another study, carbamazepine was less likely to cause cognitive impairment than was phenobarbital.[122] Vining et al.[123] found that children on phenobarbital had lower full-scale and performance IQ scores than did those on valproate.

In another comparison of valproate and phenobarbital, baseline WAIS FSIQ and WAIS performance IQ scores were lower for the phenobarbital group; the scores improved over time for the valproate group but not for the phenobarbital group.[124] Trimble[41] found that increased phenytoin and phenobarbital and decreased folic acid were the most important correlates of cognitive dysfunction. Mitchell and Chavez[125] found the toxicity of phenobarbital to be limited: Patients taking phenobarbital performed less well on digit symbol testing but on no other neuropsychological tests when compared to those taking carbamazepine. Camfield et al.[126] found, after 8–12 months of therapy, no significant differences in IQ between patients on phenobarbital and those taking placebo, but memory was affected in a serum-dependent manner and comprehension was negatively affected with longer duration of treatment. Gallassi et al.[127] found that phenytoin impairs memory and cognition and that this impairment resolves on drug withdrawal.

Comparisons of different drugs are problematic. Dodrill[47] noted that when two equally efficacious AEDs are prescribed for two patients with the same seizure type, differences between the patients likely account for different usage of medication. These patient differences include ability to deal with complex AED regimens, general intelligence, patient's financial status versus cost of medication, various emotional factors, and distance from the clinic where serial laboratory testing is conducted. Despite superficial resemblance of study groups, important intrinsic differences may exist between them that can account for different test scores.

Another issue in assessing cognitive side effects of AEDs is the role of polytherapy. Studies show that reduction of a multidrug regimen to monotherapy has beneficial effects on cognitive functioning and mood.[128] However, studies that suggest greater cognitive impairment with polypharmacy usually involve conversion to monotherapy of groups of patients doing poorly on polytherapy.[116] Dodrill[47] found that seizure frequency is positively correlated with the number and amount of prescribed AEDs, so that polypharmacy is used to treat sicker patients.

Several methodologic problems are present in the study of cognitive side effects of AEDs: lack of prospective studies, wide cognitive fluctuations in epilepsy, study of acute rather than chronic effects of the drug, use of normal volunteers rather than patients with seizures, attribution of cognitive change to AEDs by default, testing of multiple drugs simultaneously, comparison of drugs at noncomparable doses, testing of performance postictally, emphasis on statistical significance over clinical relevance, and attempts to analyze more factors than is warranted by a sample size.[129] These problems must be addressed before the role of AEDs in cognitive decline can be definitively stated.

Psychosocial Factors

Psychosocial problems affect cognitive and behavioral development in epilepsy patients. Psychological and psychiatric disorders can contribute to academic and cognitive problems. For example, depression is associated with memory impairments, sometimes mimicking dementia. Also, ongoing academic problems in children can cause an apparent progression of cognitive impairment, as healthy peers develop at an accelerated rate. Among the factors that contribute to impairment are physical disability that prevents participation in activities, side effects of medications, fatigue, feeling different from peers, impaired self-esteem, depression or

anxiety about illness, worries about the future, lack of independence, loss of sense of control, multiple hospitalizations and visits to health care professionals, restriction of social activities, and increased stressors on parents and children.[70] These psychosocial problems may have a greater impact on patients with epilepsy than was demonstrated in the past.[130,131] A study matched children with epilepsy to those with asthma and assessed them with regard to physical, psychological, social, and school functioning.[132] Children with epilepsy showed greater impairments in the psychological, social, and school categories, whereas asthmatics had a more compromised quality of life in the physical domain.

Subclinical Epileptiform Discharges

Defined as an epileptiform electroencephalographic discharge accompanied by temporary cognitive impairment as the only manifestation of seizure activity,[133] *transitory cognitive impairment* (TCI) is a controversial phenomenon. The precise electroencephalographic findings necessary to qualify a discharge as TCI are uncertain, but characteristic electroencephalographic changes of TCI include 3-Hz spike and wave discharges of greater than 3 seconds, prominent spike components, and early involvement of the frontocentral region.[134,135] Rugland,[136] however, observed that subclinical discharges impaired performance in 61% of the patients on a simple and a choice reaction time test, even though some discharges lasted only 1 second. Other studies also claimed that impairment occurs with discharges of less than 3 seconds' duration.[137,138] Proponents claim that measurements of performance such as the modified Corsi's Block Tapping Task,[134] the writing-to-dictation test,[139] and computer-based tests[136] are sensitive to TCI. These tests, however, share a complexity that is more sensitive to all types of seizure activity.[140,141]

Most TCI is found in patients who also suffer from epilepsy, causing confusion as to whether long-term changes in cognitive function result from TCI or effects of the comorbid epilepsy and the associated neuropathologic changes, seizures, and medications. Additionally, the distinction among TCI, interictal discharge in epilepsy patients, and subtle seizure is unclear. Aldenkamp et al.[140] attempted to separate these entities and found poor cognitive performance only in the group experiencing subtle seizures, thereby challenging the distinction of TCI as a separate phenomenon.

Summary

Early epileptologists understood that epilepsy caused cognitive impairment and behavioral problems. Modern researchers expanded on these findings, but progressive cognitive and behavioral decline in epilepsy remains a debated issue for several reasons. The first problem is one of methodology: No set of standards exist by which to measure behavioral, intellectual, and neuropsychological functioning in patients with epilepsy. Studies with longitudinal designs and those that use time as a variable strongly suggest cognitive and behavioral decline, but agreement is not universal. Other variables studied include etiology, type, severity, and laterality of seizures. Symptomatic epilepsy is more often associated with a severe decline than is idiopathic epilepsy. The cognitive changes caused by SE, generalized tonic-clonic seizures, and complex partial seizures must be separated from those caused by underlying structural damage. Absence seizures were traditionally considered benign, but recent studies have shown long-term cognitive and behavioral problems. The cause of these problems in patients with absence epilepsy remains unknown. Although postictal and interictal psychoses are well-documented phenomena, the issue of progression from postictal to interictal psychosis requires further exploration. Pathologic and radiologic findings demonstrate progressive cell loss and atrophy in selected cases, and further work is needed to correlate changes in neuropsychological and intellectual performance with anatomic changes. In addition, the identification of seizure, epilepsy, and individual patient characteristics that predispose individuals to progressive cell loss will be critical. AEDs are an important variable in the study of cognitive and behavioral decline: Successful control of seizures may prevent cognitive decline, but many drugs have recognized cognitive side effects. Poor psychosocial adjustment and subclinical epileptiform discharges cause subtle effects on performance, and further study of these two variables also is needed. Many potential variables that contribute to cognitive and behavioral decline in epilepsy are recognized, but their precise contributions to this decline must be the subject of further study.

References

1. Temkin O. The Falling Sickness (2nd ed). Baltimore: Johns Hopkins Press, 1971.
2. Esquirol E. Des Maladies Mentales. Paris: JB Balliere, 1838;284.
3. Romberg MH. A Manual of the Nervous Diseases of Man. (EH Sieveking, transl.) London: Syndenham Society, 1853.
4. Gowers WR. Epilepsy and Other Chronic Convulsive Diseases: Their Causes, Symptoms, and Treatment. New York: Wood & Co., 1885.
5. Lennox WG. Brain injury, drugs, and environment as causes of mental decay in epilepsy. Am J Psychiatry 1942;99:174–180.
6. Symonds C. Discussion. Proc R Soc Med 1962;55:314–315.
7. Aldenkamp AP. Effect of seizures and epileptiform discharges on cognitive function. Epilepsia 1997;38 [Suppl 1]:S52–S55.
8. Dodrill CB. Interictal cognitive aspects of epilepsy. Epilepsia 1992;33[Suppl 2]:S7–S10.
9. Wechsler D. The Wechsler Adult Intelligence Scale–Revised Manual. New York: The Psychological Corporation, 1981.
10. Cochrane HC, Marson AG, Baker GA, Chadwick DW. Neuropsychological outcomes in randomized controlled trials of antiepileptic drugs: a systematic review of methodology and reporting standards. Epilepsia 1998;39:1088–1097.
11. Golden CJ, Hammeke T, Purisch A. The Luria-Nebraska Battery Manual. Los Angeles: Western Psychological Services, 1981.
12. Reitan RM, Wolfson D. The Halstead-Reitan Neuropsychological Test Battery: Theory and Clinical Interpretation. Tucson: Neuropsychology Press, 1985.
13. Goldstein G. Comprehensive Neuropsychological Assessment Batteries. In G Goldstein, M Hersen (eds), Handbook of Psychological Assessment. New York: Pergamon, 1990;197–227.
14. Rosvold HE, Mirsky AF, Sarason I, et al. A continuous performance test of brain damage. J Consult Psychol 1956;20:343–350.
15. Dodrill CB. A neuropsychological battery for epilepsy. Epilepsia 1978;19:611–623.
16. Alpherts WCJ, Aldenkamp AP. Computerized neuropsychological assessment of cognitive functioning in children with epilepsy. Epilepsia 1990;31[Suppl 4]:S35–S40.

17. Arieff AJ, Yacorzynski GK. Deterioration of patients with organic epilepsy. J Nerv Ment Dis 1942;96:49–55.

18. Dawson S, Conn JCM. The intelligence of epileptic children. Arch Dis Child 1929;4:142–151.

19. Kugelmass IN, Poull LE, Rudnick J. Mental growth of epileptic children. Am J Dis Child 1938;55:295–303.

20. Barnes MR, Fetterman JL. Mentality of dispensary epileptic patients. Arch Neurol Psychiatry 1938;40:903–910.

21. Sullivan EB, Gahagan L. On intelligence of epileptic children. Genet Psychol Monogr 1935;17:369–376.

22. Holmes MD, Dodrill CB, Wilkus RJ, et al. Is partial epilepsy progressive? Ten-year follow-up of EEG and neuropsychological changes in adults with partial seizures. Epilepsia 1998;39:1189–1193.

23. Bourgeois BFD, Prensky AL, Palkes HS, et al. Intelligence in epilepsy: a prospective study in children. Ann Neurol 1983;14:438–444.

24. Meinardi H, Aldenkamp AP, Nunes B. Mental deterioration at epilepsy onset: a hypothesis. Acta Neurochir 1992;55:68–71.

25. Aldenkamp AP, Alpherts WCJ, De Bruine D, Dekker MJA. Test-retest variability in children with epilepsy—a comparison of WISC-R subtest profiles. Epilepsy Res 1990;7:165–172.

26. Rodin EA, Schmaltz S, Twitty G. Intellectual functions of patients with childhood-onset epilepsy. Dev Med Child Neurol 1986;28:25–33.

27. Seidenberg M, O'Leary DS, Giordani B, et al. Test-retest changes of epilepsy patients: assessing the influence of practice effects. J Clin Neuropsychol 1981;3:237–255.

28. Neyens LGJ, Aldenkamp AP, Meinardi HM. Prospective follow-up of intellectual development in children with a recent onset of epilepsy. Epilepsy Res 1999;34:85–90.

29. Ellenberg JH, Hirtz DG, Nelson KB. Do seizures in children cause intellectual deterioration? N Engl J Med 1986;314:1085–1088.

30. Dikmen S, Matthews CG, Harley JP. Effect of early versus late onset of major motor epilepsy on cognitive-intellectual performance: further considerations. Epilepsia 1977;18:31–36.

31. Dikmen S, Matthews CG, Harley JP. The effect of early versus late onset of major motor epilepsy upon cognitive intellectual performance. Epilepsia 1975;16:73–81.

32. Dodrill CB. Neuropsychological aspects of epilepsy. Psychiatr Clin North Am 1991;15:383–394.

33. Dodrill CB, Matthews CG. The role of neuropsychology in the assessment and treatment of persons with epilepsy. Am Psychol 1992;47:1139–1142.

34. Gomez MR, Kuntz NL, Westmoreland BF. Tuberous sclerosis, early onset of seizures, and mental subnormality: study of discordant homozygous twins. Neurology 1982;32:604–611.

35. O'Leary DS, Lovell MR, Sackellares JC, et al. Effects of age of onset of partial and generalized seizures on neuropsychological performance in children. J Nerv Ment Dis 1983;171:624–629.

36. Saykin AJ, Gur RC, Sussman NM, et al. Memory deficits before and after temporal lobectomy: effect of lateralization and age of onset. Brain Cogn 1989;9:191–200.

37. O'Leary DS, Seidenberg B, Berent S, et al. Effects of age of onset of tonic-clonic seizures on neuropsychological performance in children. Epilepsia 1981;22:197–204.

38. Strauss E, Loring D, Chelune G, et al. Predicting cognitive impairment in epilepsy: findings from the Bozeman epilepsy consortium. J Clin Exp Neuropsychol 1995;17:909–917.

39. Chaudhry MR, Pond DA. Mental deterioration in epileptic children. J Neurol Neurosurg Psychiatry 1961;24:213–219.

40. Farwell JR, Dodrill CB, Batzel LW. Neuropsychological abilities of children with epilepsy. Epilepsia 1985;26:395–400.

41. Trimble MR. Cognitive hazards of seizure disorders. Epilepsia 1988;29[Suppl]:S19–S24.

42. Giordani B, Sakellares JC, Miller S, et al. Improvement in neuropsychological performance in patients with refractory seizures after intensive diagnostic and therapeutic intervention. Neurology 1983;33:489–493.

43. Dodrill CB, Troupin AS. Seizures and adaptive abilities. Arch Neurol 1976;33:604–607.

44. Neimann H, Boenick HE, Schmidt RC, et al. Cognitive development in epilepsy: the relative influence of epileptic activity and of brain damage. Eur Arch Psychiatry Neurol Sci 1985;234:399–403.

45. Tomson T, Lindbom U, Nilsson BYI. Nonconvulsive status epilepticus in adults: thirty-two consecutive patients from a general hospital population. Epilepsia 1992;33:829–835.

46. Jokeit H, Ebner E. Long-term effects of refractory temporal lobe epilepsy on cognitive abilities: a cross sectional study. J Neurol Neurosurg Psychiatry 1999;67:44–50.

47. Dodrill CB. Problems in the assessment of cognitive effects of antiepileptic drugs. Epilepsia 1992;33[Suppl 6]:S29–S32.

48. Evans DA, Hebert LE, Becket LA, et al. Education and other measures of socioeconomic status and risk of incident Alzheimer disease in a defined population of older persons. Arch Neurol 1997;54:1399–1405.

49. Satz P. Brain reserve capacity on symptom onset after brain injury: a formulation and review of the evidence for threshold theory. Neuropsychology 1993;7:273–295.

50. Schmand B, Smit JH, Geerlings MI, et al. The effects of intelligence and education on the development of dementia. A test of the brain reserve hypothesis. Psychol Med 1997;27:1337–1344.

51. Stern Y, Gurland B, Tatemichi TK, et al. Influence of education and occupation on the incidence of Alzheimer's disease. JAMA 1994;271:1004–1010.

52. Timiras PS. Education, homeostasis, and longevity. Exp Gerontol 1995;30:189–198.

53. Holmes GL. The long-term effects of seizures on the developing brain: clinical and laboratory issues. Brain Dev 1991;13:393–409.

54. Collins AL, Lennox WG. The intelligence of 300 private epileptic patients. Res Publ Assoc Res Nerv Ment Dis 1947;26:586–603.

55. Dodrill CB. Correlates of generalized tonic-clonic seizures with intellectual, neuropsychological, emotional and social function in patients with epilepsy. Epilepsia 1986;27:399–411.

56. Aicardi J, Chevrie JJ. Convulsive status epilepticus in infants and children. Epilepsia 1970;11:187–197.

57. Oxbury JM, Whitty CWM. Causes and consequences of status epilepticus in adults: a study of 86 cases. Brain 1971;94:733–734.

58. Rowan AJ, Scott DF. Major status epilepticus: a series of 42 patients. Acta Neurol Scand 1970;46:573–584.

59. Aminoff MJ, Simon RP. Status epilepticus: causes, clinical features, and consequences in 98 patients. Am J Med 1980;69:657–666.

60. Lawson JS, Inglis J, Delva NJ, et al. Electrode placement in ECT: cognitive effects. Psychol Med 1990;20:335–344.

61. Maytal J, Shinnar S, Moshé SL, Alvarez LA. Low morbidity and mortality of status epilepticus in children. Pediatrics 1989;83:323–331.

62. Dodrill CB, Wilensky AJ. Intellectual impairment as an outcome of status epilepticus. Neurology 1990;40 [Suppl 2]:23–27.

63. Krumholz A. Epidemiology and evidence for morbidity of nonconvulsive status epilepticus. J Clin Neurophysiol 1999;16:314–322.

64. Drislane FW. Evidence against permanent neurologic damage from nonconvulsive status epilepticus. J Clin Neurophysiol 1999;16:323–331.

65. Cockerell OC, Walker MC, Sander JW, Shorvon SD. Complex partial status epilepticus: a recurrent problem. J Neurol Neurosurg Psychiatry 1994;57:835–837.

66. Stores G, Zaiwalla Z, Styles E, Hoshika A. Non-convulsive status epilepticus. Arch Dis Child 1995;73:106–111.

67. Krumholz A, Sung GY, Fisher RS. Complex partial status epilepticus accompanied by serious morbidity and mortality. Neurology 1995;45:1499–1504.

68. Dam M. Children with epilepsy: the effect of seizures, syndromes, and etiological factors on cognitive functioning. Epilepsia 1990;31[Suppl 4]:S26–S29.

69. Loiseau P, Pestre M, Dartigues JF, et al. Long-term prognosis in two forms of childhood epilepsy: typical absence seizures and epilepsy with Rolandic (centrotemporal) EEG foci. Ann Neurol 1983;13:642–648.

70. Wirrell EC, Camfield CS, Camfield PF, et al. Long-term psychosocial outcome in typical absence epilepsy. Arch Pediatr Adolesc Med 1997;151:152–158.

71. Rausch R, Leib JB, Crandall PA. Neuropsychological correlates of depth spike activity in epileptic patients. Arch Neurol 1978;35:699–705.

72. Glowinski H. Cognitive deficits in temporal lobe epilepsy. An investigation of memory function. J Ment Dis 1973;137:129–137.

73. Powell GE, Polkey CE, McMillan T. The new Maudsley series of temporal lobectomy: short-term cognitive effects. Br J Clin Psychol 1985;24:109–124.

74. Bridgman PA, Malamut BL, Sperling MR, et al. Memory during subclinical hippocampal seizures. Neurology 1989;39:853–856.

75. Hermann BP, Wyler AR, Richey ET, Rea JM. Memory function and verbal learning ability in patients with complex partial seizures of temporal lobe origin. Epilepsia 1987;28:547–554.

76. Hermann BP, Seidenberg M, Schoenfeld J, Davies K. Neuropsychological characteristics of the syndrome of mesial temporal lobe epilepsy. Arch Neurol 1997;54:369–376.

77. Helmstaedter C, Kemper B, Elger CE. Neuropsychological aspects of frontal lobe epilepsy. Neuropsychologia 1996;34:399–406.

78. Wieser HG. Selective amygdalohippocampectomy: indications, investigative technique and results. Adv Tech Stand Neurosurg 1986;13:39–133.

79. Smith ML, Milner B. Differential effects of frontal-lobe lesions on cognitive estimation and spatial memory. Neuropsychologia 1984;22:697–705.

80. Morel BA. Díune forme de delire, suite díune surexcitation nerveuse se rattachant à une variété non encore décrite díepilepsie (*Epilipsie larvae*). Gaz Habdom Med Chir 1860;7:773–775, 819–821, 836–841.

81. Falret JP. Memoire sur la folie circulain. Bull Acad Imp Med 1854;19:382–400.

82. Hill D. Psychiatric disorders of epilepsy. Medical Press 1953;229:473–475.

83. Trimble MR. The Psychosis of Epilepsy. New York: Raven Press, 1991.

84. Umbricht D, Degreef G, Barr WB, et al. Postictal and chronic psychoses in patients with temporal lobe epilepsy. Am J Psychiatry 1995;152:224–231.

85. Kristensen O, Sindrup EH. Psychomotor epilepsy and psychosis: III. Social and psychological correlates. Acta Neurol Scand 1979;59:1–9.

86. Mendez MF, Grau R, Doss RC, Taylor JL. Schizophrenia in epilepsy: seizure and psychosis variables. Neurology 1993;43:1073–1077.

87. Kristensen O, Sindrup EH. Psychomotor epilepsy and psychosis: I. Physical aspects. Acta Neurol Scand 1978;57:361–369.

88. Kristensen O, Sindrup EH. Psychomotor epilepsy and psychosis: II. Electroencephalographic findings (sphe-

noidal electrode recordings). Acta Neurol Scand 1978; 57:370–379.

89. Logsdail SJ, Toone BK. Post-ictal psychoses. A clinical and phenomenological description. Br J Psychiatry 1988;152:246–252.

90. Sherwin I, Peron-Magnan P, Bancaud J, et al. Prevalence of psychosis in epilepsy as a function of the laterality of the epileptogenic lesion. Arch Neurol 1982; 39:621–625.

91. Sherwin I. Psychosis associated with epilepsy: significance of the laterality of the epileptogenic lesion. J Neurol Neurosurg Psychiatry 1981;44:83–85.

92. Kanemoto K, Takeuchi J, Kawasaki J, Kawai I. Characteristics of temporal lobe epilepsy with mesial temporal sclerosis, with special reference to psychotic episodes. Neurology 1996;47:1199–1203.

93. Devinsky O, Abramson H, Alper K, et al. Postictal psychosis: a case control series of 20 patients and 150 controls. Epilepsy Res 1995;20:247–253.

94. Savard G, Andermann F, Olivier A, Remillard GM. Postictal psychosis after partial complex seizures: a multiple case study. Epilepsia 1991;32:225–231.

95. Tarulli A, Devinsky O, Alper K. Progression from postictal to interictal psychosis. Epilepsia 2001 (in press).

96. Falconer MA, Serafetinides EA, Corsellis JAN. Etiology and pathogenesis of temporal lobe epilepsy. Arch Neurol 1964;10:233–248.

97. Meyer A, Falconer MA, Beck E. Pathological findings in temporal lobe epilepsy. J Neurol Neurosurg Psychiatry 1954;17:276–285.

98. Corsellis JAN, Bruton CJ. Neuropathology of Status Epilepticus. In AV Delgado-Escueta, CG Wasterlain, DM Treiman, RJ Porter (eds), Status Epilepticus: Mechanism of Brain Damage and Treatment. New York: Raven Press, 1983;129–139.

99. Margerison JH, Corsellis JAN. Epilepsy and the temporal lobes: a clinical, electroencephalographic and neuropathological study of the brain in epilepsy, with particular reference to the temporal lobes. Brain 1966; 89:499–530.

100. Mathieson G. Pathology of Temporal Lobe Foci. In JK Penry, DD Daly (eds), Complex Partial Seizures and Their Treatment. New York: Raven Press, 1975;163–185.

101. Sass KJ, Sass A, Westerveld M, et al. Specificity in the correlation of verbal memory and hippocampal neuron loss: dissociation of memory, language, and verbal ability. J Clin Exp Neuropsychol 1992;14:662–672.

102. Mathern GW, Babb TL, Vickney BG. The clinical-pathogenic mechanisms of hippocampal neuron loss and surgical outcomes in temporal lobe epilepsy. Brain 1995;118:105–118.

103. Lencz BA, McCarthy G, Bronen RA, et al. Quantitative magnetic resonance imaging in temporal lobe epilepsy: relationship to neuropathology and neuropsychological function. Ann Neurol 1992;31:629–637.

104. O'Brien TJ, So ES, Meyer FB, et al. Progressive hippocampal atrophy in chronic intractable temporal lobe epilepsy. Ann Neurol 1999;45:526–529.

105. Lansberg MG, O'Brien MW, Norbash AM, et al. MRI abnormalities associated with partial status epilepticus. Neurology 1999;52:1021–1027.

106. Kalvianinen R, Salmenpera T, Partanen K. Recurrent seizures may cause hippocampal damage in temporal lobe epilepsy. Neurology 1998;50:1377–1382.

107. Mathern GW, Babb TL, Leite JP, et al. The pathogenetic and progressive features of chronic human hippocampal epilepsy. Epilepsy Res 1996;26:151–161.

108. Mourtitzen-Dam A. Epilepsy and neuron loss in the hippocampus. Epilepsia 1980;21:617–629.

109. Tasch E, Cendes F, Li M, et al. Neuroimaging evidence of progressive neuronal loss and dysfunction in temporal lobe epilepsy. Ann Neurol 1999;45:568–576.

110. van Paesschen W, Duncan JS, Strauss JM, Connolly A. Longitudinal quantitative hippocampal magnetic resonance imaging study of adults with newly diagnosed partial seizures: one-year follow-up results. Epilepsia 1998;39:633–639.

111. Nohria V, Lee N, Tien RD, et al. Magnetic resonance imaging evidence of hippocampal sclerosis in progression: a case report. Epilepsia 1994;35:1332–1336.

112. Wieshmann UC, Woermann FG, Lemieux L, et al. Development of hippocampal atrophy, a serial magnetic resonance imaging study in a patient who developed epilepsy after generalized status epilepticus. Epilepsia 1997;38:1238–1241.

113. Baxendale SA, Sisodiya SM, Thompson J, et al. Disproportion in the distribution of gray and white matter. Neuropsychological correlates. Neurology 1999;52:248–251.

114. Jokeit H, Seitz RI, Markowitsch HJ, et al. Prefrontal asymmetric interictal glucose hypometabolism and cognitive impairment in patients with temporal lobe epilepsy. Brain 1997;120:2283–2294.

115. Rausch R, Henry TR, Ary CM, et al. Asymmetric interictal glucose hypometabolism and cognitive performance in epileptic patients. Arch Neurol 1994;51:139–144.

116. Devinsky O. Cognitive and behavioral effects of antiepileptic drugs. Epilepsia 1995;36[Suppl 2]:S46–S65.

117. Smith DB, Craft BR, Collins J, et al. Behavioral characteristics of epilepsy patients compared with normal controls. Epilepsia 1986;27:760–768.

118. Funakoshi A, Morikawa T, Muramatsu R, et al. A prospective WISC-R study in children with epilepsy. Jpn J Psychiatry Neurol 1988;42:562–564.

119. Aldenkamp AP, Alpherts WCJ, Blennow G, et al. Withdrawal of antiepileptic medication in children—effects on cognitive function: the multicentre "Holmfrid" study. Neurology 1993;43:41–50.

120. Blennow G, Heijbel J, Sandstedt P, Tonnby B. Discontinuation of antiepileptic drugs in children who have

outgrown epilepsy. Effects on cognitive function. Epilepsia 1990;31[Suppl 4]:S50–S53.

121. Mandelbaum DE, Burack GD. The effect of seizure type and medication on cognitive and behavioral functioning in children with idiopathic epilepsy. Dev Med Child Neurol 1997;39:731–735.

122. Voorhies TM. Cognitive and behavioral effects of antiepileptic drugs. Semin Neurol 1988;8:35–41.

123. Vining EPG, Mellitis E, Dorsen MM, et al. Psychologic and behavioural effects of antiepileptic drugs in children: a double-blind comparison between phenobarbital and valproic acid Pediatrics 1987;80.165–174.

124. Calandre EP, Dominguez-Granados R, Gomez-Rubio M, Molina-Font JA. Cognitive effects of long-term treatment with phenobarbital and valproic acid in school children. Acta Neurol Scand 1990;81:504–506.

125. Mitchell WG, Chavez JM. Carbamazepine versus phenobarbital for partial onset seizures in children. Epilepsia 1987;28:56–60.

126. Camfield CS, Chaplin S, Doyle AB, et al. Side effects of phenobarbital in toddlers: behaviour and cognitive aspects. J Pediatr 1979;95:361–365.

127. Gallassi R, Morreale A, Lorusso S, et al. Carbamazepine and phenytoin. Comparison of cognitive effects in epileptic patients during monotherapy and withdrawal. Arch Neurol 1988;45:892–894.

128. Thompson PJ, Trimble MR. Anticonvulsant drugs and cognitive functions. Epilepsia 1982;23:531–544.

129. Bourgeois BFD. Antiepileptic drugs, learning, and behavior in childhood epilepsy. Epilepsia 1998;39:913–921.

130. Hertoft P. The clinical, electroencephalographic and social prognosis in petit mal epilepsy. Epilepsia 1963;4:298–314.

131. Sillanpaa M. Medico-social prognosis of children with epilepsy. Acta Pediatr Scand Suppl 1973;237:3–104.

132. Austin JK, Smith S, Risinger MW, McNelis AM. Childhood epilepsy and asthma: comparison of quality of life. Epilepsia 1994;35:608–615.

133. Schwab RS. A method of measuring consciousness in petit mal epilepsy. J Nerv Ment Dis 1939;89:690–691.

134. Aarts JHP, Binnie CD, Smit AM, et al. Selective cognitive impairment during focal and generalised epileptiform EEG activity. Brain 1984;107:293–308.

135. Aldenkamp AP, Alpherts WCJ, Dekker MCA, et al. Neuropsychological aspects of learning disabilities in epilepsy. Epilepsia 1990;31[Suppl 4]:S9–S20.

136. Rugland AL. Neuropsychological assessment of cognitive functioning in children with epilepsy. Epilepsia 1990;31[Suppl 4]:S41–S44.

137. Mendizabal JE, Nowack WJ. Transitory cognitive impairment with brief generalized spike-wave paroxysm: a clinical counterexample to the three-second rule. Clin Electroencephalogr 1996;27:215–217.

138. Sellden U. Psychotechnical performance related to paroxysmal discharges in EEG. Clin Electroencephalogr 1971;2:18–27.

139. Siebelink BM, Bakker DJ, Binnie CD, et al. Psychological effects of sub-clinical EEG discharges in children: general intelligence tests. Epilepsy Res 1988;2:117–121.

140. Aldenkamp AP, Overweg J, Gutter T, et al. Effect of epilepsy, seizures and epileptiform EEG discharges on cognitive function. Acta Neurol Scand 1996;93:253–259.

141. Martins da Silva A. Neurophysiological Aspects of Epilepsy. In AP Aldenkamp, PE Dreifuss, WO Renier, et al. (eds), Epilepsy in Children and Adolescents. New York: CRC Press, 1995;83–101.

Chapter 13

Interictal Depression in Chronic Epilepsy

Bruce P. Hermann, Michael Seidenberg,
and Brian D. Bell

Interest in the issue of interictal psychopathology in patients with epilepsy has been long-standing, particularly in localization-related forms of epilepsy. The behaviors of interest have been diverse and include aggression, personality change, schizophreniform psychoses, mood and anxiety disorders, and other behaviors. Although this field of research has been complex and controversial for a variety of reasons, little doubt remains that comorbid interictal psychopathology can serve only to increase the burden of living with epilepsy. This chapter focuses on what appears to be one of the more commonly occurring interictal behavioral problems in epilepsy, depression. We focus on this problem because of its presumed high rate of occurrence, its known additional morbidity and mortality, and its responsiveness to treatment.

The recently published "Consensus Statement on the Undertreatment of Depression"[1] pointed out that psychiatric depression is among the most frequent of all medical illnesses, with high rates of chronicity, relapse, and recurrence. It is associated with increased psychosocial and physical impairments as well as elevated morbidity and mortality, yet depression remains significantly underrecognized and undertreated in the general population. Further, depression is an extremely costly disorder, 1 of the 10 most costly illnesses in the United States, with estimated direct and indirect costs estimated to be approximately $12 billion and $31 billion per year, respectively. Of these amounts, $8 billion of the costs are said to be associated with

premature death and $23 billion to absenteeism and loss of productivity. Major depression accounts for 85% of the total costs.

To determine what is known about depression in epilepsy, we review the literature pertaining to patients with chronic epilepsy, concentrating most on those studies using contemporary psychiatric nosology (e.g., diagnoses from *Diagnostic and Statistical Manual of Mental Disorders* [*DSM*], Washington, DC: American Psychiatric Association, 1994; *International Classification of Diseases of the World Health Organization* [*ICD*], Salt Lake City: Medicode, 1998). Five issues are addressed: (1) the risk and predominant types of lifetime-to-date psychiatric comorbidity in chronic epilepsy, (2) adequacy of recognition and treatment of psychiatric comorbidity in chronic epilepsy, (3) the additional burdens that comorbid psychiatric disorders impose on patients with chronic epilepsy, (4) the etiology of these disorders, and (5) strategies for treatment. Current appreciation for these issues in epilepsy will be contrasted to the view of these issues in related fields (e.g., primary care, psychiatry, and epidemiology).

Predominant Types of Psychiatric Comorbidity in Chronic Epilepsy

Because a very limited number of studies examine current *DSM* axis I disorders in chronic epilepsy (e.g., Fiordelli et al.,[2] Manchada et al.[3]), we focus on the rate of lifetime-to-date disorders. Review of

Table 13-1. Reported Rates of *DSM* Lifetime-to-Date Major Depression in Chronic Epilepsy

Investigation	Rate of Major Depression (%)
Koch-Weser et al.[8]	8
Bromfield et al.[9]	20
Silberman et al.[5]	48
Victoroff[4]	32
Mean	29
Median	32
Wiegartz et al.[10]	32
Altshuler et al.[6]	39
Hermann et al.[7]	23

DSM = Diagnostic and Statistical Manual of Mental Disorders.

available studies suggests that mood disorders are the most common lifetime-to-date *DSM* axis I diagnosis among patients with chronic epilepsy, followed by anxiety disorders. Victoroff[4] reported a high rate of lifetime-to-date mood (63%) and anxiety (32%) disorders in his sample of 60 patients with medically intractable chronic complex partial seizures. Silberman et al.[5] reported comparable proportions of mood (62%) and anxiety (15%) lifetime-to-date disorders in a smaller sample of patients (n = 21) with mixed seizure types. Altshuler et al.[6] reported a predominance of mood (44%) as compared to anxiety (5%) lifetime-to-date disorders in their sample of 62 patients with intractable complex partial seizures. In our unpublished series of 43 patients with definite or probable temporal lobe epilepsy, mood (46%), substance abuse (22%), and anxiety (13%) lifetime-to-date *DSM-IV* disorders predominated.[7] In summary, investigations conducting comprehensive examination of *DSM* lifetime-to-date axis I disorders among patients with chronic epilepsy have consistently reported mood disorders to be the most prevalent problem.

Within the spectrum of lifetime-to-date mood disorders, major depression has been reported to be the most prevalent among epilepsy patients.[4–6] Table 13-1 provides a summary of reported prevalences of lifetime-to-date major depression.[4–10] These estimates range from 8% to 48%, with a mean and median of approximately 30%. The prevalence of lifetime-to-date major depression within the general population also has been

somewhat variable across major epidemiologic investigations (e.g., 6% and 17% in the Epidemiologic Catchment Area and National Comorbidity Surveys, respectively).[11–13] However, results from the majority of studies of patients with chronic and intractable epilepsy argue persuasively that these patients' lifetime risk of major depression is considerably elevated as compared to the general population.

Hence, on the basis of available evidence for chronic epilepsy patients, it appears that mood disorders are the most prevalent lifetime-to-date axis I disorder and that major depression is the most prevalent of the mood disorders and occurs more frequently among patients with chronic epilepsy as compared to the general population.

In any discussion of the risk of psychiatric disorder in epilepsy, one must bear in mind several points: As has been reviewed elsewhere, research is needed to determine the degree to which elevated rates of *DSM*-defined mood disorders and major depression are associated with epilepsy specifically, as compared to neurologic disorder or chronic medical illness more generally.[14–19] It should also be appreciated that rates of neurobehavioral impairment are lower in community-based samples as compared to tertiary care clinic populations, in which the epilepsy is more severe and intractable. Furthermore, although several investigators reported that the onset of depression followed the onset of epilepsy in the majority of patients investigated, evidence reveals that mood disorders may antedate the onset of epilepsy, an issue that warrants closer appreciation in the clinical literature. Finally, comparison of the expression and natural history of mood disorders and major depression in epileptic patients versus other populations has been studied only infrequently (see Robertson[14] and Lambert and Robertson[17]). Several of these issues have been examined using self-report measures of depressive symptoms but remain to be investigated in the setting of a study of depressive illness.

Recognition and Treatment of Comorbid Psychiatric Disorder in Chronic Epilepsy

An extensive literature has shown that psychiatric comorbidity in general, and depression in particular, is underrecognized and undertreated in non-epilepsy medical settings, including primary care. For example, Katon et al.[20] reported that only 55% of depressed primary care patients had been identified, and only 11% received an adequate trial of antidepressant medication. Similarly, Spitzer et al.[21] reported that 67% of primary care patients with current major depression were undetected. The degree to which psychiatric comorbidity has been underrecognized and undertreated in community settings has been documented as well. For instance, the National Comorbidity Survey reported that only 40% of patients with at least one lifetime disorder and only 20% with a current disorder had obtained professional help, with only 11% receiving that help in the mental health sector,[13] which is consistent with earlier reports of undertreatment.[12]

Although underrecognition and undertreatment of major depression have been studied in primary care, psychiatric, and epidemiologic settings, the degree to which comorbid psychiatric disorder is undertreated in epilepsy has been studied only rarely. The limited available information in the epilepsy population is consistent with that reported earlier for primary care patients and other populations.

Wiegartz et al.[10] conducted a standardized psychiatric interview—the Structured Clinical Interview for *DSM-IV*—to assess the presence and type of *DSM-IV* mood disorders in 76 patients with chronic complex partial seizures who were attending a tertiary care center. They found that 32.0% of the sample had experienced lifetime-to-date episodes of major depression, including 9.2% with current major depression, whereas 25.0% of the sample had a current minor depression. Examination of medical records and interviews with patients were conducted to determine whether patients with past or current major depression had undergone treatment (psychotherapy or antidepressant medication) for their mood disorder. Wiegartz et al.[10] reported that the depression had gone untreated in 38% of the patients with lifetime-to-date major depression and in 43% of those with current major depression.

Ettinger et al.[22] administered self-report measures of depression (Child Depression Inventory, n = 42) and anxiety (Child Manifest Anxiety Scale, n = 44) to children and adolescents with epilepsy (ages 7–18 years). Medical records were

reviewed and family members were interviewed to determine whether psychiatric comorbidity had been detected or treated and whether the patient had been referred for further evaluation or treatment. Using clinical cut-off points on the self-report measures, Ettinger et al.[22] reported that 26% of the children and adolescents exhibited elevated symptoms of depression and 16% reported significant anxiety. None of these children had been previously recognized as having experienced depression or anxiety or had been referred for further psychiatric assessment or treatment.

Paradiso et al.[23] conducted a standardized psychiatric examination of 70 consecutive patients with intractable temporal lobe epilepsy undergoing inpatient monitoring for determination of surgical candidacy. These researchers reported that, although 34% of patients were clinically depressed, none were taking antidepressant medications on presentation to the monitoring unit. The majority of these patients (85%) subsequently were started and maintained on antidepressant medications.

O'Donoghue et al.[24] conducted a survey of 109 patients with epilepsy drawn from two general practices in the United Kingdom. The patients completed self-report measures of perceived handicap (Subjective Handicap of Epilepsy Scale), quality of life (QOL; Short Form General Health Survey [SF]-36), and anxiety and depression (Hospital Anxiety and Depression [HAD] Scale). In addition, charts were audited to determine whether the general practitioner had recorded symptoms of depression, anxiety, psychosis, attempted self-harm, or other psychiatric symptoms and to determine whether antidepressant or antipsychotic medications had been prescribed. For only one-third of those who were classified as definite or borderline psychiatric cases by objective self-report (HAD Scale) was there a record of psychological symptoms in their medical notes in the last 2 years.

These findings suggest that psychiatric comorbidity is as underrecognzed and undertreated in chronic epilepsy patients as it is in primary care studies and the general population. This underrecognition and undertreatment of psychiatric comorbidity has been detected in adult and pediatric patients in specialty epilepsy centers as well as in

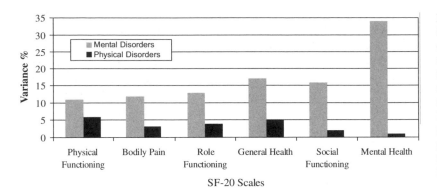

Figure 13-1. Unique variance in self-reported health quality of life due to comorbid psychiatric disorder versus physical illness. (SF-20 = Short-Form General Health Survey.) (Adapted from R Spitzer, K Kroenke, M Linzer, et al. Health-related quality of life in primary care patients with mental disorders: results from the Prime-MD 1000 study. JAMA 1995;274[19]:1511–1517.)

epilepsy patients receiving community-based care. The causes underlying this problem in epilepsy remain to be determined and should constitute a focus for future investigation.

Additional Burdens Associated with Psychiatric Comorbidity in Chronic Epilepsy

Research in primary care and other settings has demonstrated that psychiatric comorbidity is associated with additional burdens in daily life. These studies have shown that major depression is associated with significantly decreased self-reported QOL, increased disability or missed work, and increased use of the health care system and medical costs.[25–31] Further, synchrony between psychosocial disability and variations in the severity of psychiatric symptomatology has been demonstrated.[32]

Spitzer et al.[21] examined 1,000 adult patients assessed by 31 primary care physicians using PRIME-MD (Primary Care Evaluation of Mental Disorders) to make diagnoses of selected psychiatric conditions. One or more PRIME-MD disorders were identified in 39% of patients, including mood (39%), anxiety (18%), somatoform (14%), alcohol (5%) and eating disorders (3%). Twenty-six percent of patients had a psychiatric condition that met full criteria for a *DSM-III* disorder, whereas another 13% had subthreshold symptoms. Patients also were assessed with the Short-Form General Health Survey (SF-20). Psychiatric disorders, particularly mood disorders, accounted for considerably more of the impairment across all domains of QOL than did medical disorders. Whereas mood

disorders adversely affected all QOL domains, anxiety, somatoform, and eating disorders affected only selected domains. Figure 13-1 demonstrates the relative effects of mood and physical illness on the SF-20.

Other examples of psychosocial impairment associated with psychiatric comorbidity have been provided in clinical[25] and epidemiologic investigations.[33] Broadhead et al.[33] examined 3,798 community residents in the North Carolina component of the ECA study. Baseline interviews occurred in 1982–1983 (wave 1), with follow-up interviews conducted approximately 1 year later (wave 2). The results to be described here pertain to 2,980 community residents who were seen at wave 1 and who also completed wave 2. At wave 1, subjects underwent a standardized psychiatric interview (Diagnostic Interview Schedule) and were classified as exhibiting major depression, dysthymia, minor depression with mood disturbance, or minor depression without mood disturbance or were asymptomatic. Subjects were assessed with regard to the number of days in the last 3 months that they had missed work, were late to work, spent all or part of the day in bed, or were kept from their usual activities. As Figure 13-2 shows, the odds ratio for disability days or missed work is significantly elevated among subjects with major depression.

It has also been appreciated that patients with depression are more frequent users of the health care system and may incur more medical costs. Simon et al.[29,30] recently reported annual yearly medical costs for patients with depression in a large health maintenance organization as compared to controls. These

Figure 13-2. Odds ratio for one or more disability days or missed workdays in a 90-day interval. (Adapted from W Broadhead, D Blazer, L George, C Tse. Depression, disability days, and days lost from work in a prospective epidemiologic survey. JAMA 1990;264[19]:2524–2528.)

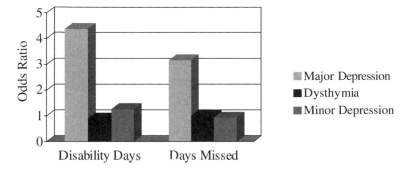

increased costs related to depression were seen across levels of chronic disease severity (Figure 13-3), with medical costs for depressed patients being significantly higher than those for controls. The increased medical costs were not limited to mental health care, which actually constituted only a fraction of total expenditures. Rather, the increased costs for depressed patients were evident across every category of medical expenditure.

What is the state of evidence regarding the additional burdens associated with comorbid psychiatric disorder among patients with chronic epilepsy? This issue has not received adequate attention to date. Wiegartz et al.[10] examined the relationship among self-reported health-related QOL in epilepsy (QOLIE-31) and *DSM-IV* diagnoses of current minor depression (n = 19), lifetime but not current major depression (n = 17), current major depression (n = 7), and no lifetime-to-date mood disorder (n = 32). Figure 13-4 shows overall QOL scores for the patient groups. Specifically, patients with current major depression reported poorer QOL on seven of eight QOLIE-31 scales as compared to nonde-

pressed controls, and patients with current minor depression also reported significantly lower QOL as compared to controls.

Similar results were reported recently by Lehrner et al.[34] These investigators examined the effects of comorbid depression on health-related QOL in 56 patients with temporal lobe epilepsy who were undergoing evaluation for epilepsy surgery. Overall, 45% of the sample exhibited significant symptoms of depression, as assessed by self-report. Comorbid depression was found to be associated with significantly reduced self-reported QOL across all scales (physical well-being, activity and capability, relations and family, independence, coping and control, emotional state and mood) after adjustment for intellectual status, demographic, and seizure-related variables.

Paradiso et al.[23] examined the neuropsychological correlates of depression in a series of 70 consecutive patients with chronic temporal lobe epilepsy. After controlling for any sociodemographic and clinical seizure variables, they found that patients with temporal lobe epilepsy and

Figure 13-3. Mean annual health care costs for primary care patients with recognized depression, controlling for chronic disease level. (Adapted from G Simon, M von Korff, W Barlow. Healthcare costs of primary care patients with recognized depression. Arch Gen Psychiatry 1995;52:850–856.)

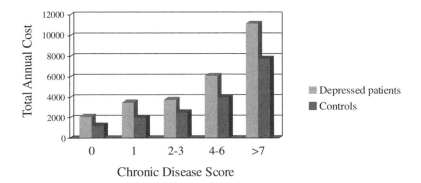

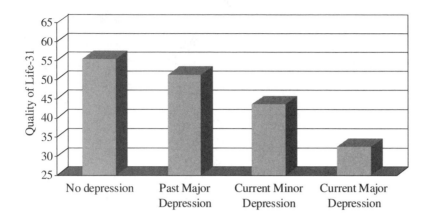

Figure 13-4. Self-reported quality of life in epilepsy as a function of depression. (Adapted from P Wiegartz, M Seidenberg, A Woodard, et al. Co-morbid psychiatric disorder in chronic epilepsy: recognition and etiology of depression. Neurology 1999;53[5]:3–25.)

depression exhibited more impairments in neuropsychological status as compared to nondepressed patients with temporal lobe epilepsy.

Finally, we recently examined the effects of comorbid depression on QOL among a sample of 54 outpatients with temporal lobe epilepsy attending a tertiary care clinic.[35] Patients completed self-report measures of psychiatric symptomatology (Symptom Checklist-90-Revised [SCL-90-R]) and a well-known measure of health-related QOL in epilepsy (QOLIE-89). Summary measures of psychiatric distress in general, and depression in particular, were examined as to their relationship with the QOLIE-89. The results, shown in Table 13-2, revealed a strong relationship between increased interictal psychopathology in general and depression in particular and significantly lower QOL.

Understanding the additional burdens posed by comorbid psychiatric disorder in chronic epilepsy is preliminary, although these burdens appear to be significant and include cognition and QOL. Within the epilepsy literature is little understanding of the temporal course or synchrony between depression and associated psychosocial disability, no information regarding use of the health care system or health care costs associated with depression in epilepsy, and only the most rudimentary understanding of the more general consequences of comorbid depression. Further, the use of paper-and-pencil measures to assess psychosocial burden (e.g., QOL measures) is problematic given the confounding effects of negative affectivity and response bias associated with depression: More objective measures of psychosocial burden are needed to address this topic in epilepsy.

Etiology of Depression in Chronic Epilepsy

Identifying reliable predictors of interictal comorbid psychiatric disorder in epilepsy is a difficult venture. As outlined previously, we reviewed 36 studies of depression in epilepsy.[35] Although these studies do not represent the entire body of epilepsy and depression literature, our purpose was to gain some preliminary insight into the factors that had been investigated as potential predictors of depression in epilepsy and to assess the degree to which reliable predictors of depression had been identified.

Across these 36 studies, a total of 60 different variables were examined in relation to depression in epilepsy. Potential predictor variables fell into four categories: (1) neuroepilepsy (e.g., age of onset, laterality, duration of disorder, etiology, seizure type); (2) psychological and social factors (e.g., adjustment to epilepsy, perceived stigma or discrimination, stressful life events); (3) medication (e.g., monotherapy vs. polytherapy, use of barbiturate medications, blood levels); and (4) socio-demographic factors (e.g., age, gender, education). Table 13-3 indicates the degree to which research activity has been devoted to these four categories of variables. It also reveals the proportion of positive findings that resulted from analyses of their relationship to depression. As can be seen, neuroepilepsy variables were the most frequently investigated predictors of interictal depression but, interestingly, they resulted in the fewest positive findings. Less commonly evaluated were psychological and social and medication variables (representing 15% and 12% of the analyses, respectively), although these variable types were more frequently associated with depression

Table 13-2. Correlations between Emotional-Behavioral Distress and Health-Related Quality of Life

	Global Severity Index	Symptom Distress Index	Depression
Health perceptions	−.54[a]	−.57[a]	−.50[a]
Overall quality of life	−.60[a]	−.52[a]	−.63[a]
Physical function	−.44[a]	−.41[a]	−.42[a]
Role limitations			
Physical	−.54[a]	−.43[a]	−.51[a]
Emotional	−.63[a]	−.55[a]	−.63[a]
Pain	−.45[a]	−.40[a]	−.42[a]
Work, driving, social	−.61[a]	−.54[a]	−.56[a]
Energy, fatigue	−.57[a]	−.62[a]	−62[a]
Emotional well-being	−.70[a]	−.67[a]	−.67[a]
Attention, concentration	−.70[a]	−.70[a]	−.63[a]
Health discouragement	−.64[a]	−.57[a]	−.59[a]
Seizure worry	−.41[a]	−.42[a]	−.38[a]
Memory	−.48[a]	−.48[a]	−.36[a]
Language	−.58[a]	−.51[a]	−.50[a]
Medication effects	−.48[a]	−.40[a]	−.46[a]
Social support	−.29[b]	−.17	−.19
Social isolation	−.64[a]	−.56[a]	−.63[a]
Total	−.84[a]	−.77[a]	−.79[a]

[a]$p < .01$.
[b]$p < .05$.

than were neuroepilepsy variables. However, the nature of the relationship between self-reported depression and several of the psychosocial measures is uncertain, owing to potential overlap of item content and response bias complications associated with depression.

Overall, the relationship between specific predictor variables and depression was examined in 196 analyses. We categorized predictor variables (regardless of type) into four categories on the basis of the degree to which they were associated with depression: (1) variables that were not reliably associated with depression in epilepsy (significant <50% of the time); (2) variables having mixed findings (significant approximately 50% of the time); (3) variables that were more reliably predictive of depression (significant >50% of the time); and (4) a group of variables that simply have not been examined sufficiently to determine their relationship to depression in epilepsy.

Table 13-4 provides examples of variables that were not reliably associated with depression across studies. For example, age of onset of epilepsy was significant in only 2 of 13 analyses (15%). At first glance, that several of the listed variables were not reliably associated with depression in epilepsy (e.g., seizure frequency, duration of epilepsy) is somewhat surprising. Variables that were mixed as to their relationship to depression included factors such as family psychiatric history or family history of depression, monotherapy versus polytherapy, and use of phenobarbital, although this topic is addressed in more detail later. Variables that were consistently associated with depression in epilepsy included factors such as the number of stressful adverse life events during the preceding year, patterns of hypometabolism and decreased blood flow, and seizure type. Some of these reliable predictors have been identified in the general psychiatry and depression literature and will be briefly mentioned.

Kendler et al.[36] recently reported findings from a large prospective investigation of the relationship between 15 classes of stressful life events and onset of *DSM-III*-R–defined major depression. The sample contained 24,648 person-months and 316 onsets of major depression, and the summary odds ratio for onset of major depression in the month of stressful life event was 5.64 for all subjects. Table 13-5 pro-

Table 13-3. Research Activity Devoted to Types of Predictor Variables and Degree to Which They Have Yielded Positive Findings

	Proportion Analyses (%)	Proportion Positive Findings (%)
Neuroepilepsy	52	6
Sociodemographic factors	20	40
Psychological and social factors	15	79
Medication	12	33

Table 13-4. Variables Not Reliably Associated with Depression in Epilepsy

Variable	Proportion of Significant Analyses (%)
Age of onset (2/13)	15
Seizure frequency	17
Socioeconomic status	17
Age	17
Lesion	17
Education	17
Etiology	20
Laterality	24
Generalized seizures	25
Gender	25
Aura type	33
Family history of epilepsy	33
Duration	36
Employment	40

vides a summary of the odds ratios for the onset of major depression within a month of the occurrence of a variety of specific adverse life events. Roth et al.,[37] in one of the few examples of structural equation modeling in epilepsy (Figure 13-5), demonstrated a significant relationship among stressful life events, seizure frequency, exercise participation, and depression in epilepsy. Stressful life events were found to be a particularly strong predictor of both depression and seizure frequency, whereas seizure frequency was not directly related to depression, consistent with the summary of findings provided previously. Wiegartz et al.[10] also reported a significant relationship between current *DSM-IV* major or minor depression and number of stressful life events in the last year.

A considerable psychiatric literature examines alterations in blood flow, metabolism, and magnetic resonance imaging volumetrics in psychiatric patients with major depression. These studies have reported abnormalities in left (mesial) and frontal regions among patients with major depression.[38–50] Similar findings have been reported in epilepsy. Bromfield et al.,[9] using positron emission tomography, and Schmitz et al.,[51] using single-photon emission computed tomography, reported that among patients with left temporal or focal left hemisphere epilepsy, depressed epilepsy patients were characterized by hypometabolism and decreased blood flow in the left inferior or lateral frontal regions. A

related pattern of findings has been suggested by neuropsychological investigations wherein patients with left temporal lobe epilepsy with concomitant depression performed especially poorly on tests of purported frontal lobe function.[52,53]

Clearly, a dire need exists for prospective (causal) modeling of depression in epilepsy. Most knowledge in the area of epilepsy and depression is based on correlational and cross-sectional data. Certain factors appear to show a closer relationship to depression than others, but demonstration of causal relationships generally remain to be determined. Further, few attempts have been made to integrate neurobiological, psychosocial, and iatrogenic factors into a comprehensive model of depression in epilepsy.

Availability of Effective Models of Treatment of Psychiatric Comorbidity

Although underrecognition of depression is a known problem, attempts to improve recognition of depression do not necessarily translate to improved treatment of depression. In the epilepsy literature, discussions of the treatment of depression usually are limited to overviews of antide-

Table 13-5. Odds Ratio for Onset of Major Depression within a Month of Specific Types of Life Events

Adverse Event	Odds Ratio
Assault	25.36[a]
Financial problems	5.85[a]
Serious housing problems	7.24[a]
Serious illness or injury	3.10[b]
Job loss	3.95[c]
Loss of confidant	3.17[c]
Serious marital problems	8.39[c]
Serious trouble getting along with individual	5.04[a]
Serious personal crisis	2.32[a]
Death	6.29[a]
Serious illness	2.50[a]

[a]$p < .001.$
[b]$p < .01.$
[c]$p < .05.$
Source: Adapted from K Kendler, L Karkowski, C Prescott. Causal relationship between stressful life events and the onset of major depression. Am J Psychiatry 1999;156(6):837–841.

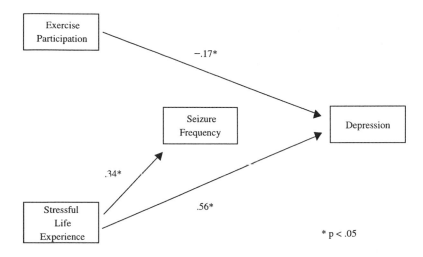

Figure 13-5. Structural equation modeling of predictors of depression. (Reprinted with permission from D Roth, KT Goode, VL Williams, E Faught. Physical exercise, stressful life experience, and depression in adults with epilepsy. Epilepsia 1994;35: 1248–1255.)

pressant medications and potential problems therein (e.g., lowering of seizure threshold with some medications). Rarely discussed is how to incorporate clinical psychiatrists and psychologists effectively into the care of patients with epilepsy, especially in light of the challenges posed by managed care schemes. Again, these issues have been examined carefully in the primary care literature. Whether the findings are applicable to epilepsy remains to be determined.

Katon et al.[54] exhibited the efficacy of one model for intervention, so-called collaborative care. Over a 12-month period, a total of 217 primary care patients, who were recognized as depressed (91 with major and 126 with minor depression) by their primary care physicians and were willing to take antidepressant medications, were randomized. The collaborative care program was three-pronged: (1) patient education (including materials on the biology of depression, how antidepressant medications work, and simple cognitive-behavioral techniques for managing depression; videos covering similar issues as well as doctor-patient vignettes; and other proactive techniques); (2) physician education (including a half-day didactic session on antidepressant and behavioral treatment of depression, monthly case conferences, and case-by-case consultation); (3) altered structure of delivery of care (consisting of alternating visits with the primary care physician [visits 1 and 3] and psychiatrist [visits 2 and 4] over 4–6 weeks); and (4) monitoring

and follow-up (psychiatrist-reviewed monthly automated pharmacy data on antidepressant refills to monitor adherence to the continuation phase [3–7 months]). In part three of the program, the initial primary care visit was expanded to provide time to discuss depression, and other aspects to this component also were included.

Table 13-6 shows the outcomes for usual and collaborative care. Collaborative care resulted in significantly better adherence to adequate dosage of antidepressant medication for 90 days or more for patients with major depression. In addition, these patients were more likely to rate the quality of care they received for depression as good to excellent, were more likely to show a 50% or more improvement on the SCL-90 depression scale, and demonstrated a greater decrease in depression severity over time. Patients with minor depression did not differentially benefit from collaborative care.

Table 13-6. Depression Outcome: Usual Care versus Collaborative Care

	Usual Care (%)	Collaborative Care (%)
Adequate trial of antidepressant	50	75
Relief of depression	43	74
Satisfaction	63	88

Katon et al.[55] also examined the impact of psychological intervention in a randomized, prospective fashion. This form of intervention also was found to be more effective than usual care for major depression. Most recently, Katon et al.[56] demonstrated the cost-effectiveness and cost savings involved in more effective collaborative care programs as well as the adequacy of stepped collaborative care—that is, subsequently initiating collaborative care for treatment-resistant usual care patients.

A need for closer involvement of psychiatrists and clinical psychologists in patient management has been noted,[16] but the most optimal and cost-effective models of care and the techniques for most effective use of mental health specialists have yet to be empirically investigated in epilepsy. Nonetheless, epileptology could benefit from the demonstration of effective models of intervention and treatment of major depression in other settings. More generally, several helpful resources are pertinent to the issue of treatment and intervention, including careful discussions of antidepressant medication treatment in epilepsy,[57-62] the "Consensus Statement on the Undertreatment of Depression,"[1] and the report from the Agency for Healthcare Policy and Research,[63] which provides guidelines for acute, continuation, and maintenance treatment of depression along with consumer information on depression. In addition, information is available concerning public screening and other public health programs for identification and awareness of depression.[64-67] Finally, the recently released surgeon general's report on mental health contains information of interest on mood and other disorders for both consumers and clinicians.[68]

Unfortunately, solid epidemiologic information regarding depression among individuals with developmental disabilities is scarce. Using conventional electronic means to search the academic literature, we were unable to locate a citation referring to the incidence and determinants of depression among individuals with intellectual limitations. Although dedicated scales for assessment of psychosocial concerns[69] and data relating to the possibility of medication-induced behavioral changes are now available,[70,71] we were unable to find a comprehensive investigation of depression in this population. We may have missed available citations, but it seems fair to suggest that the problem of psychiatric comorbidity has been understudied in the developmentally disabled population.

Summary

Psychiatric comorbidity has been, and should continue to be, of major concern in the treatment of chronic epilepsy. This review has focused on major depression, a disorder that appears to be among the predominant lifetime-to-date interictal comorbid psychiatric conditions among adult patients with chronic and intractable epilepsy. We have examined only a few of the potential key issues concerning the problem of psychiatric comorbidity in epilepsy. Through comparison of what is known about major depression in epilepsy and in other fields of investigation such as primary care, the areas requiring further investigation have been made apparent. Further, critical examinations of the existing epilepsy-depression literature have allowed us to suggest several areas for additional research; new knowledge in these areas would likely result in improved QOL for persons with epilepsy.[14-19]

Acknowledgments

This work was supported in part by National Alliances for Research on Schizophrenia and Depression and National Institutes of Health Grant NS 37738.

References

1. Hirschfeld R, Keller M, Panico S, et al. The National Depressive and Manic-Depressive Association consensus statement on the undertreatment of depression. JAMA 1997;277(4):333–340.
2. Fiordelli E, Beghi E, Bogliun G, Crespi V. Epilepsy and psychiatric disturbance: a cross-sectional study. Br J Psychiatry 1993;163:446–450.
3. Manchanda R, Schaefer B, McLachlan R, et al. Psychiatric disorders in candidates for epilepsy surgery. J Neurol Neurosurg Psychiatry 1996;61:82–89.
4. Victoroff J. DSM-III-R Psychiatric Diagnoses in candidates for epilepsy surgery:lifetime prevalence. Neuropsychiatry Neuropsychol Behav Neurol 1994;7(2):87–97.

5. Silberman E, Sussman N, Skillings G, Callanan M. Aura phenomena and psychopathology: a pilot investigation. Epilepsia 1994;35(4):778–784.
6. Altshuler L., Rausch R., Delrahim S., Kay J., Crandall P. Temporal lobe epilepsy, temporal lobectomy, and major depression. J Neuropsychiatry Clin Neurosci 11 (4):436-443.
7. Hermann BP, Seidenberg M, Bell B. Psychiatric comorbidity in chronic epilepsy: identification, consequences, and treatment of major depression. Epilepsia 2000;41:S31–S41.
8. Koch-Weser M, Garron D, Gilley D, et al. Prevalence of psychologic disorders after surgical treatment of seizures. Arch Neurol 1988;45:1308–1311.
9. Bromfield EB, Altshuler L, Liederman DB, et al. Cerebral metabolism and depression in patients with complex partial seizures. Arch Neurol 1992;49:617–623.
10. Wiegartz P, Seidenberg M, Woodard A, et al. Co-morbid psychiatric disorder in chronic epilepsy: recognition and etiology of depression. Neurology 1999;53(5):3–25.
11. Regier D, Myers J, Kramer M, et al. The NIMH Epidemiologic Catchment Area program. Arch Gen Psychiatry 1984;41:934–952.
12. Regier D, Narrow W, Rae D, et al. The de facto US mental and addictive disorders service system. Arch Gen Psychiatry 1993;50:85–94.
13. Kessler R, McGonagle K, Zhao S, et al. Lifetime and 12-month prevalence of DSM-III-R psychiatric disorders in the United States: results from the National Comorbidity Survey: Arch Gen Psychiatry 1994;51:8–19.
14. Robertson M. Mood Disorders Associated with Epilepsy. In H McConnell, P Snyder (eds), Psychiatric Comorbidity in Epilepsy. Washington, DC: American Psychiatric Press, 1998;133–167.
15. Blumer D, Altshuler L. Affective Disorders. In J Engel, T Pedley (eds), Epilepsy: A Comprehensive Textbook. Philadelphia: Lippincott–Raven, 1997; 2083–2099.
16. Blumer D, Montouris G, Hermann B. Psychiatric morbidity in seizure patients on a neurodiagnostic monitoring unit. J Neuropsychiatr Clin Neurosci 1995;7:445–456.
17. Lambert M, Robertson M. Depression in epilepsy: etiology, phenomenology, and treatment. Epilepsia 1999;40(10):21–47.
18. Altshuler L. Depression and Epilepsy. In O Devinsky, W Theodore (eds), Epilepsy and Behavior. New York: Wiley, 1991;47–65.
19. Kanner A, Nieto J. Depressive disorders in epilepsy. Neurology 1999;53(5):26–32.
20. Katon W, von Korff M, Lin E, et al. Adequacy and duration of antidepressant treatment in primary care. Med Care 1992;30(1):67–76.
21. Spitzer R, Kroenke K, Linzer M, et al. Health-related quality of life in primary care patients with mental disorders: results from the Prime-MD 1000 study. JAMA 1995;274(19):1511–1517.
22. Ettinger A, Weisbrot DM, Nolan EE, et al. Symptoms of depression and anxiety in pediatric epilepsy patients. Epilepsia 1998;39:595–599.
23. Paradiso S, Hermann BP, Blumer D, Robinson R. The impact of depressed mood on neuropsychological status in temporal lobe epilepsy. J Neurol Neurosurg Psychiatry 2001;70:180–185.
24. O'Donoghue M, Goodridge D, Redhead K, et al. Assessing the psychosocial consequences of epilepsy: a community based study. Br J Gen Pract 1999;49:211–214.
25. McQuaid J, Stein M, Laffayee C, McCahill M. Depression in a primary care clinic: the prevalence and impact of an unrecognized disorder. J Affect Dis 1999; 55:1–10.
26. Hays R, Wells K, Sherbourne C, et al. Functioning and well-being outcomes of patients with depression compared with chronic general medical illness. Arch Gen Psychiatry 1995;52:11–19.
27. Wells K, Stewart A, Hays R, et al. The functioning and well-being of depressed patients: results from the Medical Outcomes Study. JAMA 1989;262:914–919.
28. von Korff M, Ormel J, Katon W, Lin E. Disability and depression among high utilizers of health care. Arch Gen Psychiatry 1992;49:91–100.
29. Simon G, Ormel J, von Korff M, Barlow W. Health care costs associated with depressive and anxiety disorders in primary care. Am J Psychiatry 1995;152(3):352–357.
30. Simon G, von Korff M, Barlow W. Healthcare costs of primary care patients with recognized depression. Arch Gen Psychiatry 1995;52:850–856.
31. Henk H, Katzelnick D, Kobak K, Greist J. Medical costs attributed to depression among patients with a history of high medical expenses in a health maintenance organization. Arch Gen Psychiatry 1996;53:899–904.
32. Ormel J, von Korff M, van Brink W, et al. Depression, anxiety, and social disability show synchrony of change in primary care patients. Am J Pub Health 1993;83:385–390.
33. Broadhead W, Blazer D, George L, Tse C. Depression, disability days, and days lost from work in a prospective epidemiologic survey. JAMA 1990;264(19):2524–2528.
34. Lehrner J, Kalchmayr R, Serles W, et al. Health-related quality of life (HRQOL), activity of daily living (ADL) and depressive mood disorder in temporal lobe epilepsy patients. Seizure 1999;8:88–92.
35. Hermann BP, Seidenberg M, Bell B, et al. Co-morbid psychiatric symptoms in temporal lobe epilepsy: association with chronicity of epilepsy and impact on quality of life. Epilepsy Behav 2000;1:184–190.
36. Kendler K, Karkowski L, Prescott C. Casual relationship between stressful life events and the onset of major depression. Am J Psychiatry 1999;156(6):837–841.

37. Roth D, Goode KT, Williams VL, Faught E. Physical exercise, stressful life experience, and depression in adults with epilepsy. Epilepsia 1994;35:1248–1255.

38. Bench C, Frackowiak R, Dolan R. Changes in regional cerebral blood flow on recovery from depression. Psychol Med 1995;25:247–251.Bench C, Friston K, Brown R, et al. The anatomy of melancholia—focal abnormalities of cerebral blood flow in major depression. Psychol Med 1992;22:607–615.

39. Bench C, Friston K, Brown R, et al. Regional cerebral blood flow in depression measured by positron emission tomography: the relationship with clinical dimensions. Psychol Med 1993;23:579–590.

40. Biver F, Goldman S, Delvenne V, et al. Frontal and parietal metabolic disturbances in unipolar depression. Biol Psychiatry 1994;36:381–388.

41. Bremner J, Innis R, Salomon R, et al. Positron emission tomography measurement of cerebral metabolic correlates of tryptophan depletion-induced depressive relapse. Arch Gen Psychiatry 1997;54: 364–374.

42. Coffey C, Wilkinson W, Weiner R, et al. Quantitative cerebral anatomy in depression: a controlled magnetic resonance imaging study. Arch Gen Psychiatry 1993; 50:7–16.

43. Drevets W, Price J, Simpson J, et al. Subgenual prefrontal cortex abnormalities in mood disorders. Nature 1997;386:824–827.

44. Drevets W, Videen T, Price J, et al. A functional anatomical study of unipolar depression. J Neurosci 1992; 12(9):3628–3741.

45. Duman R, Charney D. Cell atrophy and loss in major depression. Bio Psychiatry 1999;45:1083–1084.

46. Mayberg H, Liotti M, Brannan S, et al. Reciprocal limbic-cortical function and negative mood: converging PET findings in depression and normal sadness. Am J Psychiatry 1999;156(5):675–682.

47. Rajkowska G, Miguel-Hidalgo J, Wei J, et al. Morphometric evidence for neuronal glial prefrontal cell pathology in major depression. Biol Psychiatry 1999; 45:1085–1098.

48. Teneback C, Nahas Z, Speer A, et al. Changes in prefrontal cortex and paralimbic activity in depression following two weeks of daily left prefrontal TMS. J Neuropsychiatry Clin Neurosci 1999;11(4): 426–435.

49. Triggs W, McCoy K, Greer R, et al. Effects of left frontal transcranial magnetic stimulation on depressed mood, cognition, and corticomotor threshold. Biol Psychiatry 1999;45:1440–1446.

50. Schmitz B, Moriarty J, Costa D, et al. Psychiatric profiles and patterns of cerebral blood flow in focal epilepsy: interactions between depression, obsessionality, and perfusion related to the laterality of the epilepsy. J Neurol Neurosurg Psychiatry 1997;62:458–463.

51. Hermann BP, Seidenberg M, Haltiner A, Wyler AR. Mood state in unilateral temporal lobe epilepsy. Bio Psychiatry 1991;30:1205–1218.

52. Seidenberg M, Hermann BP, Haltiner A, et al. Depression in temporal lobe epilepsy: interaction between laterality of lesion and Wisconsin Card Sort performance. Neuropsychiatry Neuropsychol Behav Neurol 1995;8:81–87.

53. Katon W, von Korff M, Lin E, et al. Collaborative management to achieve treatment guidelines impact on depression in primary care. JAMA 1995;273(13): 1026–1031.

54. Katon W, Robinson P, von Korff M, et al. A multifaceted intervention to improve treatment of depression in primary care. Arch Gen Psychiatry 1996;53:924–932.

55. von Korff M, Katon W, Bush T, et al. Treatment costs, cost offset, and cost-effectiveness of collaborative management of depression. Psychosom Med 1998;60:143–149.

56. Curran S, De Pauw K. Selecting an antidepressant for use in a patient with epilepsy. Drug Safety 1998;18(2): 125–133.

57. Schmitz B. Psychiatric syndromes related to antiepileptic drugs. Epilepsia 1999;40(10):65–70.

58. Trimble M. Anticonvulsant-induced psychiatric disorders the role of forced normalisation. Drug Safety 1996;15(3): 159–166.

59. Monaco F, Cicolin A. Interactions between anticonvulsant and psychoactive drugs. Epilepsia 1999;40(10):71–76.

60. Pisani F, Spina E, Oteri G. Antidepressant drugs and seizure susceptibility: from in vitro data to clinical practice. Epilepsia 1999;40(10):48–56.

61. Krishnamoorthy E., Trimble M. Forced normalization: clinical and therapeutic relevance. Epilepsia 1999;40 (10):57–64.

62. Depression in Primary Care: Treatment of Major Depression, vol 2. [Publication AHCPR 93-0511.] Rockville, MD: Agency for Health Care Research and Policy, U.S. Department of Health and Human Services, 1993.

63. Greenfield S, Reizes J, Magruder K, et al. Effectiveness of community-based screening for depression. Am J Psychiatry 1997;154(10):1391–1397.

64. Magruder K, Norquist G, Feil M, et al. Who comes to a voluntary depression screening program? Am J Psychiatry 1995;152(11):1615–1622.

65. Paykel E, Tylee A, Wright A, et al. The defeat depression campaign: psychiatry in the public arena. Am J Psychiatry 1997;154(6):59–65.

66. Regier D, Hirschfeld R, Goodwin F, et al. The NIMH depression awareness, recognition, and treatment program: structure aims and scientific basis. Am J Psychiatry 1988;145(11):1351–1357.

67. Satcher D. Mental Health: A Report of the Surgeon General. Washington, DC: Public Health Service, U.S. Department of Health and Human Services, 1999.

68. Espie CA, Paul A, Graham M, et al. The Epilepsy Outcome Scale: the development of a measure for use with carers of people with epilepsy plus intellectual disability. J Intellect Disabil Res 1998;42: 90–96.

69. Alvarez N. Barbiturates in the treatment of epilepsy in people with intellectual disability. J Intellect Disabil Res 1998;42[Suppl 1]:15–23.

70. Ylinen A. Antiepileptic efficacy of vigabitrin in people with severe epilepsy and intellectual disability. J Intellect Disabil Res 1998;42[Suppl 1]:46–49.

Chapter 14

Problem Behaviors in Individuals with Developmental Disabilities

Vicki Sudhalter

The main purpose of this chapter is to present methods for understanding the development and persistence of problem behaviors in individuals with developmental disabilities (DD). The chapter is divided into three sections. The first section defines what is meant by problem behaviors and discusses possible causes for such behaviors in people with DD. The second section presents a biopsychosocial model of the development and maintenance of problem behaviors. In the third section, some intervention strategies are discussed that result from the model of problem behavior presented herein.

Characterization of Problem Behaviors

Definition of Problem Behaviors

United Kingdom surveys of people with DD within the severe range of mental handicap suggest that approximately 20% of the child and adolescent population and 15% of the adult population exhibit some form of problem behavior.[1,2] More recently, Jacobson[3] wrote that one in four individuals with diagnosed DD also had a diagnosed mental illness or a behavioral disorder. Given these statistics, clearly the management of problem behaviors represents a great concern to the community dedicated to the care of individuals with DD.

The first step in managing difficult behavior is to recognize the point at which a behavior should be considered a problem. A behavior becomes a problem when it is harmful or noxious to the individual performing that behavior or to others.[4] Behaviors that involve self-injury and aggression are the most serious, as they can pose real threats to life and limb. Persons biting or hitting themselves or others so as to cause callusing or bleeding; gouging at their eyes so as to cause pain and tissue damage; or engaging in pica (i.e., the eating of such inedible objects as glass, paper clips, cigarettes, or coffee grounds) are illustrations of such severe problem behaviors.

A behavior also becomes a problem when its occurrence interferes with the acquisition of academic or social skills. Such behavior is exemplified by a child who begins to scream when his or her teacher tries to teach new vocabulary words. Because the lesson must be stopped so that the teacher can intervene in the screaming, the child loses the opportunity to increase verbal skills. Another example of such behavior is seen in the closing to affected persons of occasions for social interaction because their behavior is either dangerous to others or is unacceptable. This outcome effectively limits an individual's opportunity to develop and practice social skills. An example of this type of behavior is seen in a 9-year-old child with autistic disorder who removes his or her clothing in the classroom or in a shopping mall. These types of social opportunities essentially are closed to such children until they learn to remain clothed in public.

Finally, a behavior becomes a problem when its frequency, severity, or duration is significantly outside the range of what is acceptable by everyday conventions.[4] For example, we all have screamed, cried, scratched, or used unacceptable language. However, when affected individuals begin to scratch and pick at their fingers until they bleed, the intensity has escalated into a problem behavior. When someone cries constantly regardless of what is occurring, the crying has become a problem behavior.

Equally important as recognizing the point at which a behavior has become a problem is recognizing that a behavior is not a problem. For example, is it a problem when an individual with autistic disorder cannot go to sleep unless all the window shades in the group home are at a particular angle? Clinicians or caregivers have to ask themselves whether the frequency or severity of the behavior is outside the acceptable level in the particular context and whether the behavior interferes with the quality of life or infringes on the health or well-being of such a person or of other housemates. Because, in this particular case, the answer to all these questions is no, this particular behavior should not be considered a problem. Of further importance is recognizing that when individuals with DD express a personal preference, such as a desire to eat peaches rather than apples or to watch basketball rather than baseball, they are not engaging in problem behavior.

In sum, acknowledging and respecting the personal choices of individuals with DD is as important as for those without DD, as long as those choices do not cause injury or damage, do not substantially limit access to the benefits provided in academic or social settings, and are not associated with risk of physical harm.

Causes of Problem Behaviors in People with Developmental Disabilities

Many factors are associated with problem behaviors in people with DD. Such factors include neuroanatomic, physiologic, and chemical abnormalities; deficits in executive functioning; inhibitory control and communication; impoverished living conditions; and learning experiences. These factors can be grouped into two broad categories: processes that are internal to an individual and processes associated with an individual's external environment. (Seizures, a very prevalent concern in the population with DD, are not discussed here, as this topic is covered in other chapters of this book.)

The cases presented in the following sections are, of course, not all-inclusive, and, as indicated, the reasons for the emergence of any particular behavior can be very complex. To understand the origins of problem behaviors and their intended purposes well enough to create a successful plan of intervention, data must be collected very carefully. The topology (e.g., exactly what is happening) must be described precisely and objectively. This characterization, which is of primary importance, should describe the behavior and should indicate where the behavior occurred, its precipitating factors, and its consequences for the affected individual.

Internal Causes of Problem Behaviors

Cognitive Deficits. The desires, wants, and needs of individuals with DD are comparable to those of their nondisabled peers. However, all too often, individuals with DD have extreme communication difficulties that interfere with the expression of their needs and, thus, with the attainment of goals. For example, one diagnostic criterion for autistic disorder or other types of pervasive developmental disorder is the presence of impaired language capability.[5] This impairment can take the form either of inability to talk or of production of echolalic responses, stereotypic vocalizations, or limited one- or two-word utterances. Individuals with other conditions such as fragile X syndrome (FXS), Down syndrome, or mental retardation are also likely to have language difficulties that can take the form of disfluency, perseverative and tangential language[6] or limited linguistic repertoires. In fact, a sizable subpopulation of persons with DD have no functional expressive skills. Thus, individuals with DD can experience frustrating difficulty in expressing their desires, which in turn can lead to anger when those desires are not met. Anger and frustration can then lead to new forms of communication, such as self-injury or aggression, which become affected individuals' primary means of expressing dissatisfaction.

Along with communication difficulties, individuals with DD often experience deficits in impulse control and executive functioning.[7–9] Deficits in impulse control are exemplified by grabbing things that are wanted, touching things that are attractive, and generally not being able to wait until a more appropriate environment or time for fulfilling desires (e.g., masturbating during a classroom activity). Deficits in executive functioning in affected individuals can result in severe limits in problem-solving skills and in persistence of well-learned (although inefficient or inappropriate) routines. Thus, if affected individuals are confronted with a particular challenge, such as the unavailability of a favorite food, their executive functioning deficits would create great difficulty for them in conceiving of an adaptively appropriate plan or strategy for getting the food, and instead they may scream or engage in self-abuse until they receive attention.

Psychiatric Problems. Individuals with DD exhibit the full range of psychiatric disorders found in their non-DD peer population. Most estimates of the prevalence of serious psychiatric disorders, including personality disorders, range from 8–15% within the DD population.[10] These numbers probably are underestimates, however, given a documented tendency to underdiagnose psychiatric problems in individuals with DD.[11,12] In research of diagnostic overshadowing in the population with DD, Reiss[13] found that psychologists were less likely to diagnose a debilitating fear in a population of individuals with mental retardation than in a population without DD. Additionally, obsessive-compulsive disorder in individuals with DD often remains undiagnosed.[14] Some aggressive behavior problems in people with DD appear to be associated with psychiatric disorders,[13] and Barak et al.[15] and Gedye[16,17] stated that individuals with DD and obsessive-compulsive disorder may become aggressive on being prevented from engaging in their obsession.

Individuals with DD also can manifest the full range of affective disorders.[18,19] Numerous reports cite examples of both children and adults who engage in various problem behaviors (e.g., self-injurious behavior [SIB], aggression, screaming, and property destruction) and in whom bipolar disorder or depression has been diagnosed.[20]

In sum, investigators have demonstrated that such problem behaviors as SIB or aggression may be symptomatic of a wide variety of psychoses, neuroses, and affective disorders, and a very careful analysis of behavior and its associated symptoms must be performed to determine the correct course of medical treatment.[21–23]

Pain and Sensory Difficulties. Combined with the lack of communicative skill to express wants and desires and overlooked symptoms of psychiatric disorders, individuals with DD may lack the ability to verbalize the presence of pain. In such instances, affected individuals may hit themselves in the affected area (e.g., in the ears if experiencing an ear infection). In addition, such individuals may become aggressive toward other people, owing to frustration over having to endure pain or in an attempt to protect a painful area from intrusion from the outside.

Individuals with DD may have sensory difficulties that lead to an intolerance of certain environmental conditions, such as crowding, loud noises, lights, food, the touch of clothing, taking a bath, or cutting hair or nails. Thus, when confronted with subjectively aversive environmental stimuli that are acceptable to the non-DD population, individuals with sensory difficulties may begin to express aggressive or self-abusive behaviors (or both).

Lesch-Nyhan Syndrome and Riley-Day Syndrome. The Lesch-Nyhan and Riley-Day syndromes are two of several associated with SIB. Lesch-Nyhan syndrome is caused by a deficiency in the enzyme hypoxanthine guanine phosphoribosyltransferase. The lack of this enzyme is associated with mental retardation and severe self-biting, particularly of the lips, tongue, and fingers.[24] The exact mechanisms causing the self-mutilation are poorly understood. Several hypotheses have been proposed, however, ranging from a problem with pain perception[25] to a dynamic interplay between dopamine uptake, serotonin, and the neuronal systems of the basal ganglia.[26]

Riley-Day syndrome is a disorder of the autonomic nervous system with an autosomal recessive mode of inheritance.[27,28] The diagnosis is based on clinical features that include absence of tears, corneal anesthesia, keratinized conjunctiva and cornea, insensitivity to pain, poor temperature control, abolished deep tendon reflexes, postural hypotension, vomiting attacks, poor motor control, and mental retardation. The disease probably results from an as-yet unidentified enzymatic insufficiency.

Endorphin and Serotonin Models of Self-Injurious Behavior. Several systems, including the beta-endorphin and the serotonergic systems, have been implicated in the pathophysiology of treatment-resistant SIB and related behaviors, such as stereotypic behaviors. These hypotheses have been supported by the beneficial effects of treating affected individuals with the opiate antagonist naltrexone and with serotonin-modulating compounds, respectively.[23,29,30]

External Causes of Behavior Problems

Social Conditions. Children and adults with DD must cope with lives that are characterized by limited personal freedom. The situations that adults with DD may be asked to tolerate include the sharing of living environments with other people they may not like; performing activities they may not enjoy; eating food they may not savor; going places to which they may not want to go; and participating in social activities in which they may not want to participate. Thus, along with deficits in communication, impulse control, and executive functioning, such individuals often are asked to accept living situations that few of us would find very satisfying.

Environmental Conditions. Because problematic behaviors usually attract attention and the receipt of attention can be rewarding, such behaviors often result in the resolution of some personal needs that prompted them. Of course, this outcome can reinforce those behaviors and encourage their expression in the future—exactly the opposite of a desirable treatment. A few examples will clarify this point. A child who has a terrible toothache, cannot produce the words to tell his or her parents of the existence of the pain, and has not been given an alternative form of communication may begin to strike the mouth

area either as a means of alleviating the pain or as an attempt to indicate the location of the pain. In the course of producing this behavior, she or he notices that the parents become upset and provide the desired attention. In the course of trying to stop the self-injury, the parents may also discover the mouth infection and provide the appropriate treatment. When the child again wants attention, the likelihood is increased that he or she may try striking that area of the mouth, even though the initial reason for the behavior no longer pertains.

In another example, an adult with DD and impulse control limitations is asked to share a room with an individual who screams at night. The situation is highly volatile, and this adult, in an attempt to quiet the screaming, hits the roommate rather than selecting a less aggressive strategy. (The DD adult also may have executive functioning deficits that cause great difficulty in finding alternate ways of quieting the roommate or may have communication deficits that create difficulty in alerting caregivers to the dissatisfaction. Thus, aggression toward the roommate is the only method this dissatisfied adult can deduce to express dissatisfaction with the living situation.) The result of the aggression is that the adult is removed from the room to prevent injury to the roommate, and this action resolves the problem by terminating exposure to the screaming. Thus, a situation that arose because of deficits in certain skill areas can result in learning that aggression is a very effective way of having one's needs met.

Biopsychosocial Model of Problem Behaviors

The understanding of problem behaviors is complicated for many reasons, not the least of which is that behaviors that appear fairly similar across situations can serve varying functions.[31] For example, one individual may hit his head because he has a headache, another because she is having a seizure, a third because his roommate is bothering him, and a fourth because she does not want to perform the task with which she is being confronted. Mason and Iwata[32] demonstrated how one subject's SIB appeared to be an attention-getting response, a second person's SIB was suggestive of stereotypic behavior, and a third person's SIB functioned as an escape response. Additionally, Oliver and Head[33] recognized that varied problem behaviors can emerge from the same external conditions. For example, when confronted with having to perform a disliked task, one person may hit her or his head, a second may hit the teacher, a third may scream, and a fourth may try to run away. This is why a careful and individualized analysis of the behavior, affected persons, and the environment must be performed to discover effective treatments. The biopsychosocial model provides a method of analyzing behaviors and determining the functions that specific behaviors perform for individuals.

Major theorists in the area of behavioral analysis have argued that problem behaviors exhibited by individuals with DD are functional.[34] Problem behaviors serve specific purposes for affected individuals; if this were not the case, the behaviors would have been extinguished. The role of clinicians, therefore, is to identify the biological, psychological, and social factors that trigger and reinforce the behavior, so as to understand the function provided by the behavior. A biopsychosocial model of problem behavior is designed to do just that. This model divides the analysis of problem behaviors into the following components: (1) events that produce or increase the likelihood that a behavior will occur; (2) events that strengthen and maintain a behavior; and (3) events that decrease the likelihood that a behavior will occur.[35] The first two components are discussed here. Events that decrease the likelihood that a behavior will occur are presented in the Therapy section.

Events That Trigger or Increase the Likelihood That a Behavior Will Occur

Triggering events are those situations that must exist for a behavior to occur, whereas *contributing events* are additional conditions that, when present at the time of the occurrence of a triggering event, increase the likelihood that the problem behavior will occur. Triggering and contributing events can be either environmental (external) and or personal (internal).

Environmental events are those circumstances that are external to the individual exhibiting the problem behavior. In attempting to understand a behavior, many questions can be asked concerning these external conditions:

- Does the behavior occur when such individuals are being prevented from doing something they want to do?
- Does the behavior occur when such individuals are asked to do something they do not want to do?
- Does the behavior occur only at certain times of the day or only in certain environments?
- Does the behavior occur when such individuals are not provided with attention?
- Has a recent change in staff or teacher occurred?
- Is someone or something in the environment annoying such individuals?

The list of questions goes on. A complete description of the external circumstances surrounding the emergence of a behavior is necessary to understand why it occurs and what function it serves.

We have described many of the personal conditions that provide the context for problem behaviors in individuals with DD. Do such individuals have seizures? Do such individuals have a concomitant psychiatric disorder? Are such individuals prone to certain types of illnesses or susceptible to certain pains (e.g., recurrent ear infections, gastrointestinal disorders, skin rashes)? Do such individuals have a major cognitive skill deficit, such as being nonverbal or having impulse control deficits? Thus, along with a complete description of the external circumstances, a complete personal history of affected individuals must be completed to determine the contributing and triggering events of the problematic behavior.

Events That Strengthen and Maintain Problem Behaviors

If the performance of a behavior results in positive consequences from affected individuals' point of view, it will be strengthened and maintained. A few examples will illustrate this fundamental law of learning.

It is 11:45, and Anne is very hungry. She has an ulcer that begins to cause pain when she becomes very hungry. In addition, she does not like going to the cafeteria because Susan, a former classmate whom she does not like, will be there. Anne does not have the communicative ability to indicate that she is in pain and needs to eat, so she begins to scream and bite her fingers until they bleed. Consequently, she is taken out of the class and is allowed to eat her lunch alone. Anne immediately quiets and eats contentedly.

In this example, the triggering event is the prospect of meeting Susan in the cafeteria (social) and the contributing events are the pain the ulcer is causing and the hunger Anne is experiencing (biological). The problem behaviors are the screaming and the biting of fingers. The events that are maintaining and strengthening these behaviors are the removal of Anne from the classroom and her eating lunch by herself (social and biological).

John is a 10-year-old boy with FXS. He lacks the ability to adjust to auditory and visual stimulation, is very anxious, and does not like to enter new environments. When he is asked to go to a new classroom because his teacher is absent, John begins to bite the thumb and forefinger of his right hand. Consequently, he is not taken into the new environment but rather is allowed to remain in his familiar classroom with a known paraprofessional.

In this example, the triggering event is the prospect of moving to an unfamiliar environment (social). The contributing events are John's sensory defensiveness (biological) and anxiety (psychological). The problem behavior is the self-injury. The event that is maintaining and strengthening this behavior is his being allowed to remain in his known, familiar environment.

Jacqueline is a 35-year-old nonverbal woman who has severe mental retardation and is living in a group home. She has few skills with which to occupy her free time. She does not enjoy television or listening to the radio; thus, little remains for Jacqueline to do after supper. She has begun to scream and tear at her clothes while she is sitting in the living room waiting to go to bed. When this occurs, her caregivers remove her from the living room, take her into a quiet place, and engage her in some activities.

In this example, the triggering event is the boredom Jacqueline feels between supper and bedtime (psychological), and the contributing events are her lack of leisure activity skills (social) and the fact that the environment does not supply appropriate activities after supper. Jacqueline's screaming is

her problem behavior, and her removal from the living room and placement in a situation in which she is engaged are the events that maintain the screaming (psychological and social).

Therapy

In many cases, the first step in helping individuals who have DD and are demonstrating problem behaviors is to provide a complete physical and psychiatric examination so as to rule out physical and psychiatric causes. Gedye[36] compiled a guide to diagnosing the medical and psychiatric causes of many problematic behaviors in individuals with DD. Many other assessment instruments also are available for helping to diagnose psychiatric problems in children and adults with DD.[37–40] In this section are presented some nonmedical therapies that are available to psychologists and other professionals who are working with individuals with problem behaviors.

Behavior Therapy

Behavior therapy has been very effective in the elimination of problem behaviors in the population with DD. It involves the precise definition of the problem behavior, measurement of its occurrence, and a focus on antecedent and consequent events. One of its general tenets is that problematic behaviors are, to a considerable degree, learned behaviors. Behavior therapy endeavors to specify exactly how the environment may influence affected people in terms of established learning principles. Behavior therapists use the principles of learning to teach individuals new and more adaptive behaviors by modifying the environmental contingencies.

For those unfamiliar with behavioral analysis, Hurley[41] has created a very useful tool for analyzing problem behaviors. This publication describes how to use the ABC sheet (antecedent, behavior, and consequence) to analyze behavior within the applied behavior analysis context.

Skill Acquisition

Many of the causes of problem behaviors in individuals with DD are associated with deficits in important skills, such as communication, executive functioning, and impulse control. One of the methods for correcting problem behaviors in such individuals is to teach new skills that can replace the undesirable skills.

Personal Skill Therapy

Group therapy has become popular for people with DD. Elman[47] described the advantages of group therapy for individuals with speech, language, or cognitive disorders. These advantages include offering individuals the opportunity to talk and develop problem-solving skills. Group therapy promotes interaction among its members, in turn promoting pragmatic and conversational skills. The group environment can improve affected individuals' overall functioning by providing a supportive environment. Several organizations (e.g., Young Adult Institute in New York State) have been using group therapy to teach skills and personal management. The Institute has groups for individuals of all ages and intelligence levels and with all types of problem behaviors.

Additionally, counseling and psychotherapy can be very effective interventions for individuals with DD.[43,44] However, all too often, individuals with DD are thought to be unable to benefit from counseling and psychotherapy. Clearly, for these therapies to be effective, modification of the standard techniques would have to be made.[45] In general, Hurley et al.[45] have found that counseling and psychotherapy can be rendered effective for individuals with DD if the therapy materials are made simpler and more concrete.

Brier and Demb[46] described the efficacy of psychotherapeutic intervention for disabled adolescents. They also emphasized the need to consider the cognitive deficits of affected individuals. These authors stressed the utility of using a direct teaching approach, involving a great deal of behavioral rehearsal and repetition.

Alternative Forms of Communication

Problem behaviors frequently are a form of communicating wants and needs when more conventional forms of communication are closed to individuals with DD. Nonetheless, individuals with DD often are not taught alternative forms of communication. Frequently, the speech difficulties demonstrated by individuals with developmental delays are explained (and dismissed) by the fact that these persons have learning difficulties; consequently, intensive speech therapy is not attempted. Such individuals are left without an effective form of communication and, as a result, can become aggressive or self-abusive in an attempt to express themselves and gain attention.[47–49] In these cases, when maladaptive behavior is reinterpreted as an attempt to communicate and individuals are given an effective form of communication, the maladaptive behavior abates.[50,51] Several alternative forms of communication can be used in place of speech, including American sign language, picture exchange communication systems, and augmentative and alternative communication devices. Such alternatives should be explored for use with people for whom verbal expression is not an option.

Video and Role Modeling

The use of video recording and playback has recently become very popular as a method for teaching new skills to children and adults with DD. Individuals can view people performing certain target skills on the video and then try to perform these same skills in their own environments. Additionally, they can watch themselves performing already acquired skills. By performing an activity with new items, with new people, or in a new setting, affected individuals learn to generalize their newly acquired skills.

Role modeling is also a very effective means of teaching new skills. In this exercise, the therapist and the person with DD practice new conversational routines or social routines *before* the individual has to perform those skills in a real situation. The repetition of the routine lowers the anxiety that naturally accompanies the learning of novel tasks and helps in the successful learning and execution of new skills.

Environmental Modification

Caregiver Variables

Whether wittingly or unwittingly reinforced, a problem behavior must be recognized and stopped. Thus, parents or caregivers who intervene to stop or meet the demands of children or adults who have begun to hit themselves must change their own behavior to provide reinforcement for a preferred—as opposed to a nonpreferred—behavior. People often do not recognize that they inadvertently are encouraging undesirable behaviors until those behaviors have become a serious problem.

Physical Environmental Modifications

One also must consider the environment and the degree of ease or difficulty with which a person with DD can act appropriately within it. For example, people with FXS have sensory integration problems and are very distractible and impulsive. Consequently, loud, noisy, and stimulating environments cause these individuals great distress and may promote problem behaviors. As suggested by the foregoing example of the 10-year-old boy with FXS, unexpected transitions and changes also will distress such individuals. In addition, if youngsters with FXS are placed in academic environments filled with attractive items, they may not be able to sustain attention to lessons, as they will be concentrating on touching and exploring these attractive things.

Many individuals with autistic disorder do not like changes in their personal routine. When such individuals are confronted with changes in staff, living conditions, or usual routines, they may begin to engage in problem behaviors as a means of expressing their dissatisfaction with these changes.

Summary

This chapter has presented an introduction to behavior problems in individuals with DD. The causes of these problems are complex and usually entail a combination of personal (internal) and social (external) factors. The personal causes of behavior problems can include skill deficits that interfere with the meeting of personal needs and may include symptoms of unappreciated psychiatric conditions. The social causes can include interpersonal and environmental conditions that may conspire unwittingly to reinforce problem behaviors. A biopsychosocial model is offered as a way of interpreting behavior problems that provides specific guidelines for the

development of effective therapy. Several therapeutic interventions, ranging from behavior therapy to group therapy, are discussed.

It is important to appreciate that each individual's problem behavior takes place against the backdrop of a unique personal history and within a particular biopsychosocial milieu. Therefore, effective therapy to reduce an undesirable behavior cannot be developed until that behavior has been analyzed carefully and the specific circumstances that control it have been recognized.

References

1. Wing L. Severely retarded children in a London area: prevalence and provision of services. Psychol Med 1971;1:405–415.
2. Kushlik A, Cox GR. The epidemiology of mental handicap. Dev Med Child Neurol 1973;15:748–759.
3. Jacobson J. Assessing the Prevalence of Psychiatric Disorders in the Developmentally Disabled Population. In E Dibble, CD Gray (eds), Assessment of Behavior Problems in Persons with Mental Retardation Living in the Community. Rockville, MD: National Institute of Mental Health, 1990;19–70.
4. Emerson E, Barrett S, Bell C, et al. Developing Services for People with Severe Learning Difficulties and Challenging Behaviors. Canterbury, UK: University of Kent at Canterbury, Institute of Social and Applied Psychology, 1987.
5. Diagnostic and Statistical Manual of Mental Disorders (4th ed). Washington, DC: American Psychiatric Association, 1990.
6. Belser RC, Sudhalter V. Conversational characteristics of children with fragile X syndrome: repetitive speech. Am J Ment Retard 2001;106:28–38.
7. Ozonoff S, Strayer DL, McMahon WM, Filloux F. Inhibitory deficits in Tourette syndrome: a function of comorbidity and symptom severity. J Child Psychol Psychiatry 1998;39(8):1109–1118.
8. McEvoy RE, Rogers SJ, Pennington BF. Executive function and social communication deficits in young autistic children. J Child Psychol Psychiatry 1993;34(4):563–578.
9. Hughes C, Russell J, Robbins T. Evidence for executive dysfunction in autism. Neuropsychologia 1994;32(4):477–492.
10. Reiss S. Prevalence of dual diagnosis in community-based day programs in Chicago metropolitan area. Am J Ment Def 1990;14:43–50.
11. Reiss S, Levitan GW, McMally RJ. Emotionally disturbed, mentally retarded people: an underserved population. Am Psychol 1982;37:361–367.

12. Reiss S, Levitan GW, Szyszko J. Emotional disturbance and mental retardation: diagnostic overshadowing. Am J Ment Def 1982;86:567–574.

13. Reiss S. Assessment of man with dual diagnosis. Ment Retard 1992;30:1–16.

14. Rasmussen SA, Eisen JL. Epidemiology of obsessive compulsive disorder. J Clin Psychiatry 1990;51 [Suppl]:10–13.

15. Barak Y, Ring A, Levy D, et al. Disabling compulsions in 11 mentally retarded adults: an open trial of clomipramine SR. J Clin Psychiatry 1995;56·459–461.

16. Gedye A. Recognizing obsessive-compulsive disorder in clients with developmental disabilities. Ment Health Newsl 1992;11:73–77.

17. Gedye A. Issues involved in recognizing obsessive-compulsive disorder in developmentally disabled clients. Semin Clin Neuropsychiatry 1996;1:142–147.

18. Sovner R, Hurley AD. Do the mentally retarded suffer from affective illness? Arch Gen Psychiatry 1983;40: 61–67.

19. Szymanski LS, Biederman J. Depression and anorexia nervosa of persons with Down syndrome. Am J Ment Def 1984;89(3):246–251.

20. Marston GM, Perry DW, Roy A. Manifestations of depression in people with intellectual disability. J Intellect Disabil Res 1997;41[Pt 6]:476–480.

21. Pies RW, Popli AP. Self-injurious behavior: pathophysiology and implications for treatment. J Clin Psychiatry 1995;56(12):580–588.

22. Osman OT, Loschen EL. Self-injurious behavior in the developmentally disabled: pharmacologic treatment. Psychopharmacol Bull 1992;28(4):439–449.

23. Verhoeven WM, Tuinier S, van den Berg YW, et al. Stress and self-injurious behavior; hormonal and serotonergic parameters in mentally retarded subjects. Pharmacopsychiatry 1999;32(1):13–20.

24. Nyhan WL. The recognition of Lesch-Nyhan syndrome as an inborn error of purine metabolism. Inherit Metab Dis 1997;20(2):171–178.

25. Pellicer F, Buendia-Roldan I, Pallares-Trujillo V. Self-mutilation in the Lesch-Nyhan syndrome: a corporal consciousness problem? A new hypothesis. Med Hypotheses 1998;50(1):43–47.

26. Sivam SP. Dopamine, serotonin and tachykinin in self-injurious behavior. Life Sci 1996;58(26):2367–2375.

27. Francois J. The Riley-Day syndrome. Familial dysautonomy, central autonomic dysfunction. Ophthalmologica 1977;174(1):20–34.

28. Tonholo-Silva ER, Takahashi SI, Yoshinaga L. Familial dysautonomia (Riley-Day syndrome). Arq Neuropsiquiatr 1994;52(1):103–105.

29. Sandman CA. Beta-endorphin dysregulation in autistic and self-injurious behavior: a neurodevelopmental hypothesis. Synapse 1988;2(3):193–199.

30. Sandman CA, Barron JL, Colman H. An orally administered opiate blocker, naltrexone, attenuates self-injurious behavior. Am J Ment Retard 1990;95 (1):93–102.

31. Matson JL, Gardner WI. Behavioral learning theory and current applications to severe behavior problems in persons with mental retardation. Clin Psychol Rev 1991;11:175–183.

32. Mason SA, Iwata BA. Artifactual effects of sensory-integrative therapy on self-injurious behavior. J Appl Behav Anal 1990;23(3):361–370.

33. Oliver C, Head D. Self injurious behavior in people with learning disabilities: determinants and interventions. Int Rev Psychiatry 1990;2:101–116.

34. Gardner WI, Moffat CW. Aggressive behavior: definition, assessment, treatment. Int Rev Psychiatry 1990; 2:91–100.

35. Gardner WI, Graeber JL. Use of Behavioral Therapies to Enhance Personal Competence: A Multimodal Diagnostic and Intervention Model. In N Bouras (ed), Mental Health in Mental Retardation: Recent Advances and Practices. Cambridge, UK: Cambridge University Press, 1994;205–223.

36. Gedye A. Behavioral Diagnostic Guide for Developmental Disabilities. Vancouver: Canada Diagnostic Books, 1998.

37. Reiss S, Valenti-Hein D. Development of a psychopathology rating scale for children with mental retardation. Consult Clin Psychol 1994;62(1):28–33.

38. Singh NN, Sood A, Sonenklar N, Ellis CR. Assessment and diagnosis of mental illness in persons with mental retardation. Methods and measures. Behav Modif 1991;15(3):419–443.

39. Rojahn J, Helsel WJ. The aberrant behavior checklist for children and adolescents with dual diagnosis. J Autism Dev Disord 1991;21(1):17–28.

40. Kazdin AE, Matson JL, Senatore V. Assessment of depression in mentally retarded adults. Am J Psychiatry 1983;40(8):1040–1043.

41. Hurley AD. Using the ABC sheet to analyze behavior: a training guide. Habil Ment Healthcare Newsl 1997;16(5):81–89.

42. Elman RJ. Introduction to Group Treatment of Neurogenic Communication Disorders. In RJ Elman (ed), Group Treatment of Neurogenic Communication Disorders. Woburn, MA: Butterworth–Heinemann, 1999: 3–7.

43. Tomasulo D. Group Counseling for People with Mild to Moderate Mental Retardation/Developmental Disabilities: An Interactive-Behavioral Model. New York: Young Adult Institute, 1992.

44. Pfadt A. Group psychotherapy with mentally retarded adults: issues related to design, implementations and evaluations. Res Dev Disabil 1991;12:261–286.

45. Hurley AD, Pfadt A, Tomasulo D, Gardner WI. Counseling and Psychotherapy. In JW Jacobson, JA Mulik (eds),

Manual of Diagnosis and Professional Practice in Mental Retardation. Washington, DC: American Psychological Association, 1996;371–378.

46. Brier NM, Demb HB. Psychotherapy with the developmentally disabled adolescent. J Dev Behav Pediatr 1980;1(1):19–23.

47. Carr EG, Durand VM. Reducing behavior problems through functional communication training. J Appl Behav Anal 1985;18(2):111–126.

48. Durand VM, Carr EG. Functional communication training to reduce challenging behavior: maintenance and application in new settings. J Appl Behav Anal 1991;24(2):251–264.

49. Cipani E. The communicative function hypothesis: an operant behavior perspective. J Behav Ther Exp Psychiatry 1990;21(4):239–247.

50. Jayne D, Schloss PJ, Alper S, Menscher S. Reducing disruptive behaviors by training students to request assistance. Behav Modif 1994;18(3):320–338.

51. Reichle J, Wacker DP. Communicative alternatives to challenging behaviors. Baltimore: Paul H. Brookes, 1993.

Chapter 15

Nonepileptic Seizures

A. James Rowan

Paroxysmal events resembling epileptic seizures are a confounding problem for neurologists who treat people with epilepsy or those suspected of having epilepsy. Too often, the diagnosis is missed or not even entertained. This is particularly true in those patients who have known epilepsy and develop coexisting nonepileptic events of psychogenic origin. It is also true in those who have medical conditions characterized by episodic events that are true seizures and not manifestations of epilepsy or those with episodic physiologic dysfunction. Failure to recognize such events for what they are leads to inappropriate and ineffective treatment, compromising affected patients' quality of life, sometimes for years. The following discussion lays out both clinical and physiologic guidelines that will aid the alert physician to the diagnostic possibility of nonepileptic events and can provide a framework for accurate diagnosis.

Nonepileptic seizures (NES) were well described by Charcot and Gowers in the late nineteenth century.[1] In Charcot's clinic and during his well-publicized demonstrations, the classic manifestations of opisthotonos (arc de circle) were the object of great interest and were said to be characteristic in young women. Since that time, the subject surfaced in sporadic case reports, and NES were recognized as manifestations of psychiatric illness. Various treatments were prescribed, usually individual psychotherapy, with varying degrees of success. Little attention, however, was paid to NES by the neurologic and psychiatric communities until the last 25 years when, with the growth of multidisciplinary epilepsy centers both abroad and in the United States, the extent of the problem became well known. The use of intensive electroencephalographic video (EEG-video) monitoring allowed a diagnosis to be made with relative certainty and permitted the study of phenomenology of these events. We now recognize that NES are fairly common, occurring both in epileptic and nonepileptic populations. Moreover, NES comprise a rich fabric of clinical signs, far beyond those originally described. Of greater importance has been the growing understanding of the range of psychiatric problems that underlie the seizures themselves.

Definitions

The term *hysterical seizures*, by which these events were known for many years, is derived from the Greek "hustere," or womb. Hysteria itself was a psychiatric condition thought to affect women and to derive from a disorder of the uterus. These false notions have been relegated to the dustbin of history, yet some physicians still refer to *hysteria* or a *hysterical personality*. These terms should not be used.

Pseudoseizures gained popularity earlier in this century, due mainly to the concept that the observed events were not epileptic but indeed simulated epilepsy.[2] As the seizures were not "real," by definition they were false or "pseudo." The American Heritage Dictionary defines *pseudo* as false, deceptive, sham.

Like hysteria, the term *pseudoseizure* should be discarded, for patients affected by these events are ill, and deception does not underlie the often alarming and always disabling symptoms.

The term that best describes the clinical problem is *nonepileptic seizures*. This clearly defines episodic events that resemble epileptic seizures but are not manifestations of epilepsy. The patient comes to neurologic attention because of this resemblance; thus, the term recognizes the serious nature of the illness without containing an intrinsic pejorative.

NES are not always an overt manifestation of psychiatric illness. Indeed, many physiologic conditions result in clinical events that resemble epileptic seizures. To distinguish between the two, NES are classified into two main categories: psychogenic NES and physiologic NES. In this chapter, the abbreviation *NES* refers to psychogenic NES. Each category is discussed in subsequent sections.

Epidemiology

NES are more common than generally appreciated. In the absence of specialized diagnostic procedures, such as EEG-video monitoring, affected patients often receive a diagnosis of epilepsy based on descriptions provided by relatives or others or on historical data provided by the patients. Details of the events often are obscured by their often frightening manifestations, and many patients with NES understandably receive a diagnosis of epilepsy and, therefore, are treated with antiepileptic drugs (AEDs). In a recent series of 79 patients with diagnosed psychogenic NES in our EEG-video monitoring unit, 51 (65%) were taking AEDs at the time of study, and an additional 5 had been treated with AEDs in the past.[3]

Relatively few data address the prevalence or incidence of NES. Scott[4] estimated that 5% of his patients in an epilepsy clinic were affected by NES, although he did not have the benefit of EEG-video monitoring. Gates et al.[5] reported that 20% of patients entered into a comprehensive epilepsy center had NES. The coexistence of epilepsy and NES has been estimated by other authors at 10–58%.[6,7] The wide range of these figures may be explained by varying referral patterns, the availability of monitoring, and perhaps the specialized interest of the investigators. In any case, NES are common, and increased sensitivity to the possibility of NES by all neurologists can lead to more accurate diagnosis.

Classification

No widely accepted classification system categorizes psychogenic NES. The classification used most commonly follows the International Classification of Epileptic Seizures, based on the idea that NES may resemble generalized tonic-clonic convulsions, complex partial seizures, or absence attacks. Although true in a general sense, this categorization contains so many exceptions that it has little practical utility. Moreover, this system contains no recognition of the associated psychiatric conditions that are variable in their type and extent, nor does it take into account any underlying brain disease that may contribute to the overall syndrome.

A more suitable system would combine clinical manifestations and psychiatric diagnoses. Gates and Erdahl[8] suggested using psychiatric diagnoses based on the *Diagnostic and Statistical Manual of Mental Disorders,* 4th ed. (*DSM-IV*) (Wahington, DC: American Psychiatric Association, 1994) system *DSM-III-R* (now *DSM-IV*) to categorize patients with NES. NES is essentially a somatoform disorder[9] (i.e., a disorder with primarily somatic manifestations). In addition, patients with NES often meet criteria for additional disorders (e.g., depression or panic disorder).[10] Such a classification has implications for treatment and prognosis and better portrays the clinical status of affected patients. When used in conjunction with descriptive phenomenology, this schema represents an advance in our understanding of NES. It does not, however, meet the problem of attempting to match types of NES with types of epileptic seizures as defined by the International Classification.

In our review of 79 consecutive patients with NES documented by EEG-video monitoring, several general types of seizure phenomenology were observed, ranging from vigorous, chaotic motor activity to unresponsive staring.[3] Also, some events truly resembled epileptic seizures (e.g., generalized tonic-clonic convulsions), whereas many did not. Patients could be classified into two broad categories: Those who exhibited active events and those who exhibited passive events, with subdivisions of each. Conceptually, the particular phenomenology of NES may be related to the underlying psychiatric disorder. Further, the presence or absence of organic brain dysfunction may play a role in both seizure manifestations and resultant disability.[11] Thus, a multiaxial classification for NES based on symptoms, on psychiatric diagnosis, and on neurologic and neuropsychological findings may allow a broader understanding of affected individuals' illness and might improve communication among clinicians and investigators (Table 15-1).

Using axis I of the proposed classification, (see Table 15-1), we were able to classify 75 of 77 consecutive patients. With respect to active events, some form of chaotic motor activity was found in 26, minor motor activity in 30, pure ocular manifestations in 2, and events strikingly similar to epileptic seizures in only 8. Thirteen patients had passive events, and two were unclassifiable. Insufficient data were available to classify patients according to axes II and III. A prospective study will be required to determine the utility of this system for the purposes of professional communication, planning therapy, and determining prognosis.

Characteristics of Psychogenic Nonepileptic Seizures

As outlined, psychogenic NES may or may not closely resemble true epileptic seizures. Although arriving at the diagnosis may be difficult without the availability of monitoring, historical and phenomenological features can suggest the diagnosis. None, however, is pathognomonic.

Historical Features Suggestive of Psychogenic Nonepileptic Seizures

The history of patients with psychogenic NES usually contains important clues regarding the true nature of the events. If the seizures are of relatively recent onset, inquiry into any surrounding social or

Table 15-1. Proposed Multiaxial Classification of Psychogenic Nonepileptic Seizures

Axis I: Event phenomenology
   I. Active events
     A. Chaotic motor activity
      1. Bilateral
      2. Unilateral or clearly asymmetric
     B. Minor motor activity
      1. Bilateral
      2. Unilateral
      3. Wandering
     C. Oculofacial motor activity
     D. Events strikingly similar to epileptic seizures
      1. Generalized tonic-clonic; tonic; clonic
      2. Complex partial
      3. Myoclonic
     E. Unclassifiable
      1. Each of the preceding categories modified with
       a. Apparent altered consciousness
        i. Emotional
        ii. Nonemotional
       b. Without altered consciousness
        i. Emotional
        ii. Nonemotional
  II. Passive events
     A. Staring, unresponsive
     B. Sleep-like, motionless
     C. Subjective
Axis II: Underlying psychiatric disorder (partial listing)
   I. Somatoform disorder
   II. Mood disorder
   III. Anxiety disorder
   IV. Psychotic disorder
Axis III: Associated organic brain dysfunction
   I. Epilepsy
     A. Current
     B. Remote
   II. Brain dysfunction as manifested by the following:
     A. Clinical examination
     B. Electroencephalography
      1. Focal slowing (specify location)
      2. Diffuse slowing
      3. Epileptiform activity (specify)
     C. Neuroimaging
      1. Focal abnormality
      2. Diffuse abnormality
     D. Neuropsychological testing
      1. Localized abnormality (specify)
      2. Global abnormality

Source: Reprinted with permission from M Muxfeldt, HE Price, SH Dane, et al. Non-epileptic seizures: characteristics and proposed classification. Epilepsia 1995;36:1995.

emotional factors may suggest a correlation with onset of the illness. Seizures may occur only when a patient is alone or, conversely, only when a patient is in the company of others (e.g., family members). Such selectivity might be regarded with suspicion. Precipitating emotional factors for each event may or may not be present. If the patient is receiving AEDs, a careful assessment of response is required. Lack of response to AEDs, regardless of type or dose, may arouse suspicion, as may an increase in seizures as the AED dose is increased. Another clue is intolerance to any AED despite slow and careful dose escalation.

Patients with NES may experience a relatively high seizure frequency, sometimes many in the course of a day. High seizure frequency is seen also in patients with epilepsy, especially those with seizures involving the supplementary motor area. Incontinence and tongue biting are hallmarks of tonic-clonic seizures, although they do not occur invariably. Conversely, these symptoms are considered rare in patients with NES. Both are seen sometimes in NES and their absence, therefore, cannot provide definitive proof of NES. Patients with NES may reveal a history of some personal experience with seizures, whether as hospital personnel, having observed a seizure at some time, or having a family member with epilepsy. In itself, this means little, but such experience may have provided a template for a patient's events.

One may find, in a patient with known epilepsy, a change in seizure type or, after a seizure-free interval, emergence of a new type of seizure. Although such a change may suggest development of a new cerebral process, such as tumor, also possible is that NES have intervened. In addition to the recording of a careful history, such patients require EEG, imaging study, and, in doubtful cases, intensive EEG-video monitoring.

Previous sexual or physical abuse appears to be common in psychogenic NES. In our clinic, up to 70% of patients divulge such a history.[11] Alper et al.[12] found a history of sexual or physical abuse in 37.4% of patients with NES, as compared with a frequency of 8.6% in controls with complex partial epilepsy. In addition, a history of minor head trauma appears to be relatively common in patients with NES.[13]

One of the foregoing historical features by itself establishes a diagnosis of NES. For a group-ing of several items, however, the possibility of NES should be entertained. At that point, further investigations may be indicated.

Clinical Signs Suggestive of Psychogenic Nonepileptic Seizures

Certain seizures classified as NES appear to have obvious qualities of "nonorganicity" to the professional and even the casual observer. Thus, a patient observed to flail about with an excessive emotional reaction is usually thought to have NES. On the other hand, seizures with subtle manifestations, such as apparent confusion or unresponsive staring, are more likely to be thought of as epileptic. A number of particular seizure phenomena suggest the possibility of NES. NES with prominent motor characteristics often have a gradual onset, with progressively increasing vigor, unlike epileptic seizures, in which the onset is abrupt. Further, the motor activity frequently is interrupted or discontinuous, whereas epileptic seizures usually display continuity throughout. Related to this is the apparent disjointed or "nonphysiologic" progression of symptoms in NES. Epileptic seizures consisting primarily of motor activity have a progression of manifestations that adhere to physiologic and anatomic principles, good examples being the progression seen in a jacksonian march and the typical sequence of generalized tonic-clonic convulsions. The motor activity of NES is rarely so predictable or stereotypic. This is best exemplified by the chaotic, flinging, side-to-side movements often associated with NES. Out-of-phase, repetitive movements may be observed, along with intermittent dystonic posturing or pelvic thrusting.[5] Often, elements of all these phenomena coexist. Interestingly, the face rarely is involved.[14,15] A marked emotional reaction is not unusual either during or after a nonepileptic seizure event.

The duration of NES is, on average, longer than that of epileptic seizures. In a study by Gates et al.,[5] NES were approximately 20% longer on average than true tonic-clonic convulsions. Durations of up to one-half hour or more sometimes are observed, intermittent motor activity associated with unresponsiveness occurring throughout the event. The NES usually subside gradually, unlike epileptic events that usually end more abruptly. However, determining the interface between the ictal and the postictal states in patients with complex partial seizures is often difficult. Thus, in such cases, the epileptic event may appear to be prolonged, with gradual cessation of symptoms.

The foregoing signs that raise the question of NES are not specific to the diagnosis. For example, the clinical picture of seizures of frontal lobe origin often is bizarre, and the motor activity is chaotic.[16] The initial stages of the seizure, perhaps consisting of brief tonic posturing, often are not appreciated by an observer or seen by hospital staff. Thus, only the striking motor phase is reported and taken to be nonepileptic in nature. Moreover, duration of epileptic seizures may be variable, some of relatively long duration. Thus, duration in an individual case may not be helpful. Further, intermittency in epileptic seizures may be seen if brief events occur repetitively without recovery of full awareness between events. As in the case of the history, a grouping of several clinical manifestations is required to improve specificity. Even then, the diagnosis may be in doubt. Perhaps the most specific clinical sign is the ability of an examiner to provoke the patient's habitual NES using techniques of suggestion, such as intravenous saline or application of alcohol pads.[17] Epileptic seizures rarely are provoked in this manner. The role of suggestion in confirming the diagnosis of NES is outlined later.

Nonepileptic Seizures in the Context of Developmental Disability

It is well known that individuals with learning disabilities or mental retardation have a high prevalence of epileptic seizures. Some studies indicate that up to one-third of such individuals have epilepsy.[18–20] Therefore, not surprisingly, NES can be observed in this group, although reliable prevalence figures for NES in the learning disabled are not available. McDade and Brown[21] described the difficulties of classifying episodic behaviors in the learning disabled. These authors pointed out that behaviors eventually proven to be epileptic in origin are complex and that their classification is difficult. On the other hand, some behaviors that are initially regarded as epileptic

turn out to be nonepileptic in nature. Incorrect diagnosis of NES, therefore, leads to ineffective treatment with AEDs.

Neill and Alvarez[22] cited 124 mentally retarded persons who had behaviors suggestive of epilepsy and all of whom were monitored with EEG-video recording. Recorded behaviors included myoclonus, eye blinks, head drops, automatisms, and motor arrest. They classified 50 of the 124 subjects as having only nonepileptic events, 4 of whom had epileptiform EEG recordings. Eleven were classified as having both epileptic and nonepileptic events. In 43, the authors were unable to classify the behaviors. Donat and Wright[23] studied neurologically impaired children with EEG-video recordings and emphasized that episodic nonepileptic behaviors may be mistaken for epileptic seizures. Holmes et al.[24] studied 38 patients with profound mental retardation in an effort to differentiate epileptic from nonepileptic behaviors. All patients had abnormal EEG readings, but in only 39% were the recorded events epileptic in nature.

Many learning-disabled individuals may be placed on AEDs incorrectly, with the attendant danger of sedative side effects, potentially worsening the underlying cognitive deficit. Therefore, it is essential that episodic behaviors in the mentally and neurologically impaired be diagnosed correctly, using EEG-video monitoring whenever clinical doubt exists.

Donat and Wright[25] studied infants with a clinical history suggestive of infantile spasms. Of 53 patients in their series, 45 had episodic signs and symptoms that proved to be nonepileptic, including spasticity, gastroesophageal reflux, and myoclonus. These authors emphasized that correct diagnosis in these cases leads to discontinuation of inappropriate treatment.

Self-induced epileptic seizures comprise a special category among the mentally retarded, although not all such individuals are mentally or neurologically impaired. These events fall in a category best described as epileptic seizures of psychogenic origin. Although not nonepileptic, these events must be recognized, for they lead to considerable disability and should not be treated with ever-increasing doses of AEDs. Perhaps the best-known mechanism of self-induced seizures is found in photosensitive subjects. Such individuals learn to wave the outstretched fingers rapidly before a light source, often the sun, at a frequency to which they are photosensitive. Monitoring studies during such behavior demonstrate provocation of generalized spike and wave complexes, often with attendant eye blinking. The genesis of this behavior may be unclear, but probably the seizures produce psychological gratification, perhaps sexual in some cases. Other behaviors leading to self-induced seizures included eye closure with forced upward deviation of the eyes. These patients are also photosensitive and may be retarded. All display psychiatric or psychosocial problems.[26]

The author observed in a large European epilepsy center a resident patient with complex partial seizures. This individual was able to induce his typical seizures by sucking on a piece of hard candy. During an interview, the patient revealed that sucking on the candy led to a pleasant aura with sexual overtones. This was followed by loss of consciousness and typical automatisms. The true nature of these events was revealed during EEG-video monitoring.

Treatment of patients with self-induced seizures should be aimed at reducing the gratification the patients receive from their behavior. Binnie[27] suggested that the use of dopamine antagonists may be helpful in rendering these events nonrewarding. In the event that such treatment is successful, reducing AED dosage may be possible.

Physiologic Nonepileptic Seizures

A great many physiologic events mimic epileptic seizures. One of the most common is syncope, either neurogenic or cardiogenic. Syncopal attacks are diagnosed readily if an accurate history is available. The characteristic premonitory symptoms, brief loss of consciousness, and lack of a postictal confusional state immediately suggest the true diagnosis. In some cases, the syncopal event is complicated by convulsive activity, either tonic or clonic in character.[28,29] This motor phase usually is brief, and the patient recovers quickly. Convulsive syncope sometimes occurs when an affected patient does not fall down immediately. In these circumstances, the upright or sitting position prolongs the cerebral ischemic phase. The major problem lies in an observer's description, wherein the event may be reported as a tonic-clonic seizure. Details that could confirm the syncopal nature of the attack may not be forthcoming. Such patients often are treated inappropriately with AEDs. Suspicion of syncope, however, should lead to appropriate testing, including search for orthostatic hypotension, other forms of autonomic dysfunction, and intermittent cardiac arrhythmias.

A variety of sleep disorders lead to a misdiagnosis not only of epilepsy but of psychogenic NES. Nocturnal enuresis in children, and occasionally in adults, may raise the question of an unobserved seizure. The evidence shows, however, that unsuspected seizures rarely are the cause of nocturnal enuresis unless associated symptoms are present.[30]

Sleep walking is a parasomnia associated with slow-wave sleep.[31] The subject wanders about in an apparently confused state, reminiscent of ictal or postictal motor activity of a complex partial seizure. In this circumstance, misdiagnosis on either side of the NES-epilepsy border is possible. Akin to sleep walking is sleep drunkenness, which occurs at the interface of sleep and wakefulness.[32] Affected individuals may carry out complex motor activities in a confused state. Sleep drunkenness may occur after sleep deprivation or after consuming alcohol or taking hypnotics.[33] Narcolepsy, when symptoms are well described, usually is diagnosed without difficulty. Patients presenting with sudden diurnal sleep episodes, however, may be given an incorrect diagnosis of epilepsy. Polysomnography to confirm a sleep disorder should be carried out in suspicious cases. An unusual parasomnia—rapid-eye-movement behavior disorder—has dramatic manifestations that are diagnosed as either epileptic or psychiatric.[34] During rapid-eye-movement sleep, affected individuals have failure of brainstem mechanisms that normally inhibit motor activity. Thus, dreams are acted out as if real. With frightening dreams, such as those involving pursuit or struggle, the person may strike out or run, leading to injury to self or others. Deaths have even been reported due to jumping from a window in an apparent attempt to escape. The diagnosis may be suspected, even if the nocturnal events are not the chief complaint, if it is ascertained that a husband and wife have decided on separate bedrooms to avoid injury due to kicking or striking by one of the partners during sleep. Treatment with clonazepam has been tried in such cases, with some success.[34]

Migraine may be mistaken for epilepsy when associated with neurologic dysfunction and especially when headache is not a prominent symptom. A good example is the patient who presents with scintillating scotomata or other purely visual phenomena. These symptoms, common in migraine, are seen also in occipital epilepsy, the latter associated with occipital spikes and a benign prognosis.[35] EEG recording performed during the visual symptoms of a migraine attack show only occipital slowing without epileptiform discharges.

Transient global amnesia, described by Bender in 1956,[36] amplified by Fisher and Adams in 1958,[37] and more recently reviewed by Caplan,[38] presents with a confusional state that usually lasts for hours. Transient global amnesia episodes may be recurrent, although a low attack frequency is the rule. During such attacks, the EEG reading is normal.[39] If the patient cannot be examined during an attack, which is often the case, the question of complex partial seizures is raised. Transient global amnesia often occurs in older patients with a history of cerebrovascular disease. During an attack, affected patients appear to be confused although able to carry out complex activities. Because of the inability to store new information, such patients characteristically ask questions repeatedly (e.g., "What day is it?" or "What are we doing here?"). A carefully recorded history should establish the diagnosis in most cases.

Paroxysmal movement disorders, such as paroxysmal kinesigenic choreoathetosis or paroxysmal dystonia, may suggest seizure activity.[40,41] These disorders involve subcortical structures, and their etiology has been the subject of debate. Again, a carefully recorded history and observation of the attacks during EEG-video monitoring will establish the diagnosis. These conditions sometimes respond to anticonvulsant therapy, such as carbamazepine.

Transient ischemic attacks may mimic epileptic seizures, especially in the presence of a dysphasic component. During such an attack, an affected individual may appear confused and, to the casual observer, the language deficit may not be obvious. Thus, the history becomes one of episodic confusion, raising the question of complex partial seizures. In the event of associated motor deficit or if sensorimotor deficit occurs without language impairment, the nature of the attacks is more obvious in that negative motor signs (e.g., hemiparesis) are uncommon manifestations of seizures. The EEG recording does not contain epileptiform activity but may show some lateralized slowing. Appropriate tests, including noninvasive carotid studies, should be performed in doubtful cases.

Diagnostic Procedures

The diagnostic evaluation of psychogenic NES is similar to that of epilepsy. The first step includes a routine EEG workup, imaging study, and routine blood work, including assessment of AED levels, if applicable. EEG after sleep deprivation or sedation should be performed if the routine record is unrevealing.[42] A finding of interictal epileptiform activity on the EEG recording does not imply that an affected patient's spells are epileptic. Conversely, a normal record in the context of high seizure frequency, especially seizures with apparent loss of awareness, arouses suspicion of NES.

Although the foregoing evaluation provides useful information, EEG-video monitoring is the critical diagnostic procedure. The object is to record the behavioral aspects of the episodic event with a simultaneous EEG recording. If possible, more than one event should be recorded (preferably several), to look for stereotypy. Classically, epileptic seizures are stereotyped with respect to phenomenology, progression, and duration, although NES also may reveal a stereotyped pattern. During the event, the EEG recording is devoid of epileptiform activity, premonitory spikes or amplitude depression, and postictal slowing.[43] Although the EEG reading during the event may be dominated by artifact, brief windows of interpretable tracing may reveal alpha activity. The interictal record may or may not contain epileptiform discharges and cannot be considered diagnostic.

Important to note is that focal epileptiform activity underlying simple partial seizures may not be recorded with scalp electrodes.[44] Thus, a seizure recorded without any evidence of concurrent epileptiform activity is not necessarily nonepileptic in origin. A critical factor in differentiating epileptic from nonepileptic seizures, therefore, is an analysis of the video-recorded behavior during the event. Every effort should be made to record several events, and, if successful, the events should be edited to a master tape and viewed consecutively. Events that are highly stereotyped in phenomenology and duration signal a high likelihood that they are epileptic and, if more heterogeneous, nonepileptic. During monitoring, techniques of suggestion should be applied to all patients suspected of having NES. If the family recognizes an evoked event as typical, even though no other events are recorded, a nonepileptic origin is likely.[15] Despite all efforts, patients will be encountered in whom differentiation of NES from epilepsy is difficult if not impossible. In these cases, restudy may reveal the true diagnosis.

Ambulatory monitoring has limited usefulness in diagnosing NES. The lack of video recording is a severe limitation, especially if seizures are of the motor type. In some cases (e.g., in absence-type NES), useful information may be obtained if the events are recorded with an event marker. Some systems now are coupled with video monitoring, which may increase the usefulness of ambulatory monitoring. Still, currently no substitute exists for EEG-video monitoring in the presence of a trained observer.

Determination of prolactin levels has gained some favor in distinguishing patients with NES from those with epilepsy.[45] The most consistent finding is a marked elevation of prolactin after a generalized tonic-clonic convulsion in 90–100% of patients.[46] The elevation is at least twofold, often more. With complex partial seizures, the elevation is variable, ranging from 43% to 100%, depending on which deep temporal structures are maximally involved.[47] Simple partial seizures raise prolactin only slightly and absence attacks and NES not at all.[48] Thus, if the differential diagnosis lies between a generalized convulsion and NES with prominent motor activity, prolactin determination may be useful. For other seizure types, the test appears to be of lower specificity.

Neuropsychological Testing

Neuropsychological testing provides useful information in evaluating patients with NES. In partic-

ular, the Minnesota Multiphasic Personality Inventory (MMPI) has been the subject of several studies, recently reviewed by Dodrill et al.[49] In some cases, MMPI results in patients with NES were compared with those in patients with epilepsy; in others, patients with coexisting NES and epilepsy were compared with an epileptic group. Variable results were reported, although patients with NES tended to score higher in the hypochondriasis, depression, hysteria, and schizophrenia scales. Dodrill et al.[49] compared 23 patients with NES and 22 patients who had intractable epilepsy and had undergone epilepsy surgery.[49] The four scales mentioned demonstrated elevations in patients with NES, with significant findings for hypochondriasis and hysteria scales. The depression scale was lower than these scales, resulting in a characteristic V-shaped profile. Dodrill et al. analyzed four studies that compared patients with "pure" NES to those with epilepsy.[49–52] MMPI configurational rules, devised by Wilkus et al.,[50] classified epilepsy correctly in 78%, whereas the figure for NES was 65%. However, the error rate of 22% for epileptic and 35% for nonepileptic patients was significant, thus diminishing the specificity of this test.

The MMPI may have other applications in NES. Dodrill et al.[49] found that NES with prominent affect and minimal motor manifestations showed differences on the hypochondriasis, hysteria, and schizophrenia scales as compared with epileptic patients. On the other hand, those with marked motor and minimal affect manifestations showed no such differences. This lends support to the concept that a multiaxial classification system would be likely to provide greater insight into the mechanisms of NES than would a classification based on phenomenology alone.

Psychiatric Considerations

Roy[53,54] conducted an early study of NES and their psychiatric concomitants. He used standard scales of depression and anxiety in a comparative study of NES and epilepsy and found significantly higher scores for both in patients with NES. NES were regarded not as a conversion of anxiety into a physical symptom but rather as a "signal of distress." Roy considered the symptom of a nonepileptic seizure to be a ticket of admission into the health care system for a patient with a psychiatric disorder.

NES fall under the rubric of the somatoform disorders in *DSM-IV* and include conversion disorder, somatization disorder, and somatoform disorder not otherwise specified. *Conversion disorder* is successor to the term *conversion* that, as used by Freud, suggested that psychic energy was converted into somatic symptoms. Today, conversion is thought to be precipitated by psychic stress and continued as a result of secondary gain. Underlying psychiatric illness has been emphasized. Ford and Folks[55] noted that conversion should be viewed as a symptom, not a diagnosis.

Somatization disorder is successor to the term *hysteria*. It is also termed *Briquet's syndrome*, named after Pierre Briquet who, in 1859, reported 430 patients with hysteria.[56] Briquet's syndrome describes patients with multiple unexplained somatic symptoms and specific criteria for this diagnosis, which requires at least 13 unexplained medical symptoms set forth in *DSM-IV.* NES are considered among the possible features of this disorder.

Somatization disorder not otherwise specified is a broad category that can include patients who have medical disease and symptoms not explained by the illness but who do not meet criteria for somatization disorder. This may be appropriate for patients with coexisting epilepsy and NES. Such patients have difficulty in coping with stress and may use NES as a way to continue the role of illness as a coping mechanism.

Treatment and Prognosis

Too often after a diagnosis of NES is made, an affected patient is cast into limbo. Neurologists, having completed their work, feel they have little to contribute to future management. This problem is compounded by psychiatrists who often are reluctant to take on these patients because of lack of experience with NES or a lack of interest in somatoform disorders. Nonetheless, if an affected patient demonstrates evidence of depression or anxiety, psychiatrists may be willing to provide appropriate care, working closely with the referring neurologist.

Because the psychiatric backgrounds of patients with NES are diverse, the approach to management must be individualized. Some patients will require psychotropic medication, others short-term psychotherapy, and still others psychiatric support with a view toward coping with the symptom. A multidisciplinary approach to management may be best. Some epilepsy centers have programs to diagnose and manage the psychiatric problems of patients with NES. Examples are MINCEP Epilepsy Care in Minneapolis and the Minnesota Epilepsy Group in St. Paul. These groups provide a team approach to therapy, using the services of neurologists, psychiatrist, psychologists, social workers, and other personnel.[57] Team meetings comprise the forum for discussion and planning and are conducted while a patient is hospitalized at the center. After the diagnosis is presented and the patient is begun on an individualized therapy program, outpatient follow-up is arranged with a therapist in the community.

Inpatient evaluation is costly, and many patients do not have access to such centers. Outpatient management, also using a team approach, can be a viable alternative.[11,58] In this model, patients with diagnosed NES review the EEG-video monitoring tape with a significant other to ensure that the recorded event is the same as the patient's habitual seizures. The diagnosis then is presented to the patient in a positive light: Emphasis is placed on the concept that NES are as disabling as epilepsy, that a specialized clinic deals with this particular problem, and that the outlook is optimistic. During the first NES clinic visit, an affected patient meets with the NES team, at which time the patient's history is reviewed and general therapeutic goals are outlined. Appointments then are made with a psychiatrist, a psychologist, and a social worker. After interviews are completed, a therapeutic plan is formulated and presented to the NES team. The plan depends on the specific psychiatric problem and may include pharmacotherapy, supportive therapy, or short-term psychotherapy. The patient's progress is monitored by the NES team. If the patient has seen a psychiatrist outside the clinic, the team works with him or her and supplements ongoing therapy. In all cases, the continued participation by the neurologist is considered an important element in providing continuity of care and contributing to the authenticity of the treatment plan.

Overall, the prognosis of NES is favorable. Various studies report between 50% and 70% remission or marked improvement in attack frequency.[59–62] Even in the absence of formal psychiatric intervention, patients tend to improve over time. Factors considered less favorable for outcome include long duration of NES and true somatoform disorder. Those patients developing acute stress-related NES of relatively short duration appear to have a more favorable outlook.

Conclusion

Misdiagnosis of NES as epileptic seizures leads to continuing disability, puts affected patients at risk for the adverse effects of unneeded antiepileptic medication, promotes needless contact with multiple physicians, and results in frustration for physician and patient alike. On the other hand, a correct diagnosis of NES leads to exploration of the underlying psychiatric problem, allows discontinuation of AEDs with elimination of any side effects, and renders possible the application of specific treatment.

References

1. Massey EW, McHenry LC. Hysteroepilepsy in the nineteenth century: Charcot and Gowers. Neurology 1986;36:65–67.
2. Liske E, Forster FM. Pseudoseizures: a problem in the diagnosis and management of epileptic patients. Neurology 1964;14:41–49.
3. Muxfeldt M, Price HE, Dane SH, et al. Non-epileptic seizures: characteristics and proposed classification. Epilepsia 1995;36:159.
4. Scott DF. Recognition and Diagnostic Aspects of Non-Epileptic Seizures. In TL Riley, A Roy (eds), Pseudoseizures. Baltimore: Williams & Wilkins, 1982;21–34.
5. Gates JR, Ramani V, Whalen SM. Ictal characteristics of pseudoseizures. Arch Neurol 1985;42:1183–1187.
6. Desai BT, Porter RJ, Penry JF. Psychogenic seizures: a study of 42 attacks in sick patients, with intensive monitoring. Arch Neurol 1982;39:202–209.
7. Lesser RP. Psychogenic Seizures. In TA Pedley, BS Meldrum (eds), Recent Advances in Epilepsy, vol 2. Edinburgh: Churchill Livingstone, 1985;273–296.
8. Gates JR, Erdahl P. Classification of Non-Epileptic Events. In AJ Rowan, JR Gates (eds), Non-Epileptic Seizures. Boston: Butterworth–Heinemann, 1993;21–30.
9. American Psychiatric Association. Diagnostic and Statistical Manual of Mental Disorders (4th ed). Washington, DC: American Psychiatric Press, 1995.
10. Novelly RA. Cerebral Dysfunction and Cognitive Impairment in Non-Epileptic Seizure Disorders. In AJ Rowan, JR Gates (eds), Non-Epileptic Seizures. Boston: Butterworth–Heinemann, 1993;233–243.
11. Snyder S, Rosenbaum DH, Rowan AJ, Strain JJ. SCID diagnosis of panic disorder in psychogenic seizure patients. J Neuropsychiatry Clin Neurosci 1994;6:261–266.
12. Alper K, Devinsky O, Perrine K, et al. Nonepileptic seizures and childhood sexual and physical abuse. Neurology 1993;43:1950–1953.
13. Westbrook LE, Devinsky O, Geocadin R. Nonepileptic seizures after head injury. Epilepsia 1998;39:978–982.
14. Kanner AM, French JA, Rosenbaum DH, Rowan AJ. Ictal phenomena as discriminators in the diagnosis of epileptic vs. psychogenic seizures. Epilepsia 1987;28:613.
15. Kanner AM, Morris HH, Lueders H, et al. Supplementary motor area seizures mimicking pseudoseizures: some clinical differences. Neurology 1990;40:1404–1407.
16. Williamson PD, Spencer DD, Spencer SS, et al. Complex partial seizures of frontal lobe origin. Ann Neurol 1985;18:497–504.
17. French JA. The use of suggestion as a provocative test in the diagnosis of psychogenic NES. In AJ Rowan, JR Gates (eds), Non-Epileptic Seizures. Boston: Butterworth–Heinemann, 1993;111–122.
18. Payne D, Johnson RC, Abelson J. A Comprehensive Description of Institutional Retardates in the Western United States. Boulder: Western Interstate Commission for Higher Education, 1969.
19. Corbett JA. Epilepsy and Mental Retardation. In M Parsonage (ed), Proceedings of the Sixth International Symposium on Epilepsy, London. New York: Raven Press, 1983;207–214.
20. Corbett JA. Epilepsy and Mental Handicap. In J Laidlaw, A Richens, J Oxley (eds), A Textbook of Epilepsy (3rd ed). Edinburgh: Churchill Livingstone, 1988;533–538.
21. McDade G, Brown SW. Non-epileptic seizures: management and predictive factors of outcome. Seizure 1992;1:7–10.
22. Neill JC, Alvarez N. Differential diagnosis of epileptic versus pseudoepileptic seizures in developmentally disabled persons. Appl Res Ment Retard 1986;7:285–298.
23. Donat JF, Wright FS. Episodic symptoms mistaken for seizures in the neurologically impaired child. Neurology 1990;40:156–157.
24. Holmes GL, McKeever M, Russman BS. Abnormal behavior or epilepsy? Use of long-term EEG and video monitoring with severely to profoundly mentally retarded patients with seizures. Am J Ment Defic 1983;87:456–458.
25. Donat JF, Wright FS. Clinical imitators of infantile spasms. J Child Neurol 1992;7:395–399.
26. Binnie CD, Darby CE, De Korte RA, Wilkins AJ. Self-induction of epileptic seizures by eye closure: inci-

dence and recognition. J Neurol Neurosurg Psychiatry 1980;43:386–389.

27. Binnie CD. Self-induction of seizures: the ultimate non-compliance. Epilepsy Res Suppl 1988;1:153–158.

28. Dohrmann MML, Cheitlin MD. Cardiogenic syncope: seizure versus syncope. Neurol Clin 1986;4:549–562.

29. Aminoff MJ, Scheinman MM, Griffin JC, Herre JM. Electrocerebral accompaniments of syncope associated with malignant ventricular arrhythmias. Ann Intern Med 1988;108:791–796.

30. Pedley TA. Differential diagnosis of episodic syndromes. Epilepsia 1983;24[Suppl 1]:S31–S34.

31. Guilleminault C, Phillips R, Dement WC. A syndrome of hypersomnia with automatic behavior. Electroencephalogr Clin Neurophysiol 1975;38:403–413.

32. Thorpy MJ, Glovinsky PB. Parasomnias. Psychol Clin North Am 1987;10:623–639.

33. Roth B, Nevsimalova S, Rechtschaffen A. Hypersomnia with "sleep drunkenness." Arch Gen Psychiatry 1972;26:377–393.

34. Mahowald MW, Schenck CH. REM Sleep Behavior Disorder. In MH Kryger, T Roth, WC Dement (eds), Principles of Sleep Medicine. Philadelphia: Saunders, 1989;389–402.

35. Gastaut H. Benign Epilepsy of Childhood with Occipital Paroxysms. In J Roger, C Dravet, M Bureau, et al. (eds), Epileptic Syndromes in Infancy, Childhood and Adolescence. London: Hohn Libbey Eurotext, 1985; 159–170.

36. Bender MB. Syndrome of isolated episode of confusion with amnesia. J Hillside Hosp 1956;5:12–15.

37. Fisher CM, Adams RD. Transient global amnesia. Trans Am Neurol Assoc 1958;83:143–146.

38. Caplan LR. Transient Global Amnesia. In P Vinken, G Bruyn, H Klawans (eds), Handbook of Clinical Neurology. Amsterdam: Elsevier, 1985;205–218.

39. Cole AJ, Gloor P, Kaplan R. Transient global amnesia; the electroencephalogram at onset. Ann Neurol 1987; 22:771–772.

40. Kertesz A. Paroxysmal kinesigenic choreoathetosis: an entity within the paroxysmal choreoathetosis syndrome. Description of 10 cases including 1 autopsied. Neurology 1967;17:680–690.

41. Lance JW. Familial paroxysmal dystonic choreoathetosis and its differentiation from related syndromes. Ann Neurol 1977;2:285–293.

42. Rowan AJ, Veldhuisen RJ, Nagelkerke NJD. Comparative evaluation of sleep deprivation and sedated sleep EEGs as diagnostic aids in epilepsy. Electroencephalogr Clin Neurophysiol 1982;54:357–364.

43. Mattson RH. Electroencephalographic (Polygraphic) Studies in the Diagnosis of Non-Epileptic Seizures. In AJ Rowan, JR Gates (eds), Non-Epileptic Seizures. Boston: Butterworth–Heinemann, 1993;85–92.

44. Devinsky O, Nadi SN, Theodore WH, Porter RJ. Electroencephalographic studies of simple partial seizures with subdural electrode recordings. Neurology 1989; 39:527–533.

45. Trimble M. Serum prolactin in epilepsy and hysteria. BMJ 1978;2:1682.

46. Prichard PB, Wannamaker BB, Sagel J, Daniel C. Serum prolactin and cortisol levels in evaluation of pseudoepileptic seizures. Ann Neurol 1985;18:87–89.

47. Sperling MR, Pritchard PB, Engel J, et al. Prolactin in partial epilepsy: an indicator of limbic seizures. Ann Neurol 1986;20:716–722.

48. Bercovic S. Clinical and Experimental Aspects of Complex Partial Seizures. Doctor of Medicine Thesis, University of Melbourne. Quoted in J Laidlaw, A Richens, J Oxley (eds), A Textbook of Epilepsy (3rd ed). New York: Churchill Livingstone, 1988.

49. Dodrill CB, Wilkus RJ, Batzel LW. The MMPI as a Diagnostic Tool in Non-Epileptic Seizures. In AJ Rowan, JR Gates (eds), Non-Epileptic Seizures. Boston: Butterworth–Heinemann, 1993;211–219.

50. Wilkus RJ, Dodrill BV, Thompson PM. Intensive EEG monitoring and psychological studies of patients with pseudoepileptic seizures. Epilepsia 1984;25:100–107.

51. Vanderzant CW, Giordani B, Berent S, et al. Personality of patients with pseudoseizures. Neurology 1986; 36:664–668.

52. Henrichs TF, Tucker DM, Farha J, et al. MMPI indices in the identification of patients evidencing pseudoseizures. Epilepsia 1988;29:184–187.

53. Roy A. Hysterical seizures previously diagnosed as epilepsy. Psychol Med 1977;7:271–273.

54. Roy A. Hysterical seizures. Arch Neurol 1979;36:447.

55. Ford CV, Folks DG. Conversion disorders: an overview. Psychosomatics 1985;6:371–383.

56. Mai FM, Merskey H. Briquet's treatise on hysteria: a synopsis and commentary. Arch Gen Psychiatry 1980;37:1404–1405.

57. Gumnit RJ. Inpatient Multidisciplinary Management of Non-Epileptic Seizures. In AJ Rowan, JR Gates (eds), Non-Epileptic Seizures. Boston: Butterworth–Heinemann, 1993;269–274.

58. Rosenbaum DH, Snyder S, Rowan AJ, et al. Outpatient Management of Non-Epileptic Seizures. In AJ Rowan, JR Gates (eds), Non-Epileptic Seizures. Boston: Butterworth–Heinemann, 1993;279–283.

59. Ramani V, Gumnit RJ. Management of hysterical seizures in epileptic patients. Arch Neurol 1982;39:78–81.

60. Williams DT, Gold AP, Shrout P, et al. The impact of psychiatric intervention on patients with uncontrolled seizures. J Nerv Ment Dis 1979;167:626–631.

61. French JA, Rosenbaum DH, Rowan AJ. Outcome in 55 patients with documented psychogenic seizures: clinical and EEG correlates. Epilepsia 1988;29:653.

62. Lesser RP, Lueders H, Dinner DS. Evidence for epilepsy is rare in patients with psychogenic seizures. Neurology 1983;33:502–504.

Chapter 16

Attention-Deficit Hyperactivity Disorder

Glenn S. Hirsch and Harold S. Koplewicz

Attention-deficit hyperactivity disorder (ADHD) is one of the most common of all the childhood psychiatric disorders. It is also one of the most studied of all the psychiatric disorders. In mental health clinics, ADHD often represents approximately 50% of all referrals and 10% of the behavioral problems noted in general pediatric settings. In this chapter, we review the history, diagnosis, and treatment of ADHD, with special emphasis on developmentally disabled populations.

History

ADHD has a rich and long history. One of the earliest descriptions of a child with hyperactivity is in a German book of nursery rhymes first published in the mid-1800s by the physician Heinrich Hoffman, who divided his time between private practice and responsibilities in a local psychiatric hospital. The story of "fidgety Phil" came with graphic pictures of a youngster who created havoc at the dinner table. It included the following lines: "But fidgety Phil, he won't sit still; he wriggles and giggles, and then, I declare, swings backwards and forwards and tilts up his chair."[1]

In 1902, the British pediatrician, Sir George Still, gave a series of three lectures describing 20 children who were often aggressive, defiant, and resistant to discipline and who exhibited impaired attention and overactivity.[2] He described these children as having a "defect of moral control" and noted a male-female ratio of nearly 3 to 1. In the United States, interest in this disorder can be traced to the pandemic encephali-

tis in 1917. Numerous observers reported on a "post-encephalitis behavior disorder" that included "hyperkinesis" and "organic driveness." This resulted in comparisons to other brain injuries and their behavioral manifestations. Strauss[3] found that symptoms of disinhibition, hyperactivity, and distractibility differentiated brain-injured mentally retarded children from those who were not brain-injured. These comparisons led to the concept of *minimal brain damage* and, eventually in the early 1960s, to *minimal brain dysfunction* (MBD). Over time, the label *MBD* was increasingly criticized for its overinclusiveness and the increasing understanding that hyperactivity can be present in the absence of organicity. The term *MBD* eventually was dropped, giving rise to the term *hyperactive child syndrome*. In 1968, compilers of the *Diagnostic and Statistical Manual of Mental Disorders, second edition (DSM-II)*,[4] changed the term to *hyperkinetic reaction of childhood*. Research in the 1970s that examined the role of attention and impulsivity in the disorder eventually gave rise to the position taken by *DSM-III*[5] that one could have attention-deficit disorder with or without hyperactivity. *DSM-III* created three symptom lists for each of the major areas: inattention, hyperactivity, and impulsivity. A revision of the *DSM-III*[6] combined all the symptoms into a single list. Finally, in 1994, *DSM-IV*[7] was published and provides the criteria that are in current use.

Symptoms

DSM-IV modified the triad of symptoms present in *DSM-III*. Instead of three groupings—attention,

Table 16-1. Diagnostic Criteria for Attention-Deficit Hyperactivity Disorder

A. Either (1) or (2)

  (1) Six (or more) of the following symptoms of *inattention* have persisted for at least 6 months to a degree that is maladaptive and inconsistent with developmental level:

    Inattention

      (a) Often fails to give close attention to details or makes careless mistakes in schoolwork, work, or other activities

      (b) Often has difficulty sustaining attention in tasks or play activities

      (c) Often does not seem to listen when spoken to directly

      (d) Often does not follow through on instructions and fails to finish schoolwork, chores, or duties in the workplace (not due to oppositional behavior or failure to understand instructions)

      (e) Often has difficulty organizing tasks and activities

      (f) Often avoids, dislikes, or is reluctant to engage in tasks that require sustained mental effort (such as schoolwork or homework)

      (g) Often loses things necessary for tasks or activities (e.g., toys, school assignments, pencils, books, or tools)

      (h) Is often easily distracted by extraneous stimuli

      (i) Is often forgetful in daily activities

  (2) Six (or more) of the following symptoms of *hyperactivity-impulsivity* have persisted for at least 6 months to a degree that is maladaptive and inconsistent with developmental level:

    Hyperactivity

      (a) Often fidgets with hands or feet or squirms in seat

      (b) Often leaves seat in classroom or in other situations in which remaining seated is expected

      (c) Often runs about or climbs excessively in situations in which it is inappropriate (in adolescents or adults, may be limited to subjective feelings of restlessness)

      (d) Often has difficulty playing or engaging in leisure activities quietly

      (e) Is often "on the go" or often acts as if "driven by a motor"

      (f) Often talks excessively

    Impulsivity

      (g) Often blurts out answers before questions have been completed

      (h) Often has difficulty awaiting turn

      (i) Often interrupts or intrudes on others (e.g., butts into conversations or games)

B. Some hyperactive-impulsive or inattentive symptoms that caused impairment were present before age 7 years.

C. Some impairment from the symptoms is present in two or more settings (e.g., at school [or work] and at home).

D. There must be clear evidence of clinically significant impairment in social, academic, or occupational functioning.

E. The symptoms do not occur exclusively during the course of a pervasive developmental disorder, schizophrenia, or other psychotic disorder and are not better accounted for by another mental disorder (e.g., mood disorder, anxiety disorder, dissociative disorder, or a personality disorder).

Code based on type*:

314.1   *Attention-deficit hyperactivity disorder, combined type*: if both criteria A1 and A2 are met for the last 6 months

314.00   *Attention-deficit hyperactivity disorder, predominantly inattentive type*: if criterion A1 is met but criterion A2 is not met for the last 6 months

314.01   *Attention-deficit hyperactivity disorder, predominantly hyperactive-impulsive type*: if criterion A2 is met but criterion A1 is not met for the last 6 months

*Note: For individuals (especially adolescents and adults) who currently have symptoms that no longer meet full criteria, *in partial remission* should be specified.

Source: American Psychiatric Association. Diagnostic and Statistical Manual of Mental Disorders (4th ed). Washington, DC: American Psychiatric Association, 1994:83–85.

hyperactivity, and impulsivity—the symptoms of ADHD are divided into two core symptoms—inattention and impulsivity-hyperactivity (Table 16-1).[7] This revision reflects the growing understanding that hyperactivity and impulsivity probably have the same underlying biological substrate.

Nine symptoms compose each dimension. The hyperactivity-impulsivity dimension consists of six symptoms that reflect hyperactivity and three symptoms that reflect impulsivity. One of the key modifiers in each symptom description is the word *often*, which emphasizes that these are not rare or occasional symptoms but are persistent, more severe than in other children at a comparable stage of development, and result in significant functional impairment.

Meeting the criteria for ADHD requires that some impairing symptoms be present before the age of 7 years, in at least two settings, and for at least 6 months. These constraints reflect the fact that ADHD is a chronic disorder and that different environmental settings may reduce or exacerbate symptoms.

DSM-IV lists four subtypes of ADHD. For a diagnosis of the combined type of ADHD, at least six symptoms from the dimensions of both inattention and hyperactivity-impulsivity must be present. The predominantly inattentive type is characterized by the presence of six or more symptoms from the inattention category and fewer than six symptoms from the hyperactivity-impulsivity list. The predominantly hyperactive-impulsive type is defined as the presence of at least six symptoms from the hyperactivity-impulsivity dimension but fewer than six from the inattention symptoms. For patients who met full criteria for the disorder at some point but who no longer do so, the modifier *in partial remission* should be appended to the diagnosis. For patients with prominent symptoms who do not meet the criteria for the full syndrome, the diagnosis *ADHD not otherwise specified* can be used.

The core symptoms may manifest themselves differently at different stages of development. Preschoolers tend to show more hyperactive symptoms, and it is during the school years that attentional issues usually are first recognized. In the preschool years, motor restlessness, destructive play, fearlessness, temper tantrums, sleep difficulties, and noncompliance may be the predominant symptoms. Because many of these behaviors can be seen in healthy preschoolers, accurately making a diagnosis of ADHD can be difficult. For this reason, it has been suggested that symptoms be noted for at least 12 months before the diagnosis is confirmed. The *DSM-IV* field trials targeted children ages 5–12 years, and the criteria are clearest for this age group.[8] In the school-age child, difficulties with peer relationships often are present. In adolescence, high-risk behaviors, disorganization, and a feeling of inner restlessness (as opposed to hyperactivity) are prominent. The greater demands of a departmentalized school system with multiple teachers and the requirement to change classrooms throughout the day can result in increasing academic difficulties and school failure.

The differing rates of ADHD in male versus female children raises questions of what the symptoms of ADHD look like in girls. In a study of 42 girls in whom ADHD was diagnosed and the subjects were compared with ADHD-affected boys, few differences emerged. Both groups were similar in age of onset, comorbidity, parent diagnosis and response to stimulants. There was some suggestion that the female cohort had more severe symptoms, but this may have been a result of referral bias.[9]

Barkley and Biederman[10] presented some cogent arguments for doing away with the age-of-onset criteria and reviewed several studies, pointing out problems with retrospective recall and demonstrating that a subgroup of patients have ADHD onset in adolescence. Clinical lore and the *DSM-II* reported that children outgrow the symptoms of ADHD sometime during early adolescence, but we now know that up to 65% of children with ADHD have symptoms through adulthood.

Assessment

Diagnostic Interview

The diagnosis of ADHD is made clinically. A careful diagnostic interview begins with the gathering from caregivers of a comprehensive picture of the child's developmental status and symptoms. Information about the child's functioning in different settings and contexts is essential; the interviewer must understand where and under what situations symptoms occur. The intensity of symptoms in each setting must be ascertained. Questions should be asked of the caregivers about the child's academic achievement, family life, peer relationships, leisure activities, independent functioning, and self-care. Family and psychosocial histories provide information about how the family has handled the child's difficulties and clarifies a family's strengths and impediments in dealing with possible treatments. A detailed medical history can help to exclude any physical causes that may account for symptoms. A physical examination should have been completed within the previous year. Routine laboratory screening, lead levels, and thyroid function tests are not indicated and should be performed only if warranted by a clinical evaluation.

In general, information is best obtained using a combination of open-ended and focused, semistructured questions. Symptoms may not be present in a structured setting, such as during an office visit, so observing the child in a classroom and on the playground can be useful.

The American Academy of Child and Adolescent Psychiatry, National Institutes of Health, and American Academy of Pediatrics have all published useful guidelines on the evaluation and diagnosis of ADHD.[11-13]

Checklists

Behavior rating scales, long used in research, are well suited both for the initial assessment and for the ongoing treatment of children with disruptive behaviors. Rating scales or checklists allow for the gathering of information from multiple informants and enable the clinician to understand the similarities and differences in a child's behavior across settings. The clinician can use such scales to compare a youngster's behavior to a set of standardized norms, to help set treatment goals, and to follow a child's progress and change in symptoms over time.

Rating scales can either be broadband, covering a wide swath of psychopathology, or be designed to gather information about one group of symptoms or disorder. The Child Behavior Checklist (CBCL)[14] is one of the most widely used general rating scales. It comes in various versions, to be completed by teachers, parents, preschoolers, and teenagers (in self-report form). The Revised Conners' Rating Scales[15] for parents and teachers is another scale that provides information in a number of symptom areas. Narrow scales used for the evaluation of disruptive behaviors include the short forms of the Conners' Scales—the Conners' ADHD/*DSM-IV* scales, global index, and ADHD index. The Swanson, Nolan, and Pelham Rating Scale (SNAP-IV) is keyed to the diagnostic criteria for ADHD and for oppositional defiant disorder (ODD), as cited in the *DSM-II*, *DSM-IIIR*, and *DSM-IV*.

These rating scales must be used appropriately. A youngster who meets certain cutoff points on any scale is not automatically considered to have the disorder in question. Likewise, a child who does not meet certain cutoff points may still have the disorder. These checklists should function in the same way that any laboratory test might be used: That is, they provide additional useful information but do not substitute for a careful diagnostic interview. In addition, discrepancies between different informants are not unexpected, and the interview process should seek to clarify those discrepancies.

Additional Assessments

A neuropsychological evaluation is a useful tool for evaluating a youngster for a learning disorder. The behavior during the prolonged test session can sometimes reveal a variety of behaviors, including distractibility and hyperactivity. However, the absence of these behaviors in this structured setting does not preclude the diagnosis. The freedom-from-distractibility factor on the Wechsler Intelligence Scale for Children III, which includes the arithmetic and digit span subscales, cannot discriminate between youngsters with and without ADHD.[16] Other neuropsychological tests, including the Stroop Color Word Test and the Wisconsin Card Sort, which measure attentional functions, also do not successfully discriminate between youngsters with and without ADHD.

Continuous performance tests typically involve a 20-minute computerized task. Subjects need either to respond quickly or to inhibit a response to particular stimuli. Variables such as errors of commission, errors of omission, and response time measure attention, vigilance, and impulsivity. Although such tests are commercially available (e.g., Test of Variables of Attention, Gordon Diagnostic System), no evidence exists to prove that any are useful in making the diagnosis of ADHD or in consistently monitoring medication effects.

Epidemiology

The prevalence among school-age samples in multiple studies suggests that 4–12% of the school-age population meets criteria for ADHD. Depending on the sampling technique, the male-female ratio ranges from 4 to 1 to 9 to 1. ADHD accounts for up to 50% of all referrals to child mental health clinics. When similar criteria are used to make the diagnosis, rates of the disorder have generally been the same in other countries, including England.[17]

Differential Diagnosis and Comorbidity

Many disorders share morbidity with ADHD or may involve symptoms of impulsivity, hyperactivity, or inattention that must be differentiated from ADHD as a primary diagnosis. Several physical illnesses and some medications can exacerbate or cause symptoms of ADHD. Among these are hearing or vision deficits, seizures, sleep disorders, and such medications as phenobarbital, the selective serotonin reuptake inhibitors (e.g., fluoxetine and theophylline).

Attention-Deficit Hyperactivity Disorder Symptoms in Medical Disorders

Mental Retardation and Developmental Disabilities

Children with mental retardation (MR) and developmental delays experience a wide range of psychopathology.[18] Problems of definition, level of retardation, measurement, and assessment make the clarification of the nature of psychopathology in this population difficult. Prevalence studies have suggested that 7–21% of children with MR have ADHD.[19] Some of the disorders with prominent ADHD symptoms and for which there is an etiology for MR include fragile X syndrome, fetal alcohol syndrome (FAS), and Williams syndrome.

Fragile X Syndrome. Fragile X syndrome is the most common inherited cause of MR. It is the result of an excessive repetition of the nucleotide sequence CGG on the X chromosome. Children with fragile X syndrome range from those mildly affected without MR to those with severe MR and autistic features. The degree of involvement depends on the amount of fragile X mental retardation 1 (FMR1) protein that is produced. Fully affected male individuals produce no FMR1 protein. Most male patients with fragile X syndrome have distinctive physical features, including a long face, prominent ears, and macro-orchidism, which often begins to develop at age 8. Boys and men

with fragile X syndrome have a spectrum of difficulties with social relatedness. Poor eye contact, perseveration, and sensory sensitivity are prominent symptoms. Hyperactivity and attentional problems occur in most individuals with the fragile X syndrome.[20]

Fetal Alcohol Syndrome. FAS is a common cause of MR. First noted in the early 1970s, children with FAS have a characteristic facial appearance, including an elongated midface, thin upper lip, flattened maxilla, and microcephaly.[21] In addition, they often have growth retardation. Children with FAS are prone to a variety of developmental delays, along with symptoms of ADHD, and memory and abstraction difficulties.[22,23]

Williams Syndrome. Williams syndrome is caused by a microdeletion on chromosome 7 that includes the elastin locus. The syndrome is characterized by congenital facial and cardiovascular abnormalities and MR. Children with Williams syndrome often are socially disinhibited and are seen as outgoing and friendly. Inattention, impulsivity, and hyperactivity are commonly associated features. Unlike typical youngsters with ADHD, however, these children have a marked degree of persistent fears, phobias, and anticipatory anxiety.[24]

Generalized Resistance to Thyroid Hormone

A rare, autosomal dominant, genetic disorder, generalized resistance to thyroid hormone is characterized by reduced responsiveness of pituitary and peripheral tissues to the action of thyroid hormone. Children with this disorder have a variety of cognitive difficulties. They appear clinically euthyroid or mildly hypothyroid. Laboratory measures indicate elevated triiodothyronine and thyroxine levels without thyroid-stimulating hormone suppression. In a recent study, 70% of affected children were found to have ADHD.[25] Because generalized resistance to thyroid hormone is extremely rare, thyroid testing of children with ADHD is not recommended as part of a routine evaluation.[26,27]

Lyme Disease

Lyme disease is caused by a spirochete transmitted to humans by the deer tick. Common first signs include a distinctive rash followed by flulike symptoms. Fallon et al.[28] reported a case of Lyme disease in a 7-year-old girl who first presented with complaints of problems focusing in school. She met criteria for ADHD–inattentive type but demonstrated additional symptoms of lethargy, irritability, forgetfulness, and headaches, along with poor coordination, joint pain, word-finding difficulties, and light and sound sensitivity. Symptoms resolved with antibiotic treatment.

Closed-Head Injuries

Brown et al.[29] studied 31 children with severe closed-head injuries (CHI) over the course of 2.25 years. A new psychiatric disorder developed in fewer than half the subjects. Five of the subjects developed symptoms resembling a "frontal lobe syndrome," including excessive talking, carelessness, and impulsiveness. Psychiatric sequelae were limited to the group of patients whose injury resulted in a post-traumatic amnesia of at least 7 days. Brown et al.[29] found that psychosocial adversity was a good predictor of psychiatric disorder. Max et al.[30] studied 42 patients with CHI. New psychiatric disorders developed in 36% of their subjects over the course of 2 years, and six of these subjects met criteria for ADHD.

Gerring et al.,[31] using structured interviews, examined 99 children and adolescents who had experienced moderate to severe CHI. Nineteen of the subjects met criteria for ADHD prior to injury, suggesting that children with ADHD are disproportionately represented in the CHI population. At re-evaluation 1 year after the injury, an additional 15 children who did not have a premorbid diagnosis met criteria for ADHD. The number of new cases is higher than in the general population. Consistent with the findings of Brown et al.,[29] Gerring et al.[31] found that subjects who developed secondary ADHD had a higher level of psychosocial adversity than those subjects who did not.

Psychiatric Comorbidity

Nearly 70% of children with ADHD have at least one other comorbid psychiatric condition. These comorbid conditions can affect treatment decisions and prognosis and pose special challenges to the psychopharmacologist treating these patients. In addition, some of these disorders have symptoms that overlap those of ADHD, which may make diagnosis difficult.

Disruptive Behavior Disorders

ODD, conduct disorder (CD), and ADHD are part of the spectrum of disorders that *DSM-IV* designates as *disruptive behavior disorders*. Up to 50% of youngsters with ADHD also meet criteria for ODD, and between 30% and 50% meet criteria for CD.

Children with ODD have a pattern of negativistic, defiant, disobedient, and hostile behavior toward authority figures.[7] They often actively resist and refuse to comply with requests by parents and teachers. This contrasts with children with ADHD, who may not comply because of impulsive or distractible symptoms.

Youngsters with CD often violate the basic rights of others or of societal norms, displaying such behaviors as aggressiveness, destruction of property, deceitfulness or theft, and serious violation of rules (e.g., running away, school truancy). Although CD and ADHD are independent disorders, in clinic settings one rarely sees a youngster with CD who does not have a history of ADHD. Hinshaw et al.,[32] in a review of the literature, concluded that youngsters with combined CD and ADHD have more severe and persistent difficulties. In a study of 84 children recruited for a study of CD, Klein et al.[33] found that 69% also met criteria for ADHD. Several studies found that the risk of substance abuse disorders in patients with ADHD is increased only if comorbid CD is present.[34,35]

Learning Disorders

Learning disorders or *learning disabilities* (LDs) are defined by achievement that is substantially below a youngster's intelligence quotient (IQ). A *substantial difference* has been defined in *DSM-IV* as two standard deviations between IQ and achievement. Prevalence rates are affected by the degree of discrepancy used to define the disorder. Conservative estimates suggest that between 20% and 30% of children with ADHD have a comorbid LD. One study examining the overlap between ADHD and LDs found that 50% of children with ADHD also had an LD, with the overwhelming majority having a specific reading disability.[36]

Anxiety Disorders

The childhood anxiety disorders include several subtypes. Children with separation anxiety disorder have excessive concerns about separating from a close attachment figure from home. They may have morbid concerns about something bad happening to a parent or about being kidnapped. These symptoms can cause the youngster to avoid leaving the home, to refuse to go to school, and to experience nightmares and problems getting to sleep.

Youngsters with generalized anxiety disorder have excessive worries about a wide range of events, including school and competence. Social phobia may cause a child to avoid any situation in which he or she feels that others may judge him or her. Finally, obsessive-compulsive disorder may result in a wide variety of ritualistic behaviors or uncomfortable, involuntary thoughts that impair one's ability to function.

Because some anxiety symptoms such as restlessness, difficulties with concentration, and irritability can also occur in ADHD, any youngster presenting with ADHD symptoms should be evaluated for anxiety disorders. The comorbidity between ADHD and the anxiety disorders combined is approximately 25%.

Mood Disorders

Major depressive disorder is characterized by a persistently depressed mood or loss of pleasure and interest. In children, the mood can often be irritable. Other symptoms of depression include appetite or sleep disturbances, psychomotor retardation or agitation, decreased concentration, fatigue, feelings of worthlessness, and suicidal thoughts.

Adult patients in the manic phase of a bipolar disorder often exhibit a euphoric, expansive, or irritable mood. In its severest form, grandiose or paranoid delusions may be present. In many children, an explosive, irritable mood may be the most prominent symptom. Associated symptoms include grandiosity, decreased need for sleep, increased talkativeness, racing thoughts, distractibility, psychomotor agitation, and excessive pleasure-seeking activities. The relationship and comorbidity between ADHD and bipolar disorder in children currently is one of the most debated diagnostic areas in child and adolescent psychiatry.[37,38] One

controversial issue is symptom overlap, which may confuse the diagnosis. In addition, it has been suggested that the manic disorder in children often does not have the cyclical quality that is seen in classic bipolar disorder and that children are more irritable than euphoric. Biederman et al.[39] found that in a sample of 6- to 17-year-old children with ADHD, 11% also met criteria for the diagnosis of bipolar disorder, a finding that is higher than that in most other samples.

Gilles de la Tourette's Syndrome

The prevalence of tics in ADHD is unclear. Some studies fail to distinguish between youngsters with and without preexisting tics, other studies differ on how tics are rated, and some evidence exists of a genetic link between Gilles de la Tourette's syndrome and ADHD in a subset of youngsters.[40,41] As many as two-thirds of children with a diagnosis of Gilles de la Tourette's syndrome also have symptoms of ADHD and obsessive-compulsive disorder.[42]

Pervasive Developmental Disorders

Children with pervasive developmental disorders (e.g., autism, Asperger's syndrome) frequently exhibit a wide variety of difficulties, including attentional problems and impulsivity.[43] In a study evaluating the pattern of medication use in a population of higher-functioning patients with pervasive developmental disorders, Martin et al.[44] found that 20% were taking stimulants. In addition, the concern has been raised that the diagnosis of pervasive developmental disorder may be missed and ADHD may be misdiagnosed in patients with severe behavioral problems.[45]

Outcome

ADHD is classified in *DSM-IV* as being among those disorders that begin in childhood. Although *DSM-II* suggested that this disorder tends to improve in adolescence, as many as 70% of children continue to meet criteria for ADHD during adolescence. These adolescents tend to show significant behavior problems, CD symptoms, increasing difficulties with peers, and school problems (e.g., poor academic performance, school suspensions). Long-term follow-up studies of children with ADHD reveal that 50% continue to have a significant degree of psychopathology, including antisocial behaviors and drug use.[46]

Etiology

The etiology of ADHD is unknown, although the disorder probably results from the interplay of genetic and environmental factors. In the first half of the twentieth century, ADHD was considered a form of brain damage. The encephalitis epidemic beginning in 1917 produced ADHD symptoms in some children. In contrast, *DSM-II*'s use of the term *hyperkinetic reaction of childhood* suggested a psychodynamic or early environmental cause.

A number of theories related to environmental causes suggest that food additives[47] and excessive sugar[48] have a role in the genesis of ADHD, but these theories have not been supported by the majority of scientific studies. Excessive lead is toxic in high doses, and early studies suggested that high lead levels could lead to marked distractibility.[49] However, later studies found that the effects of lead were greatest in the lowest socioeconomic groups and were correlated with prenatal exposure to alcohol.[50] Prenatal exposure to alcohol also is highly correlated with ADHD symptoms.[51] Several studies examining the effect of other prenatal or perinatal events on the risk of developing ADHD found minimal evidence that these factors are contributing.[52]

A variety of family and social environmental factors have been implicated as risk factors for developing or modifying the course of childhood psychiatric disorders, including marital distress and family dysfunction. However, no clear-cut evidence links these factors specifically to ADHD.[53]

Genetic factors, too, have been implicated as a cause of ADHD. Goodman and Stevenson[54,55] examined 570 twin pairs and, based on questionnaire data, found that concordance with ADHD was 51% in monozygotic twins and 33% in dizygotic twins. In a study of twins using *DSM* criteria, structured interviews, and parent and teacher ratings, similar conclusions were reached.[56] Adoption studies in conjunction with twin studies suggest that the heritability of ADHD is between 0.60 and 0.80. Increasing evidence implicates polymorphisms of the dopamine receptor genes DRD2 and DRD4 and the dopamine transporter gene DAT1 in the genesis of ADHD.[57]

A variety of neuroimaging studies have investigated the pathophysiology of ADHD. Many of these have been structural computed tomography or magnetic resonance imaging studies. These studies have implicated abnormalities in the right frontal cortex and smaller subcortical structures.[58] Functional brain imaging studies, including positron emission tomography and regional cerebral blood flow studies, generally also implicate the frontosubcortical system. The positive response of the core symptoms of ADHD to medications suggests a biochemical basis for the disease. The effectiveness of a variety of different compounds in reducing symptoms suggests an etiology in more than one neurotransmitter system. Changes in the dopaminergic and noradrenergic systems are necessary for clinical efficacy of medications in this disorder.

Treatment

Environmental Interventions

Family- and Child-Centered Interventions

Environmental interventions include psychoeducation, parent training, organizational management, psychotherapy, and classroom-based behavior modification and social skills training. Many of these psychosocial interventions can help to alleviate some of the secondary symptoms and sequelae of the core ADHD symptoms, including ODD, poor peer relationships, and school failure; however, they have no established efficacy in managing the core symptoms of ADHD.[59]

Psychoeducational interventions involve the parents, school personnel, and other significant adults in the child's world. The psychoeducational process includes providing an understanding of the illness, its effects in different settings, and its course, prognosis, and treatment strategies. It involves ongoing support of the family and advocacy with schools, camps, and other organizations.[60] Parent training uses a behavioral approach to help parents deal with oppositional symptoms and other problematic behaviors. Parents are taught principles of positive reinforcement, the appropriate use of consequences, and how and when to use "time out." Such training often involves teachers in establishing a daily report card that provides feedback to parents on the child's performance at school. This daily report provides additional information to parents so that they can provide appropriate rewards and consequences. This behavioral work can be done with parents individually or in multiparent groups. In addition to psychoeducation and parent training, parent support groups can provide helpful resources, a sense of empowerment, and mutual support.

One of the more debilitating aspects of ADHD is its effect on a youngster's social life. Children with ADHD often are stigmatized and teased by peers. Attempts at using interpersonal problem-solving skills therapy, cognitive training, or social skills therapy have had minimal impact on social behavior.[61]

School-Based Interventions

Children with ADHD often require accommodations in the classroom to optimize their learning environment and potential. Two pieces of federal legislation can help parents and professionals to advocate better for the special needs of these children. The Individuals with Disabilities Education Act (IDEA) Amendments of 1997 (Public Law 105-17), constitute the fifth set of amendments to the Education for All Handicapped Children Act (Public Law 94-142). The IDEA has several principles: free appropriate public education, appropriate evaluation, individualized education programming, least restrictive environment, parent and student participation in decision making, and procedural safeguards. Many children with ADHD qualify for special education services under the "other health impairment" category within the IDEA.

Section 504 of the Rehabilitation Act of 1973 prohibits discrimination on the basis of handicap by recipients of federal funds. This civil rights law has the potential to be more liberal in obtaining services for children within the regular classroom. Taken together, section 504 and IDEA are powerful weapons for parents and professionals working with children with ADHD, to maximize the possibility of academic success for these youngsters.

Multimodal Interventions

It has been suggested that children with ADHD generally require multimodal treatment, combining environmental interventions and medication. The expectation is that a carefully tailored approach that deals with the core symptoms and with a youngster's secondary and comorbid symptoms would provide increased benefits. Satterfield et al.[62] treated 117 youngsters with hyperactivity who were assigned to a multimodal treatment study that individualized treatment for each subject. Youngsters were assigned a combination of therapeutic interventions, including methylphenidate (MPH), individual therapy, family therapy, educational remediation, and group therapies. Children receiving the combined treatments showed major improvements in the form of increased academic performance and decreased antisocial behaviors. Limitations of this and other multimodal studies led to the National Institute of Mental Health Collaborative Multisite Multimodal Treatment Study of Children with ADHD (MTA),[63] which included six geographic sites. In the MTA, 576 children, ages 7–9 years, were randomly assigned to one of four treatment groups: a medication-only group; a behavioral treatment group that included parent training, child-focused treatment, school-based interventions, and an 8-week all-day summer program; a combined group that received both treatments; and a group treated in the community but assessed periodically by the research staff. This study demonstrated the clear-cut superiority of medication over behavior therapy. Behavior therapy applied in conjunction with medication did not augment the robust effects of medication alone on the core symptoms of ADHD. Nonetheless, behavioral treatments may provide some improvements for non-ADHD and anxiety symptoms.

The medication-only group was also superior to the community treatment group in the MTA. This superiority appeared to be related to three factors. First, the patients in the study were getting MPH three times daily and were receiving a higher total daily dose than were subjects in the community. In the community, patients were often getting medication only twice daily. Second, the frequency of evaluative visits for the community treatment group was much less than that for the other subjects, who were seen monthly. Finally, a teacher contact was made before each evaluative visit of subjects in the medication-only group.[64,65]

Medications

A large number of studies, including the MTA, have documented the powerful and clear-cut effi-

Table 16-2. Stimulants

Generic Name	Brand Name	Dose (mg/pill)	Maximum Approved FDA Dosage	Duration of Behavioral Effects (hrs)
Methylphenidate	Ritalin	5, 10, 20	60	2–4
Methylphenidate SR	Ritalin SR, Metadate ER	10, 20	60	
ER methylphenidate	Concerta	18, 36	54	10–12
	Metadate CD	20	60	8–10
Dextroamphetamine	Dexedrine, DextroStat	5, 10	45	4–5
Dextroamphetamine SR	Dexedrine Spansules	5, 10, 15	45	
Amphetamine salts	Adderall	5, 10, 20, 30	45	5–7
Cylert	Pemoline	18.75, 37.50, 75.00	112.5	7–9

ER = extended release; FDA = U.S. Food and Drug Administration; SR = sustained release.

cacy of medications, especially the stimulants, on the core symptoms of ADHD. These medications also improve oppositional behaviors; increase appropriate interactions with family members, peers, and teachers; and improve participation in extracurricular and leisure activities. Because ADHD is a disorder that affects most children throughout their waking hours, medications should not be limited to school hours only.

Before a child is placed on a medication regimen, his or her baseline target symptoms should be established, and these symptoms should be monitored throughout the course of treatment. One of the checklists used during the evaluation process should be used to monitor efficacy of treatment at home and at school. As ADHD medications still are associated with some stigma and are relatively short-acting, compliance can be a major problem. Even a few missed doses in a week can cause a teacher to report no changes or worsening behavior during a medication trial. A critical component of any psychoeducational session is to underscore the importance of medication regimen compliance and to find mechanisms for enhancing and monitoring compliance.

Stimulants

The use of stimulants has a long history, starting with Charles Bradley,[66] who reported on the successful use of benzedrine—a racemic mixture of d- and l-isomers of amphetamine—in 30 school-

age children with behavioral problems. His keen clinical observations on the first use of a stimulant in children remain relevant today. Most children with ADHD have a robust response to the stimulants, and most clinicians agree that one of the stimulants should be the first pharmacologic treatment of choice. Currently available stimulants and their U.S. Food and Drug Administration–approved dose ranges are summarized in Table 16-2.

The therapeutic effects of the stimulants are related to their ability to enhance catecholaminergic transmission.[67] All stimulants are rapidly absorbed and metabolized and demonstrate low plasma protein binding. The immediate-release preparations generally begin to act 30 minutes after ingestion, and their effects last 3–5 hours. Although the sustained-release preparations of dextroamphetamine (Dexedrine [DEX]), MPH, and pemoline are longer-acting, they rarely cover a child for the entire school day. The traditional sustained-release version of MPH is erratically absorbed and performs poorly. Pharmaceutical companies are working to develop longer-acting stimulants, including a d-isomer of and a patch delivery system for MPH.

Adderall consists of equal portions of four salts: dl-amphetamine sulfate, dl-amphetamine aspartate, dextroamphetamine sulfate, and dextroamphetamine saccharate. Several studies have shown that Adderall is as effective as MPH, that the duration of action is longer than immediate-release MPH, and that the duration of action increases as the dose increases.

Pemoline is used infrequently, in part because it was less extensively studied but also because it appeared to take 3–4 weeks to become effective and periodic liver function testing was required. More recent studies indicate that pemoline is as effective as MPH and has the advantage of a longer half-life. In addition, its titration can be accomplished much more quickly than can that for MPH, resulting in clinical efficacy within a short period.[68] However, liver toxicity, liver failure, and deaths were associated with pemoline treatment,[69] resulting in newly revised guidelines for its use by the manufacturer. These guidelines include obtaining serum alanine aminotransferase levels every 2 weeks during pemoline therapy and obtaining written consent for use of this agent.

The newest additions to the stimulants are Concerta and Metadate CD, which are MPHs in unique, controlled-release delivery system. These systems appear to give a steady release of MPH throughout the day, resulting in up to 12 hours of efficacy.

The choice of stimulant is dictated by such issues as duration of action and slight differences in adverse effects. All the stimulants have similar effects on target symptoms. One study testing the efficacy of MPH and DEX in boys found that 75% of subjects improved on one of the stimulants. However, a majority of the nonresponders to one stimulant responded to the other. As a result, 96% of the subjects showed improvement.[70]

Successful treatment improves the core symptoms of ADHD. In addition, improvements in fine motor control, decreased aggression, improvements in social relationships, reductions in oppositional and rule-breaking behaviors, and improved accuracy in schoolwork are seen. In patients with comorbid CD, treatment with MPH resulted in marked reduction not only in aggressive symptoms but also in covert symptoms such as cheating and stealing. No evidence exists for the development of tolerance with these medications. The effective use of stimulant medication is not specific to ADHD but can extend to other disorders of attention and behavior.

The stimulants have often been titrated on the basis of a youngster's body mass. Rapport and Denney,[71] in their study of 76 children treated with MPH under double-blind crossover conditions,

found no evidence that body mass predicted the appropriate medication dose or distinguished between responders and nonresponders. It appears that this practice should be abandoned. For most children, U.S. Food and Drug Administration guidelines for maximum daily dose of a particular stimulant can be followed. A subgroup of children require higher dosages or more frequent doses to bring symptoms under effective control.

All stimulants have similar side effects. They tend to be mild and short-lived. They occasionally cause decreased appetite, mild stomachache, headaches, and initial insomnia in susceptible individuals. Patients on high dosages have rarely exhibited perseverative behaviors or hallucinatory phenomena. Generally, no additional sleep delays are seen with an afternoon dose of MPH.[72] Many side effects are time-limited and can often be reduced or eliminated by manipulating the timing, dose, form, or kind of stimulant.

Several side effects, including growth suppression and tics, have historically been more worrisome. The effects of stimulants on the rate of growth and final height have been controversial. Studies examining this issue have found that, in cases in which growth suppression did occur, generally modest deficits of 1–3 cm over a several-year period were identified. Approximately one-third of the studies found no evidence of growth suppression. Follow-up studies of adults treated for ADHD in childhood found no difference in the height of these adults as compared to controls.[73] A study by Spencer et al.[74] of 124 subjects with ADHD found that, whether or not the subjects were treated with stimulants, their rate of growth during childhood was slower than that of non-ADHD children, and their rate of growth normalized by late adolescence.

Whether the development or exacerbation of tics is related to MPH and other stimulants is a long-standing and controversial issue. A concern persists that stimulants can precipitate tics in individuals without tics,[75] worsen tics in individuals with preexisting tics, and precipitate the full picture of Gilles de la Tourette's syndrome in susceptible individuals.[76–78] Recently, however, several studies suggested that stimulants can be a useful and powerful treatment in patients with ADHD and comorbid Gilles de la Tourette's syndrome.[79–81]

Gadow et al.[81] studied boys with ADHD and moderately severe tics who were taking MPH and found no worsening of tics at doses of 0.1–0.5 mg/kg twice daily. Castellanos et al.[82] examined 20 children with ADHD and Gilles de la Tourette's syndrome in a 9-week, placebo-controlled, double-blind crossover trial involving MPH and DEX. Doses ranged from 15 to 45 mg twice daily for MPH (means of 0.43–1.20 mg/kg per dose) and from 7.5 to 22.5 mg twice daily for DEX (means of 0.20–0.64 mg/kg per dose). At the lowest doses, no significant effects on tic severity were observed, whereas with increasing doses, tic exacerbation became evident. In most patients on MPH, these exacerbations were only temporary. However, for most of the patients on DEX, tic severity did not decrease while subjects remained on the medication. During follow-up, clear-cut advantages for MPH over DEX remained. Two-thirds of the patients remained on stimulant medication at the 4-year follow-up, whereas a subgroup was unable to tolerate such treatment. Interestingly, transient obsessive-compulsive symptoms were noted in five subjects on MPH and in one subject on DEX. In a long-term follow-up by Gadow et al.,[83] subjects demonstrated high acceptance for continued use of MPH.

Law and Schacher[84] studied 91 children with ADHD who had received no previous medical treatment. The children, who had a mean age of 8 years, participated in a 1-year, randomized, placebo-controlled trial of MPH titrated to an effective dose. Thirty percent of the subjects had preexisting tics. The mean MPH dose was 0.5 mg/kg twice daily. Over the course of the study, 60% of the placebo-treated subjects were switched to active medication because of lack of improvement of their ADHD. The results indicated that, regardless of whether they were on active medication or placebo, approximately 19% of children without preexisting tics developed tics. Sixty-seven percent of children with preexisting tics experienced no change in or improvement of their tics. The majority of those whose preexisting tics worsened were managed with a reduction in dose. The current data indicate that for patients with Gilles de la Tourette's syndrome or tic disorder and ADHD, MPH is an appropriate medication.

Stimulants and Preschoolers. The use of stimulant medication for preschool children has been controversial for several reasons. First, making the diagnosis of ADHD in this age group is difficult. Second, the public has concerns about administering medication to very young children[85]; in fact, the early literature suggested that the medication was either unhelpful or caused unacceptable side effects. Musten et al.[86] studied 31 children, ages 4–6 years, in whom ADHD had been diagnosed and found that preschoolers' symptoms responded to both 0.3 mg/kg and 0.5 mg/kg in a fashion similar to both that in school-age children and that side effects were relatively mild.[87]

Stimulants and Seizures. The *Physicians' Desk Reference* entry for Ritalin states: "There is some clinical evidence that [MPH] Ritalin may lower the convulsive threshold in patients with prior history of seizures, with prior [electroencephalographic] EEG abnormalities in absence of seizures and, very rarely, in absence of history of seizures and no prior EEG evidence of seizures."[88] This caution appears to be largely unsubstantiated.

Gross-Tsur et al.[89] studied 30 children with epilepsy and ADHD who were on antiepileptic medications. All children were monitored for a 2-month period and then given a morning dose of MPH of 0.3 mg/kg for 2 months. All children who were seizure-free on antiepileptics alone remained seizure-free. Of the five subjects whose seizure activity was incompletely controlled by the antiepileptics, three showed an increase in seizures, one showed no change, and one was seizure-free. These investigators also found no significant changes in antiepileptic levels or electroencephalographic findings. On parent reports, 70% of all the subjects showed a positive response to MPH.

Feldman et al.,[90] in a double-blind crossover study, evaluated 10 children having a variety of seizure disorders. All were on antiepileptic drugs and seizure-free. The addition of MPH twice daily (0.3 mg/kg per dose) in a double-blind, placebo-controlled manner did not result in significant changes in electroencephalographic findings. None of the children had seizures while on MPH, and 70% of youngsters while on MPH showed improvement of their ADHD symptoms.

A single case report describes two children who developed dyskinesia and bruxism when MPH was added to a maintenance dose of valproic acid.[91]

Stimulants in Mental Retardation and Pervasive Developmental Disorders. Several studies have evaluated the use of stimulants in school-age children who have MR.[92,93] Generally, these studies reported some improvement in core symptoms, but most subjects continued to have a significant level of symptoms and a greater level of adverse effects than subjects without MR.

Studies of stimulant use in preschoolers with MR have tended to be complicated because of the difficulty in determining the appropriateness of these youngsters' behavior as it relates to their mental age. Small studies and case reports have generally revealed improvement of some symptoms, but almost half the subjects experience significant side effects. Handen et al.[94] treated 11 preschool-age children who were mentally retarded. The study was a double-blind crossover design using placebo and two doses of MPH (0.3 mg/kg and 0.6 mg/kg). The study found that 73% of subjects responded positively. Although the positive response was greater at the 0.6-mg dose, adverse events also increased with the higher dose. Adverse events were reported in 45% of the sample. The most commonly reported side effect was social withdrawal.

A double-blind study of patients with fragile X syndrome found that subjects improved while on stimulants.[95] Birmaher et al.[96] found significant improvement of all ADHD symptoms with use of MPH in a group of autistic children. Given their ease of use, stimulants should be the first line of treatment for ADHD symptoms in these children.

Nonstimulant Medications

Alternatives to stimulants may be used when stimulants cause unacceptable side effects or provide an incomplete response or when comorbid disorders are present. These medications include alpha-adrenergic agonists, tricyclic antidepressants (TCAs), and the antidepressant bupropion. The U.S. Food and Drug Administration has not approved these medications for use in ADHD, so their use in that setting is considered "off-label."

Alpha$_2$-Adrenergic Agonists. Clonidine, an alpha$_2$-adrenergic agonist, has been used in the treatment of ADHD,[97] Gilles de la Tourette's syndrome,[98] and sleep disturbances secondary to the use of stimulants in children with ADHD.[99] Connor et al.[100] reviewed 39 studies of the use of clonidine in ADHD. Eleven studies included sufficient information to permit a meta-analysis, with eight having some form of methodological control. Connor's group[100] concluded that clonidine can be a useful second-line medication in ADHD. Recently, four fatalities were reported in youngsters taking a combination of MPH and clonidine.[101,102] However, the data are incomplete and unclear. In a recent review, Wilens et al.[103] point out that although the combination of MPH and clonidine has not been evaluated in double-blind trials, the effectiveness of this combination in clinical work and the complicating issues in the deaths reported make this a reasonable treatment option in appropriate children.

Guanfacine, another alpha$_2$-adrenergic agonist with less sedative effects than clonidine, has also been used in the treatment of ADHD and Gilles de la Tourette's syndrome. Unlike clonidine, guanfacine may also improve attention in ADHD.[104]

Tricyclic Antidepressants. All TCAs inhibit reuptake of norepinephrine and, to some degree, serotonin. They are the second most frequently studied medication for treating ADHD. The most common medicines in this class used for ADHD include imipramine, desipramine, amitriptyline, and nortriptyline. Several studies have found that TCAs are effective in ADHD.[105] Their main disadvantage is the potential for serious cardiac side effects that require careful monitoring. Seven deaths have been reported in youngsters taking desipramine, which may be more cardiotoxic than other TCAs. Although these medications can be given once daily, twice-daily dosing is appropriate to reduce adverse effects. As with the stimulants, no relationship exists between effective dose and body weight. Maximum dose should be no higher than 5 mg/kg, except in the case of nortriptyline, the maximum dose of which should be 2.5 mg/kg. Cardiac and blood level monitoring should accompany dose changes. Although immediate effectiveness may be obvious, most studies suggest a 2-week period before one should expect to see changes. The TCAs are more effective for the impulsive-hyperactive symptoms than for inattention. The most common side effects include fatigue and dry mouth.

Other Antidepressants.   Bupropion is a novel antidepressant that possesses both dopaminergic and noradrenergic effects. Although bupropion appears to have some positive effects on the symptoms of ADHD, the magnitude of the effect is much less than that of the stimulants.[106] This agent's main adverse effects are dermatologic reactions and the potential to lower seizure threshold. Dosing usually is up to 6 mg/kg per day in divided doses.

Venlafaxine is an antidepressant with noradrenergic and serotoninergic properties. Open-label trials in children and adults with ADHD suggest some efficacy in reducing symptoms but with a fair degree of adverse effects, including worsening of hyperactivity.[107]

The monoamine oxidase inhibitors have been used with some efficacy in adults and children with ADHD.[108] However, use of these agents is severely limited in this population whose impulsivity may preclude following a rigid diet.

Combining Medications

For several reasons, more than one medication may have to be used to treat ADHD patients. Among these reasons are partial response to one medication, the need to improve early-morning and late-evening behaviors, and the need to address comorbid conditions. For example, children with comorbid anxiety or depression may require the addition of a selective serotonin reuptake inhibitor. A youngster who exhibits aggressive symptoms along with ADHD or who has early-morning symptoms may benefit from the combination of a stimulant and an alpha$_2$-adrenergic agonist. When a patient is being treated with more than one medication, only one medication at a time should be manipulated before changing to or adding another medication. With combined pharmacotherapy, the possibility of increased side effects always must be considered.

Conclusion

ADHD is a diagnosis that has historically generated controversy but, in recent years, has gained increasing acceptance. For some children, the diagnosis is clear and the treatment approach straightforward. However, for many children, the diagnosis is complicated by comorbid medical and psychiatric disorders and developmental disabilities. For these youngsters, treatment is often complex and challenging. The field of pediatric psychopharmacology is gaining new scientific knowledge at an exponential rate and is increasingly studying subjects with comorbid conditions.

References

1. Hoffman H. Struwwelpeter: in English Translation. New York: Dover, 1995;20–23.
2. Still GF. The Goulstonian lectures on some abnormal psychical conditions in children. Lancet 1902;1:1008–1012, 1077–1082, 1163–1168.
3. Strauss AA, Lehitinen V. Psychopathology and Education of the Brain-Injured Child, vol 1. New York: Grune & Stratton, 1947.
4. American Psychiatric Association. Diagnostic and Statistical Manual of Mental Disorders (2nd ed). Washington, DC: American Psychiatric Association, 1968.
5. American Psychiatric Association. Diagnostic and Statistical Manual of Mental Disorders (3rd ed). Washington, DC: American Psychiatric Association, 1980.
6. American Psychiatric Association. Diagnostic and Statistical Manual of Mental Disorders (3rd ed rev). Washington, DC: American Psychiatric Association, 1987.
7. American Psychiatric Association. Diagnostic and Statistical Manual of Mental Disorders (4th ed). Washington, DC: American Psychiatric Association, 1994.
8. Lahey BB, Applegate B, McBurnett K, et al. *DSM-IV* Field trials for attention deficit hyperactivity disorder in children and adolescents. Am J Psychiatry 1994;151:1673–1685.
9. Sharp WS, Walter JM, Marsh WL, et al. ADHD in girls: clinical comparability of a research sample. J Am Acad Child Adolesc Psychiatry 1999;38:40–47.
10. Barkley RA, Biederman J. Toward a broader definition of the age-of-onset criterion for attention-deficit hyperactivity disorder. J Am Acad Child Adolesc Psychiatry 1997;36:1204–1210.
11. Dulcan M. Practice parameters for the assessment and treatment of children, adolescents, and adults with attention-deficit/hyperactivity disorder. J Am Acad Child Adolesc Psychiatry 1997;36[Suppl]:85S–121S.
12. Diagnosis and treatment of attention deficit hyperactivity disorder (ADHD). NIH Consensus Statement 1998;16(2):1–37.

13. Clinical practice guideline: diagnosis and evaluation of the child with attention-deficit/hyperactivity disorder. Pediatrics 2000;105:5.

14. Achenbach TM. Integrative Guide to the 1991 CBCL, YSR and TRF Profiles. Burlington: University of Vermont, 1991.

15. Conners CK. Conners' Rating Scales–Revised. New York: Multi-Health Systems, 1997.

16. Reinecke MA, Beebe DW, Stein MA. The third factor of the WISC-III: it's (probably) not freedom from distractibility. J Am Acad Child Adolesc Psychiatry 1999;38:322–328.

17. Prendergast M, Taylor E, Rapoport JL, et al. The diagnosis of childhood hyperactivity. A U.S.–U.K. cross-national study of *DSM-III* and ICD-9. J Child Psychol Psychiatry 1988;29:289–300.

18. Bregman JD. Current developments in the understanding of mental retardation: II. Psychopathology. J Am Acad Child Adolesc Psychiatry 1991;20:861–872.

19. Dykens EM. Annotation: psychopathology in children with intellectual disability. J Child Psychol Psychiatry 2000;41:407–417.

20. Baumgardner TL, Reiss AL, Freund LS, Abrams MT. Specification of the neurobehavioral phenotype in males with fragile X syndrome. Pediatrics 1995;95:744–752.

21. Jones KL, Smith DW, Ulleland CN, et al. Pattern of malformation in offspring of chronic alcoholic mothers. Lancet 1973;1(7815):1267–1271.

22. Streissguth A. Fetal Alcohol Syndrome. Baltimore: Paul H. Brookes, 1997.

23. Autti-Ramo I. Twelve-year follow-up of children exposed to alcohol in utero. Dev Med Child Neurol 2000;42(6):406–411.

24. Dykens EM, Rosner BA. Refining behavioral phenotypes: personality-motivation in Williams and Prader-Willi syndromes. Am J Ment Retard 1999;104(2):158–169.

25. 25.Hauser P, Zametkin A, Martinez P, et al. Attention deficit-hyperactivity disorder in people with generalized resistance to thyroid hormone. N Engl J Med 1993;328:997–1001.

26. Elia J, Gulotta C, Rose SR, et al. Thyroid function and attention-deficit hyperactivity disorder. J Am Acad Child Adolesc Psychiatry 1994;33:169–172.

27. Spencer T, Biederman J, Wilens T, et al. ADHD and thyroid abnormalities: a research note. J Child Psychol Psychiatry 1995;36:879–885.

28. Fallon BA, Kochevar JM, Gaito A, Nields JA. The underdiagnosis of neuropsychiatric Lyme disease in children and adults. Psychiatr Clin North Am 1998;21:693–703.

29. Brown G, Chadwick O, Shaffer D, et al. A prospective study of children with head injuries: III. Psychiatric sequelae. Psychol Med 1981;11:63–78.

30. Max JE, Robin DA, Lindgren SD, et al. Traumatic brain injury in children and adolescents: psychiatric disorders at two years. J Am Acad Child Adolesc Psychiatry 1997;36:94–102.

31. Gerring JP, Brady KD, Chen A, et al. Premorbid prevalence of ADHD and development of secondary ADHD after closed head injury. J Am Acad Child Adolesc Psychiatry 1998;37:647–654.

32. Hinshaw S, Lahey B, Hart E. Issues of taxonomy and comorbidity in the development of conduct disorder. Dev Psychopathol 1993;5:31–49.

33. Klein RG, Abikoff H, Klass E, et al. Clinical efficacy of methylphenidate in conduct disorder with and without attention deficit hyperactivity disorder. Arch Gen Psychiatry 1997;54(12):1073–1080.

34. Biederman J, Wilens T, Mick E, et al. Is ADHD a risk factor for psychoactive substance use disorders? Findings from a four-year prospective follow-up study. J Am Acad Child Adolesc Psychiatry 1997;36:21–29.

35. Disney ER, Elkins IJ, McGue M, Iacono WG. Effects of ADHD, conduct disorder, and gender on substance use and abuse in adolescence. Am J Psychiatry 1999;156:1515–1521.

36. Dykman RA, Ackerman PT. Attention deficit disorder and specific reading disability: separate but often overlapping disorders. J Learn Disabil 1991;24:96–103.

37. Carlson GA. Juvenile mania versus ADHD. J Am Acad Child Adolesc Psychiatry 1999;38:353–354.

38. Biederman J, Klein RG, Pine DS, Klein DF. Resolved: mania is mistaken for ADHD in prepubertal children. J Am Acad Child Adolesc Psychiatry 1998;37:1091–1096.

39. Biederman J, Faraone SV, Mick E, et al. Attention deficit hyperactivity disorder and juvenile mania: an overlooked comorbidity? J Am Acad Child Adolesc Psychiatry 1996;35:997–1008.

40. Comings DE, Comings BG. Tourette's syndrome and attention deficit disorder with hyperactivity: are they genetically related? J Am Acad Child Psychiatry 1984;23:138–146.

41. Knell ER, Comings DE. Tourette's syndrome and attention-deficit hyperactivity disorder: evidence for a genetic relationship. J Clin Psychiatry 1993;54:331–337.

42. Kadesjo B, Gillberg C. Tourette's disorder: epidemiology and comorbidity in primary school children. J Am Acad Child Adolesc Psychiatry 2000;39:548–555.

43. Practice parameters for the assessment and treatment of children, adolescents, and adults with autism and other pervasive developmental disorders. J Am Acad Child Adolesc Psychiatry 1999;38[Suppl]:32S–54S.

44. Martin A, Scahull L, Klin A, Volkmar F. Higher-functioning pervasive developmental disorders: rates and patterns of psychotropic drug use. J Am Acad Child Adolesc Psychiatry 1999;38:923–931.

45. Perry R. Misdiagnosed ADD/ADHD; rediagnosed PDD. J Am Acad Child Adolesc Psychiatry 1998;37:113–114.

46. Klein R, Mannuzza S. Long-term outcome of hyperactive children: a review. J Am Acad Child Adolesc Psychiatry 1991;30:383–387.

47. Conners CK. Food Additives and Hyperactive Children. New York: Plenum, 1980.

48. Wender EH, Solanto MV. Effects of sugar on aggressive and inattentive behavior in children with attention deficit disorder with hyperactivity and normal children. Pediatrics 1991;88:960–966.

49. Needleman HL, Gunnoe C, Leviton A, et al. Deficits in psychologic and classroom performance of children with elevated dentine lead levels. N Engl J Med 1979;300:689–695.

50. Ernhart CB, Morrow-Tlucak M, Marler MR, et al. Low level lead exposure in the prenatal and early preschool periods: early preschool development. Neurotoxicol Teratol 1987;9:259–270.

51. Nanson JL, Hiscock M. Attention deficits in children exposed to alcohol parentally. Alcohol Clin Exp Res 1990;14:656–661.

52. Werner EE, Smith RS. An epidemiological perspective on some antecedents and consequences of childhood mental health problems and learning disabilities. J Am Acad Child Psychiatry 1979;18:292–306.

53. Faraone SV, Biederman J. Neurobiology of attention-deficit hyperactivity disorder. Biol Psychiatry 1988;44:951–958.

54. Goodman R, Stevenson J. A twin study of hyperactivity: II. The aetiological role of genes, family relationships and perinatal adversity. J Child Psychol Psychiatry 1989;30:691–709.

55. Goodman R, Stevenson J. A twin study of hyperactivity: I. An examination of hyperactivity scores and categories derived from Rutter teacher and parent questionnaires. J Child Psychol Psychiatry 1989;30: 671–689.

56. Sherman DK, Iacono WG, McGue MK. Attention-deficit hyperactivity disorder dimensions: a twin study of inattention and impulsivity-hyperactivity. J Am Acad Child Adolesc Psychiatry 1997;36:745–753.

57. Winsberg BG, Comings DE. Association of the dopamine transporter gene (DAT1) with poor methylphenidate response [see comments]. J Am Acad Child Adolesc Psychiatry 1999;38(12):1474–1477.

58. Castellanos FX, Giedd JN, Marsh WL, et al. Quantitative brain magnetic resonance imaging in attention-deficit hyperactivity disorder. Arch Gen Psychiatry 1996;53:607–616.

59. Richters JE, Arnold LE, Jensen PS, et al. NIMH collaborative multisite multimodal treatment study of children with ADHD: I. Background and rationale. J Am Acad Child Adolesc Psychiatry 1995;34:987–1000.

60. Weiss M. Psychoeducational intervention with the family, school, and child with attention-deficit hyperactivity disorder. Child Adolesc Psychiatr Clin North Am 1992;1(2):467–479.

61. Abikoff H. An Evaluation of Cognitive Behavior Therapy for Hyperactive Children. In BB Lahey, AE Kazdin (eds), Advances in Clinical Child Psychology, vol 10. New York: Plenum 1987;171–216.

62. Satterfield JH, Satterfield BT, Cantwell DP. Three-year multimodality treatment study of 100 hyperactive boys. J Pediatr 1981;98:650–655.

63. Arnold LE, Abikoff HB, Cantwell DP, et al. National Institute of Mental Health Collaborative Multimodal Treatment Study of Children with ADHD (the MTA): design challenges and choices. Arch Gen Psychiatry 1997;54:865–870.

64. Moderators and mediators of treatment response for children with attention-deficit/hyperactivity disorder: the Multimodal Treatment Study of Children with Attention-Deficit/Hyperactivity Disorder. Arch Gen Psychiatry 1999;56:1088–1096.

65. A 14-month randomized clinical trial of treatment strategies for attention-deficit/hyperactivity disorder. The MTA Cooperative Group, Multimodal Treatment Study of Children with ADHD. Arch Gen Psychiatry 1999;56:1073–1086.

66. Bradley C. The behavior of children receiving benzedrine. Am J Psychiatry 1937;94:577–585.

67. Solanto MV. Neuropsychopharmacologic mechanisms of stimulant drug action in attention-deficit hyperactivity disorder: a review and integration. Behav Brain Res 1998;94:127–152.

68. Pelham WE Jr, Swanson JM, Furman MB, Schwindt H. Pemoline effects on children with ADHD: a time-response by dose-response analysis on classroom measures. J Am Acad Child Adolesc Psychiatry 1995; 34(11):1504–1513.

69. Shevell M, Schreiber R. Pemoline-associated hepatic failure: a critical analysis of the literature. Pediatr Neurol 1997;16:14–16.

70. Elia J, Borcherding BG, Rapoport JL, Keysor CS. Methylphenidate and dextroamphetamine treatments of hyperactivity: are there true nonresponders? Psychiatry Res 1991;36:141–155.

71. Rapport MD, Denney C. Titrating methylphenidate in children with attention-deficit/hyperactivity disorder: is body mass predictive of clinical response? J Am Acad Child Adolesc Psychiatry 1997;36:523–530.

72. Kent JD, Blader JC, Koplewicz HS, et al. Effects of late-afternoon methylphenidate administration on behavior and sleep in attention-deficit hyperactivity disorder. Pediatrics 1995;96:320–325.

73. Gittelman R, Mannuzza S. Hyperactive boys almost grown up: III. Methylphenidate effects on ultimate height. Arch Gen Psychiatry 1988;45:1131–1134.

74. Spencer T, Biederman, J, Harding M, et al. Growth deficits in ADHD children revisited: evidence for disorder associated growth delays? J Am Acad Child Adolesc Psychiatry 1996;35:1460–1467.

75. Lowe TL, Cohen TJ, Detlor J, et al. Stimulant medications precipitate Tourette's syndrome. JAMA 1982; 247:1729–1731.

76. Denckla MB, Bemporad JR, MacKay MC. Tics following methylphenidate administration: a report of 20 cases. JAMA 1976;235:1349–1351.

77. Shapiro AK, Shapiro E. Do stimulants provoke, cause or exacerbate tics and Tourette's syndrome? Compr Psychiatry 1981;22:265–273.

78. Erenberg G, Cruse RP, Rothner AD. Gilles de la Tourette's syndrome: effects of stimulant drugs. Neurology 1985;35:1346–1348.

79. Gadow KD, Nolan E, Sprafkin J, Sverd J. School observations of children with attention-deficit hyperactivity disorder and comorbid tic disorder: effects of methylphenidate treatment. J Dev Behav Pediatr 1995;16:167–176.

80. Gadow KD, Sverd J. Stimulants for ADHD in child patients with Tourette's syndrome: the issue of relative risk. J Dev Behav Pediatr 1990;11:269–271.

81. Gadow KD, Sverd J, Sprafkin J, et al. Efficacy of methylphenidate for attention deficit hyperactivity disorder in children with tic disorder. Arch Gen Psychiatry 1995;52:444–455.

82. Castellanos FX, Giedd JN, Elia J, et al. Controlled stimulant treatment of ADHD and comorbid Tourette's syndrome: effects of stimulant and dose. J Am Acad Child Adolesc Psychiatry 1997;36:589–596.

83. Gadow KD, Sverd J, Sprafkin J, et al. Long-term methylphenidate therapy in children with comorbid attention-deficit hyperactivity disorder and chronic multiple tic disorder. Arch Gen Psychiatry 1999;56:330–336.

84. Law SF, Schachar RJ. Do typical clinical doses of methylphenidate cause tics in children treated for attention-deficit hyperactivity disorder? J Am Acad Child Adolesc Psychiatry 1999;38:944–951.

85. Zito JM, Safer DJ, dosReis S, et al. Trends in the prescribing of psychotropic medications to preschoolers. JAMA 2000;283(8):1025–1030.

86. Musten LM, Firestone P, Pisterman S, et al. Effects of methylphenidate on preschool children with ADHD: cognitive and behavioral functions. J Am Acad Child Adolesc Psychiatry 1997;36:1407–1415.

87. Firestone P, Musten LM, Pisterman S, et al. Short-term side effects of stimulant medication are increased in preschool children with attention-deficit/hyperactivity disorder: a double-blind placebo-controlled study. J Child Adolesc Psychopharmacol 1998;8:13–25.

88. Physicians' Desk Reference (53rd ed). Montvale, NJ: Medical Economics, 1999.

89. Gross-Tsur V, Manor O, van der Meere J, et al. Epilepsy and attention deficit hyperactivity disorder: is methylphenidate safe and effective? J Pediatr 1997;130:670–674.

90. Feldman H, Crumrine P, Handen BL, et al. Methylphenidate in children with seizures and attention-deficit disorder. Am J Dis Child 1989;143:1081–1086.

91. Gara L, Roberts W. Adverse response to methylphenidate in combination with valproic acid. J Child Adolesc Psychopharmacol 2000;10:39–43.

92. Handen BL, Feldman H, Gosling A, et al. Adverse side effects of methylphenidate among mentally retarded children with ADHD. J Am Acad Child Adolesc Psychiatry 1991;30:241–245.

93. Handen BL, Janosky J, McAuliffe S, et al. Prediction of response to methylphenidate among children with ADHD and mental retardation. J Am Acad Child Adolesc Psychiatry 1994;33:1185–1193.

94. Handen BL, Feldman HM, Lurier A, Murray PJ. Efficacy of methylphenidate among preschool children with developmental disabilities and ADHD. J Am Acad Child Adolesc Psychiatry 1999;38:805–812.

95. Hagerman RJ, Murphy M, Wittenberg M. A controlled trial of stimulant medication in children with fragile X syndrome. Am J Med Genet 1988;33:513–518.

96. Birmaher B, Quintana H, Greenhill LL. Methylphenidate treatment of hyperactive autistic children. J Am Acad Child Adolesc Psychiatry 1988;27:248–251.

97. Hunt RD, Minderaa RB, Cohen DJ. Clonidine benefits children with attention deficit disorder and hyperactivity: report of a double-blind placebo-crossover therapeutic trial. J Am Acad Child Adolesc Psychiatry 1985;24:617–629.

98. Leckman JF, Hardin MT, Riddle MA, et al. Clonidine treatment of Gilles de la Tourette's syndrome. Arch Gen Psychiatry 1991;48:324–328.

99. Prince JB, Wilens TE, Biederman J, et al. Clonidine for sleep disturbances associated with attention-deficit hyperactivity disorder: a systematic chart review of 62 cases. J Am Acad Child Adolesc Psychiatry 1996;35:599–605.

100. Connor DF, Fletcher KE, Swanson JM. A meta-analysis of clonidine for symptoms of attention-deficit hyperactivity disorder. J Am Acad Child Adolesc Psychiatry 1999;38:1551–1559.

101. Swanson J, Flockhart D, Udrea D, et al. Clonidine in the treatment of ADHD: questions about safety and efficacy. J Child Adolesc Psychopharmacol 1995;5:301–304.

102. Fenichel RF. Combining methylphenidate and clonidine: the role of post-marketing surveillance. J Child Adolesc Psychopharmacol 1995;5:155–156.

103. Wilens TE, Spencer TJ, Swanson JM, et al. Combining methylphenidate and clonidine: a clinically sound medication option. J Am Acad Child Adolesc Psychiatry 1999;38:614–619.

104. Hunt RD, Arnsten AF, Asbell MD. An open trial of guanfacine in the treatment of attention-deficit hyperactivity disorder. J Am Acad Child Adolesc Psychiatry 1995;3:50–54.

105. Spencer T, Biederman J, Wilens T, et al. Pharmacotherapy of attention deficit disorder across the life cycle. J Am Acad Child Adolesc Psychiatry 1996;35:409–432.

106. Conners CK, Casat CD, Gualtieri CT, et al. Bupropion hydrochloride in attention deficit disorder with hyperactivity. J Am Acad Child Adolesc Psychiatry 1996;35:1314–1321.

107. Olvera RL, Pliszka SR, Luh J, Tatum R. An open trial of venlafaxine in the treatment of attention-deficit/hyperactivity disorder in children and adolescents. J Child Adolesc Psychopharmacol 1996;6:241–250.

108. Zametkin A, Rapoport JL, Murphy DL, et al. Treatment of hyperactive children with monoamine oxidase inhibitors: I. Clinical efficacy. Arch Gen Psychiatry 1985;42:962–966.

Chapter 17

Psychotropic Drug Use in Patients with Epilepsy and Developmental Disabilities

John J. Barry and Nga Huynh

For in Diseases of the mind, as well as in all other ailments, it is an art of no little importance to administer medicines properly.

—Philippe Pinel (1745–1826), *A Treatise on Insanity*[1]

The rate of epilepsy in patients with developmental disabilities (DDs) and mental retardation (MR) appears to be related to the level of cognitive impairment.[2] Those individuals with mild impairment may have rates approximating 30%. In contrast, severely disabled and institutionalized patients have been found to have a prevalence of up to 50%.[2] The symptomatic epilepsies are over-represented in this population.

Fifty percent to 60% of individuals with DDs and MR will have at least mild psychological dysfunction, and 10–15% will have severe psychiatric disorders.[2] In comparison with the general population, this rate may be up to seven times higher.[3] As with epilepsy, the frequency of psychiatric disease is correlated with the severity of cognitive compromise.[2] The common DDs with prominent psychiatric presentations include Prader-Willi, fragile X, Down, Angelman's, and fetal alcohol syndromes and autism.[4] These disorders frequently coexist with symptoms of epilepsy.

The purpose of this chapter is to explore the most frequent psychiatric syndromes seen in patients with DDs. This discussion is followed by an examination of diagnostic issues and a general approach to using psychotropic drugs in the DD population. The major portion of this chapter specifically focuses on psychopharmacologic issues in patients with DDs comorbid with psychiatric dysfunction and epilepsy. The side effects of the psychotropic agents used in these patients is discussed in general. Because almost all these medications decrease the seizure threshold, the issue of seizure exacerbation is analyzed more specifically.

Psychiatric Disorders in Developmental Disabilities

Patients with DDs are not a uniform population. Therefore, they present with varied psychiatric signs and symptoms, probably because of unique neurotransmitter dysfunction.[2] Regardless of the neuroanatomic dysfunction involved, symptoms tend to cluster. The most frequent reason for psychiatric consultation is for the management of aggressive and impulsive symptoms. Stereotyped and self-injurious behaviors (SIBs) are also frequent,[4] in addition to affective, psychotic, attention deficit, and anxiety disorders.

Aggression and Impulse Control Dysfunction

Aggression and impulse control dysfunction can be viewed as having a cacophonous presentation, which may color intervention. Patients who display uncontrolled outbursts because of overwhelming arousal can be discriminated from patients with affective irritability often associated with ictal causes or exacerbations. Other patients may present with more goal-directed behavior and may be candidates for behavioral treatments.[4] Self-injurious and stereotypic behavior is diagnosed more easily and may be particular to the underlying organic disorder (e.g., Lesch-Nyhan syndrome). Overarousal has been associated with serotonin dysfunction along with excessive dopaminergic and opioid activity.[2,4]

Affective Disorders

Affective disorders commonly are underdiagnosed in those individuals with DDs. Prevalence rates show frequencies from three to seven times that found in the general population.[5] In the mildly impaired, the diagnosis of depression can be made with the *Diagnostic and Statistical Manual of Mental Disorders* criteria, but a reliance on exacerbations of irritability and psychomotor agitation aid in evaluating the more severely handicapped.[6] Mania also can be found and usually is exhibited by increased motor activity, decreased sleep, and aggression.[5]

Psychosis

Diagnosing psychosis often is difficult in the DD population. A thought disorder generally is not obvious because of language impairment. Likewise, evaluating the presence of delusions, hallucinations, and illusions is difficult in the setting of general perceptual compromise. However, response to hallucinations or catatonic behavior can provide some objective evidence of a psychotic process.[7] "Voices" whose content is derogatory may be suggestive of a psychotic depression, in which case treatment would focus on the mood disorder as well as on the psychosis. Lovell et al.[5] suggested using the acronym ADMITTING (*a*natomic, *d*egenerative, *m*etabolic, *i*nfectious, *t*oxic, *t*raumatic, *i*mmunologic, *n*eoplastic, *g*enetic) to evaluate the many organic causes of psychosis.[5]

Attention-Deficit Hyperactivity Disorders

Attention-deficit hyperactivity disorders (ADHD) also can be seen with the developmentally disabled. The diagnosis of the disorder is the same as in the general population. The frequency of ADHD

in individuals with MR (approximately 11%) is from two- to threefold greater than expected in a cognitively normal population.[5] Behavioral dysfunction can accrue from the disorder in much the same way as in others with ADHD, and the treatment should be directed toward behavioral and pharmacologic modalities.[5]

Anxiety Disorders

Anxiety disorders can be extremely prevalent in patients with MR and can appear as social and behavioral neediness, avoidance, and separation agitation. As with the aforementioned disorders, the lack of verbal abilities may render a reliance on behavioral features a necessity for correct diagnosis.[5]

Diagnostic Issues

The diagnosis of the aforementioned disorders in an individual with DDs can be an extremely difficult challenge. Adherence to the following principles can simplify the diagnostic process.

Before the implementation of pharmacologic interventions, a thorough investigation of the affected patients' overall psychosocial milieu should be assessed carefully. DD patients are extremely sensitive to their surroundings and have a limited behavioral repertoire of response. Thus, they may verbalize their distress somatically.[2] Even minor changes or fluctuations of a valued routine can present with problematic behavior. In addition, assessment also must involve the patients' family and any group or agency involved.

Regardless of these facts, however, psychiatric disorders seen in the general population are seen also in patients with DDs. However, the level of disability often will determine the manifestation of these disorders. Several factors that have been described influence the evaluation of psychiatric symptoms.[5] These factors include "intellectual distortion" limiting verbalization, poor social skills, and cognitive deterioration exacerbating preexisting deficits.[5] Because much of a psychiatric evaluation is predicated on verbal reports of internal states, an evaluator may be extremely hampered and in unfamiliar territory. As a result, a process of "diagnostic overshadowing" may take place. Individuals with a DD and a coexistent mental disorder may be less likely to be labeled with a psychiatric diagnosis, even though they display the same manifestations as does an individual without a cognitive impairment.[3] In general, evaluators need to rely more on ancillary and collateral information about affected patients and to pay more attention to neurovegetative signs of mental illness.[5]

Approach to Patients with Comorbid Epilepsy

There are special considerations in pharmacologic intervention for patients with developmental disorders, mental illness, and epilepsy. Before administration of a psychotropic drug is undertaken, several caveats idiosyncratic to an epileptic patient must be considered. First, the epileptic seizure itself can present with psychiatric manifestations. Separation of the seizure into intervals—2–3 days before the event (prodrome), the peri-ictal period (aura, ictus, and postictal interval), and the time between events (interictal interval)—allows ascribing of psychiatric manifestations to the epileptic event itself. Treatment of psychiatric manifestations attributable to the prodromal and peri-ictal periods should be directed toward maximizing antiepileptic medication intervention. The following examples illustrate this important point.

Affective Symptoms

Both manic and, more commonly, depressive symptoms can be seen related to an epileptic event itself. This phenomenon was noted first in the 1800s by Burrows and later by Falret.[8] Depressive symptoms were noted by Blanchet and Frommer,[9] who observed mood changes before a seizure that took up to 3 days postictally to resolve. Williams[10] found fear and, rarely, depression during the ictus and also noted peri-ictal elation. Although rare, peri-ictal manic symptoms have been reported as well.[11–14]

Psychotic Symptoms

Ictal psychosis can result from simple partial or complex partial status, with consciousness main-

tained in the former and impaired in the latter. In nonconvulsive status, the symptoms of psychosis appear in the context of a delirium.[15]

Postictal psychosis can develop 12–72 hours after seizure activity, often occurring in conjunction with a flurry of complex partial seizures. Predisposing factors are unclear but may include bitemporal epileptic activity, structural lesions, and the like.[15] Treatment of emergent symptoms includes neuroleptics, often given parenterally. The author (J. J. B.) frequently uses intravenous haloperidol (Haldol) because of its ease of administration and, although the evidence is sparse, fewer extrapyramidal side effects than are associated with the oral preparation.[16] (Effects on seizure induction are discussed in the section Antipsychotics.) A gradual dosage reduction then ensues, usually over the next several weeks, as tolerated by the patient. In approximately 15%, interictal psychotic symptoms may occur after an episode of postictal psychosis. A subsequent shift to a more atypical neuroleptic can then be made.[15] (These issues also are covered later.)

Aggressive Symptoms

Aggression also may be a manifestation of seizure activity. Aggression associated with epilepsy can be discriminated from a nonictally related event by its directionality.[17] Planned and focused aggression is not of ictal origin. Postictal delirium that is being forcibly contained might be a situation in which aggression ensues. In epilepsy, interictal aggression may be associated with a low intelligence quotient, early onset of seizures, and a dominant-hemisphere electroencephalographic focus.[17]

After determination that psychiatric manifestations are not part of, or related to, an ictal event itself, other possible risk factors should be evaluated prior to the institution of a psychotropic drug. These factors include the phenomenon of "forced normalization" reviewed by Trimble et al.[18] Folic acid deficiency has been associated with the use of antiepileptic drugs (AEDs), possibly catalyzing depressive features.[19–22] Also, side effects of AEDs themselves include hypomania,[23] depression,[24–27] and behavioral disturbances with the use of gabapentin and lamotrigine in the developmentally disabled (discussed in Chapter 18). AED polypharmacy also has been associated with psychiatric symptoms.[28] (Contributing psychosocial factors were discussed previously in this chapter.)

After a thorough assessment of these factors, if a salient psychiatric symptom persists or the instigating AED cannot be changed, psychotropic initiation should ensue. Although side effects of each class of psychotropic medication exist, the major cause for their underuse is a fear of seizure exacerbation. Nearly all the medications used for the aforementioned psychiatric conditions decrease the seizure threshold.

Therapeutic Options

Antidepressants

Antidepressants have been the mainstay of treatment of patients presenting with the symptoms of a major depressive disorder (MDD) or major dysthymic disorder. The features of an MDD include persistent depressed mood (>2 weeks) with anhedonia, weight loss or gain, sleep dysfunction, agitation or psychomotor retardation, guilt, concentration difficulty, and recurrent thoughts of death or suicide. Five or more such symptoms must be present at any one time for this diagnosis to be made.[29] Dysthymic disorder is a low-grade chronic depression with many of the same features of an MDD but without the severity. Many practitioners who deal frequently with epileptic patients have emphasized the pleomorphic quality of the patients' depressive symptoms. Blumer[30] coined the term *interictal dysphoric disorder* to describe patients with these symptoms, emphasizing especially their irritability, mood variability, and anxiety. Regardless of the criteria used, issues of efficacy, seizure induction, and potential drug interactions remain of paramount importance.

Behavioral dyscontrol also can be a significant problem in patients with DDs and comorbid epilepsy. In particular, overarousal and dysfunctioning of the serotonin system have been implicated as frequent primary factors. Beta-blockers may be useful for modulating overstimulation (see the section Beta-Blockers). Aggression may be another area in which antidepressants may be useful.[31]

Antidepressants constitute a wide variety of medications. The "classic" agents were discovered in the 1950s and include tricyclic antidepressants (TCAs) and monoamine oxidase inhibitors (MAOIs). The TCAs used most frequently include amitriptyline, nortriptyline, imipramine, desipramine, doxepin, and clomipramine. In addition, this class includes two tetracyclic antidepressants: amoxapine and maprotiline. The MAOIs include phenelzine, selegiline, tranylcypromine, and isocarboxazid.[32]

In 1988, the introduction of the selective serotonin reuptake inhibitors (SSRIs) provided a new class of antidepressants with a unique and advantageous side effect profile. Among the SSRIs are fluoxetine, paroxetine, sertraline, citalopram, and fluvoxamine. In addition, the combined serotonin-norepinephrine reuptake inhibitor (SNRI) venlafaxine and the noradrenergic-dopaminergic compound bupropion also have been added to the armamentarium. The 5-hydroxytryptamine-2 antagonists nefazodone and trazodone and the new noradrenergic antidepressant mirtazapine also are available.[32]

The efficacy of antidepressants to treat depression in patients with epilepsy has scant substantiation in the literature. However, the data that do exist appear very encouraging. Anecdotal studies by Blumer[30] corroborate the utility of antidepressants in low dosages, an observation that has mirrored the author's experience as well (J. J. B.). Blumer frequently used the TCA imipramine in dosages up to 150 mg per day and, for more refractory cases, added SSRIs.[30] (Concerns about this combination are discussed later in this section.)

Ojemann et al.[33,34] performed two retrospective studies on the use of psychotropics in patients with epilepsy. The first focused on epilepsy patients with depressive symptoms treated with the TCA doxepin. Depressive symptoms decreased by 89%, and seizure frequency improved in 79%, with the suggestion of a link between both effects.[33] In the second review, a wide variety of psychiatric syndromes and psychotropic drugs were evaluated but with a similar finding (i.e., 86% improvement and 58% decrease in seizure frequency).[34]

Robertson and Trimble[35] conducted a double-blind, placebo-controlled study using amitriptyline and nomifensine. All patients improved somewhat. In the second part of the study, in which all nonresponders were enrolled without a control group and in which antidepressant dosages were increased, a 65% response rate resulted.[35]

Favale et al.[36] used fluoxetine (20 mg per day) to treat 17 epileptic patients with symptoms of depression. Of significant interest was the complete remission of seizure activity in six patients, with the remaining patients having a 30% reduction in seizure frequency.[36] In addition, no increase in carbamazepine levels occurred during the study.

A wide variety of side effects are associated with the use of antidepressants, depending on the specific group of medications employed. MAOIs have the most serious restrictions, including dietary and drug interactions, along with hypotension, weight gain, and the like. The TCAs as a group and the tertiary amines in particular (amitriptyline-imipramine) cause tachycardia, hypotension, dry mouth, and constipation and have a rather low therapeutic index. SSRIs and SNRIs have a more benign side effect profile, occasionally causing headache, gastrointestinal effects, akathisia, agitation, hypomania and, possibly, sexual dysfunction, but they are considerably safer in the event of overdosage.[32]

The single most disconcerting factor in the use of antidepressants in patients with concomitant epilepsy is their potential to exacerbate seizure control. All these medications decrease the seizure threshold to varying degrees. Evaluating the extent of this problem is difficult and extremely complex, given the many methodologies used to determine the frequency of seizure induction.

One method often used includes recording the incidence of seizures seen in patients after overdose. Extrapolation to the risk in patients whose levels are in the therapeutic range is suspect at best. Other methods involve the use of animal models and may not allow generalization to humans. For example, a drug such as maprotiline in animal studies was thought to be relatively safe but, when marketed, was found to be one of the more epileptogenic antidepressant compounds.[17]

Finally, the base rate of the natural occurrence of a seizure in the general population must be factored into the discussion. From a population-based study in Rochester, Minnesota, the overall incidence of a first seizure was calculated to be approximately 0.086%.[37] Any drug considered to be a severe risk for seizure induction would, therefore, have to demonstrate a rate higher than that anticipated to occur spontaneously.

Other risk factors are listed in Table 17-1.[17,37] Inclusion of patients exhibiting these factors has confounded the data in assessing the seizure

Table 17-1. Predisposing Risk Factors for Seizure Induction

Previous history of a seizure
Central nervous system trauma
Neoplasia
Cerebrovascular disease
Mental retardation
Dementia
Drug abuse
Withdrawal states
Psychiatric illness (e.g., bulimia, obsessive-compulsive disorder)

Source: DL Rosenstein, JC Nelson, JC Jacobs. Seizures associated with antidepressants: a review. J Clin Psychiatry 1993;54: 216, 289–299; and H McConnell, D Duncan. Treatment of Psychiatric Comorbidity in Epilepsy. In H McConnell, PJ Snyder (eds). Psychiatric Comorbidity in Epilepsy: Basic Mechanisms, Diagnosis, and Treatment. Washington, DC: American Psychiatric Press, 1998.

induction potential of these antidepressants. The process of choosing an antidepressant for a patient with concomitant epilepsy must take into consideration three major factors. The first is the age of the patient. The phenomenology of depression in children and adolescents is thought to be similar to that found in adults. However, children appear to respond differently to antidepressants.[38,39] TCAs in general have not been shown to ameliorate depressive symptoms in double-blind studies of children, and sudden unexplained death has been reported with the use of desipramine in this patient population.[40] Thus, the use of TCAs in children and adolescents is of concern. The SSRIs are showing more promise with efficacy and safety. To date, however, only two of the SSRIs—fluvoxamine and sertraline—have been approved by the U.S. Food and Drug Administration for use in children, and both for symptoms of obsessive-compulsive disorder. In double-blind studies, the data on safety and utility of fluoxetine and paroxetine were positive for symptoms of MDD in children, data that may result in eventual U.S. Food and Drug Administration approval.[38–40]

The second factor concerns the seizure induction potential of antidepressants, and the third, possible drug-drug interactions. Table 17-2 summarizes the clinical reports regarding these

Table 17-2. Antidepressants: Seizure Incidence and Drug Interactions[41–64]

	Seizure Incidence (%)
TCAs[a] and tetracyclic antidepressants	
Amitriptyline	<0.1–0.3
Amoxapine	24.5–36.4
Clomipramine	0.7–3.0
Desipramine	<0.1
Doxepin	<0.1
Imipramine	<0.1–0.9
Maprotiline	0.4–15.6
Nortriptyline	<0.1
Protriptyline	<0.1
SSRI and SNRI	
Citalopram	<0.1
Fluoxetine[b]	<0.1–0.2
Fluvoxamine[b]	<0.2
Paroxetine[b]	<0.1
Sertraline[b]	<0.1
Venlafaxine	<0.26
Other antidepressants	
Bupropion	0.6–1.0
>450 mg/day	0.6–2.19
SR 400 mg/day	0.4
SR 300 mg/day	0.1
Mirtazapine	<0.1
Nefazodone	NA
Trazodone	<0.1

NA = limited information; SNRI = serotonin-norepinephrine reuptake inhibitor; SR = sustained-release formula; SSRI = selective serotonin reuptake inhibitor; TCAs = tricyclic antidepressants.
[a]General reduction of TCA levels with induction of antiepileptic drugs (i.e., carbamazepine, phenytoin, phenobarbital, and primidone). Valproic acid inhibits TCA metabolism and, therefore, may increase TCA serum levels.
[b]Case reports provide evidence of interactions between carbamazepine and phenytoin that have resulted in an increase in serum antiepileptic drug levels.
Source: Adapted from JJ Barry, A Lembke, N Huynh. Affective Disorders in Epilepsy. In AB Ettinger, AM Kanner (eds), Psychiatric Issues in Epilepsy: A Practical Guide to Diagnosis and Treatment (in press). Philadelphia: Lippincott Williams & Wilkins, 2001;45–71.

issues.[12,41–59] Relative rates of seizures in patients administered antidepressants and most frequently drug interactions with AEDs are displayed.

The TCAs have an overall seizure induction potential of 0.1–4.0%.[37] The primary factor involved appears to be serum levels. In the experience of Preskorn and Fast[60] and in their review of the literature, they noted that only those TCA levels exceeding the therapeutic range were associated with seizure induction.

Also important is that TCAs are metabolized via the 2D6 cytochrome and that some patients may have congenital deficiencies of this enzyme.[32] Therefore, even though a patient is taking an adequate dose of a TCA, elevated serum levels may result. In addition, drugs that inhibit the 2D6 cytochrome (e.g., paroxetine and fluoxetine) will cause TCA serum level increases.[32] Thus, serum levels must be followed carefully. The rapidity of dosage escalation is another factor; gradual increase in antidepressant dosages in epileptic patients is recommended.[37]

Amitriptyline and imipramine have a seizure induction potential (approximately 0.1–0.6%) that is documented to be higher than that of their respective metabolites nortriptyline and desipramine (approximately 0.1%). However, in overdose, the incidence of seizures with desipramine and nortriptyline increases to 17.9% and 22.0%, respectively.[17,52] Experience with doxepin was discussed earlier in conjunction with Ojemann's study.[33]

The TCA clomipramine and the tetracyclic antidepressants amoxapine and maprotiline have an unacceptable rate of seizure induction (see Table 17-2). They are, therefore, considered contraindicated in patients with epilepsy.

The SSRIs (fluoxetine, paroxetine, sertraline, fluvoxamine, citalopram) and the SNRI venlafaxine constitute the drugs of choice for patients with comorbid depression and epilepsy. They have an overall seizure induction potential of between 0.10% and 0.26%,[17,37,49] except in overdosage, in which case the rate can be higher.[61,62] SSRIs appear to be relatively safe, especially considering the aforementioned rate of spontaneous seizure occurrence (0.086%). Fluoxetine, however, may cause more seizure induction than do other SSRIs.

Of the other antidepressants available, bupropion remains the most controversial for use in patients with epilepsy. As noted, drug dosage remains one of the most critical issues in determining seizure induction. Bupropion provides an excellent example of this fact. In dosages exceeding 450 mg per day, the rate was 0.60–2.19%.[50] This is reduced to 0.4% with the sustained-release preparation at 400 mg per day and can be decreased even further to 0.1% when 300 mg per day of the sustained-release preparation is used. Given these facts and the variety of antidepressants from which to choose in patients with epilepsy, other alternatives are recommended.

The remaining antidepressants available probably are safe for use in comorbid epilepsy patients and include trazodone and nefazodone. Few data are available regarding seizure induction by mirtazapine and reboxetine, in contrast to the MAOIs, which also appear relatively safe.[17] Phenytoin and carbamazepine may hypothetically lower mirtazapine levels. Cases of agranulocytosis or neutropenia have been associated with mirtazapine.[17] Combining it with another bone marrow–suppressing drug, such as carbamazepine, should be avoided until more data are available.[17]

Other concerns regarding the use of antidepressants in patients with epilepsy focus on potential drug interactions with AEDs. Both classes of drugs undergo hepatic metabolism. Biotransformation at the hepatic microsomal cytochrome P450 oxidases appears to be the process most responsible for drug-drug interactions. Antidepressants and AEDs share several common cytochrome P450 enzymes (3A4, 1A2, 2C19, 2C9, and, possibly, 2B6)[12,63–68] and also influence the 2D6 cytochrome. Drugs can influence these enzymes by inducing or inhibiting them. The serum levels of medications that act as a substrate for the cytochrome may be decreased if an inducing agent is added, whereas an inhibitory compound has the opposite effect.[59]

The AEDs most commonly responsible for interactions with antidepressants are the cytochrome-inducing drugs carbamazepine, phenytoin, and phenobarbital[12,69–79] and the inhibitory agent valproic acid. Table 17-3 further clarifies these relationships. Clinically significant elevations of these AEDs have been observed when used in combination with fluoxetine, although available data are conflicting.[36] Other SSRIs have been implicated as well, but less frequently and with less clinical relevance. For this reason, fluoxetine usage in combination with the aforementioned AEDs should be avoided or, at the least, requires serum monitoring.

Finally, the SSRIs—in particular fluoxetine, paroxetine and, to a lesser extent, scrtraline—interact with TCAs, increasing their levels by as much as threefold.[80] Caution and careful moni-

Table 17-3. Antipsychotics and Seizure Induction

Antipsychotic	Incidence of Seizures (%)	Sources
Chlorpromazine		
<900 mg/day	0.3–5.0	94,98,99
>1 g/day	10	94
Clozapine		
All doses	1–10	90,91,93–97
<300 mg/day	1–2	89,92,95
300–600 mg/day	0.8–4.0	89,92,95
>600 mg/day	2.1–14.0	89,92,95
Fluphenazine	<1.0–1.2	92,94,97
Haloperidol	No reports of incidence	
Mesoridazine	<1.0–1.2	92,94,97
Loxapine	19	99
Molindone	No reports of incidence	
Olanzapine[a]	0.88	92
Perphenazine	<1.0–1.2	92,94,97
Pimozide	No reports of incidence	
Prochlorperazine	<1.0–1.2	92,94,97
Quetiapine[b]	<1	
Risperidone[c]	0.3	88
Thioridazine	<1.0–1.2	92,94,97
Thiothixene	No reports of incidence	
Trifluoperazine	<1.0–1.2	92,94,97
Triflupromazine	<1.0–1.2	92,94,97

[a]Product information. Olanzapine (Zyprexa). Eli Lilly Company, Indianapolis, IN, 1997.
[b]Product information. Quetiapine (Seroquel). Zeneca Pharmaceuticals, Wilmington, DE, 1997.
[c]Product information. Risperidone (Risperdal). Jansen Pharmaceutica, Inc., Titusville, NJ, 1997.

toring of drug levels are recommended with these combinations.

The serotonin syndrome, a rare disorder consisting of symptoms of restlessness, myoclonus, hyperthermia, convulsions, and possible death, may result from drug interactions.[81,82] It is caused by excessive serotoninergic stimulation. Most reports have documented the interaction between SSRIs and an MAOI, but similar results have been documented with TCAs, in particular imipramine and clomipramine. Treatment is symptomatic and, with the offending agent removed, syndrome resolution usually takes place in 24 hours.[83] Notably, some of the AEDs have serotonin effects and theoretically can cause this syndrome, as has been reported with carbamazepine.[84]

Antipsychotics

Neuroleptics have two common uses in patients with DDs and epilepsy. They are the primary pharmacologic intervention for patients with a psychotic disorder resulting from a primary psychiatric or an organic etiology. They also are used frequently to ameliorate both acute and chronic aggression and SIB.

The antipsychotic drugs can be divided into typical and atypical categories, depending on their affinity for blocking the dopamine D2 receptor site. The typical neuroleptics function almost exclusively at this site. In contrast, the atypical antipsychotics additionally block other dopamine subtypes and serotonin receptors. The significantly decreased rate of extrapyramidal (EPR) side effects and tardive dyskinesia (TD) associated with the atypical agents probably stems from these unique factors.[85]

The typical neuroleptics include the phenothiazines (chlorpromazine, fluphenazine, trifluoperazine, perphenazine, thioridazine), the butyrophenones (haloperidol), thioxanthenes (thiothixene), dihydroindolones (molindone), and dibenzoxazepines (loxapine). These drugs were discovered in the 1950s and revolutionized the treatment of schizophrenia. They were found to be especially useful for the positive symptoms of the disease (e.g., hallucinations, delusions). However, negative symptoms (e.g., withdrawal, flattened affect) remained less effected. In addition, side effects of these medications have limited their utility.[32]

EPRs are the most common side effects of typical antipsychotic drugs. The most frequent EPR is akathisia, described as a feeling of anxiety that can result in pacing, aggression, and suicide. It is seen in 25–75% of patients treated with these drugs.[85] Dystonia is seen—especially in young male patients—in up to 21%. Drug-induced parkinsonism can occur in approximately 30% of patients treated chronically with these drugs. EPRs are treated with anticholinergic drugs, propranolol, or amantadine. Prolactin elevation, weight gain, and cardiovascular effects also may be seen.[86]

The most disturbing associated complications of traditional antipsychotics are TD and neuroleptic malignant syndrome (NMS). The 1-year incidence of TD is 5% but steadily increases in ensuing years, with nearly 70% of patients becoming symptomatic by 25 years. Patients who are especially susceptible include those who have manifested EPR side effects, patients with an affective disorder, and the elderly. NMS has a frequency of 0.01–2.40% and manifests as muscle rigidity, autonomic instability, hyperthermia, and changing level of consciousness. It carries a mortality rate of 20–30% in patients with florid symptoms.[86]

The atypical antipsychotic agents have largely supplanted their older relatives, except in more acute circumstances in which parenteral forms are required (e.g., postictal psychosis). Clozapine was the first to be approved in 1990 and has a unique mechanism of action, with greater D1 than D2 and increased D3 and D4 antagonism. Its effects on serotonin receptors, however, has heralded other atypical agents as well. However, as is discussed later, clozapine has a dose-dependent decrease on the seizure threshold.[87] Thus, its utility in treating epilepsy patients is low.

Conversely, risperidone, olanzapine, and the newest atypical agent, quetiapine, may offer significant advantages in patients with comorbid epilepsy. Like clozapine, these drugs have potent serotoninergic activity and sparing effects on the nigrostriatal dopaminergic neurons. Thus, the incidence of EPR side effects, TD, and NMS would be expected to be substantially lower than that associated with traditional antipsychotics.[87] However, the atypical neuroleptics do have idiosyncratic side effects. Clozapine is associated with agranulocytosis, with an incidence of 1% in the first year and a maximal risk in the initial 4–18 weeks of treatment.[86] Risperidone has been associated with QT interval prolongation and olanzapine with hepatic transaminase enzyme elevations, especially in the first few weeks of treatment, which eventually may normalize.[86] Lens changes have been associated with quetiapine, requiring intermittent ocular examinations.[86] All of these antipsychotic medications decrease the seizure threshold to varying degrees. Table 17-3 illustrates available data regarding this topic.[88–99]

The possible mechanisms by which antipsychotics lower the seizure threshold include disruption of the dopaminergic-cholinergic balance and depletion of γ-aminobutyric acid. Seizure potential is dose-related; high-dose therapy and rapid upward dose titration of antipsychotics should be avoided. Prophylactic use of an anticonvulsant may be necessary. Clozapine has been associated with a dose-related and plasma drug level increase in the incidence of seizures.

As illustrated previously, several caveats apply to the use of antipsychotics in patients with comorbid epilepsy. The rate of potential seizure induction is dose-dependent and prohibitive for the antipsychotics clozapine, loxapine, and chlorpromazine. Fluphenazine, thioridazine, perphenazine, and trifluoperazine have an intermediate range of less than 1.0–1.2%. Of the typical agents, haloperidol, molindone, and pimozide have the least activity for seizure induction. The atypical agents risperidone, olanzapine, and quetiapine seem to be the antipsychotics of choice on the basis both of epileptogenesis and of the side effect profiles mentioned.

Most antipsychotics are metabolized by the 2D6 and CYP3A subfamilies of the cytochrome P450 system; thus, drug-drug interactions are a significant possibility. Fluoxetine, therefore, can increase antipsychotic serum levels, whereas such drugs as the barbiturates and carbamazepine can lower them.[85,87] For example, carbamazepine can decrease haloperidol levels by as much as 50–60% and similarly can decrease risperidone and olanzapine levels.[59] Therefore, the addition of carbamazepine to a stable antipsychotic regimen may aggravate psychosis, and the discontinuation of the drug after prolonged use may result in NMS.[59]

Aggression and SIB may be a significant problem in patients with developmental disorders. Several studies have confirmed the unique safety and effectiveness of the atypical antipsychotics for these target symptoms. Risperidone has been evaluated in a double-blind, placebo-controlled fashion in patients with pervasive developmental disorders and in adults with autism and was found to reduce repetitive behaviors, anxiety, irritability, and aggression significantly. The response rate was 60% with a mean dosage of 2.9 ± 1.4 mg per day with no evidence of EPR side effects or seizures.[100] Risperidone was found to be useful also in controlling explosive aggression in autistic patients[101] (at 0.5 mg twice daily) and in patients with behavioral disturbances associated with MR[102] (1–8 mg per day).

Likewise, olanzapine has been evaluated in a pilot study involving children, adolescents, and adults with pervasive developmental disorders. Significant decreases in aggression, irritability, SIB,

and depression were found, with a comparable increase in social relatedness.[103] Weight gain and sedation were the most significant side effects. Quetiapine also might be useful for the same target symptoms. The high 5-hydroxytryptamine-2:D2 ratio has been postulated to underlie the low frequency of EPR side effects for the atypical agents.[87]

Buspirone

Buspirone is a nonbenzodiazepine that currently is marketed as an antianxiety agent. It appears to exert partial agonist activity at the 5-hydroxytryptamine-1A receptor. Perhaps because of this activity, buspirone has been found also to exert antiaggressive activity. At low dosages, it has been found to be useful for ameliorating aggression in patients with MR and autism.[104] It does not appear to interact with anticonvulsants.[104]

Buspirone, however, has been shown in animal models to be proconvulsant.[17,105] The drug is contraindicated in Britain for use in patients with epilepsy because of these findings.[17] In addition, one case report cites a patient who sustained a seizure after an overdose of buspirone.[106] Other authors recommend this drug's use for anxiety in patients with epilepsy.[107] Therefore, careful observation is recommended for the use of buspirone in this patient population until more information is available.

Beta-Blockers

Beta-blockers, in particular nadolol and propranolol, have been used in the DD population for the treatment of aggression. Both medications decrease hyperarousal, restlessness, and tension. They also cause little cognitive compromise and, therefore, by decreasing anxiety, may help patients with MR increase their ability to integrate different elements in their environment and to shift cognitive sets. Nadolol works peripherally, whereas propranolol is more lipophilic and exerts more central nervous system effects.[32] Both medications—but especially propranolol—may require titration to obtain an effective dosage. Hypotension and bradycardia limit utility, and the agents are contraindicated in asthmatic patients and in those with Raynaud's disease.[32] Depression is a rare side effect of propranolol.[31,32] In addition, propranolol should not be combined with thioridazine, as the former may increase the serum level of thioridazine significantly.[31]

Propranolol has been noted to be associated with seizure activity in overdosage.[108] In contrast, in some animal models it appears to increase the seizure threshold.[109–111] It is metabolized via the cytochromes 1A2, 2D6, and 2C19; thus, it may interact with psychotropic agents. SSRIs may increase serum levels of beta-blockers, whereas carbamazepine may have the opposite effect.[32]

Amphetamines

Amphetamines are the mainstay of therapy for those patients displaying impulsivity, distractibility, and motor overactivity in the constellation of a diagnosis of ADHD. The prevalence rate of this disorder in patients with MR can be up to 11%, although making the diagnosis often is difficult at best. Amphetamines can exacerbate stereotypies, but they remain the drugs of choice for this disorder.[5]

Comorbid epilepsy in patients with ADHD may complicate the use of amphetamines. Methylphenidate has been evaluated in children with ADHD and epilepsy. Those patients in whom the epilepsy was well controlled had no increase in seizure activity (n = 25). However, three of the five children with continued seizure activity experienced an increase in seizure rate.[112] In contrast, in patients with a seizure disorder secondary to brain injury, reduced seizure frequencies were seen with the use of methylphenidate.[113] Amphetamines in high dosages certainly can be associated with seizure activity; therefore, low dosages are recommended, as is slow medication titration.[17]

Mood Stabilizers

Mood stabilizers include the AEDs (discussed in Chapter 18). Lithium has taken a secondary place in the treatment of bipolar affective disorder and MDD, especially in patients with epilepsy. Lithium is considered proconvulsant but has been used safely in patients with epilepsy and bipolar affective disorder.[114] It has been associated also with encephalopathy when used in combination with carbamazepine.[32] Lithium may be very useful in augmenting AED effects for these disorders but should be used with caution in the epileptic patient.

Summary

This chapter has focused on the use of psychotropic agents in patients with DDs and a comorbid psychiatric disorder and epilepsy. Diagnostic issues were reviewed in an attempt to establish a treatment focus with clear target symptoms, differentiating diagnostic issues prior to the use of psychotropic agents.

The major classes of psychotropic agents useful in this population include the antidepressants, antipsychotic drugs, and those agents useful for controlling overall aggression. Side effects of these drugs, particularly those affecting the seizure threshold, were reviewed.

It is hoped that this chapter has provided a template for the diagnosis and effective psychotropic treatment of this very specialized population. Although side effects are many, effective use of these medications can significantly ameliorate the considerable difficulties associated with psychiatric illness.

References

1. Koran LM. Medical Conditions Associated with Obsessive Compulsive Symptoms. In LM Koran, Obsessive-Compulsive and Related Disorders in Adults: A Comprehensive Clinical Guide. New York: Cambridge University Press, 1999;81.
2. Ratey JJ, Dymek MP. Neuropsychiatry of Mental Retardation and Cerebral Palsy. In BS Fogel, RB Schiffer, SM Rao (eds), Neuropsychiatry. Baltimore: Williams & Wilkins, 1996;549–571.
3. Borthwick-Duffy SA. Epidemiology and prevalence of psychopathology in people with mental retardation. J Consult Clin Psychol 1994;62(1):17–27.
4. Duffy JD. The Management of Patients with Developmental Disabilities. Advances in Neuropsychiatry course. Presented at the one hundred fifty-first annual meeting of the American Psychiatric Association. Toronto, Ontario, Canada, May 30–June 4, 1998.
5. Lovell RW, Reiss AL. Dual diagnosis: psychiatric disorders in developmental disabilities. Pediatr Clin North Am 1993;40(3):579–592.
6. Meins W. Symptoms of major depression in the mentally retarded adults. J Intellect Disabil Res 1995;39:41–45.

7. King BH, DeAntonio C, McCracken JT, et al. Psychiatric consultation in severe and profound mental retardation. Am J Psychiatry 1994;151(12):1802–1808.
8. Schmitz B, Trimble M. Epileptic equivalents in psychiatry: some nineteenth century views. Acta Neurol Scand Suppl 1992;140:122–126.
9. Blanchet P, Frommer GP. Mood change preceding epileptic seizures. J Nerv Ment Dis 1986;174:471–476.
10. Williams D. The structure of emotions reflected in epileptic experiences. Brain 1956;79:29–67.
11. Barczak P. Hypomania following complex partial seizures. Br J Psychiatry 1988;152:137–139.
12. Barry JJ, Lembke A, Huynh N. Affective Disorders in Epilepsy. In AB Ettinger, AM Kanner (eds), Psychiatric Issues in Epilepsy: A Practical Guide to Diagnosis and Treatment (in press). Philadelphia: Lippincott Williams & Wilkins, 2001;45–71.
13. Hypomania following complex partial seizures (letter). Br J Psychiatry 1988;152:571–572.
14. Byrne A. Hypomania following increased epileptic activity. Br J Psychiatry 1988;153:573–574.
15. Sachdev P. Schizophrenia-like psychosis and epilepsy: the status of the association. Am J Psychiatry 1998;155(3):325–336.
16. Menza MA, Murray GB, Holmes VF, Rafuls WA. Controlled study of extrapyramidal reactions in the management of delirious, medically ill patients: intravenous haloperidol versus intravenous haloperidol plus benzodiazepines. Heart Lung 1988;17:238–241.
17. McConnell H, Duncan D. Treatment of Psychiatric Comorbidity in Epilepsy. In H McConnell, PJ Snyder (eds), Psychiatric Comorbidity in Epilepsy: Basic Mechanisms, Diagnosis, and Treatment. Washington, DC: American Psychiatric Press, 1998;245–362.
18. Trimble MR, Ring HA, Schmitz B. Neuropsychiatric Aspects of Epilepsy. In BS Fogel, RB Schiffer, SM Rao (eds), Neuropsychiatry. Baltimore: Williams & Wilkins, 1996.
19. Reynolds EH, Chanarin I, Milner G, Matthews DM. Anticonvulsant therapy, folic acid and vitamin B_{12} metabolism and mental symptoms. Epilepsia 1966;7:261–270.
20. Trimble MR, Corbett JA, Donaldson D. Folic acid and mental symptoms in children with epilepsy. J Neurol Neurosurg Psychiatry 1980;43:1030–1034.
21. Charney MN. Psychiatric Aspects of Folate Deficiency. In MI Botez, EH Reynolds (eds), Folic Acid in Neurology, Psychiatry, and Internal Medicine. New York: Raven Press, 1979;475–482.
22. Froscher W, Maier V, Laage M, et al. Folate deficiency, anticonvulsant drugs, and psychiatric morbidity. Clin Neuropharmacol 1995;18:165–182.
23. Charney DS, Berman RM, Miller HL. Treatment of Depression. In AF Schatzberg, CB Nemeroff (eds), Textbook of Psychopharmacology (2nd ed).Washington, DC: American Psychiatric Press, 1998;705–732.
24. Robertson MM, Trimble MR, Townsend DRA. Phenomenology of depression in epilepsy. Epilepsia 1987;28:364–372.
25. Brent DA, Crumrine PK, Varma RR, et al. Phenobarbital treatment and major depressive disorder in children with epilepsy. Pediatrics 1987;80:909–917.
26. Brent DA, Crumrine PK, Varma RR, et al. Phenobarbital treatment and major depressive disorder in children with epilepsy: a naturalistic follow-up. Pediatrics 1990;85:1086–1091.
27. Trimble MR. New antiepileptic drugs and psychopathology. Neuropsychobiology 1998;38:149–151.
28. Ring HA, Trimble MR. Depression in Epilepsy. In SE Starkstein, RG Robertson (eds), Depression in Neurologic Disease. Baltimore: Johns Hopkins University Press, 1993.
29. Diagnostic and Statistical Manual of Mental Disorders (4th ed). Washington, DC: American Psychiatric Press, 1994.
30. Blumer D. Antidepressant and double antidepressant treatment for the affective disorder of epilepsy. J Clin Psychiatry 1997;58:3–11.
31. Yudofsky SC, Silver JM, Hales RE. Treatment of Agitation and Aggression. In SC Yudofsky, RE Hales (eds), The American Psychiatric Press Textbook of Neuropsychiatry. Washington, DC: American Psychiatric Press, 1997;881–900.
32. Schatzberg AF, Cole JO, DeBattista C. Manual of Clinical Psychopharmacology (3rd ed). Washington, DC: American Psychiatric Press, 1997.
33. Ojemann LM, Friel PN, Trejo WJ, et al. Effect of doxepin on seizure frequency in depressed epileptic patients. Neurology 1982;33(5):646–648.
34. Ojemann LM, Baugh-Bookman C, Dudley DL. Effect of psychotropic medications on seizure control in patients with epilepsy. Neurology 1987;37:1525–1527.
35. Robertson MM, Trimble MR. The treatment of depression in patients with epilepsy. A double-blind trial. J Affect Discord 1985;9:127–136.
36. Favale E, Rubino V, Mainardi P, et al. Anticonvulsant effect of fluoxetine in humans. Neurology 1995;45:1926–1927.
37. Rosenstein DL, Nelson JC, Jacobs SC. Seizures associated with antidepressants: a review. J Clin Psychiatry 1993;54:289–299.
38. Labellarte MJ, Walkup JT, Riddle MA. The new antidepressants: selective serotonin reuptake inhibitors. Child Adolesc Psychopharmacol 1998;45(5):1137–1155.
39. Ryan ND, Varma D. Child and adolescent mood disorders—experience with serotonin-based therapies. Biol Psychiatry 1998;44:336–340.
40. McConville BJ, Chaney RO, Browne KL, et al. Newer antidepressants: beyond selective serotonin reuptake inhibitor antidepressants. J Child Adolesc Psychopharmacol 1998;45(5):1157–1171.
41. Cohn JB, Shrivastava R, Mendels J, et al. Double-blind, multicenter comparison of sertraline and

amitriptyline in elderly depressed patients. J Clin Psychiatry 1990;51:28–33.

42. Davidson J. Seizures and bupropion: a review. J Clin Psychiatry 1989;50:256–261.

43. Horne RL, Ferguson JM, Pope HG Jr, et al. Treatment of bulimia with bupropion: a multicenter controlled trial. J Clin Psychiatry 1988;49(7):262–266.

44. Jabbari B, Bryan GE, Marsh EE, Gunderson CH. Incidence of seizures with tricyclic and tetracyclic antidepressants. Arch Neurol 1985;42:480–481.

45. Jick SS, Jick H, Knauss TA, et al. Antidepressants and convulsions. J Clin Psychopharmacol 1992;12:241–245.

46. Johnston JA, Lineberry CG, Ascher JA, et al. A 102-center prospective study in association with bupropion. J Clin Psychiatry 1991;52:450–456.

47. Leonard BE. Safety of amoxapine. Lancet 1989;2:808.

48. Milne RJ, Goa KL. Citalopram: a review of its pharmacodynamic and pharmacokinetic properties, and therapeutic potential in depressive illness. Drugs 1991;41:450–477.

49. Montgomery SA. Novel selective serotonin reuptake inhibitors (part 1). J Clin Psychiatry 1992;53:107–112.

50. Peck AW, Sterm WC, Watkinson C. Incidence of seizures during treatment of tricyclic antidepressants and bupropion. J Clin Psychiatry 1983;44:197–201.

51. Tasini M. Complex partial seizures in a patient receiving trazodone. J Clin Psychiatry 1986;47:318–319.

52. Wedin GP, Oderda GM, Klein-Schwartz W, Gormun RL. Relative toxicity of cyclic antidepressants. Ann Emerg Med 1986;15:797–804.

53. Wernicke JF. The side effect profile and safety of fluoxetine. J Clin Psychiatry 1985;46:59–67.

54. Litovitz TL, Troutman WG. Amoxapine overdose. Seizures and fatalities. JAMA 1983;250(8):1069–1071.

55. Merigan KS, Browning RG, Leeper KV. Successful treatment for amoxepine-induced refractory status epilepticus with propofol. Acad Emerg Med 1995;2(2):128–133.

56. Dunner DL, Zisok S, Billow AA, et al. A prospective safety surveillance study for bupropion sustained-release in the treatment of depression. J Clin Psychiatry 1998;59(7):366–373.

57. Phillips S, Brent J, Kulig K, et al. Fluoxetine versus tricyclic antidepressants: a prospective multicenter study of antidepressant drug overdoses. The Antidepressant Study Group. J Emerg Med 1997;15(4):439–445.

58. Feeney DJ, Klykylo M. Medication-induced seizures. J Am Acad Child Adolesc Psychiatry 1997;36(8):1018–1019.

59. Monaco F, Cicolin A. Interactions between anticonvulsant and psychoactive drugs. Epilepsia 1999;40[Suppl 10]:S71–S76.

60. Preskorn SH, Fast GA. Tricyclic antidepressant-induced seizures and plasma drug concentration. J Clin Psychiatry 1992;53:160–162.

61. Personne M, Persson H, Sjoberg G. Citalopram toxicity. Lancet 1997;350:519.

62. Setzer SC, Anderson DA, Lawler RJ, et al. Acute venlafaxine overdose—a multicenter study. J Toxicol Clin Toxicol 1995;33:496–497.

63. Harvey AT, Preskorn SH. Cytochrome P450 enzymes: interpretation of their interactions with selective serotonin reuptake inhibitors (part 1). J Clin Psychopharmacol 1996;16(4):273–285.

64. Nemeroff CB, DeVane CL, Pollock BG. New antidepressants and the cytochrome P450 system. Am J Psychiatry 1996;153(3):311–320.

65. Michalets EL. Update: clinically significant cytochrome P-450 drug interaction. Pharmacotherapy 1998;18(1):84–112.

66. Mullen WJ, North DS, Weiss MA. Pharmaceuticals and the cytochrome P450 isoenzymes: a tool for decision making. Pharm Pract News 1998;25:20–23.

67. Pham Z, Anderson PO. Cytochrome P450 in drug metabolism and interactions. Discourse 1996;18(1):1–4.

68. Riesenman C. Antidepressant drug interactions and the cytochrome P450 system: a critical appraisal. Pharmacotherapy 1995;15:84S–99S.

69. Spina E, Pisani F, Perucca E. Clinically significant pharmacokinetic drug interactions with carbamazepine: an update. Clin Pharmacokinet 1996;31(3):198–214.

70. Droulers A, Bodak N, Oudjhani M, et al. Decrease of valproic acid concentration in the blood when coprescribed with fluoxetine. J Clin Psychopharmacol 1997;17:139.

71. Fritze J, Unsorg B, Lanczik M. Interaction between carbamazepine and fluvoxamine. Acta Psychiatr Scand 1991;84:583–584.

72. Gernaat HBPE, van de Woude J, Touw DJ. Fluoxetine and parkinsonism in patients taking carbamazepine. Am J Psychiatry 1991;148:1604–1605.

73. Grimsley SR, Jann MW, Carter G, et al. Increased carbamazepine plasma concentrations after fluoxetine coadministration. Clin Pharmacol Ther 1991;50:10–15.

74. Haselberger MB, Freedman LS, Tolbert S. Elevated serum phenytoin concentrations associated with coadministration of sertraline. J Clin Psychopharmacol 1997;17:107–109.

75. Jalil P. Toxic reaction following the combined administration of fluoxetine and phenytoin: two case reports. J Neurol Neurosurg Psychiatry 1992;55:412–413.

76. Lucena MI, Blanco E, Corrales MA, et al. Interaction of fluoxetine and valproic acid. Am J Psychiatry 1998;155:575.

77. Pearson HJ. Interaction of fluoxetine with carbamazepine. J Clin Psychiatry 1990;51:126.

78. Weber SW. Drug interactions with antidepressants. CNS [Special Ed] 1999;Spring:47–55.

79. Baldessarini RJ, Teicher MH, Cassidy JW, et al. Anticonvulsant cotreatment may increase toxic metabolites of antidepressants and other psychotropic drugs. J Clin Psychopharmacol 1998;8(5):381–382.

80. Nelson JC. Augmentation strategies with serotonin-noradrenergic combinations. J Clin Psychiatry 1998;59(S5):65–69.

81. Thompson GA. Serotonin syndrome. Drug Consults 1999, vol. 99. Micromedex, Inc.

82. Steinbach H. The serotonin syndrome. Am J Psychiatry 1991;148:705–713.

83. Brown TM, Skop BP, Mareth TR. Pathophysiology and management of the serotonin syndrome. Ann Pharmacother 1996;30:527–533.

84. Dursun SM, Mathew VM, Reveley MA. Toxic serotonin syndrome after fluoxetine plus carbamazepine. Lancet 1993;342:442–443.

85. Marder S. Antipsychotic Medications. In AF Schatzberg, CB Nemeroff (eds), Textbook of Psychopharmacology (2nd ed). Washington, DC: American Psychiatric Press, 1998;309–322.

86. PCS Rx Reviews. Antipsychotics: emphasis on side effects. CNS Disorders–Schizophrenia 1998.

87. Owens MJ, Risch SC. Atypical Antipsychotics. In AF Schatzberg, CB Nemeroff (eds), Textbook of Psychopharmacology (2nd ed). Washington, DC: American Psychiatric Press, 1998;323–348.

88. Lane HY, Chang WH, Chou JC. Seizure during risperidone treatment in an elderly woman treated with concomitant medications. J Clin Psychiatry 1998;59(2):81–82.

89. Casey DE. The relationship of pharmacology to side effects. J Clin Psychiatry 1997;58[Suppl 10]:55–62.

90. Wilson WH, Claussen AM. Seizures associated with clozapine treatment in a state hospital. J Clin Psychiatry 1994;55(5):184–188.

91. Umbricht D, Kane JM. Medical complications of new antipsychotic drugs. Schizophr Bull 1996;22(3):475–483.

92. Lee JW, Crismon ML, Dorson PG. Seizure associated with olanzapine. Ann Pharmacother 1999;33:554–556.

93. Denney D, Stevens JR. Clozapine and seizures. Biol Psychiatry 1995;37:425–426.

94. Toth P, Frankenburg FR. Clozapine and seizures: a review. Can J Psychiatry 1994;39:236–238.

95. Pacia SV, Devinsky O. Clozapine-related seizures. Neurology 1994;44:2247–2249.

96. Lieberman JA, Safferman AZ. Clinical profile of clozapine: adverse reactions and agranulocytosis. Psychiatr Q 1992;63:51–70.

97. Marks RC, Luchins DJ. Antipsychotic medications and seizures. Psychiatr Med 1991;9(1):37–51.

98. Markowitz JC, Brown RP. Seizures with neuroleptics and antidepressants. Gen Hosp Psychiatry 1987;9:135–141.

99. Cold JA, Wells BG, Froemming JH. Seizure activity associated with antipsychotic therapy. DICP 1990;24:601–606.

100. McDougle J, Holmes JP, Carlton DC, et al. Double-blind, placebo-controlled study of risperidone in adults with autistic disorder and other pervasive developmental disorders. Arch Gen Psychiatry 1998;55:633–641.

101. Horrigan JP, Barnhill LJ. Risperidone and explosive aggressive autism. J Autism Dev Disord 1997;27(3):313–323.

102. Lott RS, Kerrick JM, Cohen SA. Clinical and economic aspects of risperidone treatment in adults with mental retardation and behavioral disturbance. Psychopharmacol Bull 1996;32(4):721–729.

103. Potenza MN, Holmes JP, Kanes SJ, et al. Olanzapine treatment of children, adolescents, and adults with pervasive developmental disorders: an open-label pilot study. J Clin Psychopharmacol 1999;19(1):37–44.

104. Ninan TN, Cole JO, Yonkers KA. Nonbenzodiazepine Anxiolytics. In AF Schatzberg, CB Nemeroff (eds), Textbook of Psychopharmacology (2nd ed). Washington, DC: American Psychiatric Press, 1998;287–300.

105. Peroutka SJ, Gonzales DA, Shapiro M. Modulation of postdecapitation convulsions in rats by alpha-adrenergic and 5-hydroxytryptamine 1A agents. Exp Neurol 1987;96(2):344–351.

106. Catalano G, Catalano MC, Hanley PF. Seizures associated with buspirone overdose: case report and literature review. Clin Neuropharmacol 1998;21(6):347–350.

107. Goldberg RS, Posner DA. Anxiety in the Medically Ill. In A Stoudemire, B Fogel (eds), Psychiatric Care of the Medical Patient. New York: Oxford University Press, 1993;87–104.

108. Reith DM, Dawson AH, Epid D, et al. Relative toxicity of beta blockers in overdose. J Toxicol Clin Toxicol 1996;34(3):273–278.

109. Raju SS, Gopalakrishna HN, Venkatadri N. Effect of propranolol and nifedipine on maximal electroshock-induced seizures in mice: individual and in combination. Pharmacol Res 1998;38(6):449–452.

110. Akkan AG, Yillar DO, Eskazan E, et al. The effect of propranolol on maximal electroshock seizures in mice. Int J Clin Pharmacol Ther Toxicol 1989;27(5):255–257.

111. Muller M, Schramek J. Combined application of propranolol and local anesthetics: enhanced anticonvulsant action. Biomed Biochim Acta 1989;48(4):333–336.

112. Gross-Tsur V, Manor O, van der Meere J, et al. Epilepsy and attention deficit hyperactivity disorder: is methylphenidate safe and effective? J Pediatr 1997;130:670–674.

113. Wroblewski BA, Leary JM, Phelan AM, et al. Methylphenidate and seizure frequency in brain injured patients with seizure disorders. J Clin Psychiatry 1992;53(3):86–89.

114. Shukla S, Mukherjee S, Decina P. Lithium in the treatment of bipolar disorders associated with epilepsy: an open study. J Clin Psychopharmacol 1988;8(3):201–204.

Chapter 18

Psychotropic Properties of Antiepileptic Drugs in Patients with Developmental Disabilities

Alan B. Ettinger, William B. Barr, and Sanford P. Solomon

Epilepsy is a common comorbid condition among patients with developmental disabilities (DDs),[1] estimated to occur in 30–50% of cases. Having seizures appears to raise the risk for psychiatric disturbances among DD patients, perhaps reflecting more widespread and severe underlying brain pathology and postictal and interictal psychiatric complications.[2] Therefore, in the treatment of epilepsy in DD individuals, psychiatric issues are an important consideration.

Antiepileptic Drug Administration in Developmentally Disabled Patients

In a recent review of antiepileptic drug (AED) use in epilepsy patients with mental retardation, Coulter[3] summarized the typical selection of AEDs on the basis of relative efficacy of the drug against specific seizure type. Phenytoin (PHT) and carbamazepine (CBZ) commonly are used to treat partial seizures, whereas valproic acid (VPA), gabapentin (GPN), lamotrigine (LTG), tiagabine (TGB), and topiramate (TPM) also are effective. Ethosuximide (ESM) is indicated in the treatment of absence seizures, although VPA and LTG also may be considered. Generalized myoclonic, tonic, and atonic seizures (all features of the Lennox-Gastaut syndrome commonly encountered in this population) may be treated with VPA, LTG, felbamate (FBM), or TPM.

Generalized tonic-clonic seizures can be treated with PHT, CBZ, FBM, LTG, or TPM. Use of barbiturates is discussed later.

In the selection of AED therapy, clinicians must consider drug side effects, including favorable or adverse AED psychotropic effects. Although only very few studies focus on these concerns in DD patients, lessons from our experience with AEDs in other populations can be applied in the management of epileptic DD patients.

AED effects on behavior may relate to their variable effects on different groups of cortical neurons. AEDs may alter neurotransmitter levels (e.g., norepinephrine and γ-aminobutyric acid [GABA]) or ion channel function, which in turn may have an impact on both seizures and mood.[4] For example, the mood instability of bipolar disorder has been theorized to occur on the basis of decreased GABA-ergic neurotransmission or by altered sodium channel function. Some AEDs may improve mood instability by increasing GABA and modifying sodium channels.

Ketter et al.[5] classified AEDs into two categories on the basis of their psychotropic properties and mechanisms of action. Animal models and evidence from clinical experience are used to support this classification. One group is considered to be "sedating" in association with fatigue, cognitive slowing, and possible anxiolytic and antimanic effects. These actions are speculated to be related to a predominance of potentiation of GABA-inhibitory neurotransmission and occur with barbiturates, benzodiazepines, VPA, GPN, TGB, and vigabatrin (VGB). A second group is thought to be "activating" with possible anxiogenic and antidepressant effects. The second group is associated with attenuation of glutamate excitatory neurotransmission and includes FBM and LTG. TPM, which possesses both GABA-ergic and antiglutamatergic actions, is said to have a mixed profile.

Clinical Assessment of Psychotropic Effects

Assessment of AED psychotropic effects in DD patients poses a challenge to both clinicians and researchers. Many DD patients experience unusual reactions to drugs as a result of idiosyncratic physiologic and metabolic responses resulting from their underlying conditions. DD patients may be unable to convey the subtleties of these effects, owing to reduced awareness or impaired communication. As a result of reduced cerebral functioning, many patients are sensitive to sedating drug effects, which may in turn alter mood, behavior, and cognitive functioning. Psychiatric symptoms as outlined in the fourth edition of *Diagnostic and Statistical Manual of Mental Disorders* (Washington, DC: American Psychiatric Association, 1994) are not manifested in the same manner in patients with DDs as they are in the general population but are represented alternatively by maladaptive behaviors, including aggression, antisocial conduct, and self-mutilation.

Higher rates of behavioral disturbance exist in DD patients both with and without epilepsy. Many strictly behavioral symptoms may resemble features of different seizure types. Therefore, both epileptic seizures and drug effects should be considered in the differential diagnosis of aberrant behaviors. If the clinical evaluation and routine electroencephalography (EEG) do not clarify the diagnosis sufficiently, capturing behaviors on continuous video-EEG monitoring should be considered. In the general population, drug-induced mood alterations can be assessed through self-report. In most studies examining drug effects, this can be conducted through routine contact with affected patients, aided by structured interviews or with such self-report instruments as the Beck Depression Inventory or the Profile of Mood States.

These instruments are not employed readily in the DD population as a result of restrictions in patients' intellectual capacities or restrictions in their ability to communicate. Although some clinicians' rating scales have been developed,[6] direct observation and quantification of these behaviors often are required.[7,8] This may include a thorough analysis of baseline behavior, determination of factors influencing the behavior, and regular monitoring of these features after initiation or discontinuation of a drug.[9] Because many patients are supervised closely, caregiver assessments also can be useful measures of drug effects in this population.

Similar issues arise in assessing cognitive effects of AEDs. Although decreases in concentration and memory may be assessed through self-report, this method often is unreliable. Many of the side effects of AEDs are subtle in nature and can be documented only through the use of sensitive neuropsychological measures of attention, motor speed, and memory. Use of these measures in a DD population can be problematic, as the validity and reliability of a particular instrument may be affected by general reductions in intellectual functioning. Use of these tests in DD populations also often leads to "floor effects," whereby test sensitivity and the ability to assess changes in functioning are obscured by reduced variance in the measure. In many cases, caregiver ratings or a systematic analysis of target behaviors is recommended in place of neuropsychological assessment of subtle cognitive deficits.[10]

Many reports of AED psychotropic effects are anecdotal, some fail to examine premorbid psychiatric status, and many are based on cases with very high anticonvulsant levels.[4] Clinicians are very likely to encounter DD epilepsy patients who are receiving more than one medication, including AEDs and psychotropic drugs. This confounds the determination of which agent is specifically responsible for the positive or negative effects on behavior. Recent consensus among epileptologists on the value of striving for AED monotherapy in the treatment of the non-DD epilepsy patient should also apply to DD patients. Numerous studies have demonstrated that reduction in AED polypharmacy does not necessarily lead to seizure exacerbation, and patients may enjoy improvements in cognition and behavior when they receive a smaller number of medications.[11–13]

Other methodologic pitfalls in the drug literature include (1) association of mood changes with the introduction of a new AED and ignoring potential effects of discontinuing the current agent; (2) disregard of the positive effects on mood achieved by reducing seizures; (3) failure to address the complex relationship of drug-induced cognitive impairment with mood; (4) poor recognition of important inequities in drug trial comparison groups (e.g., groups with noncomparable drug levels); (5) analysis of limited samples; (6) selection bias; (7) the negative effect of polytherapy irrespective of the specific agent; and (8) failure to apply correction methods in statistical analysis of large numbers of variables.[14] Other confounding variables include reliance on retrospective data, focus on transient acute drug effects, and inappropriate extrapolation to epilepsy patients of data on drug effects in normal volunteers.[15] Significantly lower rates of psychotropic effects on mood and behavior also may be noted in general drug trial reports as compared to studies that specifically target these factors.

For most AEDs, numerous conflicting reports abound concerning both positive and negative psychotropic effects, and the reader of the medical literature must remember that mean tendencies may differ from individual patient experience.

Another challenge in analyzing the psychotropic effect of AEDs relates to our inability to assess these effects as completely independent variables. Patients who experience a reduction or resolution of seizures as a result of AED therapy may experience associated elevations in mood and improvements in quality of life. Conversely, the stigma of taking AEDs or reactions to the experience of side effects (e.g., cosmetic effects, fatigue, cognitive impairments) may adversely affect mood and behavior.[16]

Individual Antiepileptic Drugs

Benzodiazepines

Such benzodiazepines as chlorazepate, clobazam, clonazepam, diazepam, lorazepam, and nitrazepam may be used in epileptic patients with DDs as antiepileptic, anxiolytic, or sedative hypnotic drugs.[17] Benzodiazepines also appear to have limited antidepressant[18] and antimanic[19] properties. Because of their broad-spectrum antiepileptic properties, they have been used to treat Lennox-Gastaut syndrome, an epileptic syndrome characterized by generalized seizures (typically tonic, atonic, myoclonic, and atypical absence), characteristic spike and wave complexes and, usually, cognitive dysfunction.[20] Their tendency to cause sedation, cognitive impairment, tolerance, and addiction limit their utility as chronic antiepileptic therapy.[21] Further, intravenous benzodiazepines administered to patients with the Lennox-Gastaut syndrome (common in the DD epilepsy population) rarely may induce generalized status epilepticus[22] or convert absence status to generalized tonic status epilepticus.[23] Adverse psychotropic effects among DD patients include behavioral abnormalities (e.g., hyperactivity, restlessness, reduced attention span, irritability, disruptiveness, or aggressiveness).[4,17] Anecdotal experience suggests that clobazam may have fewer adverse effects than does clonazepam, with less impairment of attention, less mood disturbance, and diminished drooling. One study noted no difference in cognitive impairment among patients receiving clobazam and those receiving CBZ.[24] Special care should be taken in withdrawing benzodiazepines, as delirium, psychosis, and withdrawal seizures have been reported with excessively rapid withdrawal of these drugs.[25]

Barbiturates

Despite the current availability of more AEDs than were available in the past, such barbiturates as phenobarbital and primidone continue to be prescribed frequently for DD epilepsy patients. This is not necessarily because of superior drug efficacy but may be owing to physician discomfort with the newer and less familiar AEDs. This is unfortunate, as the barbiturates may impair cognition significantly in the general population and in patients with already compromised intellectual abilities.[4,26] The risk of withdrawal seizures also may render barbiturates a less-than-optimal AED for use in this population. Cognitive impairment due to barbiturates may be subtle, occur in the absence of frank sedation and, anecdotally, may not be obvious to affected patients until they notice an improvement on withdrawal from the drug.[27] Reduction in the use of barbiturates in DD patients may be accompanied by significant behavioral improvements.[28]

Although barbiturates have been used in the past to treat anxiety and insomnia,[29] and scattered reports even suggest modest efficacy against bipolar disorder,[30] most attention has been placed on their adverse psychotropic profile. Barbiturates are associated with a significant risk of eliciting depressive symptomatology.[31] A classic study by Brent et al.[32] of patients receiving phenobarbital as compared to CBZ demonstrated a statistically significant increase in the risk of depression and suicidal ideation in the former group, particularly among those with a personal or family history of affective disorder. In patients with documented depression, avoiding barbiturates is advisable.[33]

Barbiturates also may cause paradoxical hyperactivity,[34–36] conduct problems,[37] behavioral agitation, and irritability[38,39] in children, adolescents, and patients with mental retardation.[27] Identifying these potential side effects is crucial, as an optimal approach to their treatment would be to remove the responsible agent rather than adding a psychotropic drug to control these behaviors.

Phenytoin

PHT is used commonly in patients with partial and generalized tonic-clonic seizures but is not effective for absence seizures.[40] Variable reports cite a relation between depressive symptoms and PHT, although some of this relationship may involve reactive symptoms from experiencing the stigma associated with cosmetic side effects of the drug.[41] Although a dose-related sedation may occur, a paradoxical excited delirium may be seen with either therapeutic or toxic PHT levels.[42]

PHT's mild effects on cognition are well-known. Some studies have demonstrated PHT-induced memory impairments, and others have shown impairments in complex reaction time or motor speed.[43,44] An older literature describes a chronic cumulative encephalopathy that has an impact on both behavior and global cognition[4] and an acute reversible encephalopathy accompanying toxic PHT levels (manifested by increased seizures, drowsiness, and cognitive impairment, sometimes with ataxia).[42] These encephalopathic syndromes should be considered in evaluating DD patients who have shown declines in cognition or coordination. Switching of AEDs should be considered if this potentially reversible syndrome is suspected.

Ethosuximide

ESM is used commonly as a first-line therapy for typical absence seizures occurring in primary generalized epilepsy syndromes. However, atypical absence is more common in the DD population. Although ESM may be effective against atypical absence, the common association with other seizures (e.g., atonic, myoclonic, generalized tonic-clonic) that do not respond to ESM renders it a less-than-optimal choice for treating such patients. Although ESM usually is considered to be a benign treatment for absence seizures in primary generalized epilepsies, it can cause confusion, sleep disturbances, and a wide assortment of behavioral changes, such as aggressive activity, depression, hostility, and even psychosis.[33] The controversial entity of "forced normalization"[45] has been invoked as a potential explanation for ESM-related behavioral abnormalities, in which ESM-induced "normalization" of the EEG recording results in a paradoxical behavioral abnormality.[46]

Valproic Acid

Valproic acid (VPA) has broad-spectrum anticonvulsant properties, including antiepileptic effects against many seizure types common to the DD population (e.g., atonic, myoclonic, atypical absence, and generalized tonic-clonic seizures).[47] In one recent series, VPA was the AED prescribed most commonly in a population-based cohort of adults with a learning disability and epilepsy.[48] Like CBZ, VPA now is used commonly to treat bipolar affective disorder, particularly in patients who do not respond adequately to lithium; therefore, it is speculated to have mood-stabilizing properties in epilepsy patients as well.[49,50] VPA may be useful also in the treatment of panic and, possibly, of obsessive-compulsive disorder.[51] Agitation and mood problems in association with central nervous system neurologic abnormalities, such as head trauma or seizures, may be particularly responsive to VPA therapy.[52] VPA has been suggested also to lessen irritability and aggressive or self-injurious behavior among nonepileptic DD patients, including patients with dementia.[53,54] Notable adverse effects include weight gain, gastrointestinal upset, hyperandrogenism, polycystic ovary disease, and neural tube defects in the offspring of pregnant patients.[55]

Although, for most patients, VPA has minimal cognitive side effects,[56,57] it may cause somnolence and rare acute toxic encephalopathies.[58,59] In children with learning disabilities and complex partial seizures, VPA has been reported to induce or exacerbate hyperactivity and aggressive behavior.[60] However, similar kinds of reports have been noted with other AEDs, such as GPN (described in the section Gabapentin).

Carbamazepine

CBZ, a widely prescribed AED for both partial and generalized tonic-clonic seizures, has structural properties similar to those of the tricyclic antidepressant imipramine. Few reports cite negative behavioral effects associated with CBZ, although one notable retrospective study of patients who had mental retardation and were treated with CBZ for mood disorders found adverse behavioral reactions in nearly 10% of cases.[61] For the most part, CBZ-related behavioral problems occur in patients with preexisting behavioral difficulties.[62] Other studies have shown behavioral improvement in this population when the drug was removed.[10]

Numerous reports suggest that CBZ may have utility also in treating impulse control disorders, including borderline personality traits with aggression and dyscontrol syndromes.[63] Therefore, on the basis of antimanic and mood-stabilizing properties similar to those described with VPA, CBZ may be considered also for use in epilepsy patients who demonstrate both behavioral difficulties and seizures. However, absence, myoclonic, and atonic seizures that may occur commonly among DD patients do not respond to CBZ and actually may worsen in severity.[64,65] Other AEDs with similar spectra of action, such as PHT and phenobarbital, may have similar effects on these seizure types. Therefore, CBZ may be useful for patients with DD, epilepsy, and behavioral disturbances, but careful consideration should be given to seizure type.

Gabapentin

A number of reports from the epilepsy literature suggest that GPN may promote an improved sense of well-being independent of seizure reduction.[66–70] However, separating these two effects may be difficult. For example, in a recent open-label study, Harden et al.[71] contended that epilepsy patients receiving GPN demonstrated significant reduction in depressive scores on a dysthymia rating scale independent of seizure reduction. However, sample size was limited, and no significant differences were recorded on other depression or anxiety measures.

GPN has been demonstrated to be effective in treating mood disturbance in patients with partial epilepsy. Some studies showed increases in ratings of quality of life and well-being when patients were switched to this drug.[72,73] The results of most studies have demonstrated minimal cognitive side effects associated with GPN.[72–74]

Open-label and case reports suggest that GPN has efficacy in treating mania[75–78] and the depressive phase of bipolar disorder.[79,80] Anecdotally, it may reduce agitation and improve sleep patterns in manic patients. It is being evaluated also in behavioral dyscontrol,[81] agitation in senile dementia,[82] anxiety states,[83] social phobia,[84] and self-injurious behaviors in neurologic syndromes.[85] If further validated with clinical experience and more rigorous studies, these reports may have important relevance for the treatment of DD epilepsy patients with comorbid psychiatric syndromes. The absence of protein binding or serious metabolic interactions gives GPN an excellent safety profile when used in combination therapy.

GPN may not be the optimal AED for treating some common seizure types encountered in this population, such as absence and myoclonic and atonic seizures. Further, anecdotal experience in DD adults suggests that some patients may develop agitation. Also, several reports have cited the development or exacerbation of aggressive and agitated behaviors in epileptic children, most of whom had some degree of intellectual impairment.[86,87] Clinicians, therefore, should watch carefully for behavioral side effects in treating DD patients with GPN.

Lamotrigine

LTG is a broad-spectrum AED with efficacy against both partial and generalized seizures. Anecdotal experience in epilepsy patients suggests that LTG may enhance alertness. After the discovery of serious adverse effects associated with the use of FBM (including bone marrow dyscrasias and hepatitis), many considered LTG to be an important alternative treatment for refractory generalized epilepsies in DD epilepsy patients. In a double-blind, placebo-controlled trial of LTG in treating the Lennox-Gastaut syndrome,[88] 33% of patients receiving LTG experienced a reduction in seizure frequency of at least 50%. This study noted minimal behavioral effects, whereas two subsequent series found significant effects, both positive and negative, among DD epilepsy patients treated with LTG. Beran and Gibson[89] noted the development of aggressive or violent behavior (or both) in 14 of 19 patients who received LTG, and one patient demonstrated behavioral improvement. Ettinger et al.[90] cited 3 of 20 mentally retarded epilepsy patients receiving LTG who developed new or worsened hyperactivity, irritability, and stereotypy. Conversely, another four patients exhibited positive psychotropic effects, including reduction in irritability and hyperactivity, decreased lethargy, diminished perseverative speech, or improvement in cooperation and better social engagement. Although behavioral improvements may have represented a mood-stabilizing effect of LTG in some, with increased alerting leading to irritability in others, the reasons for these disparate effects was unclear. Serum LTG levels did not predict who developed positive versus negative symptoms.

LTG now is being used for treatment-resistant bipolar disorder.[91–93] Although more published double-blind trials address the use of CBZ and VPA than of the newer AEDs in the treatment of this disorder, the arguably more favorable side effect profiles of GPN and LTG may render the latter two drugs more optimal choices for mood stabilization in bipolar disorder. A positive psychotropic effect of LTG is supported by the observation that several epilepsy patients who were entered in a randomized double-blind study of LTG and experienced only slight reductions in seizure severity still elected to remain in the drug trial and demonstrated elevated mood on quality-of-life measures.[94] Meador and Baker[95] also have shown LTG to possess favorable behavioral and cognitive effects. DD patients receiving LTG should be observed for the development of allergic reactions, including pruritus and rash, which can progress to potentially life-threatening Stevens-Johnson syndrome.[96]

Tiagabine

TGB, approved as adjunctive therapy for partial seizures, is a generally well-tolerated AED with a central nervous system side effect spectrum similar to that of most AEDs, including dizziness, headache, ataxia, and nervousness.[97] One study of its use in treating intractable epilepsy patients demonstrated mood improvements among patients converted to TGB monotherapy. Mood elevation was not correlated with seizure reduction, suggesting that positive psychotropic benefits may be independent of antiepileptic effects.[98] Limited case series also note potential benefits against bipolar disorder.[99] Other series have noted TGB-related emotional lability and depression.[100]

TGB-induced absence status epilepticus recently was reported in patients with partial seizure disorders[101] to be a rare cause of personality changes and behavioral abnormalities in patients receiving this drug. The literature regarding the use of TGB in the DD population is sparse, perhaps because of the agent's limited utility in generalized seizure disorders. Some have suggested that significant numbers of patients left TGB drug trials as a result of developing depressive symptoms.[102] However, Dodrill et al.[103] demonstrated improved mood and psychosocial adjustment when patients were switched from other AEDs to TGB monotherapy.[98] Studies of TGB in DD populations have shown no obvious deleterious cognitive side effects.[103,104]

Vigabatrin

VGB, which has been prescribed extensively outside the United States, appears to have a significant risk of inducing adverse psychiatric events, particularly psychosis.[105] Patients at risk for such outcomes may include those with severe epileptic disorders, a sudden reduction in seizure frequency, or a history of psychosis. In children with static encephalopathies or hyperactive behavior, VGB (especially in high doses) may exacerbate hyperkinesia.[106,107] Caution is advised, therefore, in using VGB in patients with established psychopathology or static encephalopathies. Doses should be advanced slowly, and acute withdrawal of the drug should be avoided.[108] Alternatively, reports of favorable psychotropic effects also have been published, such as its utility in treating posttraumatic stress disorder.[109] Recent concerns about VGB-associated restriction of visual field function may limit its widespread use in epilepsy patients.[110]

Felbamate

When introduced several years ago, FBM was greeted with great enthusiasm as the first in a series of drugs termed the *new AEDs*. FBM was particularly welcome for its potential contribution to the treatment of refractory epilepsy syndromes in the DD population, including Lennox-Gastaut syndrome. Subsequent discoveries about its association with fatal hepatitis and aplastic anemia have restricted its use greatly. If factors are determined that can predict which patients are at risk for these dreaded complications and which are not, FBM may re-emerge as an important tool in the treatment of refractory epilepsy syndromes. In such cases, knowledge of FBM's psychotropic properties will be of great importance. Anecdotal experience with FBM suggests that it has stimulantlike properties that may be experienced favorably or unfavorably by patients. Although some patients have experienced increased alertness, improved attention, and enhanced concentration abilities (in contrast to the commonly encountered sedation associated with other AEDs), other patients have reported anorexia, insomnia, and anxiety.[111-113] Numerous reports of mania, psychosis, and behavioral disturbances also have been noted with FBM administration.[114,115]

Topiramate

Recently approved by the U.S. Food and Drug Administration, TPM is an AED with broad-spectrum antiepileptic properties. TPM-induced attentional disturbances and psychomotor slowing have been reported commonly.[116] In double-blind,

placebo-controlled, and open-label trials of TPM for partial seizures, the most common adverse effects observed in greater than 10% of subjects included somnolence, psychomotor slowing, difficulty with memory, difficulty with concentration or attention, and speech or language problems (Dr. Natalie Addi, Ortho-McNeil Pharmaceuticals, personal communication, November 1999).[117] Slow escalation of TPM dose and reduction of polypharmacy may improve tolerance of the drug.[118,119]

Among healthy young adults randomly assigned in blinded fashion to receive TPM, GPN, or LTG,[74] only the TPM group demonstrated statistically significant declines in measures of attention and word fluency at acute doses and persisting at 2- and 4-week intervals. Although TPM acute dosing was higher and chronic administration was escalated more rapidly than in current clinical practice, this study supports previous experience with TPM. Self-reported ratings on the anger-hostility subscales of the Profile of Mood States inventory also were elevated in the TPM group.

A recent, double-blind, randomized trial of TPM in treating Lennox-Gastaut syndrome found 33% of patients experiencing at least a 50% reduction in seizures.[120] In this study, 42% of patients experienced somnolence, 40% had anorexia, 21% experienced nervousness, and 21% demonstrated behavioral problems. Although no patients discontinued therapy because of an adverse event, one wonders whether this population may have been too cognitively impaired to communicate about the severity of their distress from side effects. At this time, unclear for the clinician considering using TPM in this population is whether cognitive function is compromised only mildly or compromised severely beyond baseline and how much impact this outcome should have on the drug's risk-benefit ratio.

Anecdotal experience and several reports also suggest that TPM may cause symptoms of depression,[121-124] although this may be due in part to a reaction to the cognitive side effects. Anxiety, irritability, behavioral problems, and even symptoms of psychosis also have been noted in patients treated with TPM.[5,125] Acute psychotic symptoms have been shown to be associated with initiation of TPM.

In contrast, a few recent reports indicate that TPM may be useful in treating both the manic and depressive phases of bipolar disorder.[126-128] As weight gain often is a serious side effect of the medications used to treat bipolar disorder, TPM's promotion of weight loss may be an advantage of this drug over other mood stabilizers.[129] Patients using TPM should be advised to drink plenty of fluids, as TPM may be associated with a two- to fourfold increased risk for nephrolithiasis.[121,130]

Vagal Nerve Stimulation

Vagal nerve stimulation (VNS)—a novel therapy for partial and generalized epilepsy—involves the repetitive stimulation of the left vagus nerve via connections from a programmable neurocybernetic prosthesis implanted in the left upper chest region.[131] Intermittent vagal nerve stimulation may be supplemented by additional activation of the neurocybernetic prosthesis at the time of a seizure by holding a magnet over the left chest wall region. The mechanism of the antiepileptic effect of VNS is unclear, but animal studies suggest that stimulated vagal nerve afferent fibers terminating on the nucleus of the solitary tract (NTS) in the brainstem experience increased GABA transmission or decreased glutamate transmission at the NTS, resulting in inhibition of ascending outputs from the NTS on numerous forebrain structures and other brainstem nuclei known to play a role in seizure control.[132] Projections from the NTS on limbic structures also may play a role in potential mood-elevating effects of VNS.

VNS is a generally well-tolerated treatment, with adverse events including hoarseness, tingling sensations in the neck, or intermittent alterations in voice, all of which usually abate significantly over time. Although VNS therapy is more invasive than the administration of AEDs, it is associated also with a number of advantages over typical AED treatment. Although most AEDs (particularly when used in polytherapy) are associated with central nervous system side effects (e.g., sedation and impairment of cognition), VNS potentially offers antiepileptic effect in the absence of such adverse events.

Although VNS has been studied more extensively in the non-DD epilepsy population with partial seizures, the process is a welcome addition to the therapeutic armamentarium against refractory generalized epilepsy syndromes common to the DD population, such as Lennox-Gastaut syndrome.[133] Preliminary reports of VNS experience

in this population have been impressive, with reductions in seizures and increased attention and alertness reported.[134] In one report of 15 children with the Lennox-Gastaut syndrome or myoclonic epilepsies of infancy,[135] more than 25% of patients demonstrated greater than a 50% seizure reduction, although the methods for supporting the claim that behavioral improvements seen were independent of seizure reduction were not clarified.

Many clinicians may be concerned about implanting devices in DD patients, fearing that patients will pull at the operative site in the chest wall. Recent experience with VNS has defied these concerns, with good tolerance of the neurocybernetic prosthesis implant. Nevertheless, watching such patients carefully is advisable in the immediate postoperative period (Paul Devereaux, Cyberonics Corporation, personal communication, November 1999).

Animal models and recent human studies suggest that VNS may enhance memory. Electrical stimulation of the vagus nerve delivered after an aversive learning experience has been shown to improve later retention performance in rats.[136] In non-DD epilepsy patients, a protocol administering electrical stimulation of the vagus nerve versus sham stimulation demonstrated statistically significant higher recognition memory resulting from the former protocol.[137] These studies offer hope for patients with the cognitive impairments so common among epilepsy patients.

Preliminary evidence from two recent studies suggests that VNS may reduce depressive symptomatology in adult epilepsy patients.[138,139] The former study found a trend toward statistically significant reduction of dysthymic symptoms on the Cornell Dysthymia Rating Scale as compared to symptoms in control patients, although notably no significant differences were noted on other mood inventories. No correlation was seen between seizure reduction and mood improvements, but specifics of this analysis must be clarified further. Studies also are under way examining the potential role of VNS in treating primary depression in nonepilepsy patients.

Little information is available about the psychotropic effects of VNS in DD epilepsy patients. However, the aforementioned studies in nonepilepsy patients and the potential to reduce the dosage or number of AEDs administered in such patients offer optimism for improving mood and cognition in this population.

References

1. Sunder TR. Meeting the challenge of epilepsy in persons with multiple handicaps. J Child Neurol 1997;12[Suppl 1]:S38–S43.
2. Lund J. Epilepsy and psychiatric disorder in the mentally retarded adult. Acta Psychiatr Scand 1985;72:557–562.
3. Coulter DL. Comprehensive management of epilepsy in persons with mental retardation. Epilepsia 1997;38[Suppl 4]:S24–S31.
4. Rivinus TM. Psychiatric effects of the anticonvulsant regimens. J Clin Psychopharmacol 1982;2:165–192.
5. Ketter TA, Post RM, Theodore WH. Positive and negative psychotropic effects of antiepileptic drugs in patients with seizure disorders. Neurology 1999;53[Suppl 1]:S52–S66.
6. Aman MG, Singh NN. Aberrant Behavior Checklist. East Aurora, NY: Slosson Educational Publications, 1994.
7. Sturmey P, Carlsen A, Crisp AG, Newton JT. A functional analysis of multiple aberrant responses: a refinement and extension of Iwata et al.'s (1982) methodology. J Ment Defic Res 1988;32:31–46.
8. Iwata BA, Wong SE, Riordan MM, et al. Assessment and training of clinical interviewing skills: analogue analysis and field replication. J Appl Behav Anal 1982;15:191–203.
9. Einfeld SL. Guidelines for the use of psychotropic medication in individuals with developmental disabilities. Aust N Z J Dev Disabil 1990;16:71–73.
10. Kalachnik JE, Hanzel TE, Harder SR, et al. Antiepileptic drug behavioral side effects in individuals with mental retardation and the use of behavioral measurement techniques. Ment Retard 1995;33:374–382.
11. Bates ER, Wilder BJ, Brown R, et al. Antiepileptic drug reduction program at a center for the developmentally disabled (abstract). Epilepsia 1991;32[Suppl 3]:3.
12. Schmidt D. Reduction of two-drug therapy in intractable epilepsy. Epilepsia 1983;24:368–376.
13. Bennet HS, Dunlop T, Ziring PR. Reduction of polypharmacy for epilepsy in an institution for the retarded. Dev Med Child Neurol 1983;25:735–737.
14. Devinsky O. Cognitive and Behavioral Effects of AEDs. Annual Course of the American Epilepsy Society: New Developments in Antiepileptic Drug Therapy. New Orleans: American Epilepsy Society, 1994;E1–E50.
15. Bourgeois BFD. Antiepileptic drugs, learning, and behavior in childhood epilepsy. Epilepsia 1998;39:913–921.
16. Ettinger AB, Weisbrot DM, Krupp LB, et al. Fatigue and depression in epilepsy. J Epilepsy 1998;11:105–109.
17. Ko DY, Rho JM, DeGiorgio CM, Sato S. Benzodiazepines. In JJ Engel, TA Pedley (eds), Epilepsy: A Comprehensive Textbook. Philadelphia: Lippincott–Raven,
    1997;1475–1489.
18. Rickels K, Chung HR, Csanalosi IB, et al. Alprazolam, diazepam, imipramine, and placebo in outpatients with major depression. Arch Gen Psychiatry 1987;44:862–866.
19. Bradwejn J, Shriqui C, Koszycki D, Meterissian G. Double-blind comparison of the effects of clonazepam and lorazepam in acute mania. J Clin Psychopharmacol 1990;10:403–408.
20. Farrell K. Symptomatic Generalized Epilepsy and Lennox-Gastaut Syndrome. In E Wyllie (ed), The Treatment of Epilepsy (2nd ed). Baltimore: Williams & Wilkins, 1996;530–539.
21. Schoch P, Moreau JL, Martin JR, Haefely WE. Aspects of benzodiazepine receptor structure and function with relevance to drug tolerance and dependence. Biochem Soc Symp 1993;59:121–134.
22. Bittencourt PRM, Richens A. Anticonvulsant-induced status epilepticus in Lennox-Gastaut syndrome. Epilepsia 1981;22:129–134.
23. Prior PF, Maclaine GN, Scot DF, Laurance BM. Tonic status epilepticus precipitated by intravenous diazepam in a child with petit mal status. Epilepsia 1982;13:467–472.
24. Bawden HN, Camfield CS, Camfield PR, et al. The cognitive and behavioural effects of clobazam and standard monotherapy are comparable. Epilepsy Res 1999;33:133–143.
25. Hauser P, Devinsky O, DeBellis M, et al. Benzodiazepine withdrawal delirium with catatonic features. Arch Neurol 1989;46:696–699.
26. Meador KJ, Loring DW, Moore EE, et al. Comparative cognitive effects of phenobarbital, phenytoin, and valproate in healthy adults. Neurology 1995;45:1494–1499.
27. Stoudemire A, Fogel BS. Psychiatric Care of the Medical Patient. New York: Oxford University Press, 1993;475–476.
28. Poindexter AR, Berglund JA, Kolstoe PD. Changes in antiepileptic drug prescribing patterns in large institutions: preliminary results of a five-year experience. Am J Ment Retard 1993;98:34–40.
29. Rickels K, Pereira-Ogan JA, Chung HR, et al. Bromazepam and phenobarbital in anxiety: a controlled study. Curr Ther Res Clin Exp 1973;15:679–690.
30. Schaffer LC, Schaffer CB, Caretto J. The use of primidone in treatment of refractory bipolar disorder. Ann Clin Psychiatry 1999;11:61–66.
31. Robertson MM. Depression in Patients with Epilepsy: An Overview and Clinical Study. In MR Trimble (ed), The Psychopharmacology of Epilepsy. Chichester, UK: Wiley, 1985.
32. Brent DA, Crumrine PK, Varma R, et al. Phenobarbital treatment and major depressive disorder in children with epilepsy. Pediatrics 1987;80:909–917.
33. Perrine K, Congett S. Neurobehavioral problems in epilepsy. Neurol Clin 1994;12:129–152.

34. Ounsted C. The hyperkinetic syndrome in epileptic children. Lancet 1955;2:203.

35. Wolf S, Forsythe A. Behavioral disturbance, phenobarbital and febrile seizures. Pediatrics 1978;61:728–731.

36. Thorn I. A controlled study of prophylactic long-term treatment of febrile convulsions with phenobarbital. Acta Neurol Scand 1975;60[Suppl]:67–73.

37. Corbett JA, Trimble MR, Nichol TC. Behavioral and cognitive impairments in children with epilepsy: the long-term effects of anticonvulsant therapy. J Am Acad Child Psychiatry 1985;24:17–23.

38. Camfield C, Chaplin S, Doyle AB, et al. Side effects of phenobarbital in toddlers: behavioral and cognitive aspects. J Pediatr 1979;95:361–365.

39. Ferrari M, Barabas G, Matthews W. Psychologic and behavioral disturbance among epileptic children treated with barbiturate anticonvulsants. Am J Psychiatry 1983;140:112–113.

40. Wilder BJ. Phenytoin: Clinical Use. In RH Levy, RH Mattson, BS Meldrum (eds), Antiepileptic Drugs. New York: Raven Press, 1995;334–344.

41. Weisbrot DM, Ettinger AB. Epilepsy and behavior: controversies and caveats. Neurologist 1997;3:155–172.

42. Dam M. Phenytoin: Toxicity. In DM Woodbury, JK Penry, CE Pippenger (eds), Antiepileptic Drugs. New York: Raven Press, 1982;247–256.

43. Dodrill CB, Troupin AS. Neuropsychological effects of carbamazepine and phenytoin: a reanalysis. Neurology 1991;41:141–143.

44. Meador KJ, Loring DW, Allen ME, et al. Comparative cognitive effects of carbamazepine and phenytoin in healthy adults. Neurology 1991;41:1537–1540.

45. Landolt H. Serial electroencephalographic investigations during psychotic episodes in epileptic patients and during schizophrenic attacks. In L deHass (ed), Lectures on Epilepsy. London: Elsevier, 1958.

46. Wolf P. Acute Behavioral Symptomatology at Disappearance of Epileptiform EEG Abnormality: Paradoxical or "Forced" Normalization. In D Smith, D Treiman, M Trimble (eds), Neurobehavioral Problems in Epilepsy. Advances in Neurology. New York: Raven Press, 1991;127–142.

47. Delgado-Escueta AV, Treiman DM, Walsh GO. The treatable epilepsies. N Engl J Med 1983;308:1508–1514.

48. Deb S, Joyce J. The use of antiepileptic medication in a population-based cohort of adults with learning disability and epilepsy. Int J Psychiatry Clin Pract 1999;3:129–133.

49. Small JG, Klapper MH, Milstein V, et al. Carbamazepine compared with lithium in the treatment of mania. Arch Gen Psychiatry 1991;48:915–921.

50. Freeman TW, Clothier JL, Pazzaglia P, et al. A double-blind comparison of valproate and lithium in the treatment of acute mania. Am J Psychiatry 1992;149:108–111.

51. Post RM, Ketter TA, Denicoff K, et al. The place of anticonvulsant therapy in bipolar illness. Psychopharmacology 1996;128:115–129.

52. Stoll AL, Banov M, Kolbrener M, et al. Neurologic factors predict a favorable valproate response in bipolar and schizoaffective disorders. J Clin Psychopharmacol 1994;14:311–313.

53. Kastner T, Finesmith R, Walsh K. Long-term administration of valproic acid in the treatment of affective symptoms in people with mental retardation. J Clin Psychopharmacol 1993;13:448–451.

54. Gupta S, O'Connell RO, Parekh A, et al. Efficacy of valproate for agitation and aggression in dementia: case reports. Int J Geriatr Psychopharmacol 1998;1: 244–248.

55. Knowles SR. Adverse effects of antiepileptics. Can J Clin Pharmacol 1999;6:137–148.

56. Prevey ML, Delaney RC, Cramer JA, et al. Effect of valproate on cognitive functioning: comparison with carbamazepine. Arch Neurol 1996;53:1008–1016.

57. Duncan JS, Shorvon SD, Trimble MR. Effects of removal of phenytoin, carbamazepine, and valproate on cognitive function. Epilepsia 1990;31:584–591.

58. Zaret BS, Cohen RA. Reversible valproic acid-induced dementia: a case report. Epilepsia 1986;27:234–240.

59. Marescaux C, Warter JM, Micheletti G, et al. Stuporous episodes during treatment with sodium valproate: report of seven cases. Epilepsia 1982;23: 297–305.

60. Husain SB, Wical BS. Adverse behavioral effects of valproate therapy in children with complex partial seizures (abstract). Epilepsia 1998;39[Suppl 6]:162.

61. Friedman DL, Kastner T, Plummer AT. Adverse behavioral effects in individuals with mental retardation and mood disorders treated with carbamazepine. Am J Ment Retard 1992;96:541–546.

62. Reid AH, Naylor GJ, Kay DS. A double-blind placebo-controlled crossover trial of carbamazepine in overactive severely mentally handicapped patients. Psychol Med 1981;11:109–113.

63. Silver JM, Yudofsky SC, Hurowitz GI. Psychopharmacology and Electroconvulsive Therapy. In RE Hales, SC Yudofsky, JA Talbott (eds), Textbook of Psychiatry (2nd ed). Washington, DC: American Psychiatric Press, 1994;897–1007.

64. Snead OC. Exacerbation of seizures in children by carbamazepine. N Engl J Med 1985;313:916–921.

65. Shields WD, Saslow E. Myoclonic, atonic and absence seizures following institution of carbamazepine therapy in children. Neurology 1983;33:1487–1489.

66. Ojemann LM, Wilensky AJ, Temkin NR, et al. Long-term treatment with gabapentin for partial epilepsy. Epilepsy Res 1992;13:159–165.

67. Dimond KR, Pande AC, Lamoreaux L, Pierce MW. Effect of gabapentin (Neurontin) on mood and well-being in patients with epilepsy. Prog Neuropsychopharmacol Biol Psychiatry 1996;20:407–417.

68. Harden C, Pick L. Alterations in mood and anxiety in epilepsy patients treated with gabapentin (abstract). Epilepsia 1996;37[Suppl 5]:137.

69. Brodie MJ, Richens A, Yuen A. Double-blind comparison of lamotrigine and carbamazepine in newly diagnosed epilepsy. Lancet 1995;345:468–476.

70. Handforth A, Treiman DM. Efficacy and tolerance of long-term, high-dose gabapentin: additional observations. Epilepsia 1994;35:1032–1037.

71. Harden CL, Lazar LM, Pick LH, et al. A beneficial effect on mood in partial epilepsy patients treated with gabapentin. Epilepsia 1999;40:1129–1134.

72. Dodrill CB, Arnett JL, Hayes AG, et al. Cognitive abilities and adjustment with gabapentin: results of a multisite study. Epilepsy Res 1999;35:109–121.

73. Mortimore C, Trimble M, Emmers E. Effects of gabapentin on cognition and quality of life in patients with epilepsy. Seizure 1998;7:359–364.

74. Martin R, Kuzniecky R, Ho S, et al. Cognitive effects of topiramate, gabapentin, and lamotrigine in healthy young adults. Neurology 1999;52:321–327.

75. McElroy SL, Soutullo CA, Keck PE, Kmetz GF. A pilot trial of adjunctive gabapentin in the treatment of bipolar disease. Ann Clin Psychiatry 1997;6:99–103.

76. Ryback RS, Brodsky L, Manasifi F. Gabapentin in bipolar disorder (letter). J Neuropsychiatry Clin Neurosci 1997;9:301.

77. Knoll J, Stegman K, Suppes T. Clinical experience using gabapentin adjunctively in patients with a history of mania or hypomania. J Affect Disorder 1998;49:229–233.

78. Schaffer CB, Schaffer LC. Gabapentin in the treatment of bipolar disorder. Am J Psychiatry 1997;154: 291–292.

79. Young LT, Robb JC, Patelis-Siotis I, et al. Acute treatment of bipolar depression with gabapentin. Biol Psychiatry 1997;42:851–853.

80. Ghaemi SN, Katzow JJ, Desai SP, Goodwin FK. Gabapentin treatment of mood disorders: a preliminary study. J Clin Psychiatry 1997;59:426–429.

81. Ryback R, Ryback L. Gabapentin for behavioral dyscontrol (letter). Am J Psychiatry 1995;152:1399.

82. Sheldon LJ, Ancill RJ, Holliday SG. Gabapentin in geriatric psychiatry patients. Can J Psychiatry 1998;43:422–423.

83. Pollack MH, Matthews J, Scott EL. Gabapentin as a potential treatment for anxiety disorders (letter). Am J Psychiatry 1998;155:992.

84. Pande AC, Davidson JRT, Jefferson JW, et al. Treatment of social phobia with gabapentin: a placebo controlled study. J Psychopharmacol 1999;19:341–348.

85. McManaman J, Tam DA. Gabapentin for self-injurious behavior in Lesch-Nyhan syndrome. Pediatr Neurol 1999;20:381–382.

86. Wolf SM, Shinnar S, Kang H, et al. Gabapentin toxicity in children manifesting as behavioral changes. Epilepsia 1995;36:1203–1205.

87. Lee DO, Steingard RJ, Cesena M, et al. Behavioral side effects of gabapentin in children. Epilepsia 1996;37:87–90.

88. Motte J, Trevathan E, Arvidsson JFV, et al. Lamotrigine for generalized seizures associated with the Lennox-Gastaut syndrome. N Engl J Med 1997;337:1807–1812.

89. Beran RG, Gibson RJ. Aggressive behaviour in intellectually challenged patients with epilepsy treated with lamotrigine. Epilepsia 1998;39:280–282.

90. Ettinger AB, Weisbrot DM, Saracco J, et al. Positive and negative psychotropic effects of lamotrigine in epilepsy patients with mental retardation. Epilepsia 1998;39:874–877.

91. Kotler M, Matar MA. Lamotrigine in the treatment of resistant bipolar disorder. Clin Neuropharmacol 1998;21:65–67.

92. Calabrese JR, Fatemi SH, Woyshville MJ. Antidepressant effects of lamotrigine in rapid cycling bipolar disorder (letter). Am J Psychiatry 1996;153:1236.

93. Kusumakar V, Yatham LN. An open study of lamotrigine in refractory bipolar depression. Psychiatr Res 1997;72:145–148.

94. Smith D, Davies G, Dewey M, Chadwick DW. Outcomes of add-on treatment with lamotrigine in partial epilepsy. Epilepsia 1993;34:312–322.

95. Meador KJ, Baker GA. Behavioral and cognitive effects of lamotrigine. J Child Neurol 1997;12:S44–S47.

96. Besag FMC. Lamotrigine in the management of subtle seizures. Rev Contemp Pharmacother 1994;5:123–131.

97. Rowan AJ, Uthman B, Ahmann P, et al. Safety and efficacy of three dose levels of tiagabine HCl versus placebo as adjunctive treatment for complex partial seizures. Epilepsia 1994;35[Suppl 8]:54.

98. Dodrill CB, Arnett JL, Shu V, et al. Effects of tiagabine monotherapy on abilities, adjustment, and mood. Epilepsia 1998;39:33–42.

99. Kaufman KR. Adjunctive tiagabine treatment of psychiatric disorders: three cases. Ann Clin Psychiatry 1998;10:181–184.

100. Leppik IE. Tiagabine: the safety landscape. Epilepsia 1995;36:S10–S13.

101. Ettinger AB, Bernal OG, Andriola MR, et al. Two cases of nonconvulsive status epilepticus in association with tiagabine therapy. Epilepsia 1999;40:1159–1162.

102. Brodie MJ. Tiagabine in the management of epilepsy. Epilepsia 1997;38:S23–S27.

103. Dodrill CB, Arnett JL, Sommerville KW. Cognitive and quality of life effects of differing dosages of tiagabine in epilepsy. Neurology 1997;48:1025–1031.

104. Sveinbjornsdottir S, Sander JWAS, Patsalos PN, et al. Neuropsychological effects of tiagabine, a potential new antiepileptic drug. Seizure 1994;3:29–35.

105. Sander JWAS, Hart YM, Trimble MR, Shorvon SD. Vigabatrin and psychosis. J Neurol Neurosurg Psychiatry 1991;54:435–439.

106. Dulac O, Chiron C, Luna D, et al. Vigabatrin in childhood epilepsy. J Child Neurol 1991;6:2S30–2S37.

107. Appelton R. The role of vigabatrin in the management of infantile epileptic syndromes. Neurology 1993;43: S21–S23.

108. Ben-Menachem E, French J. Vigabatrin. In J Engel, TA Pedley (eds), Epilepsy: A Comprehensive Textbook. Philadelphia: Lippincott–Raven, 1997;1609–1618.

109. Macleod AD. Vigabatrin and posttraumatic stress disorder. J Clin Psychopharmacol 1996;16:190–191.

110. Eske T, Talbot JF, Lawden MC. Severe persistent visual field constriction associated with vigabatrin. Br Med J 1997;314:180–181.

111. Ketter TA, Malow BA, Flamini R, et al. Felbamate monotherapy has stimulant-like effects in patients with epilepsy. Epilepsy Res 1996;23:129–137.

112. Asconape JJ, Brotherton TA, Lauve LM, et al. Felbamate: efficacy and tolerability in patients with refractory epilepsies (abstract). Epilepsia 1994;35[Suppl 8]:114.

113. Ettinger AB, Jandorf L, Berdia A, et al. Felbamate-induced headache. Epilepsia 1996;37:503–505.

114. King JA. Increased incidence of adverse behavioral side effects associated with the addition of felbamate (FBM) to antiepileptic drug (AED) regimens in the mentally retarded (MR) population (abstract). Epilepsia 1994;35[Suppl 8]:94.

115. Woodhams KA, Bennett B, Bronstein KS, et al. Behavioral changes in individuals treated with felbamate (abstract). Epilepsia 1994;35[Suppl 8]:160.

116. Crawford P. An audit of topiramate use in a general neurology clinic. Seizure 1998;7:207–211.

117. Biton V, Montouris GD, Ritter F, et al. A randomized, placebo-controlled study of topiramate in primary generalized tonic-clonic seizures. Neurology 1999;52:1330–1337.

118. Faught E, French J, Harden C. Postmarketing Antiepileptic Drug Survey Group (PADS). Adverse effects of TPM: results from a large post-marketing survey (abstract). Epilepsia 1997;38[Suppl 8]:97.

119. Faught E, Kuzniecky R, Gilliam F. Cognitive effects of TPM (abstract). Neurology 1997;48:A336.

120. Sachdeo RC, Glauser TA, Ritter F, et al. A double-blind, randomized trial of topiramate in Lennox-Gastaut syndrome. Neurology 1999;52:1882–1887.

121. Shorvon SD. Safety of topiramate: adverse events and relationships to dosing. Epilepsia 1996;37[Suppl 2]:S18–S22.

122. Tassanari CA, Michelucci R, Chauvel P, et al. Double-blind, placebo-controlled trial of topiramate (600 mg daily) for the treatment of refractory partial epilepsy. Epilepsia 1996;37:763–768.

123. Abou-Khalil B, Fakhoury T. Neuropsychiatric profile of high-dose topiramate (abstract). Epilepsia 1997;38[Suppl 8]:207.

124. Betts T, Smith K, Khan G. Severe psychiatric reactions to topiramate (abstract). Epilepsia 1997;38[Suppl 3]:64.

125. Dohmeier C, Kay A, Greathouse N. Neuropsychiatric complications of topiramate therapy (abstract). Epilepsia 1998;39[Suppl 6]:189.

126. Marcotte TD. Topiramate in the Treatment of Mood Disorders (abstract 115). Presented at the one hundred fifty-first annual meeting of the American Psychiatric Association. Toronto, Ontario, Canada, May 30–June 4, 1998.

127. Calabrese JR, Shelton MD III, Keck PE Jr, et al. Pilot Study of Topiramate in Acute Severe Treatment-Refractory Mania. Presented at the one hundred fifty-first annual meeting of the American Psychiatric Association. Toronto, Ontario, Canada, May 30–June 4, 1998.

128. Suppes T, Brown ES, McElroy SL, et al. A Pilot Trial of Adjunctive Topiramate in the Treatment of Bipolar Disorder: Application of the Stanley Foundation Bipolar Network (SFBN) Prospective Protocol (abstract). Proceedings of the Thirty-Seventh Annual Meeting of the American College of Neuropsychopharmacology. Las Croabas, Puerto Rico, 1998;306.

129. Sherman C. Topiramate may curb bingeing in bipolar patients. Clin Psychiatry News 1999;27:4.

130. Curry WJ, Kulling DL. Newer antiepileptic drugs: gabapentin, lamotrigine, felbamate, topiramate and fosphenytoin. Am Fam Physician 1998;57:513–520.

131. Reid SA. Surgical technique for implantation of the neurocybernetic prosthesis. Epilepsia 1990;31[Suppl 2]:S38–S39.

132. Walker BR, Easton A, Gale K. Regulation of limbic motor seizures by GABA and glutamate transmission in nucleus tractus solitarius. Epilepsia 1999;40:1051–1057.

133. Ben-Menachem E, Hellstrom K, Waldton C, Augustinsson LE. Evaluation of refractory epilepsy treated with vagus nerve stimulation for up to 5 years. Neurology 1999;52:1265–1267.

134. Helmers SL, Al-Jayyousi M, Madsen J. Adjunctive treatment in Lennox-Gastaut syndrome using vagal nerve stimulation (abstract). Epilepsia 1998;39[Suppl 6]:169.

135. Parker APJ, Polkey CE. Vagal nerve stimulation in epileptic encephalopathies. Pediatrics 1999;103:778–782.

136. Clark KB, Krahl SE, Smith DC, Jensen RA. Post-training unilateral vagal stimulation enhances retention performance in the rat. Neurobiol Learn Mem 1995;63:213–216.

137. Clark KB, Naritoku DK, Smith DC, et al. Enhanced recognition memory following vagus nerve stimulation in human subjects. Nature Neurosci 1999;2:94–98.

138. Harden CL, Pulver MC, Nikolov B, et al. Effects of vagus nerve stimulation on mood in adult epilepsy patients (abstract). Neurology 1999;52[Suppl 2]:A238.

139. Ettinger AB, Nolan E, Vitale S, et al. Changes in mood and quality of life in adult epilepsy patients treated with vagal nerve stimulation (abstract). Epilepsia 1999;40:62.

Chapter 19

Spasticity

Vicky Bassi, Mariko Kita, David S. Feldman,
and Orrin Devinsky

Spasticity is a motor disorder characterized by a velocity-dependent increase in tonic muscle tone with exaggerated tendon jerks, resulting from hyperexcitability of the tonic stretch reflex. Spasticity is a component of the upper motor neuron syndrome, is characterized by increasing resistance to more rapid passive movements,[1] and results from interruption of inhibitory descending spinal motor control. A clasp-knife phenomenon, marked by a sudden reduction in tone as the limb is flexed or extended passively, may occur when resistance dissipates during stretch. Additional signs associated with spasticity include weakness, increased muscle tone, impaired dexterity and coordination, hyperreflexia, extensor plantar responses, and spontaneous muscle spasms and contractures.[2]

Spasticity complicates such neurologic disorders as cerebral palsy (CP), spinal cord injury, stroke, multiple sclerosis (MS), and degenerative disorders. Patients with spasticity experience increased muscle tone in the setting of noxious stimuli such as infection, urolithiasis, bladder or bowel retention, decubitus ulcers, and tight or ill-fitting clothing or orthotics. Thus, the symptoms of spasticity can greatly interfere with a patient's functional capacity and quality of life.

Pathophysiology

The pathophysiology of spasticity is poorly understood, but the final common pathway underlying the mechanism is over-reactivity of the alpha motor neuron. Descending spinal pathways (corticospinal, reticulospinal, vestibulospinal) exert control over alpha motor neurons via monosynaptic and polysynaptic pathways. Complete destruction or partial interruptions of these descending pathways from cortical and brainstem structures can reduce the inhibitory tone on the spinal cord alpha motor neurons. This disinhibition can increase the resting tone of motor neurons. However, the most severe pathologic effect may be the excessive and exaggerated response to peripheral excitatory input.

The muscle spindle consists of several bundles of intrafusal muscle fibers surrounded by a connective tissue capsule. It represents the most complex sensory structure of the muscle and conveys information about muscle length. The central part of this specialized structure is composed of a noncontractile nuclear bag region. Spindles lie in parallel with extrafusal fibers, large muscle fibers that effect gross movement. Stretching the noncontractile bag region, or stretching the extrafusal fibers, constitutes the mechanical stimulus to fire the primary afferent or group Ia fiber. Group Ia afferents from the muscle spindle make synaptic contact with the cells of the dorsal nucleus of the spinal cord and with alpha motor neurons. Shortening of the extrafusal muscle shortens the spindle and silences the Ia afferents. The intrafusal muscle fibers of the spindle complex are innervated by gamma motor neurons in the anterior horns of the spinal cord, which increase the tension of the intrafusal fiber when it is shortened. This resets the spindle after shortening, so that it is again sensitive to changes in muscle length.[3]

When the muscle is lengthened by tendon tap or stretch, Ia afferents produce excitatory postsynaptic potentials on agonist motoneurons. Although this monosynaptic connection plays a role in the reflex, most excitatory activity in the stretch reflex is mediated by oligosynaptic and polysynaptic pathways.[2] Interneurons play a major role in the reflex arc. Antagonist muscle spindles also send Ia afferents to produce excitatory postsynaptic potentials on agonist inhibitory interneurons, which then evoke inhibitory postsynaptic potentials on motoneurons. The firing of the motoneuron depends on the summation of excitatory and inhibitory postsynaptic potentials. Additional inhibitory interneurons act on Ia afferents to inhibit the afferent signal presynaptically. γ-Aminobutyric acid (GABA) is the neurotransmitter mediating this selective presynaptic inhibition.[4]

The spinal segmental reflexes require the participation of muscle spindles, fusimotor innervation (gamma motor neurons), Ia primary afferents, and alpha motor neurons, as well as Renshaw recurrent inhibition, disynaptic reciprocal inhibition, nonreciprocal autogenic Ib inhibition, presynaptic inhibition, and remote inhibition-excitation of alpha motor neurons.[2] Spasticity results from prolonged disinhibition of components of this system, but the exact mechanism remains unclear.

Spasticity in Central Nervous System Disorders

MS and CP are two central nervous system disorders in which spasticity is a classic feature. MS is the most common demyelinating disease and affects primarily young adults. It is characterized by the dissemination of demyelinating events in time and space. After demyelination occurs, destroyed myelin is phagocytosed by macrophages, and gliosis ensues. In most patients, the course is characterized by exacerbations and remissions, but a pattern of steady or stepwise progression can occur. In MS, spasticity results from plaques of demyelination in the upper motor neuron fibers (i.e., pyramidal tract) in the brain or spinal cord.[4]

Paroxysmal neurologic disturbances of spinal cord origin, so-called spinal cord seizures, can also result from demyelinating lesions and can be difficult to distinguish from spasticity. However, they have also been associated with intravenous dye placement, transverse myelitis, and traumatic spinal cord injury.[5] These seizures are characterized by tonic spasm in the extremities, often accompanied by painful dysesthesia, and are transient, usually lasting no more than 2 minutes. Although they may occur spontaneously, these seizures commonly are precipitated by tactile stimulation or movement of the extremity. Clinical differentiation from spasticity is critical, as seizures may respond to antiepileptic drug (AED) therapy (e.g., carbamazepine).[6] Spinal cord seizures may limit rehabilitation of patients with idiopathic transverse myelopathy unless the disorder is recognized and appropriate AED therapy is initiated.[7]

CP is a persistent but dynamic disorder of movement and posture, resulting from brain lesions or anomalies arising in early development. It is a symptom complex, not a specific disease.[8] CP can result from in utero brain malformations or hemorrhagic-ischemic insults, from perinatal insults, or from postnatal insults (e.g., meningitis, trauma, ischemia) that occur before age 5 years.[9] CP is more likely to result from antepartum causes than from birth asphyxia.[10–13]

CP is classified on the basis of the predominant movement abnormality (spasticity, dystonia, athetosis, chorea, ataxia, hypotonia, or mixed forms) and by the extremities affected (monoplegic, diplegic, triplegic, hemiplegic, and quadriplegic). Dystonia, athetosis, chorea, and dyskinesia are hyperkinetic movement disorders, also known as *dyskinetic movements*. In contrast, spasticity is a hypertonic but isokinetic movement disorder. *Dystonia* is characterized by sustained muscle contractions that result in twisting and repetitive movements or abnormal postures. Dystonia is present in 15–25% of patients with CP and begins at 3–5 years of age or older.[14] It persists throughout life but, because it causes continuous motion, it rarely causes contractions or deformities (e.g., scoliosis).[8] *Athetosis* is a nonrhythmic, involuntary movement of the limbs, trunk, or vocal muscles, producing dysarthrias. Approximately 25% of CP patients develop athetosis, usually owing to basal ganglia injury in the full-term brain.[15] *Chorea* is characterized by involuntary, abrupt, rapid, brief, unsustained, irregular movements. Choreiform movements in CP usually develop at between 3 and 5 years of age.[8] *Spasticity* occurs in approximately two-thirds of CP patients and typically affects the lower more than the upper extremities. In the legs, flexors, adductors, and internal rotators are more prominently involved than are their antagonists.

Epilepsy in Patients with Cerebral Palsy

Patients with CP have problems beyond motor control. Epilepsy is commonly associated with CP and can further impair the affected individual's quality of life. The risk of epilepsy varies in different subtypes of CP, being most frequent in quadriplegics (50%) and least frequent in diplegic patients (27%).[16,17] Therefore, epilepsy is likely related to the type of brain lesion. The relationship between epilepsy and a specific type of brain lesion, however, is not fully understood.

Okumura et al.[18] studied the relationship between epilepsy in the first 5 years of life in patients with CP and the type of brain lesions found on magnetic resonance imaging. Fourteen patients had congenital anomaly, and 116 had perinatal injury. Epilepsy occurred in 37 of the 130 patients (31%), similar to other studies in which epilepsy incidence ranges from 25% to 45%.[16–19] Twelve patients had partial seizures, 20 had infantile spasms, and 5 had generalized seizures. Patients with congenital anomaly had a significantly higher incidence and an earlier age of onset of epilepsy than did those with perinatal injury. Among perinatal injury patients, those with term injury (with or without preterm injury) showed a higher incidence and a later onset of epilepsy than did those with only preterm injury.[18] Thus, the percentage of patients with epilepsy and the time course for development of epilepsy differ according to the type of brain lesion in CP.

Rationale for Treatment of Spasticity

The goal of therapy for spasticity is to increase functional capacity and relieve discomfort. Before initiating treatment, one must first evaluate the functional consequences of reducing spasticity. For some patients with proximal leg weakness, increased extensor tone in the legs offers necessary stability and support during transferring and walking. For other patients, hyperreflexia and clonus interfere with normal ambulation. In nonambulatory patients, flexor spasms may be painful and debilitating. Patients with spasticity may exhibit further increase in tone or spontaneous spasm in the setting of an underlying infection (e.g., urinary tract) or other noxious stimuli. Such causes should be excluded before a given therapeutic regimen is altered.

Treatment for spasticity should be multimodal. Physical therapy is an essential component and, in the most refractory cases, surgical intervention (e.g., posterior rhizotomy or tendon release procedures) may help. This review focuses on pharmacologic and surgical treatments of spasticity.

Pharmacotherapeutic Options

Medications used in the treatment of spasticity include baclofen, benzodiazepines, tizanidine, clonidine, dantrolene, gabapentin, botulinum toxin, and 4-aminopyridine. Of these, only baclofen, diazepam, tizanidine, and dantrolene are approved for treating spasticity. Generally, treatment is initiated at low doses and increased gradually to avoid adverse effects. The lowest effective dose for an individual patient is considered optimal. Table 19-1 outlines the administration of frequently used oral antispasticity agents.

Baclofen

Baclofen (Lioresal) is a structural analog of GABA and inhibits monosynaptic and polysynaptic spinal reflexes. It binds the GABA(B) receptor, which is coupled to calcium and potassium channels and occurs both pre- and postsynaptically.[20] Presynaptic binding hyperpolarizes the membrane, restricting calcium influx into presynaptic terminals and thereby decreasing neurotransmitter release in excitatory spinal pathways and decreasing alpha motor neuron activity.[21] Postsynaptic binding on the Ia afferent terminal increases potassium conductance and hyperpolarizes the membrane, thus enhancing presynaptic inhibition. Activation of GABA(B) receptors may also inhibit gamma motor neuron activity and decrease muscle spindle sensitivity.[22,23]

Table 19-1. Commonly Used Oral Antispasticity Agents

Agent	Starting Dose	Maximum Recommended Dosage	Side Effects	Monitoring	Special Cautions
Baclofen	5 mg/day, increasing to tid	80 mg/day in divided doses	Muscle weakness, sedation, fatigue, dizziness, nausea	Periodic liver function tests	Abrupt cessation associated with seizures
Diazepam	2 mg bid or 5 mg qhs	40–60 mg/day in divided doses	Sedation, cognitive impairment, depression	Dependence potential	Withdrawal syndrome
Tizanidine	2–4 mg/day	36 mg/day in divided doses	Drowsiness, dry mouth, dizziness, reversible dose-related elevated liver transaminases	Periodic liver function tests	Not to be used with antihypertensives or clonidine
Clonidine	0.1 mg/day	Not approved for spasticity. In hypertensive patients, doses as high as 2.4 mg/day in divided doses have been studied but rarely employed; usual dose in hypertension, 0.2–0.6 mg/day	Bradycardia, hypotension, dry mouth, drowsiness, constipation, dizziness, depression	—	Add-on agent; hypotension may result; not to be used with tizanidine
Dantrolene	25 mg/day	400 mg/day in divided doses	Hepatotoxicity (potentially irreversible), weakness, sedation, diarrhea	Periodic liver function tests	Hepatotoxicity
Gabapentin	100 mg tid	3,600 mg/day in divided doses	Stomach upset	—	—
4-Aminopyridine	10 mg bid or tid	Not approved for spasticity	Light-headedness	—	—

In the MS population, studies reveal that baclofen effectively reduces spasticity, decreasing frequency and severity of sudden painful spasms and improving range of joint movement.[24–26] However, increased weakness was commonly reported. In patients with spinal cord lesions, baclofen is very helpful in reducing flexor spasms, whereas for stroke patients, baclofen is less beneficial.[27,28] Such patients often had a modest decrease in muscle tone that was interpreted subjectively as slightly reduced stiffness. No effect was noted on hyperreflexia or clonus.[23,28]

Baclofen is rapidly absorbed after oral administration, but central nervous system penetration is relatively limited. The mean half-life is short, averaging 3.5 hours. Because it is partially metabolized by the liver (15%) and excreted by the kidney,

the dose should be decreased in patients with hepatic or renal impairment. Elevated liver enzymes can result from baclofen therapy. Thus, baseline liver function tests should be performed before and shortly after initiating treatment and every 6 months thereafter. Doses often are initiated at 5 mg daily, increasing to three times daily as tolerated. Thereafter, doses can be increased slowly at increments of 5 mg per day as needed. It may be helpful to initiate doses and increases at night to minimize side effects. The highest recommended dosage is 80 mg daily in divided doses but, for some patients, this dose may be insufficient to relieve symptoms. Higher doses may be attempted cautiously, as side effects are likely to be more prominent.[23]

Side effects are related mainly to central nervous system depression and include drowsiness, fatigue, weakness, dizziness, and nausea. Abrupt cessation of sustained treatment should be avoided, because sudden withdrawal of baclofen may cause hallucinations, psychosis, visual disturbances, and seizures.[29,30]

Diazepam

Benzodiazepines act by coupling to the benzodiazepine–GABA(A) receptor–chloride ionophore complex.[31] Binding of benzodiazepine to the GABA(A) receptor increases chloride conductance, resulting in presynaptic inhibition in the spinal cord.[32,33] Diazepam (Valium) is the most commonly used benzodiazepine in the treatment of spasticity, having efficacy in patients with spinal cord injury, hemiplegia, and MS.[34–37]

From and Heltberg[38] studied 17 patients with MS in a double-blind crossover trial with baclofen and diazepam. Each patient received 4 weeks of therapy with each drug. No differences were seen in efficacy of reducing spasticity, clonus, and flexor spasms or improving gait or bladder function. Side effect profiles differed slightly, with more patients reporting sedation while on diazepam, but the severity of side effects was similar in both groups. When patients still masked to treatment assignment were asked which agent they preferred, baclofen was significantly favored.[38] Other studies confirmed comparable antispasticity effects of baclofen and diazepam in reducing muscle tone and frequency of spasms, but baclofen was not necessarily favored by these patients over diazepam.[39,40]

Diazepam frequently is used as an adjunct to baclofen in treating spasticity[41] but is less commonly used as a single agent. Diazepam is well absorbed orally and reaches a peak level in approximately 1 hour. It is 98% protein-bound and is metabolized by the liver to active compounds nordiazepam and oxazepam. In patients with hepatic dysfunction, doses should be titrated carefully. Total half-life can range between 20 and 80 hours. Doses may be initiated at 2 mg twice daily and may be increased as needed to a desired effect. Alternatively, single 5-mg doses at night may be effective for nocturnal symptoms. Side effects include sedation and cognitive impairment, and there is a potential for dependence. The benzodiazepine withdrawal syndrome is characterized by anxiety, dysphoria, tremor, and sympathetic activa-

tion. Seizures can occur in susceptible patients (i.e., those with a low seizure threshold) or in those who undergo rapid withdrawal after chronic use.[23]

Tizanidine

Tizanidine (Zanaflex) is an imidazole derivative and is a centrally acting alpha-adrenergic agonist that inhibits the release of excitatory amino acids in spinal interneurons. It may also act by facilitating the action of glycine. Tizanidine has potent muscle-relaxing properties in animal models of spasticity[42] and, in spine-transected cats, suppresses polysynaptic reflexes.[43,44] Also, tizanidine enhances vibratory inhibition of the H-reflex in humans and reduces abnormal cocontraction, which may partly contribute to antispasticity effects.[45] In placebo-controlled trials, tizanidine reduces muscle tone and frequency of muscle spasms in patients with MS and spinal cord injury.[46–48] Similar efficacy was found in open-label trials for stroke patients.[49] In MS, tizanidine reduced spasticity without altering muscle strength, but no consistent positive effect was noted on functional measures (e.g., timed ambulation, upper-extremity function, or movements necessary in activities of daily living).[46] When compared to baclofen or diazepam in early trials, tizanidine demonstrated similar efficacy and better tolerability.[44,47,50–57] However, night-time insomnia and weakness are more frequent with tizanidine than baclofen.[50] No controlled trials have investigated tizanidine in combination with baclofen or tizanidine therapy in patients with developmental delays such as CP.

Tizanidine undergoes first-pass hepatic metabolism and subsequently is eliminated by the kidney. Its half-life is approximately 2.5 hours, and peak effect is seen 1–2 hours after dosage. Liver function tests should be checked at baseline, months 1, 3, and 6 of treatment, and periodically thereafter. Doses are initiated at 2–4 mg daily and are increased every 3 days by 2–4 mg. Total dose should not exceed 36 mg per day in three divided doses. Little experience has been reported with single doses greater than 8 mg. Side effects—including dry mouth (45%), drowsiness (54%), and dizziness—are seen primarily when doses exceed 24 mg per day. Visual hallucinations (3%) and elevated liver function tests (5%) are reversible with dose reduction.[46] Tizanidine does not affect blood pressure but, because central alpha-adrenergic agonists may cause hypotension, concomitant use of antihypertensive agents should be monitored closely, and clonidine should be avoided.[23]

Clonidine

Clonidine is a centrally acting alpha-adrenergic agonist used mainly to treat hypertension but can reduce symptoms of opiate withdrawal, impulsivity in children, and other behavioral problems. Central alpha activation reduces sympathetic outflow. Clonidine decreases the vibratory inhibition index in spinal cord patients[58] and reduces muscle tone in brain-injured patients (stroke, trauma, hematoma, CP).[59] It can be effective as a supplement to baclofen[60] but rarely is used as a single agent to treat spasticity. It is available in 0.1-mg tablets, but the Catapres patch (0.1 mg and 0.2 mg) is designed to deliver the specified dose daily and must be changed every 7 days. Side effects include bradycardia, hypotension, dry mouth, drowsiness, constipation, dizziness, and depression.[23]

Dantrolene Sodium

Dantrolene sodium (Dantrium) is a hydantoin derivative. It acts directly on muscle contractile elements, decreasing the release of calcium from skeletal muscle sarcoplasmic reticulum and thereby interfering with the excitation-contraction coupling needed to contract muscles.[61-63] The effect is most pronounced on extrafusal fibers, but a minor effect also is seen on intrafusal fibers. Whether this effect may alter spindle sensitivity is unclear.[64] Dantrolene has a greater effect on fast-twitch fibers (those that produce rapid contraction and high tension but fatigue relatively easily) than on slow-twitch fibers (those that contract tonically, producing less tension, but are more resistant to fatigue).[65]

Placebo-controlled trials of dantrolene demonstrated significant reduction of muscle tone and hyperreflexia.[63,66-68] In a double-blind crossover design in 42 MS patients, both dantrolene and diazepam decreased spasticity, clonus, hyperreflexia, muscle stiffness, and cramping.[69] In children with CP[70] and in patients with spasticity due

to various cerebral and spinal disorders,[71] studies found that spasticity was slightly better controlled and side effects more tolerable with dantrolene than with diazepam.

The half-life for oral dantrolene is approximately 15 hours, with peak concentrations occurring in 3–6 hours. It is metabolized mainly by the liver. Dantrolene is initiated at 25 mg per day and should be increased slowly, in increments of 25 mg per day every 5–7 days, with a recommended maximum of 400 mg per day in divided doses. Because its site of action is peripheral, the most common side effect is weakness, the mechanism by which it mediates its antispasticity action. For this reason, dantrolene may be most appropriate for nonambulatory patients with severe spasticity. Other side effects include drowsiness, diarrhea, and malaise. Because hepatotoxicity—which can be irreversible—is the major concern with dantrolene sodium, in those patients who are being considered for therapy, liver function tests should be evaluated prior to the initiation of therapy and every 3 months thereafter.[23]

Gabapentin

Gabapentin (Neurontin) was first introduced in 1994 to treat partial epilepsy.[72] It is structurally similar to GABA, possibly exerting GABA-ergic activity by binding to receptors in neocortex and hippocampus. However, it does not bind conventional GABA(A), GABA(B), glycine, glutamate, benzodiazepine, or N-methyl-D-aspartate receptors.[73,74] It is well absorbed, reaching peak plasma concentrations in 2–3 hours, is not protein-bound, does not undergo metabolism, and is excreted unchanged in the urine. Gabapentin is well-tolerated in doses of 1,800–3,600 mg.[75] Preliminary reports suggested that it can reduce spasticity,[75,76] but further studies are needed.[23]

Botulinum Toxin

Botulinum toxin is a product of *Clostridium botulinum*, and ingestion of the organism or its spores results in botulism. Botulinum toxin blocks presynaptic release of acetylcholine from the nerve terminal. Seven immunologically distinct toxins (types A–G) have been purified. Local intramuscular injection of botulinum toxin A (Botox) was approved to treat strabismus and blepharospasm associated with dystonia. When injected, the agent spreads through muscle and fascia approximately 30 mm, binding presynaptic cholinergic nerve terminals and resulting in a chemical denervation.[23]

Botulinum toxin injection effectively reduces muscle tone and spasms in patients with severe spasticity due to stroke, traumatic brain injury, and other causes.[77–80] Snow et al.[81] studied botulinum toxin A in nine patients with advanced MS (wheelchair- or bed-bound) in a randomized, crossover, double-blind study. Muscle tone, frequency of spasms, and hygiene and self-care scores were used to assess efficacy. Botulinum toxin injection produced a significant reduction in spasticity and improvement in ease of nursing care, with no adverse effects. Botulinum toxin injection is promising therapy for the treatment of spasticity in children with CP.[82,83] Judicious use of botulinum toxin can delay surgery until children reach a more suitable age.

Although botulinum toxin injection is off-label for treatment of spasticity, it may be an appropriate option for selected patients with severe localized spasms. Physicians who inject it should be trained in the use of Botox, with attention to relevant topical anatomy and kinesiology. Onset of focal muscle fiber paralysis begins in 24–72 hours, with a maximal effect seen at 5–14 days. Localizing specific muscles with electromyographic guidance may be necessary to produce optimal effects. The paralysis is transient, lasting 12–16 weeks. Injection site reactions can occur and antibodies may develop to specific immunologic strains, limiting efficacy. Because the delivery of toxin is not entirely contained, the paralysis of muscles may not be exact. Excessive weakness, although ultimately reversible, may result.[23]

4-Aminopyridine

4-Aminopyridine (4-AP) is a voltage-gated, fast potassium channel blocker capable of improving axonal conduction by facilitating the propagation of action potentials in demyelinated nerve fibers.[84] 4-AP is well absorbed and reaches peak concentrations in 2–4 hours.[85] Preclinical trials of orally administered 4-AP found transient improvements in neurologic function in patients with long-standing spinal cord

injury.[86] Administration of 4-AP led to marked and sustained reductions in upper- or lower-extremity spasticity due to cervical cord lesions. Other clinical benefits included reduced pain, restored muscle strength, improved sensation, voluntary control of bowel function, and sustained penile tumescence. The patients also exhibited improved hand function, enhanced mobility in transfers and gait, and improved endurance and energy.[86]

Segal et al.[84] studied long-term safety and efficacy of orally administrated, immediate-release 4-AP. They found that in patients receiving 6 mg per day (low-dose) or 30 mg per day (high-dose) over a period of 3 months, each patient who received the high-dose regimen displayed improvement and recovery of sensory and motor function and diminished spasticity. Oral 4-AP was well tolerated during this 3-month study. However, side effects can include dizziness, nausea, restlessness and anxiety, paresthesias, abdominal pain, and obstipation.[86] Other investigations evaluating the effects of 4-AP in patients with spinal cord injury report enhanced gait,[87] improved motor control and sensory ability below the injury site, and reduction in chronic pain and spasticity.[88] One study using intravenous 4-AP to treat pain and spasticity in spinal cord injury found that benefits did not outweigh adverse effects.[89] 4-AP is not approved by the U.S. Food and Drug Administration.

Epileptogenic effects of 4-AP are documented in experimental studies and by clinical observations. Application of 4-AP on hippocampal slices produced several patterns of epileptiform discharges and seizurelike events.[90] In studies of 4-AP to treat spinal cord injury in rats, all animals that received a dose of 6 mg/kg had generalized seizures.[7] New onset of seizures can complicate 4-AP therapy in MS patients.[91]

Additional Pharmacotherapeutic Option: Intrathecal Baclofen

When oral medication fails in a patient with persistent severe spasticity, intrathecal administration of baclofen should be considered. A pump with reservoir is surgically implanted in the subcutaneous tissue or subfascial tissue on the abdominal wall. Then, a catheter is threaded into the subarachnoid space, allowing delivery of baclofen directly into the cerebrospinal fluid. This allows as much as four times the level of drug to be delivered at only 1% of the oral dose, without concomitant elevation of serum levels, thereby reducing unwanted cerebral side effects, such as lethargy.

Penn et al.[92] conducted a double-blind, placebo-controlled 3-day crossover study in 20 patients— 10 with MS and 10 with spinal cord injury. All patients had decreased muscle tone and frequency of spasms while being treated with baclofen. All patients were subsequently enrolled in a long-term open trial of continuous baclofen infusion, with a mean follow-up period of 19 months. Using a standardized scale to assess spasticity, these researchers found that all patients exhibited normal tone and that spasm frequency was diminished to the point that spasms no longer interfered with activities of daily living.[93] In seven of eight patients, bladder function also improved.[92] Other investigators have found equally dramatic results.[94–96] Safety and efficacy on long-term follow-up was documented in patients for up to 84 months.[97]

Intrathecal baclofen can effectively treat spasticity in two groups of CP patients. First are spastic diplegics or spastic quadriplegics who can ambulate with or without assistance but who have weak legs and use their spasticity to stand or walk. The ability to ambulate might be lost if spasticity were eliminated completely by rhizotomy but, because of underlying leg weakness, excessive spasticity limits ambulation. The goal of treatment for these patients is to allow them to walk with less effort. Second are nonambulatory patients with tetraplegia and severe spasticity in whom the goal of treatment is to facilitate their care and relieve discomfort.[98]

The efficacy and tolerability of continuous intrathecal infusion of baclofen can be tested by administering a trial bolus of baclofen by intrathecal injection.[99,100] In studies of CP patients, intrathecal baclofen injections in the 25- to 100-μg range led to significant reductions in muscle tone within 2 hours. The effects persisted for 6 hours. Long-term follow-up in CP patients revealed that spasticity remains almost 50% improved after more than 3 years of continuous intrathecal baclofen therapy.[101]

Intrathecal baclofen may improve medically refractory dystonia. Continuous intrathecal baclofen infusion was used with modest success in a case of hereditary generalized dystonia refractory to multiple medications and thalamotomy.[102] After pump implantation, baclofen dosage was gradually increased to 450 μg per day. The patient displayed significant improvement on the right side of her body and moderate improvement on the left side. On an average daily dose of 575 μg per day of intrathecal baclofen, 10 of 12 patients with generalized dystonia had significant reduction in scores for overall dystonia and the extremities, trunk, and cervical regions.[103] One-year follow-up studies of dystonic patients support the long-term efficacy of intrathecal baclofen for dystonia.[104]

After a patient undergoes a trial of intrathecal baclofen to establish responsiveness, pump implantation can be considered. Starting doses are 25 μg per day up to an average of 400–500 μg per day, although doses as high as 1,500 μg per day have been reported.[105] The half-life of intrathecal baclofen is approximately 5 hours. Many patients require increased dosing in the first 6 months due to tolerance.[106,107] Most side effects tend to occur during the titration phase and include drowsiness, headache, nausea, weakness, and hypotension. Reversible coma can result from baclofen overdosing.[108] Other complications may be due to mechanical problems (dislodgment, disconnection, kinking, blockage), pump failure, or infection. Intrathecal baclofen is costly and, although useful, should be considered only in patients with severe functional limitations who have not responded satisfactorily to other therapeutic options.

Epileptogenic Effects of Antispasticity Drugs

Early clinical studies suggested that baclofen might be a proconvulsant and could exacerbate epilepsy. However, two prospective studies found that baclofen neither increased seizure frequency in epilepsy patients[109] nor provoked paroxysmal activity on electroencephalography.[110] Baclofen may suppress epileptiform activity in the hippocampus at concentrations below those that suppress normal synaptic transmission. Several reports suggest that baclofen may reduce myoclonus in epilepsy patients.[111–113] Baclofen is not contraindicated in epilepsy patients but should be tapered gradually in these patients. As described earlier, 4-AP may provoke epileptiform discharges and seizures.

Antispasticity Effects of Antiepileptic and Other Drugs

Phenytoin and chlorpromazine were preliminarily investigated in open and controlled studies to treat spasticity. In both types of studies, most patients exhibited objective and subjective improvement to each drug.[114] Tone was reduced in spastic muscles, and functional status was improved. The combination of phenytoin and chlorpromazine was most effective. Lethargy and somnolence were the most common side effects. These drugs may exert their action by suppressing fusimotor efferent as well as afferent discharges from muscle spindles.[113] Notably, phenytoin toxicity can worsen spasticity.[115]

Tiagabine, a GABA uptake inhibitor developed as an AED, may reduce spasticity. In an open-label study, 14 children with congenital or acquired spastic quadriplegia and intractable epilepsy were treated with tiagabine. Tiagabine dosage gradually was titrated upward until seizures ceased, adverse effects supervened, or the maximum dose of 1.1 mg/kg daily was reached. The mean improvement in motor function was approximately 50%. Other findings included improved muscle tone, strength, coordination, range of motion, and relaxation of extremities, with less ataxia and wobbling.[116]

In one patient, baclofen and sodium valproate were used successfully to relieve writer's cramp. Writer's cramp may result from striatal dopaminergic hyperactivity. Both sodium valproate and baclofen can increase GABA-ergic activity.[117] The two drugs may act synergistically to reduce activity in the nigrostriatal dopaminergic pathway and inhibit release of dopamine in the striatum.[118]

Baclofen and carbamazepine combined therapy can reduce spasticity and improve muscle tone, range of motion, and coordination in patients with brainstem and other supraspinal injuries.[119] Bittencourt and Silvado[120] observed that in several epilepsy patients who also exhibited spasticity, oxcarbazepine reduced both seizure frequency and spasticity throughout the study. Minor side effects included nausea and dizziness. These authors subsequently assessed two MS patients and one transverse myelitis patient with lower-extremity spasticity. The antispastic effect of oxcarbazepine occurred at doses between 600 and 1,200 mg daily, usually below that which produced nausea, dizziness, and somnolence.[121]

Combined baclofen and clonazepam therapy may also be successful in treating spasticity. Cendrowski and Sobzcyk[122] studied 25 patients with MS and other spastic disorders, 33 MS patients without other spastic disorders, and 10 control patients, all of whom were given clonazepam, baclofen, or placebo. Clonazepam and baclofen were significantly more effective than placebo for spasticity; clonazepam and baclofen monotherapy were equally effective. However, trends were apparent that suggested that clonazepam was more effective in patients with slight muscle hypertonia mainly of cerebral origin and that baclofen was better suited to patients with severe spinal spasticity. The combination of both drugs was most effective in treating some MS patients.[122]

Drug Interactions between Antiepileptic Drugs and Antispasticity Agents

No chemical interactions between antispasticity drugs and AEDs are well documented. In vitro studies of cytochrome P450 isoenzymes suggest that none of the following drugs are likely to affect hepatic metabolism of AEDs (or other drugs): baclofen, diazepam, dantrolene, clonidine, botox, gabapentin, 4-AP, and their metabolites. Thus, spasticity drugs do not interact pharmacokinetically with AEDs. None of the drugs used to treat spasticity lower the seizure threshold. However, rapid withdrawal or abrupt discontinuation of baclofen or benzodiazepines should be avoided, as these changes could provoke seizures. In therapeutic doses, AEDs do not worsen spasticity and, in some cases, the AEDs (e.g., phenytoin, tiagabine, carbamazepine, oxcarbazepine) may actually reduce spasticity.

Surgical Treatment

Central Procedures

Spinal Cord Procedures

The spinal stretch reflex arc can be interrupted at the level of the spinal cord. McCarty and Kiefer[123] first described the cordotomy procedure in 1949. Because this radical procedure often had undesirable effects such as sensory loss and worsened bladder function, it is no longer preformed to treat spasticity. The longitudinal myelotomy was introduced in 1951 by Bischof.[124] To avoid damaging descending motor pathways, he later modified this procedure from a lateral to a dorsal longitudinal myelotomy.[125] Laitinen et al.[126] used this procedure in patients with spinal cord injury, CP, and MS, noting relief of spasticity in eight of nine patients but recurrence of spasticity over time. Transient bladder dysfunction and permanent sensory deficits also occurred. Moyes[127] reported that 19 of 21 patients who underwent longitudinal myelotomy had good results. This procedure has been recommended for patients with severe spinal cord injuries or diseases with severe intractable, bilateral, lower-extremity spasticity.[128]

In 1986, Sindou et al.[129] modified the selective dorsal rhizotomy such that afferent fibers were divided as they entered the spinal cord in the dorsal root entry zone (DREZ). This DREZotomy consists of a 3-mm–deep microsurgical incision directed at a 45-degree angle in the posterolateral sulcus at the involved spinal levels. This incision destroys nociceptive and myotatic fibers but spares the lemniscal fibers, thus interrupting the spinal reflex arc and nociceptive pathways. Although originally performed in adult hemiplegic patients with severe upper-extremity spasticity, favorable results were reported in 121 patients treated with microsurgical DREZotomy for lower-extremity spasticity.[128,130]

Stereotactic Procedures

Such stereotactic procedures as pallidotomy, pulvinolysis, and ventrolateral thalamotomy are used to treat extrapyramidal disorders characterized by involuntary movements and fluctuations in tone. The basal ganglia modulates motor activity, forming the center of a looping circuit between cortical motor areas and thalamus. Basal ganglia diseases may release inhibition and thereby result in abnormal movements. Stereotactic thalamotomy can reduce unilateral tremor, athetosis, and chorea, but it is not effective for spasticity.[128,131–133]

Stereotactic cerebellar lesions that interrupt outflow from the dentate nucleus (dentatomy) can diminish muscle tone by reducing the unbalanced facilitatory influences on the ventral horn cells. Gornall et al.[133] reported improvement in five of

six children with spastic CP who underwent stereotactic dentatomy. However, Guidetti and Fraioli[134] reported a series of dentatomies in 47 patients and noted some improvement in dystonias but little effect on spasticity. Siegfried et al.[135] observed that dentatomy may reduce spasticity in some cases. Overall, stereotactic procedures have not proven very effective in spastic conditions.[128]

Implanted Stimulators

Electrical stimulation of the cerebellum was initially reported by Cooper et al.[136] in 1976 to increase inhibitory outflow on the ventral motor neurons. Cooper's group implanted a subdural stimulator on the surface of the cerebellum as a "pacemaker" to decrease the extensor hypertonia in patients with spastic CP. In 1980, Davis et al.[137] reported on a series of 262 patients, 230 of whom had spastic CP and underwent chronic cerebellar stimulator implantation. Primary effect was a lowering of spastic muscle tone in 90% of patients. Six months postoperatively, 25 patients were out of their wheelchairs and another 47 had improved ambulation. Davis's group[138] later conducted a double-blind trial in 33 patients, of whom 75% enjoyed qualitative improvement in spasticity and function. Other groups, however, could not demonstrate consistent successful reductions in spasticity with chronic cerebellar stimulation.[136,138–141] Harris et al.[142] recently reported a series of 13 children with CP with up to 14 years of follow-up and concluded that cerebellar stimulation was initially effective in reducing hypertonicity but that effectiveness decreased significantly after 3–5 years. Although some groups still advocate chronic cerebellar stimulation,[143,144] this procedure rarely is used to manage spasticity.[128]

Dorsal spinal cord stimulation was introduced to treat chronic pain disorders but was found also to improve motor function in a patient with MS and to reduce painful spasticity in a patient with metastatic spinal disease.[145] Subsequent experience with chronic epidural spinal cord stimulation varies. Quantitative measures of spasticity improved in a series of 48 patients with spinal cord injury[146] but, in another series of 17 patients, only 1 patient gained long-term relief of spasticity.[147] Cervical spinal cord stimulation can reduce spasticity on functional, neurophysiologic, and subjective measures,[148,149] but its rare use suggests that clinically significant benefits are uncommon.

Peripheral Procedures

Dorsal Rhizotomy

Dorsal rhizotomy was performed first by Abbe in the late nineteenth century to relieve pain,[150] and Sherrington[151] pioneered the use of this procedure to improve spasticity in decerebrate cats. Fifteen years later, Foerster[152] reported decreased spasticity and improvement in posture and function after the division of complete dorsal nerve roots in 159 patients, 88 of whom had congenital spastic paraplegia. Foerster[152] divided the entire dorsal nerve roots from L2 to S2, sparing L4 to preserve knee extension for standing. He used intraoperative electrical stimulation to identify the nerve roots associated with knee extension and to distinguish between ventral and dorsal roots. Because this procedure caused disabling sensory deficits, it was modified such that only four-fifths of the dorsal lumbosacral nerve rootlets were sectioned. However, this revision still caused troublesome sensorimotor deficits. Intraoperative electrical stimulation and electromyography allowed rootlets innervating functionally important muscles to be spared and rootlets innervating the most dysfunctional muscle groups (e.g., hip adductors and flexors) to be cut.[153,154]

Selective Dorsal Lumbosacral Rhizotomy

During the 1970s, Fasano et al.[155] found that certain dorsal rootlets displayed an abnormal response to stimulation in spastic patients. In a selective dorsal lumbosacral rhizotomy surgical procedure, rootlets that responded to electrical stimulation with expected brief muscular contraction were spared, whereas those that evoked abnormally prolonged contractions that often spread to adjacent muscle groups were divided.[155] This Fasano procedure then was modified to identify better the sacral nerve roots involved in sphincter control. By performing a more caudal laminectomy, the surgeon can better expose the cauda equina and roots exiting the neural foramina, improving verification of nerve root levels and ventral versus dorsal rootlets. On completion of an L2 through S1 laminectomy, the dorsal nerve rootlets between L2 and S2 are electrically stimulated and selectively divided on the basis of intraoperative electromyography and visual observation and palpation of muscle responses. Between 25% and 50% of rootlets usually are divided, but more may be divided in treating a severely affected individual. Care must be taken to ensure that not all rootlets of a particular level are divided.[128]

Selective dorsal rhizotomy improves spasticity only and is indicated for patients in whom spasticity is the main physical handicap. Clinical evaluation focuses on muscle tone, tendon reflexes, range of motion, movement patterns, posture, gait, and functional capacity. The muscle disturbance must be due to spasticity, not dystonia or athetosis. The ideal patient is a spastic diplegic child without significant weakness or fixed contractures who ambulates independently with a scissoring gait, flexed hips and knees, and an equinus foot posture.[156,157]

Potential neurosurgical complications include increased weakness, sensory loss, sexual dysfunction, and spinal instability or deformity. Other adverse effects include wound infection, urinary tract infection or cystitis, hemorrhage, cerebrospinal fluid leakage, and respiratory complications.

Dorsal Cervical Rhizotomy

Dorsal cervical rhizotomy is rarely used, being reserved primarily for severe upper-extremity spasticity, dyskinesis, or athetosis. McCouch et al.[158] found that the afferent endings for tonic neck reflexes were in the joints between the occiput, atlas, and axis. By performing complete dorsal rhizotomies of the C1 through C3 nerve roots, Kottke[159] reported functional improvement in the upper extremities and more coordinated facial movement; in addition, reflex grimacing and symmetric and asymmetric tonic neck reflexes were abolished. Other groups, however, reported reduced upper-extremity spasticity but limited functional improvement.[160–162]

Anterior Rhizotomy

In 1945, Munro[163] described the technique of anterior rhizotomy to relieve painful spasticity in 10 patients with complete spinal cord injuries. The procedure is no longer performed owing to flaccid paralysis and atrophy that resulted.

Smyth and Peacock[128] performed anterior rhizotomy on three patients with incapacitating upper-extremity choreoathetoid movements. Intraoperative electrical stimulation and electromyography identified the ventral rootlets of the fifth through seventh cervical nerves. These rootlets were divided, paralyzing the abductors of the shoulder and flexors and extensors of the elbows but preserving distal sensorimotor function. The violent arm movements ceased, but only partial function was preserved.[128]

Peripheral Neurectomy

Peripheral neurectomy involves sectioning the peripheral nerve or motor nerve branch to reduce overactivity of a muscle or muscle group. Because peripheral nerves contain motor and sensory fibers, division can cause sensory loss, weakness, and atrophy.

In the upper extremities, neurectomy of the musculocutaneous nerve can relieve spastic elbow flexion.[164] Microneurosurgical ablation of fascicles in 52 spastic patients produced complete relief for 63% and some degree of improvement for 37%.[165] Selective peripheral neurectomy of collateral motor branches of the brachial plexus has been shown to relieve spasticity in the shoulder in five patients.[166]

Peripheral neurectomies in the lower limbs can improve spastic calf muscles. Feve et al.[167] noted clinical and electrophysiologic improvement in spasticity. They also reported abolition of ankle clonus and improved ankle angular variations in a large series of patients undergoing posterior tibial nerve collateral branch neurectomy. Tibial neurectomy improved gait significantly in some patients.[168] However, Berard et al.[169] found that symptoms recurred in 8 of 13 children (61%) with spastic hemiplegia who underwent unilateral tibial neurectomy.

Peripheral Nerve and Motor Point Block

Motor points are well-defined areas of the muscle that produce maximum contraction when the motor nerve branch passing through the muscle is stimulated. To relieve spasticity, motor blocks can be performed by injection of anesthetic agents or phenol into the peripheral nerve or muscle belly near the motor point and may last up to 6 months.[167,170,171] Alcohol blocks provide a shorter duration of relief of spasticity, lasting 1–6 weeks, and may be helpful in evaluating responses in spastic children without fixed contractures before more permanent procedures are undertaken.[172] A needle electrode is used to inject phenol and alcohol into the muscle belly after the motor point has been initially defined with a surface electrode. Spastic forearm flexors, hip adductors, and foot plantar-flexors can be injected to reduce scissoring and equinus deformity.[128] The peripheral nerve can also be injected either interneurally or perineurally, with both procedures risking damage to afferent pathways.

Common injection sites include the median and ulnar nerves for wrist and finger spasticity, the musculocutaneous nerve for elbow spasticity, the obturator nerve for scissoring, and the posterior tibial nerve for relief of equinus deformity. Complications include causalgia and dysesthesias, cardiac arrhythmias, and permanent neurologic deficits.[173]

Conclusion

As in any symptomatic therapy, the treatment of spasticity should be individualized. Goals for therapy and realistic expectations should be established by both care provider and patient. Conservative measures should be incorporated in antispasticity regimens. Stretching, massage, and passive range-of-motion exercises are extremely important in preventing muscle shortening and the formation of contractures. Guidance on proper positioning and posture and on how to avoid specific positions that may elicit clonus or spasms can result in increased function.

Patients should be evaluated for adaptive equipment such as ambulatory aids, reachers, and other devices and should be instructed in the appropriate use of these tools. Direct effects of muscle relaxation from physiotherapy often are short-lived and, for many patients, these conservative measures alone are insufficient to treat their symptoms. Most patients experience symptomatic improvement with physiotherapy in combination with one or more antispasticity agents. Patients whose condition is refractory to these treatment options may respond to a variety of neurosurgical procedures to relieve severe spasticity. A practitioner's understanding of the mechanisms of these therapies should aid in developing individualized regimens for patients.

References

1. Lance JW. Symposium Synopsis. In RG Feldman, RR Young, WP Koella (eds), Spasticity: Disordered Motor Control. Chicago: Yearbook Medical, 1980;485–494.
2. Young RR. Spasticity: a review. Neurology 1994;44[Suppl 9]:S12–S20.
3. Carpenter MB. Core Text of Neuroanatomy (4th ed). Baltimore: Williams & Wilkins, 1991;101–110.
4. Curtis BA, Jacobson S, Marcus EM. An Introduction to the Neurosciences. Philadelphia: Saunders, 1972;200–206.
5. Meythaler JM, Tuel SM, Cross LL. Spinal cord seizures: a possible cause of isolated myoclonic activity in traumatic spinal cord injury: a case report. Paraplegia 1991;29(8):557–560.
6. Cherrick AA, Ellenberg M. Spinal cord seizures in transverse myelopathy: report of two cases. Arch Phys Med Rehabil 1986;67(2):129–131.
7. Haghighi SS, Clapper A, Johnson GC, et al. Effect of 4-aminopyridine and single dose methylprednisolone on functional recovery after a chronic spinal cord injury. Spinal Cord 1998;36(1):6–12.
8. Albright AL. Spasticity and movement disorders in cerebral palsy. J Child Neurol 1996;11[Suppl 1]:S1–S4.
9. Kyllerman M, Baber B, Billie B. Dyskinetic cerebral palsy. Acta Paediatr Scand 1982;71:543–550.
10. Kuben KCK, Leviton A. Cerebral palsy. N Engl J Med 1994;330:188–195.
11. The Australian and New Zealand Perinatal Societies. The origins of cerebral palsy—a consensus statement. Med J Aust 1995;162:85–90.
12. Bax M, Nelson KB. Birth asphyxia: a statement. Dev Med Child Neurol 1993;35:1022–1024.
13. Sugimoto T, Woo M, Nishida N. When do brain abnormalities in CP occur? An MRI study. Dev Med Child Neurol 1995;13:67–78.
14. Fahn S, Marsden CD, Calne DB. Classification and Investigation of Dystonia. In CD Marsden, S Fahn (eds), Movement Disorders 2. London: Butterworth, 1987;332–358.
15. Albright AL. Cerebral palsy. Pediatr Ann 1997;26:592–598.
16. Aicardi J. Epilepsy in brain-injured children. Dev Med Child Neurol 1990;32:191–202.
17. Hadjipanayis A, Hadjichristodoulou C, Youroukos S. Epilepsy in patients with cerebral palsy. Dev Med Child Neurol 1997;39:659–663.
18. Okumura A, Hayakawa F, Kato T, et al. Epilepsy in patients with spastic cerebral palsy: correlation with MRI findings at 5 years of age. Brain Dev 1999;21: 540–543.
19. Aksu F. Nature and prognosis of seizures in patients with cerebral palsy. Dev Med Child Neurol 1990;32: 661–668.
20. Bormann J. Electrophysiology of GABA(A) and GABA(B) receptor subtypes. Trends Neurosci 1988;11:112–116.
21. Davidoff RA. Antispasticity drugs: mechanism of action. Ann Neurol 1985;17:107–117.
22. van Hemet JCJ. A Double-Blind comparison of Baclofen and Placebo in Patients with Spasticity of Cerebral Origin. In RG Feldman, RR Young, WP Koella (eds), Spasticity: Disordered Motor Control. Chicago: Yearbook Medical, 1980.
23. Mariko K, Goodkin DE. Drugs used to treat spasticity. Drugs 2000;59(3):487–495.
24. Jerusalem F. A double-blind study on the antispastic action of beta-(4-chlorophenyl)-gamma-amino butyric acid in multiple sclerosis. Nervenarzt 1968;39:515.
25. Jones RF, Burke D, Morasszeky JE, Gillies DJ. A new agent for the control of spasticity. J Neurol Neurosurg Psychiatry 1970;33:464–468.
26. Hudgson P, Weightman D. Baclofen in the treatment of spasticity. BMJ 1971;4:15–17.
27. Pedersen E, Arlien-Soborg P, Mai J. The mode of action of the BAGA derivative baclofen in human spasticity. Acta Neurol Scand 1974;50:665–680.
28. Milanov IG. Mechanisms of baclofen action on spasticity. Acta Neurol Scand 1992;85:305–310.
29. Rivas DA, Chancellor MB, Hill K, Freedman MK. Neurological manifestations of baclofen withdrawal. J Urol 1993;150:1903–1905.
30. Kofler M, Leis A. Prolonged seizure activity after baclofen withdrawal. Neurology 1992;42:697–680.
31. Costa E, Guidotti A. Molecular mechanisms in the receptor action of the benzodiazepines. Annu Rev Toxicol 1979;19:531–545.
32. Schwarz M, Turski L, Janiszewski W, Sontag K-H. Is the muscle relaxant effect of diazepam in spastic mutant rats mediated through GABA-independent benzodiazepine receptors? Neurosci Lett 1983;36:175–180.
33. Pedersen E. Clinical assessment and pharmacologic therapy of spasticity. Arch Phys Med Rehabil 1974;55:344–354.
34. Kendall PH. The use of diazepam in hemiplegia. Ann Phys Med 1964;7:225–228.
35. Neill RW. Diazepam in the relief of muscle spasm resulting from spinal-cord lesions. Ann Phys Med 1964;[Suppl]:33–38.
36. Nathan PW. The action of diazepam in neurological disorders with excessive motor activity. J Neurol Sci 1970;10:33–50.
37. Corbett M, Frankel HL, Michaelis L. A double blind cross-over trial of Valium in the treatment of spasticity. Paraplegia 1972;10:19–22.

38. From A, Heltberg A. A double-blind trial with baclofen and diazepam in spasticity due to multiple sclerosis. Acta Neurol Scand 1975;51:158–166.
39. Roussan M, Terrence C, Fromm G. Baclofen versus diazepam for the treatment of spasticity and long-term follow-up of baclofen therapy. Pharmatherapeutica 1987;4(5):278–284.
40. Cartlidge NEF, Hudgson P, Weightman D. A comparison of baclofen and diazepam in the treatment of spasticity. J Neurol Sci 1974;23:17–24.
41. Mitchell G. Update on multiple sclerosis therapy. Med Clin North Am 1993;77:231–249.
42. Coward DM. Selective muscle relaxant properties of tizanidine and an examination of its mode of action. Triangle 1981;20:151–158.
43. Davies J. Selective depression of synaptic transmission of spinal neurones in the cat by a new centrally acting muscle relaxant, 5-chloro-4-(2-imidazolin-2-yl-amino)-2,1,3-benzothiadazole (DS 103 282). Br J Pharmacol 1982;76:473–481.
44. Newman PM, Nogues M, Newman PK, et al. Tizanidine in the treatment of spasticity. Eur J Clin Pharmacol 1982;23:31–35.
45. Delwaide PJ. Electrophysiological Testing of Spastic Patients: Its Potential Usefulness and Limitations. In PJ Delwaide, RR Young (eds), Clinical Neurophysiology in Spasticity. Amsterdam: Elsevier, 1985;185–203.
46. The United Kingdom Tizanidine Study Group. A double-blind placebo-controlled trial of tizanidine in the treatment of spasticity caused by multiple sclerosis. Neurology 1994;44[Suppl 9]:70–79.
47. Lapierre Y, Bouchard S, Tansey C, et al. Treatment of spasticity with tizanidine in multiple sclerosis. Can J Neurol Sci 1987;14:513–517.
48. Nance PW, Bugaresti J, Shellenberger K, et al. Efficacy and safety of tizanidine in the treatment of spasticity in patients with spinal cord injury. Neurology 1994;[Suppl 9]:S44–S52.
49. Milanov I, Georgiev D. Mechanisms of tizanidine action on spasticity. Acta Neurol Scand 1994;89:274–279.
50. Bass B, Weinshenker B, Rice GPA, et al. Tizanidine versus baclofen in the treatment of spasticity in patients with multiple sclerosis. Can J Sci 1988;15(1):15–19.
51. Stein R, Nordal HJ, Oftendal SI, Slebetto M. The treatment of spasticity in multiple sclerosis: a double-blind clinical trial of a new anti-spasticity drug tizanidine compared with baclofen. Acta Neurol Scand 1987;75:190–194.
52. Smolenski C, Muff S, Smolenski-Kauts S. A double-blind comparative trial of a new muscle-relaxant, tizanidine (DS102-282), and baclofen in the treatment of chronic spasticity in multiple sclerosis. Curr Med Res Opin 1981;7(6):374–383.
53. Hoorgstraten MC, van der Ploeg RJO, van der Burg W, et al. Tizanidine versus baclofen in the treatment of multiple sclerosis patients. Acta Neurol Scand 1988;77:224–230.
54. Eyssette M, Rohmer F, Serratrice G, et al. Multi-centre, double-blind trial of a novel antispastic agent, tizanidine, in spasticity associated with multiple sclerosis. Curr Med Res Opin 1988;10(10):699–708.
55. Pagano MA, Ferreiro ME, Herskovits E. Comparative study of tizanidine and baclofen in patients with chronic spasticity. Rev Neurol Argent 1988;14(4):268–276.
56. Rinne UK. Tizanidine treatment of spasticity in multiple sclerosis and chronic myelopathy. Curr Ther Res 1980;28(6):827–836.
57. Bes A, Eyssette M, Pierrot-Deseilligny E, et al. A multi-centre, double-blind trial of tizanidine, a new anti-spastic agent, in spasticity associated with hemiplegia. Curr Med Res Opin 1988;10:709–718.
58. Nance PW, Shears AH, Nance DM. Reflex changes induced by clonidine in spinal cord injured patients. Paraplegia 1989;4:296–301.
59. Dall JT, Harmon RL, Quinn CM. Use of clonidine for treatment of spasticity arising from various forms of brain injury: a case series. Brain Inj 1996;10(6):453–458.
60. Donovan WH, Carter RE, Rossi CD, Wilkerson MA. Clonidine effect on spasticity: a clinical trial. Arch Phys Med Rehabil 1988;69(3):193–194.
61. Herman R, Mayer N, Mecomber SA. Clinical pharmaco-physiology of dantrolene sodium. Am J Phys Med 1972;51:296–311.
62. Ellis KO, Carpenter JF. Mechanisms of control of skeletal muscle contraction by dantrolene sodium. Arch Phys Med Rehabil 1974;55:362–369.
63. Pinder RM, Brogden RN, Speight TM, Avery GS. Dantrolene sodium: a review of its pharmacological properties and therapeutic efficacy in spasticity. Drugs 1977;13:3–23.
64. Whyte J, Robinson KM. Pharmacologic Management. In M Glenn, J Whyte (eds), The Practical Management of Spasticity in Children and Adults. Philadelphia: Lea & Febiger, 1990.
65. Monster AW, Tamai Y, McHenry J. Dantrolene sodium in spasticity. Acta Neurol Scand 1979;59:309–316.
66. Gelenberg AJ, Poskanzer DC. The effect of dantrolene sodium on spasticity in multiple sclerosis. Neurology 1973;23:1313–1315.
67. Tolosa ES, Soll RW, Loewenson R. Treatment of spasticity in multiple sclerosis with dantrolene. JAMA 1975;233(10):1046.
68. Katrak PH, Cole A, Poulos CJ, McCauley JCK. Objective assessment of spasticity, strength and function with early exhibition of dantrolene sodium after cerebrovascular accident: a randomized double-blind study. Arch Phys Med Rehabil 1992;73:4–9.
69. Schmidt RT, Lee RH, Spehlman R. Comparison of dantrolene sodium and diazepam in the treatment of spasticity. J Neurol Neurosurg Psychiatry 1976;39:350–356.

70. Nogen AG. Medical treatment for spasticity in children with cerebral palsy. Childs Brain 1976;2:304–308.

71. Glass A, Hannah A. A comparison of dantrolene sodium and diazepam in the treatment of spasticity. Paraplegia 1974;12:170–174.

72. The US Gabapentin Study Group. The long-term safety and efficacy of gabapentin (Neurontin) as add-on therapy in drug-resistant partial epilepsy. Epilepsy Res 1994;18(1):67–73.

73. Fromm GH. Gabapentin. Epilepsia 1995;36[Suppl 5]:S77–S80.

74. McLean MJ. Gabapentin. Epilepsia 1995;36[Suppl]: S73–S86.

75. Priebe MM, Sherwood AM, Graves DE, et al. Effectiveness of gabapentin in controlling spasticity: a quantitative study. Spinal Cord 1997;35:171–175.

76. Dunevsky A, Perel A. Gabapentin for relief of spasticity associated with multiple sclerosis. Am J Phys Med Rehabil 1998;77:451–454.

77. Yablon SA, Agana BT, Ivanhoe CB, Boake C. Botulinum toxin in severe upper extremity spasticity among patients with traumatic brain injury: an open label trial. Neurology 1996;47:939–944.

78. Simpson DM, Alexander DN, O'Brien CF, et al. Botulinum toxin type A in the treatment of upper extremity spasticity: a randomized, double-blind, placebo-controlled trial. Neurology 1996;46:1306–1310.

79. Burbaud P, Wiart L, Dubos JL, et al. A randomized, double-blind placebo-controlled trial of botulinum toxin in the treatment of spastic foot in hemiparetic patients. J Neurol Neurosurg Psychiatry 1996;61:265–269.

80. Das TK, Park DM. Effect of treatment with botulinum toxin on spasticity. Postgrad Med J 1989;65:208–210.

81. Snow BJ, Tsui JKC, Bhatt MH, et al. Treatment of spasticity with botulinum toxin: a double-blind study. Ann Neurol 1990;28:512–515.

82. Cosgrove AP, Lorry IS, Graham HK. Botulinum toxin in the management of the lower limb in cerebral palsy. Dev Med Child Neurol 1994;36(5):386–396.

83. Koman LA, Mooney JF III, Smith BP, et al. Management of spasticity in cerebral palsy with botulinum-A toxin: report of a preliminary, randomized, double-blind trial. J Pediatr Orthop 1994;14(3):299–303.

84. Segal JL, Pathak MS, Hernandez JP, et al. Safety and efficacy of 4-aminopyridine in humans with spinal cord injury: a long-term, controlled trial. Pharmacotherapy 1999;19(6):713–723.

85. Segal JL, Hayes K, Brunnemann SR, et al. Absorption characteristics of sustained-release 4-aminopyridine (fampridine SR) in patients with chronic spinal cord injury. J Clin Pharmacol 2000;40:402–409.

86. Potter PJ, Hayes KC, Hsieh JT, et al. Sustained improvements in neurological function in spinal cord patients treated with oral 4-aminopyridine: three cases. Spinal Cord 1998;36(3):147–155.

87. Segal JL, Brunnemann SR. 4-Aminopyridine alters gait characteristics and enhances locomotion in spinal cord injured humans. J Spinal Cord Med 1998;21 (3):200–204.

88. Hansebout RR, Blight AR, Fawcett S, Reddy K. 4-Aminopyridine in chronic spinal cord injury: a controlled, double-blind, cross-over study in eight patients. J Neurotrauma 1993;10(1):1–18.

89. Donovan WH, Halter JA, Graves DE, et al. Intravenous infusion of 4-AP in chronic spinal cord injured subjects. Spinal Cord 2000;38(1):7–15.

90. Bruckner C, Heinemann U. Effects of standard anticonvulsant drugs on different patterns of epileptiform discharges induced by 4-aminopyridine in combined entorhinal cortex-hippocampal slices. Brain Res 2000;859(1):15–20.

91. Bever CT Jr, Anderson PA, Leslie J, et al. Treatment with oral 3,4-diaminopyridine improves leg strength in multiple sclerosis patients: results of a randomized, double-blind, placebo-controlled, crossover trial. Neurology 1996;47(6):1457–1462.

92. Penn RD, Savoy SM, Corcos D, et al. Intrathecal baclofen for severe spinal spasticity. N Engl J Med 1989;320:1517–1521.

93. Lee KC, Carson L, Kinnin E, Patterson V. The Ashworth Scale: a reliable and reproducible method of measuring spasticity. J Neurol Rehabil 1989;3:205–209.

94. Ochs G, Struppler A, Meyerson BA, et al. Intrathecal baclofen for long-term treatment of spasticity: a multicentre study. J Neurol Neurosurg Psychiatry 1989;52:933–939.

95. Albright AL, Barron WB, Fasick MP, et al. Continuous intrathecal baclofen infusion for spasticity of cerebral origin. JAMA 1993;270:2475–2477.

96. Dralle D, Muller H, Zierski J, Klug N. Intrathecal baclofen for spasticity. Lancet 1985;8462:1003.

97. Penn RD. Intrathecal baclofen for spasticity of spinal origin: seven years' experience. J Neurosurg 1992;77: 236–240.

98. Albright AL. Baclofen in the treatment of cerebral palsy. J Child Neurol 1996;11:77–83.

99. Wiens HD. Spasticity in children with cerebral palsy: a retrospective review of the effects of intrathecal baclofen. Issues Compr Pediatr Nurs 1998;21(1):49–61.

100. Albright AL, Cervi A, Singletary J. Intrathecal baclofen for spasticity in cerebral palsy. JAMA 1991;265:1418–1422.

101. Gilmartin R, Bruce D, Storrs B, et al. Intrathecal baclofen for management of spastic cerebral palsy: multicenter trial. J Child Neurol 2000;15:71–77.

102. Grande MA, Chacon J, Trujillo J, et al. Intrathecal perfusion pump with baclofen in generalized dystonia. Rev Neurol 2000;30(2):138–140.

103. Albright AL, Barry MJ, Shultz B. Infusion of intrathecal baclofen for generalized dystonia in cerebral palsy. J Neurosurg 1998;88(1):73–76.

104. Meythaler JM, Guin-Renfroe S, Grabb P, Hadley MN. Long-term continuously infused intrathecal baclofen for spastic-dystonic hypertonia in traumatic brain injury: 1-year experience. Arch Phys Med Rehabil 1999;80(1):13–19.

105. Nance PW, Schryvers OI, Schmidt BJ, et al. Intrathecal baclofen therapy for adults with spinal spasticity: therapeutic efficacy and effect on hospital admission. Can J Neurol Sci 1995;22:122–129.

106. Ashworth B. Preliminary trial of carisprodol in multiple sclerosis. Practitioner 1964;192:540–542.

107. Nanninga JB, Frost F, Penn R. Effect of intrathecal baclofen on bladder and sphincter function. J Urol 1989;142:101–105.

108. Siegfried J, Rea GL. Intrathecal application of drugs for muscle hypertonus. Scand J Rehab Med 1988;17 [Suppl]:145–148.

109. Terrance CF, Fromm GH, Roussan MS. Baclofen: its effects on seizure frequency. Arch Neurol 1983;40:28–29.

110. Badr GG, Matousek M, Frederiksen PK. A quantitative EEG analysis of the effects of baclofen on man. Neuropsychobiology 1983;10:13–18.

111. Coletti A, Mandelli A, Minoli G, Tredici G. Post-anoxic action myoclonus (Lance-Adams syndrome) treated with levodopa and GABA-ergic drugs. J Neurol 1980;223:67–70.

112. Pedersen E, Grynderup V, Kissmeyer-Nielsen F, et al. Familial progressive myoclonic epilepsy. J Neurol 1982;53:305–320.

113. Rosen I, Fehling C, Sedgwick M, Elmqvist D. Focal reflex epilepsy with myoclonus: electrophysiological investigation and therapeutic implications. Electroencephalogr Clin Neurophysiol 1977;42:95–106.

114. Cohen SL, Raines A, Panagakos J, Armitage P. Phenytoin and chlorpromazine in the treatment of spasticity. Arch Neurol 1980;37:360–364.

115. Stark RJ. Spasticity due to phenytoin toxicity. Med J Aust 1979;1(5):156.

116. Holden KR, Titus MO. The effect of tiagabine on spasticity in children with intractable epilepsy: a pilot study. Pediatr Neurol 1999;21(4):728–730.

117. Hill DR, Bowery N. H-1 Baclofen and H-1-GABA bind to bicuculline-insensitive GABA(B) sites in rat brain. Nature 1981;290:149–152.

118. Sandyk R. Treatment of writer's cramp with sodium valproate and baclofen. S Afr Med J 1983;63:702–703.

119. Fodstad H, Ljunggren BCA. Baclofen and carbamazepine in supraspinal spasticity. J R Soc Med 1991;84:100–101.

120. Bittencourt PR, Silvado CE. Oxcarbazepine, GP4-7779, and spasticity. Lancet 1985;2(8456):676.

121. Bittencourt PR. Oxcarbazepine and spasticity: further observations. Arq Neuropsiquiatr 1988;46(4):382–384.

122. Cendrowski W, Sobczyk W. Clonazepam, baclofen and placebo in the treatment of spasticity. Eur Neurol 1977;16:257–262.

123. McCarty CS, Kiefer EJ. Thoracic lumbar and sacral spinal cordectomy. Proc Staff Meet Mayo Clin 1949;24:108.

124. Bischof W. Die longitudinale myelotomie. Zentralbl Neurochir 1951;11:79–88.

125. Bischof W. Zur dorsalen longitudinalen myelotomie. Zentralbl Neurochir 1967;28:123–126.

126. Laitinen L, Nilsson S, Fugl-Myer AR. Selective posterior rhizotomy for treatment of spasticity. J Neurosurg 1983;58:895–899.

127. Moyes PD. Longitudinal myelotomy for spasticity. J Neurosurg 1969;31:615–619.

128. Smyth MD, Peacock WJ. The surgical treatment of spasticity. Muscle Nerve 2000;23:153–163.

129. Sindou M, Misfud JJ, Boisson D, Goutelle A. Selective posterior rhizotomy in the dorsal root entry zone for treatment of hyperspasticity and pain in the hemiplegic upper limb. Neurosurgery 1986;18:587–595.

130. Mertens P, Sindou M. Microsurgical DREZotomy for the treatment of spasticity of the lower limbs. Neurochirurgie 1998;44:209–218.

131. Balasubramaniam V, Kanaka TS, Ramanujam PB. Stereotaxic surgery for cerebral palsy. J Neurosurg 1974;40:577–582.

132. Broggi G, Angelini L, Bono R. Long-term results of stereotaxic thalamotomy for cerebral palsy. Neurosurgery 1983;12:195–202.

133. Gornall P, Hitchcock E, Kirkland IS. Stereotaxic neurosurgery in the management of cerebral palsy. Dev Med Child Neurol 1975;17:279–286.

134. Guidetti B, Fraioli B. Neurosurgical treatment of spasticity and dyskinesias. Acta Neurochir Suppl (Wien) 1977;24:27–39.

135. Siegfried J, Lazorthes Y, Broggi G, et al. La neurochirurgie fonctionnelle delíinfirmite motrice cerebrale. Neurochirurgie 1985;31:1–118.

136. Cooper IS, Riklan M, Amin I, et al. Chronic cerebellar stimulation in cerebral palsy. Neurology 1976;26:744–753.

137. Davis R, Schulman J, Delehanty A. Cerebellar stimulation for cerebral palsy—five-year study. Acta Neurochir Suppl (Wien) 1980;30:317–332.

138. Schulman JH, Davis R, Nanes M. Cerebellar stimulation for spastic cerebral palsy: preliminary report. Ongoing double blind study. Pacing Clin Electrophysiol 1987;10:226–231.

139. Nomura Y, Fukuuchi A, Iwade M, et al. A case of spasticity following spinal cord injury improved by epidural spinal cord stimulation. Masui 1995;44:732–734.

140. Gottlieb GL, Myklebust BM, Stefosk D. Evaluation of cervical stimulation for chronic treatment of spasticity. Neurology 1985;35:699–704.

141. Hugenholtz H, Humphreys P, McIntyre WM, et al. Cervical spinal cord stimulation for spasticity in cerebral palsy. Neurosurgery 1988;22:707–714.

142. Harris GF, Millar EA, Hemmy DC, Lochner RC. Neuroelectric stimulation in cerebral palsy: long-

term quantitative assessment. Stereotact Funct Neurosurg 1993;61(2):49–59.

143. Bensman AS, Szegho M. Cerebellar electrical stimulation: a critique. Arch Phys Med Rehabil 1978;59:485–487.

144. Ivan LP, Ventureyra EC, Wiely J, et al. Chronic cerebellar stimulation in cerebellar palsy. Surg Neurol 1981;15:81–84.

145. Ivan LP, Ventureyra EC. Chronic cerebellar stimulation in cerebral palsy. Childs Brain 1982;9:121–125.

146. Barolat G, Singh-Sahni K, Staas WE Jr, et al. Epidural spinal cord stimulation in the management of spasms in spinal cord injury: a prospective study. Stereotact Funct Neurosurg 1995;64(3):153–164.

147. Midha M, Schmitt JK. Epidural spinal cord stimulation for the control of spasticity in spinal cord injury patients lacks long-term efficacy and is not cost-effective. Spinal Cord 1998;36(3):190–192.

148. Galanda M, Hovath S. Different effect of chronic electrical stimulation of the region of the superior cerebellar peduncle and the nucleus ventralis intermedius of the thalamus in the treatment of movement disorders. Stereotact Funct Neurosurg 1997; 69:116–120.

149. Galanda M, Mistina L, Zoltan O. Behavioural responses to cerebral stimulation in cerebral palsy. Acta Neurochir Suppl (Wien) 1989;46:37–38.

150. Abbe R. Resection of the posterior roots of spinal nerves to relieve pain, pain reflex, and spastic paralysis—Dana's operation. Med Record (NY) 1911; 79:377–381.

151. Sherrington CS. Decerebrate rigidity and reflex coordination of movements. J Physiol (Lond) 1898; 22:319–337.

152. Foerster O. On the indications and results of the excision of posterior spinal nerve roots in man. Surg Gynecol Obstet 1913;16:463–474.

153. Geos C, Ouknine G, Vlahovitch B, Frerebeau P. La radicotomie selective posterieure dans le traitement neurochirurgical de l'hypertonie pyramidale. Neurochirurgie 1967;13:505–518.

154. Privat JM, Benezech J, Frerebeau P, Gros C. Sectorial posterior rhizotomy, a new technique of surgical treatment for spasticity. Acta Neurochir (Wien) 1976;35:181–195.

155. Fasano VA, Broggi G, Barolat-Romana G, Sguazzi A. Surgical treatment of spasticity in cerebral palsy. Childs Brain 1978;4:289–305.

156. Baker LD, Hill LM. Foot alignment in the cerebral palsy patient. J Bone Joint Surg 1964;40:577–582.

157. Banks HH, Green WT. The correction of equinus deformity in cerebral palsy. J Bone Joint Surg 1958; 40:1359–1379.

158. McCouch GP, Deering ID, Ling TH. Location of receptors for tonic neck reflexes. J Neurophysiol 1951;14:191–195.

159. Kottke FJ. Modification of athetosis by denervation of the tonic neck reflexes. Dev Med Child Neurol 1981;15:81–84.

160. Benedetti A, Carbonin C, Colombo F. Extended posterior cervical rhizotomy for severe spastic syndromes with dyskinesias. Appl Neurophysiol 1977; 40:41–47.

161. Peacock WJ, Staudt LA. Central and peripheral neurosurgical management of cerebral palsy. Semin Orthop 1987;4:229–235.

162. Fraioli B, Nicci F, Baldassarree L. Bilateral cervical rhizotomy: effects on dystonia and athetosis, on respiration and other autonomic functions. Appl Neurophysiol 1977;40:26–40.

163. Munro D. The rehabilitation of patients totally paralyzed below the waist: anterior rhizotomy of spastic paraplegia. N Engl J Med 1945;233:453–461.

164. Garland DE, Thompson R, Waters R. Musculocutaneous neurectomy for spastic elbow flexion in nonfunctional upper extremities in adults. J Bone Joint Surg 1981;63A:767–772.

165. Purohit AK, Raju BS, Kumar KS, Mallikarjun KD. Selective musculocutaneous fasciculotomy for spastic elbow in cerebral palsy: a preliminary study. Acta Neurochir (Wien) 1998;140:473–478.

166. Decq P, Filipetti P, Feve A. Peripheral selective neurectomy of the brachial plexus collateral branches for treatment of the spastic shoulder: anatomical study and clinical results in five patients. J Neurosurg 1997;86:648–653.

167. Feve A, Decq P, Filipetti P. Physiological effects of selective tibial neurotomy on lower limb spasticity. J Neurol Neurosurg Psychiatry 1997;63:575–578.

168. Caillet F, Mertens P, Rabaseda S, Boisson D. The development of gait in the hemiplegic patient after selective tibial neurotomy. Neurochirurgie 1998;4:183–191.

169. Berard C, Sindou M, Berard J, Carrier H. Selective neurotomy of the tibial nerve in the spastic hemiplegic child: an explanation of the recurrence. J Pediatr Orthop 1998;7B:66–70.

170. Helweg-Larsen J, Jacobsen E. Treatment of spasticity in cerebral palsy by means of phenol nerve block of peripheral nerves. Dan Med Bull 1969;16:20–25.

171. Spira R. Management of spasticity in cerebral palsied children by peripheral nerve block with phenol. Dev Med Child Neurol 1971;13:164–173.

172. Carpenter EB. Role of nerve blocks in the foot and ankle in cerebral palsy. Foot Ankle 1983;4:164–166.

173. Garland DE, Lucie RS, Waters RL. Current uses of open phenol nerve block for adult acquired spasticity. Clin Orthop 1982;165:217–222.

Chapter 20

Management of Adults with Cerebral Palsy

Lawrence M. Samkoff

Cerebral palsy (CP) is not a single disease but a group of disorders characterized by motor, sensory, and cognitive deficits associated with a brain injury sustained early in life. Timely intervention and treatment during childhood and adolescence have greatly enhanced the quality of life for patients with CP. Nevertheless, during adulthood, patients with CP frequently develop problems not encountered previously. Some of these issues are related to normal aging; however, apparently CP itself may have an impact on the life cycle as well. This chapter discusses some of the unique medical issues facing adults with CP.

General Considerations

Few studies have examined the health status of adults with CP. Turk et al.[1] interviewed 63 community-based women with CP (mean age, 37.7 ± 12.7 years) and reported that 87% of subjects perceived themselves as healthy despite their disability. Forty-four women (73%) visited a physician at least once in the previous year, although only 18% and 22% had recent gynecologic and breast examinations, respectively. Tobacco and alcohol use was infrequent, cited by 2% and 5% of women, respectively. Fifty-two percent of study participants maintained a balanced diet, and 83% engaged in regular physical activity.

Murphy et al.[2] found that more than 90% of 101 adults with CP (mean age, 42.6 years) did not receive regular health maintenance services; however, no serious medical comorbidities were reported. Ninety percent of women did not have periodic breast examinations or Papanicolaou smears; fewer than 10% of men had routine prostate examinations. Fewer than 10% of subjects had cardiovascular risk factor assessment or electrocardiography. Possible explanations for decreased quality of preventive care in this population include lack of accessible medical services, insensitivity of medical personnel to the special needs of the chronically disabled, and the relative absence of information about the influence of aging on CP.[2]

The 30-year survival rate for individuals with CP is estimated to be 87%.[3] Factors adversely affecting life expectancy include epilepsy, presence of severe mental retardation, and severity of motor deficit.[3,4] Early mortality in such individuals is likely due to compromise of basic functional skills, such as mobility and feeding.[4] In addition to addressing general preventive medical care, the management of associated and secondary conditions of adult CP is critical to ensure both survival and quality of life in this growing population.

Associated Conditions in Adult Cerebral Palsy

Associated conditions in adults with CP are those disorders that are related directly to brain pathology. These disorders include epilepsy, mental retardation, learning disabilities, hearing and visual impairment, and pseudobulbar dysarthria.[1,2] (See

Chapters 2, 10, 25, 30–35 for details concerning management of these entities.)

Secondary Conditions in Adult Cerebral Palsy

Secondary conditions in adults with CP are disorders or illnesses that occur as a result of the primary disability. Secondary neuromuscular anomalies include chronic pain, spasticity, cervical myeloradiculopathy, musculoskeletal deformities, compressive neuropathies, dystonia and movement disorders, and bowel and bladder dysfunction. Nonneurologic entities in adult CP consist of dental abnormalities and gastroesophageal reflux.[1,2,5–7] These issues are discussed in detail.

Chronic Pain

Pain in adult CP is prevalent, ranging from an incidence of 67%[5] to 84%[1] in different studies. Turk et al.[1] reported that the most frequent sites of pain in women with CP were the head (28%), back (26%), and arm (23%). Pain-limited activity of daily living occurs in 56% of women.

In a study by Schwartz et al.[5] of 93 adults with CP, two-thirds of participants claimed to have one or more areas of pain of greater than 3 months' duration. Pain involved mostly the lower extremity (66%) and back (63%); other regions of pain included the neck and shoulder (45%), upper extremities (44%), buttock and hip (39%), head (24%), and abdomen (16%). Mean pain duration ranged from 7.5 to 15.0 years, and 56% of subjects reported having daily pain. Pain intensity was classified as low disability in 90% of individuals and as high disability in 10%. Most subjects reported that pain caused little interference with their activities, but a small subgroup did report impairment in daily activity (18%), social activity (10%), and ability to work (13%). Cognitive deficits may explain some of the discrepancy between presence of pain and experience of pain in this patient population.[1,5]

The etiology of chronic pain in adult CP is likely multifactorial. Murphy et al.[2] reported that cervical pain occurred in 75% of individuals with dyskinetic CP and in 54% of patients younger than age 50. Degenerative joint disease of the cervical spine was cited as the most frequent cause of neck pain. The high incidence of neck pain in dyskinetic CP probably is related to premature development of spondylosis resulting from continuous twisting and tortuous cervical dyskinesias.[2,6,7]

Back pain is another common problem affecting individuals with CP. It was especially prevalent in nonambulatory individuals (43%) in one survey.[2] Factors associated with back pain include inadequate wheelchair seating[2] and presence of kyphosis[1] or scoliosis.[8] Additionally, spasticity may aggravate back pain in ambulatory individuals.[9]

The optimal treatment of chronic pain in CP has not been investigated fully. Physiotherapy and exercise may reduce symptoms in some individuals.[1,5] Nonambulatory patients may derive benefit from improved positioning while seated.[2] Management of underlying sources of pain, including osteoarthritis, spasticity, and dystonia, also is essential. The use of tricyclic antidepressants (e.g., amitriptyline, nortriptyline), anticonvulsants (e.g., gabapentin), and opioids in chronic pain in CP has not been evaluated but can be considered in selected patients.

Spasticity

Spasticity is defined as a velocity-dependent increase in muscle tone with hyperactive deep-tendon and nociceptive reflexes.[10] Spasticity is one component of the upper motor neuron syndrome, which also includes muscle weakness, loss of dexterity, asynergy of voluntary movement, limb flexor and extensor spasms, and the Babinski sign. Spasticity of cerebral origin, resulting from stroke, CP, or head injury, for example, is in part due to loss of supraspinal inhibitory control on alpha motoneurons and spinal γ-aminobutyric acid (GABA) interneurons in the spinal cord. This leads to enhanced excitatory activity of alpha motoneurons by Ia-afferent fibers from muscle spindles.

Spasticity is a common cause of morbidity in the CP population, interfering with gait, positioning, and hygiene. Untreated spasticity can produce chronic pain and fibrous contractures of the limbs.[11] In one study, 35% of women with CP reported that their spasticity increased during menstruation.[1] Spasticity in individuals with CP must be managed aggressively to optimize neuromuscular function and to minimize occurrence of complications.[11] Several pharmacologic agents are available to ameliorate CP-related spasticity.

Baclofen

Baclofen, a GABA(B) agonist, acts in the spinal cord to reduce monosynaptic and polysynaptic segmental reflex activity.[11] Oral baclofen at dosages from 20 to 120 mg daily is only moderately beneficial in the treatment of cerebral spasticity because of its poor lipid solubility and low penetration into the cerebrospinal fluid.[12] Because of this, effective oral doses for cerebral spasticity are large and produce intolerable adverse effects, such as sedation and muscle weakness.

Alternatively, baclofen may be delivered through an implantable intrathecal pump.[11,12] Continuous intrathecal baclofen infusion (CIBI) produces a greater than 10-fold increase in cerebrospinal fluid concentration as compared with oral administration; however, plasma levels are substantially lower. In patients with CP, CIBI dosages varying from 27 to 800 µg daily reduce upper- and lower-extremity spasticity, leading to improvement of function.[12] As total daily CIBI is a fraction of the orally administered agent, side effects are minimal. Patients selected for CIBI must receive a therapeutic response from an intrathecal test injection (25–100 µg) before pump implantation. Complications of CIBI occur in 20% of patients and include pump malfunction, catheter disruption, and infection.[12]

Tizanidine

Tizanidine, a central alpha$_2$-adrenergic agonist, is a newer antispastic agent. Its mechanism of action is the reduction of polysynaptic reflexes through facilitation of descending supraspinal inhibitory pathways from the brainstem.[13,14] Tizanidine at dosages from 2 to 36 mg daily has been demonstrated to reduce muscle tone, spasm frequency, and clonus significantly in patients with spasticity of both spinal and cerebral origin[13,14]; however, its efficacy in CP has not been investigated thoroughly. The antispastic action of tizanidine does not affect muscle strength adversely, and subjective muscle weakness is reported less frequently by patients.[13] Somnolence, dry mouth, and orthostatic hypotension are the most common side effects of

tizanidine,[13] which can be minimized with a low initial dose (e.g., 2 mg at bedtime) followed by slow escalation over 2–4 weeks.[13]

Botulinum Toxin

Botulinum toxin (BTX), one of the most potent neurotoxins known, has been used therapeutically for many conditions associated with muscle hypertonicity.[15] BTX, a polypeptide consisting of a light chain and heavy chain bridged by a disulfide bond, is produced by the bacterium *Clostridium botulinum*. Seven distinct antigenic types of BTX (A–G) have been isolated. The majority of clinical studies have used BTX-A. When injected into muscle, BTX prevents presynaptic release of acetylcholine at the neuromuscular junction by impeding the protein-dependent fusion of acetylcholine-containing synaptic vesicles with the nerve terminal membrane.[15] With doses of BTX-A used clinically, therapeutic reduction in muscle tone can be achieved without producing excessive muscle weakness[15]; thus, voluntary muscle control and function can be maintained.

BTX-A has been demonstrated to ameliorate limb spasticity due to a variety of neurologic disorders, such as multiple sclerosis, stroke, and CP.[15–17] In CP, reduction of limb spasticity with BTX-A enhances function and minimizes development of joint contractures.[17] For example, Wissel et al.[16] found that injection of 200 units of BTX into several muscles in each lower extremity produced improvement of dynamic deformities and equina varus gait pattern in young adults with spastic CP. In nonambulatory children with CP, reduction of spastic muscle tone with BTX-A improved range of motion, hygiene, positioning, and pain in both the upper and lower extremities.[18,19] The use of BTX in adults with CP must be confirmed with further investigation.

Doses of BTX vary from 10 to 200 units, depending on muscle size and degree of muscle weakness desired.[15] Side effects are attributed mostly to local diffusion of toxin and are limited to excessive weakness of treated and nearby muscles; these usually are transient in duration but can last up to 2 weeks.[15] Systemic adverse effects are uncommon, but generalized muscle weakness rarely can occur when high doses of BTX are used.[15] The duration of action of BTX is approximately 3–4 months, and repetitive injections often are necessary to maintain a therapeutic response. Development of antibodies to BTX occurs in up to 4–6% of patients.[11,20]

Other Agents

The benzodiazepines diazepam and clonazepam also are moderately effective for the treatment of cerebral spasticity.[11] These drugs bind to distinct central nervous system receptors to facilitate GABA(A)-mediated inhibitory neurotransmission. Adverse effects include sedation and muscle weakness. Dantrolene reduces muscle contractility by preventing release of calcium from the sarcoplasmic reticulum, thereby uncoupling calcium-dependent cross-bridging of actin and myosin.[11] Excessive muscle weakness and hepatotoxicity may occur with dantrolene, so its use requires periodic monitoring of liver function tests.[11] Phenol nerve blocks can be helpful in also reducing focal limb spasticity; the most common adverse effect is dysesthetic pain in the sensory distribution of the injected peripheral nerve.[21]

Cervical Myeloradiculopathy

Physicians caring for adults with developmental disabilities need to recognize functional deterioration in this population to offer optimal medical care. In particular, the onset of new neurologic symptomatology and declining neurologic function in individuals with CP presents a difficult situation for the practitioner. Cervical spondylosis with myelopathy is one of the best-described complications of both dyskinetic and spastic CP (Figure 20-1).[6,7,22–24]

Anderson et al.[22] first reported delayed occurrence of cervical myelopathy in two patients with dyskinetic CP. These authors suggested that abnormal neck movements aggravated underlying cervical spondylosis, leading to spinal cord compression. Levine et al.[25] found a high prevalence of cervical spondylosis in 21 patients with cervical dyskinesias of various etiologies. Subsequently, Mikawa et al.,[6] Ko and Park-Ko,[7] and Pollak et al.[24] described eight patients (ages 31–61 years; average, 42.5 years) who had dyskinetic CP and developed late-onset neurologic deterioration due to cervical spondylosis with myelopathy. Clinical fea-

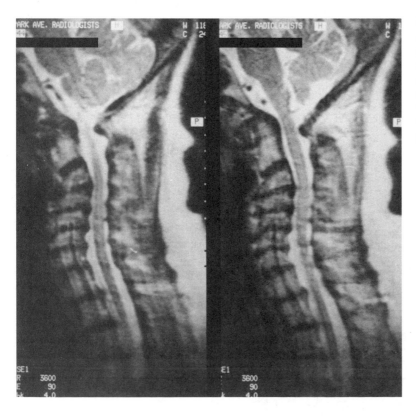

Figure 20-1. T2-weighted magnetic resonance images of cervical spine demonstrate severe spondylosis and degenerative disk changes at multiple levels in a patient with dyskinetic-spastic cerebral palsy who developed upper-extremity wasting and progressive spastic paraparesis after the age of 60.

tures in all these cases included choreoathetosis and dystonia of cervical and upper girdle muscles; radiating pain in the neck and upper extremities also was prominent. Additional findings included progressive lower-extremity weakness and spasticity, worsening of gait, wasting and weakness of upper-extremity muscles, sensory disturbances in the arms and hands, and urinary incontinence. Magnetic resonance imaging or computed tomographic myelography identified cervical cord compression due to cervical spondylosis with or without disk herniation in all patients. Seven patients underwent surgery with anterior spinal decompression, resulting in clinical improvement in all cases.

Acquired cervical myelopathy with functional neurologic deterioration has been reported to occur also in patients with spastic CP.[7,23] Reese et al.[23] described three mentally retarded patients who had spastic CP and experienced slowly progressive motor dysfunction. Two previously ambulatory patients became unable to walk and developed urinary incontinence; a nonambulatory patient lost his ability to use his hands independently to propel his wheelchair. Computed tomographic myelography demonstrated discogenic cervical cord compression in each case. The two patients who were previously ambulatory underwent posterior spinal decompression, with partial recovery of neurologic function; however, neither regained independent ambulation. Ko and Park-Ko[7] performed anterior cervical diskectomy and intervertebral fusion on a patient with spastic CP and myelopathy due to discogenic cervical cord compression at C3-4; the patient improved after 2 months.

The prevalence of acquired cervical myelopathy in individuals with CP is unknown, as no prospective studies have been done. In dyskinetic CP, cervical spondylosis and myelopathy have been postulated to be caused by accelerated and premature degeneration of intervertebral disks and ligaments owing to the presence of chronic, repetitive cervical rotatory dyskinesias.[6,7,24,25] This condition should be considered in all CP patients with neurologic decline, particularly with disturbances in ambulation, upper-extremity function, and sphincter control.[6,7,23–25]

Dystonia and Movement Disorders

Dystonia and choreoathetosis frequently are associated with CP. These adventitious movements

may be painful and can cause postural abnormalities, muscle contractures, and loss of musculoskeletal integrity.[2] Compressive neuropathies, such as carpal tunnel syndrome, also may result from repetitive limb dyskinesias.[2] Focal dystonia is managed best with BTX injections.[20] Preliminary evidence suggests that CP-associated generalized dystonia may be reduced with intrathecal baclofen.[26] Further investigation is needed before this treatment can be recommended.

Bladder and Bowel Disorders

The prevalence of bladder and bowel disturbances in adults with CP has not been well studied. Murphy et al.[2] found that 22% and 50%, respectively, of nonambulatory adults with CP had frequent urinary tract infection and urinary incontinence. Turk et al.[1] reported that 49% of women with CP had bladder disturbances, and 56% had bowel problems.

Detailed studies of bladder function in adults with CP have not been performed; however, the incidence of neurogenic bladder is well recognized in children with CP.[27–29] Both detrusor hyperreflexia and detrusor-sphincter dyssynergia have been reported.[27–29] In patients with bladder disturbances, urinalysis and urine cultures should be performed to evaluate for the presence of urinary tract infection. Persistence of symptoms warrants further urologic evaluation with sonography and urodynamics before definitive therapy can be initiated.[30]

Conclusion

In their study of adult individuals with CP, Murphy et al.[2] reported that 26 of 60 (41%) previously ambulatory patients lost their ability to walk between the ages of 11 and 68; however, the causes of gait decline were not evaluated in detail. This finding raises the intriguing question of the possible existence of a post-CP syndrome analogous to that seen in patients previously afflicted with polio. The impact of CP on aging neuromuscular and musculoskeletal systems requires further prospective studies. The literature appears to substantiate that many adults with CP develop a combination of neurologic and musculoskeletal disorders that were not present earlier in life. Some of these entities (e.g., cervical myelopathy, spasticity, and chronic pain) are at least partially amenable to medical and surgical therapy. Astute clinicians must be vigilant in evaluating developmentally disabled patients and must avoid attributing new problems to an untreatable static encephalopathy.

References

1. Turk MA, Gerenski CA, Rosenbaum PF, Weber RJ. The health status of women with cerebral palsy. Arch Phys Med Rehabil 1997;78[Suppl 5]:S10–S17.
2. Murphy KP, Molnar GE, Lankasky K. Medical and functional status of adults with cerebral palsy. Dev Med Child Neurol 1995;37:1075–1084.
3. Crichton JU, Mackinnon M, White CP. The life expectancy of persons with cerebral palsy. Dev Med Child Neurol 1995;37:567–576.
4. Strauss D, Shavelle R. Life expectancy of adults with CP. Dev Med Child Neurol 1998;40:369–375.
5. Schwartz L, Engel JM, Jensen MP. Pain in persons with cerebral palsy. Arch Phys Med Rehabil 1999;80:1243–1246.
6. Mikawa Y, Watanabe R, Shikata J. Cervical myeloradiculopathy in athetoid cerebral palsy. Arch Orthop Trauma Surg 1997;116:116–118.
7. Ko HY, Park-Ko I. Spinal cord injury secondary to cervical disc herniation in ambulatory patients with cerebral palsy. Spinal Cord 1998;36:288–292.
8. Majd ME, Muldoway DS, Holt RT. Natural history of scoliosis in the institutionalized adult cerebral palsy population. Spine 1997;22:1461–1464.
9. Gormley ME, O'Brien CE, Yablon SA. A clinical overview of treatment decisions in the management of spasticity. Muscle Nerve 1997;20[Suppl 6]:S14–S20.
10. Meyer NH. Clinicophysiologic concepts of spasticity and motor dysfunction in adults with an upper motoneuron lesion. Muscle Nerve 1997;20[Suppl 6]:S1–S13.
11. Albright AL. Spastic cerebral palsy: approaches to drug treatment. CNS Drugs 1995;4:17–27.
12. Albright AL. Baclofen in the treatment of cerebral palsy. J Child Neurol 1996;11:77–83.
13. Wagstaff AJ, Bryson HM. Tizanidine: a review of its pharmacology, clinical efficacy and tolerability in the management of spasticity associated with cerebral and spinal disorders. Drugs 1997;53:435–452.
14. Lataste X, Emre M, Davis C, Groves L. Comparative profile of tizanidine in the management of spasticity. Neurology 1994;11[Suppl 9]:S53–S59.
15. Hallett M. One man's poison—clinical applications of botulinum toxin (editorial). N Engl J Med 1999;341:118–120.
16. Wissel J, Heinen F, Schenkel A, et al. Botulinum toxin A in the management of spastic gait disorders in children and young adults with cerebral palsy: a randomized, double-blind study of "high-dose" versus "low-dose" treatment. Neuropediatrics 1999;30:120–124.
17. Russman BS, Tilton A, Gormsley ME Jr. Cerebral palsy: a rational approach to a treatment protocol, and the role of botulinum toxin in treatment. Muscle Nerve Suppl 1997;6:S181–S193.
18. Cosgrove AP, Corry IS, Graham HK. Botulinum toxin in the management of the lower limb in cerebral palsy. Dev Med Child Neurol 1994;36:386–396.
19. Corry IS, Cosgrove AP, Walsh EG, et al. Botulinum toxin A in the hemiplegic upper limb: a double-blind trial. Dev Med Child Neurol 1997;39:185–193.
20. Brin MF, Lew MF, Adler CH, et al. Safety and efficacy of NeuroBloc (botulinum toxin type B) in type A–resistant cervical dystonia. Neurology 1999;53:1431–1438.
21. Yadav SL, Singh U, Dureja GP, et al. Phenol block in the management of spastic cerebral palsy. Indian J Pediatr 1994;61:249–255.
22. Anderson WW, Wise BL, Itabashi HH, Jones M. Cervical spondylosis in patients with athetosis. Neurology 1962;12:410–412.
23. Reese ME, Msall ME, Owen S, et al. Acquired cervical spine impairment in young adults with cerebral palsy. Dev Med Child Neurol 1991;33:153–158.
24. Pollak L, Schiffer J, Klein C, et al. Neurosurgical intervention for cervical disk disease in dystonic cerebral palsy. Move Disord 1998;13:713–717.
25. Levine RA, Rosenbaum AE, Waltz JM, Scheinberg LC. Cervical spondylosis and dyskinesias. Neurology 1970;20:1194–1199.
26. Walker RH, Swope DM, Danisi FO, et al. Intrathecal baclofen therapy for dystonia (abstract). Neurology 1999;52[Suppl 2]:A521.
27. Drigo P, Seren F, Artibani W, et al. Neurogenic vesicourethral dysfunction in children with cerebral palsy. Ital J Neurol Sci 1988;9:151–154.
28. Decter RM, Bauer SB, Khoshbin S, et al. Urodynamic assessment of children with cerebral palsy. J Urol 1987;138:1110–1112.
29. McNeal DM, Hawtrey CE, Wolraich ML, Mapel JR. Symptomatic neurogenic bladder in a cerebral-palsied population. Dev Med Child Neurol 1983;25:612–616.
30. Boone TB. The Bladder and Genitourinary Tract in the Cerebral Palsies. In G Miller, GD Clark (eds), The Cerebral Palsies: Causes, Consequences, and Management. Boston: Butterworth–Heinemann, 1998;299–308.

Chapter 21

Special Issues for Women with Developmental Disabilities

Debra Shabas

As of 1992, 27 million U.S. women had disabilities, according to the U.S. Bureau of the Census. Despite the large number of women affected, the focus on women's issues relevant to this population has been inadequate.[1-3] These issues include basic medical research, preventive health care, and psychosocial consequences of disability. Only over the last decade has women's health become a concern of the American political, economic, and health care systems. However, interest in health issues for women with disabilities has lagged significantly behind.

Disability is experienced very differently in women and men. The impact on the ability to function in society varies by gender. No public health focus has been directed to preventive health care for women with disabilities. Minimal research has addressed the effects of hormones, menopause, and menstruation on diverse disabilities. Little information has been made available regarding fertility, pregnancy, and delivery or the pros and cons of hormone replacement therapy in women with diverse disabilities. Despite abundant information about male sexuality in disabling conditions, scant information is available regarding female sexuality in the same underlying conditions.

Specific Concerns of Women with Epilepsy

The importance of health issues for women with developmental disabilities can be exemplified in epilepsy. Epilepsy is a condition that affects both men and women, although special concerns apply to women with epilepsy. Approximately 800,000 such women are of childbearing age. Drugs used most commonly for epilepsy were released prior to 1978, before analysis of drug efficacy by gender was mandated by the U.S. Food and Drug Administration.

Significant hormonal influences affect epileptic activity. Thirty to fifty percent of women with epilepsy experience changes in seizure patterns around the time of hormonal fluctuations.[4-6] Catamenial exacerbations of seizures occur just before or at the onset of menstruation and at ovulation. The cause is not understood completely but may be related to estrogen and progesterone levels and their effects on neuronal excitability.[7] Very little is known about the effects of menopause on epilepsy.

The effects of hormonal contraception (birth control pills) on seizure frequency also are unclear and variable. The hormonal contraceptives may not be as effective in epileptic women who are taking certain antiepileptic medications.[8] This limitation is related to the increased metabolism of contraceptive hormones by the cytochrome P450 system, which is enhanced by antiepileptic medications, including carbamazepine, phenytoin, barbiturates, and topiramate.[9] The minipill also may not be adequate for certain women with epilepsy.

With regard to sexuality, people with epilepsy appear to have a higher incidence of sexual dysfunction.[10,11] In women, this dysfunction includes a high incidence of dyspareunia and vaginismus and lack of vaginal lubrication. The cause probably is multifactorial and may be related to the antiepilepsy medications.

Fertility rates are 25–35% lower than average in women with epilepsy,[12] the precise reasons for which are unclear. Menstrual irregularities are common. Reproductive conditions, including polycystic ovarian syndrome and hypothalamic hypopituitary dysfunction, are more common in such women.[13,14] These conditions occur whether or not a woman is taking antiepileptic medications. However, some medications might alter the risk for specific reproductive disturbances.

Pregnancy usually is uncomplicated, although women taking antiepileptic drugs are at greater risk for miscarriage and preterm delivery.[9] Frequency of seizures during pregnancy may be increased, owing to changes in the metabolism of antiepileptic drugs, hormone levels, and other factors.[12,13] Drug levels need to be monitored, and dosages should be adjusted when necessary.

More than 90% of women with epilepsy will have normal healthy infants. However, infants of such women are at higher risk for major and minor congenital malformations and neurodevelopmental disability.[9,15,16] The incidence of major congenital malformations in affected women taking anticonvulsant drugs is 4–8%, which is significantly higher than the 2–4% in the general population.[6] Many questions remain unanswered, but polypharmacy and high drug levels are associated with an increased risk of malformations. Folic acid prior to conception and during pregnancy is believed to lower the risk of neural tube defects.[9,15,16] The newborn also carries an increased risk of bleeding disorders, requiring vitamin K supplementation.

Antiepileptic drugs, particularly phenytoin, carbamazepine, and phenobarbital, can cause bone loss.[17,18] The mechanisms are unclear but result partly from increased vitamin D metabolism. Again, polytherapy and long-term use appear to be particular risk factors. The effects of the newer drugs on bone health are unknown.

The special concerns for women with epilepsy are shared by women having other developmental disabilities. The risks and side effects of medications for each diverse underlying condition are different for women and men. Hormonal influences on disease and the relative risks of pregnancy and delivery are important considerations for women with developmental disabilities. Research and information are scarce regarding these women's issues. These special issues highlight the differing impacts of diverse disabilities and gender on overall health.

Preventive Health Care

Even as recently as 1997, literature about the health care practices of women with disabilities was sparse. A few small studies did reveal that the health care practices of women with disabilities were inadequate. One San Francisco study of 101 adults with cerebral palsy (CP) noted that more than 90% of the women with CP did not have regular Papanicolaou smears or pelvic or breast examinations.[19] Another study that included 55 women with disabilities, including CP, spina bifida, and spinal muscular atrophy, revealed that women with paralysis, impaired motor function, or obvious physical deformity were not offered contraceptive counseling. Fewer than one-half of the pregnancies noted in this study were initiated by choice.[20] A British study of a diverse group of disabled young adults found that more than one-half had untreated health problems that required medical intervention.[21]

Several reasons account for this lack of adequate health care. Unlike the organized systems of care that have been established for children with disabilities, no such system exists for adults. Care changes dramatically when these disabled adolescents graduate to the adult medical system. Interest in basic health promotion for these women has been eclipsed by the narrowed focus on treating their underlying conditions. In addition, women with disabilities face many barriers when attempting to get proper health care.[3] These barriers include access, information, attitudes, finances, and personal assistance.[22]

Access is the most obvious barrier. This includes architectural barriers, accessibility of the office and the examination room, and the ability to get onto the examination table. Less obvious are the attitudinal barriers. With regard to gynecologic and obstetric care, this barrier includes the attitude that women with disabilities are asexual and, therefore, do not need information regarding reproductive health care. An additional assumption is that disabled girls will not want to or be able to have children. Clearly, this is not true: Many women with disabilities have the desire to become parents. Society's attitude is that a disabled woman will have significant difficulty in being a good mother. The courts often agree; as a consequence, many disabled women will stay in a bad marriage for fear of losing custody of their children.[23]

Attitudinal issues are a significant barrier both to general health care and to the doctor-patient relationship. In a national study, 31% of physically disabled women were turned away by physicians, solely owing to their disability.[23] The medical community displays a lack of expertise in the examination of and sensitivity toward women with physical limitations. Many disabled women who want to become pregnant have difficulty in finding an obstetrician with experience in caring for a pregnant disabled woman.

Women with disabilities are women first. General women's health concerns are as important as the treatment for each diverse underlying condition. Women with disabilities face several specific health risks. A recent study revealed that osteoporosis, heart disease, depression, and chronic urinary tract infections occurred more often and at younger ages in women with physical disabilities as compared to nondisabled women.[23]

Osteoporosis

Osteoporosis in women with disabilities is a different disease than in nondisabled women. Although the physiology of loss of bone density and the increased risk of fractures are the same, the disease occurs much earlier and is more severe in women with disabilities.[23] The current guidelines for the prevention, evaluation, and treatment of osteoporosis in nondisabled women do not apply to women with disabilities. Despite the overwhelming coverage of osteoporosis for nondisabled women, no guidelines cover bone-density testing in disabled women, and no universally prescribed bone-saving practices are specific to them. The most serious consequence of osteoporosis is fracture. Often in women with disabilities, a fracture due to minor trauma is the first evidence of osteoporosis. Many women with developmental disabilities are more prone to falls. The potential consequence of an osteoporotic fracture is far more serious in a woman who already has a physical disability.

Physical activity is important in the development and maintenance of bone density. If a woman with a disability has been inactive since childhood, adequate bone density and mass may not have developed properly. With aging and hormonal changes, such a woman is likely to experience an accelerated loss of bone density and mass. Women with spinal cord injury experience most of the bone loss early after their injuries. This outcome results from decreased physical activity and possibly also from alterations in the autonomic and circulatory systems.

Medications—including steroids and, for women with epilepsy, antiepileptic drugs—can accelerate bone loss. Proper nutrition, including adequate vitamin D and calcium, is necessary to prevent osteoporosis. Often, women who rely on caregivers for meals may not have adequate intake of vitamin D and calcium. Therefore, supplementation may be essential.

Bone-density screening (dual-energy x-ray absorptiometry) for the early identification of those at risk for osteoporosis and fracture is not prescribed routinely for women with physical disabilities. The present perimenopausal guidelines for this test in nondisabled women are not relevant to many disabled women, who develop osteoporosis in their twenties and thirties.

Preventing osteoporosis as early as possible is of utmost importance in women with disabilities, so as to avoid a potentially life-altering osteoporotic fracture. All women with disabilities should be asked about genetic, lifestyle, medical, and iatrogenic risk factors for premature osteoporosis. Exercises that are recommended for nondisabled women, including strengthening and weight-bearing exercises, can be performed with special adaptations by women with disabilities. Balance and flexibility exercises also can help to reduce falls. Adequate intake of calcium and vitamin D in the diet or as supplements is essential. Compounding risk factors, such as smoking cigarettes and drinking excessive amounts of alcohol, must be corrected. Any medications that increase the risk of osteoporosis should be discussed and monitored by the prescribing physician. The pros and cons of hormone replacement therapy at menopause should be discussed with a gynecologist. Bone-density testing should be performed early to assess the risks for the development of premature osteoporosis. Treatment with bone resorption inhibitors or other medications can be instituted early before the loss of bone density is at a critical level.

Heart Disease

Many potential reasons can explain premature heart disease in women with disabilities, including the lack of exercise. One reason is that despite all the attention to exercise programs for nondisabled women, minimal information and minimal programming are designed specifically for women with physical disabilities. Other reasons include nutritional factors and obesity and the lack of routine medical checkups. The difficulties in accessing routine preventive medical checkups could result in undetected hypertension, diabetes, and hyperlipidemia.

Breast Cancer

Early detection of breast cancer depends on education, patient self-examination, regular primary care or gynecologic preventive checkups, and mammography. Many women with physical disabilities are unable to perform breast self-examination owing to sensory loss, spasticity, difficulty with coordination, contractures, or orthopedic abnormalities. Mammography is difficult for many disabled women. This is due either to issues of access to the facility or the mammography room or to the inability of the machine to accommodate women with certain types of disabilities. The need for several assistants and difficulty with positioning contribute to rendering mammography an even more unpleasant experience. In view of all this difficulty, a disabled woman who does manage to obtain a mammogram may not have a complete, optimal reading performed. One could reasonably assume that the impact of mammogram inaccessibility, the lack of regularly scheduled primary medical and gynecologic visits, and the physical inability to perform breast self-examination would lead to an increase in breast cancer deaths in disabled women whose breast cancers are discovered at advanced stages. No studies have addressed this hypothesis.

Psychosocial Issues

Many gender-related psychosocial issues for disabled women relate to self-esteem, parenting, and social opportunity. Employment opportunities are far fewer for women with disabilities as compared to nondisabled women.[3] In addition, abuse is a particularly significant concern for women with disabilities. Physicians and health care professionals should ask specifically about abuse, as this information usually is not volunteered.

Statistics vary, but between 62% and 85% of women with disabilities have experienced emotional, physical, or sexual abuse,[23–25] whereas 25–50% of a comparable group of nondisabled women experienced abuse.[24,25] The Disabled Women's Network in Canada found that 66% of women with disabilities experienced domestic violence before puberty, twice the number of instances found in the general population.[24]

The types of abuse that disabled women experience is similar to that of nondisabled women. However, women with disabilities are abused also by withholding needed orthotic equipment, wheelchairs, medications, transportation, or essential assistance with personal tasks.[23] Women with disabilities also experience abuse for longer periods of time than do nondisabled women.[23]

Women with disabilities have significant difficulty in resolving abusive situations. Assailants are usually family but also include caregivers, medical personnel, institutional and residential school staff. Most shelters and rape crisis centers are not accessible, and staff there are not knowledgeable about disability issues. Of the 1,000 domestic violence shelter beds in New York City, the State Department of Social Services has reported that only four beds are fully wheelchair-accessible.[25]

Conclusion

Women with disabilities have been neglected by the health care system. Preventive health care practices provided to these women have been inadequate despite the fact that they are at particular risk for certain medical conditions, including heart disease and osteoporosis. Health care professionals and women with disabilities need to be aware of these special risks. Understanding the barriers to adequate health care for women with disabilities is the first step toward improving access to this care. The rise in interest in women's health issues will benefit all women. Research is necessary to provide more information on women's issues—including pregnancy, delivery, menstruation, and menopause—in diverse disabling conditions. Hormonal influences and medication side effects need to be explored. This information will improve general and reproductive health care for women with disabilities. In addition, psychosocial issues have a great impact on quality of life. Health care professionals need to address these issues as part of a general health maintenance program.

References

1. Thierry J. Promoting the health and wellness of women with disabilities. J Womens Health 1998; 7:505–507.
2. Robert Wood Johnson Foundation. Survey finds U.S. Health Care system not meeting needs of people with disabilities. RWJF Advances 1994;1:B11.
3. Nosek M. Primary care issues for women with severe physical disabilities. J Womens Health 1992;1:245–258.
4. Herzog AG, Klein P. Three patterns of catamenial epilepsy. Epilepsia 1996;37:83.
5. Duncan S, Read CL. How common is catamenial epilepsy? Epilepsia 1993;34:827–831.
6. Herzog AG, Klein P. Endocrine Aspects of Partial Seizures. In SC Schachter, DL Schomer (eds), The Comprehensive Evaluation and Treatment of Epilepsy. Boston: Academic Press, 1997;207–232.
7. Bonuccelli U, Melis G. Unbalanced progesterone and estradiol secretion in catamenial epilepsy. Epilepsy Res 1989;3:100–106.
8. Mattson RH, Cramer JA, Darney PD, Naftolin F. Use of oral contraceptives by women with epilepsy. JAMA 1986;256(2):238–240.
9. Morrell MJ. Seizures and Epilepsy in Women. In P Kaplan (ed), Neurologic Disease in Women. New York: Demos, 1998;189–203.
10. Morrell MJ. Sexual dysfunction in epilepsy. Epilepsia 1991;32[Suppl 5]:S38–S45.
11. Morrell MJ. Sexuality in Epilepsy. In J Engel, TA Pedley (eds), Epilepsy. Philadelphia: Lippincott–Raven, 1997;2021–2026.
12. Morrell MJ. Hormones, Reproductive Health and Epilepsy. In E Wyllie (ed), The Treatment of Epilepsy. Baltimore: Williams & Wilkins, 1996;179–187.
13. Isojarvi JIT, Laatikainen TJ, Pakarinen AJ, et al. Polycystic ovaries and hyperandrogenism in women taking valproate for epilepsy. N Engl J Med 1993;329:1383–1388.
14. Herzog AG, Seibel MM, Schomer DL, et al. Reproductive endocrine disorders in women with partial seizures of temporal lobe origin. Arch Neurol 1986;43:341–346.
15. Morrell MJ. Pregnancy and Epilepsy. In RJ Porter, D Chadwick (eds), The Epilepsies 2. Boston: Butterworth–Heinemann, 1997;313–332.
16. Yerby M. Treatment of Epilepsy During Pregnancy. In E Wyllie (ed), The Treatment of Epilepsy. Baltimore: Williams & Wilkins, 1996;785–798.
17. Morrell MJ. The new antiepileptic drugs and women: efficacy, reproductive health, pregnancy and fetal outcome. Epilepsia 1996;37[Suppl 6]:S34–S44.
18. Valimaki MJ, Tiihonon M. Bone mineral density measured by dual-energy x-ray absorptiometry and novel markers of bone formation and resorption in patients on antiepileptic drugs. J Bone Miner Res 1994;9:631–637.
19. Murphy K, Molnaar GE, Lankasky K. Medical and functional status of adults with cerebral palsy. Dev Med Child Neurol 1995;37:1075–1084.
20. Beckmann CR, Gittler M, Barzansky BM, Beckmann CA. Gynecological health care of women with disabilities. Obstet Gynecol 1989;74(1):75.
21. Bax M, Smyth DP, Thoma AP. Health care of physically handicapped young adults. BMJ 1988;296:1153–1155.
22. Nosek M, Young ME, Rintala DH, et al. Barriers to reproductive health maintenance among women with physical disabilities. J Womens Health 1995;4:505–518.
23. Nosek M, Rintala DH, Young ME, et al. National Study of Women with Physical Disabilities. Houston: Baylor College of Medicine, Center for Research on Women with Disabilities, 1997.
24. Disabled Women's Network (DAWN). Abilities. Kingston, Ontario, Canada: DAWN, 1995;22.
25. Feuerstein PB. Domestic violence and women and children with disabilities. New York: Milbank Memorial Fund, 1997.

Part IV

Epilepsy: Diagnosis and Treatment

Chapter 22

Malformations of Cortical Development and Epilepsy

Ruben Kuzniecky

Developmental malformations increasingly are being recognized as causing developmental delay and epilepsy. Any disruption of the mechanisms responsible for the formation of the cerebrum will result in malformations of cortical development (MCDs).[1] A wide variety of genetic and environmental factors can cause disturbance in these developmental processes and, therefore, can lead to an abnormality in the mature brain. In general, MCDs often are associated with developmental delay, abnormal intelligence, neurologic deficits, and epilepsy. However, as explained in this chapter, the clinical presentation varies even among similar pathologic entities, underscoring the importance of a syndromic approach that, it is hoped, will lead to a correct diagnosis and treatment. This chapter presents a summary of the current knowledge regarding the most common clinical MCDs associated with epilepsy.

Classification

Many different malformations (more than 35) involving the cerebrum have been recognized, especially after the introduction of high-resolution magnetic resonance imaging (MRI). However, not all MCDs are associated with epilepsy, and epilepsy is not the most prominent disorder in some syndromes. This has led to many classification models that have different emphases and that have created havoc among investigators. In addition, the nomenclature

of these disorders has been evolving. Although often described as "neuronal migration disorders," many such disorders involve abnormal cell formation in the ventricular zone prior to neuronal migration or involve abnormal cortical organization after migration has been largely completed. To address these concerns, a new classification system was introduced, based on fundamental embryologic and genetic principles plus a combination of pathologic, histologic, and neuroimaging criteria.[1] This classification system is presented in Table 22-1.

Cortical Malformations and Malformation Syndromes

In this overview, only the most common MCDs associated with epilepsy are described. However, the classification as illustrated in Table 22-1 includes all the disorders.

Malformations of Neuronal and Glial Proliferation

Malformations in neuronal and glial proliferation are characterized by an increase or decrease in the number of neurons and, often, glia; proliferation of abnormal cell types; or both. The most common types of microcephaly and macrocephaly are not included in this classification because, in these cases, brain structure appears normal. Malformations of neuronal and glial proliferation may be diffuse or localized.

Table 22-1. Classification System for Malformations of Cortical Development

Malformations due to abnormal neuronal and glial proliferation
  Generalized
    Decreased proliferation
      Microcephaly with simplified gyral pattern or microlissencephaly with thin cortex
      Microlissencephaly with thick cortex
    Increased proliferation (none known)
    Abnormal proliferation (none known)
  Focal or multifocal
    Decreased proliferation (none known)
    Increased and abnormal proliferation
      Megalencephaly and hemimegalencephaly
    Abnormal proliferation
      Focal cortical dysplasia
      Neoplastic (but associated with disordered cortex)
Malformations due to abnormal neuronal migration
  Generalized
    Classical lissencephaly and subcortical band heterotopia (agyria-pachygyria-band spectrum)
    Cobblestone lissencephaly
    Lissencephaly, other types
    Heterotopia
      Periventricular nodular heterotopia
      Subcortical cortical heterotopia
  Focal or multifocal malformations of neuronal migration
    Focal or multifocal heterotopia
    Focal or multifocal heterotopia with organizational abnormality of the cortex
    Excessive single ectopic white-matter neurons
Malformations due to abnormal cortical organization
  Generalized
    Bilateral diffuse polymicrogyria
  Focal or multifocal
    Schizencephaly-polymicrogyria complex
    Focal or multifocal cortical dysplasia (no balloon cells)
    Microdysgenesis
Malformations of cortical development, not otherwise classified

---

Microcephaly and Microlissencephalies

Several entities have been described, including microlissencephaly (MLIS) with thin cortex. Microcephaly with simplified gyral pattern consists of extreme microcephaly (defined as birth head circumference at or below –3 standard deviations [SD]), relative frontal lobe hypoplasia, diffusely simplified gyral pattern with shallow sulci, and normal or thin cortex.[2] This group of malformations was classified first as MLIS, but the name was changed to *microcephaly with simplified gyral pattern* (group 1), as the brain surface is thin rather than thick and is not smooth.[3] This classification also avoids confusion with true MLIS. In some patients, microcephaly may result from premature exhaustion of the germinal zone.[4] In others, both the thickness and the lamination of the cerebral cortex are normal, even though the number of neurons in the brain is greatly reduced.[5] Some groups have delayed myelination or other congenital anomalies. Most or all patients with microcephaly with simplified gyral pattern previously would have been classified as having primary microcephaly, or "microcephaly vera," but MRI studies do show abnormal brain structure. Patients in group 1 rarely have seizures, but those in other groups often have intractable epilepsy.[2] The last subgroup overlaps MLIS, as the brain surface is relatively smooth. However, the cortex is thin despite the smooth brain surface. Developmental delay varies but often is moderate to severe. All these syndromes are characterized by autosomal recessive inheritance.

Conversely, MLIS consists of extreme microcephaly, agyria, and a thick cortex.[6] The brainstem and cerebellum are hypoplastic in some subtypes but not in others. In one group, brain abnormalities resemble classic lissencephaly, except for the small size, whereas the brainstem and cerebellum appear relatively normal. This malformation probably corresponds to what has been called *Norman-Roberts syndrome*.[6,7] The other group consists of several patients with a thick cortex and severe hypoplasia of both brainstem and cerebellum.[8] Some have died at birth and others have not, which suggests further heterogeneity. Developmental delay is severe in most patients in this group. Most, if not all, of these malformations are characterized by autosomal recessive inheritance. Epilepsy has not been defined well in this group of patients.

Hemimegalencephaly

Hemimegalencephaly (HMEG) is defined by the presence of an enlarged hemisphere. The abnormal region may involve part of one hemisphere or one entire hemisphere with partial involvement of the other side. Patients with HMEG typically have mental retardation and epilepsy but usually no other associated congenital anomalies. HMEG may be observed in some syndromes, such as in Klippel-Trénaunay syndrome, in the epidermal nevus syndrome (sebaceous nevus),[9] and in hypomelanosis of Ito.[10] Pathologic changes include cortical dysplasia, white-matter abnormalities, polymicrogyria, pachygyria, and dysplastic cell types.

The clinical presentation in patients with HMEG with or without associated dermatologic disorders almost always includes seizures.[11] Most often, seizures start within the first 6 months of life, typically arising from the enlarged and dysplastic hemisphere. The seizures are partial, with secondary generalization, and often are intractable to medical therapy. Infantile spasms and drop attacks may present in early childhood. Unilateral neurologic sign, such as hemiparesis and hemianopia, are common. However, minimal neurologic dysfunction with normal cognitive abilities has been reported in some patients.

The appearance on MRI is characteristic, with enlargement of at least one lobe but, in more than one-half of patients, the entire hemisphere appears to be enlarged. The underlying hemispheric white matter usually is abnormal, with abnormal signal characteristics on MRI and diminished white matter in some individuals (Figure 22-1). Heterotopia are seen commonly, and the ventricular system is enlarged in most patients, with the frontal horn typically straight. Electroencephalographic (EEG) abnormalities often are extensive throughout the abnormal hemisphere. Prognostic indicators for poor outcome include severity of hemiparesis, smoothness of the cortical surface on MRI, and predominance of beta-activity on EEG scanning.

Focal Cortical Dysplasia

In 1971, Taylor et al.[12] first reported focal cortical dysplasia (FCD) with "balloon cells" in patients with focal intractable seizures. The balloon cells probably are the result of proliferation of abnormal cells in the germinal zone rather than the result of local effects on the migrating cells within the intermediate zone. Focal transmantle dysplasia consists of a streak or column of abnormal cells extending from the ependyma to the pial surface, but the

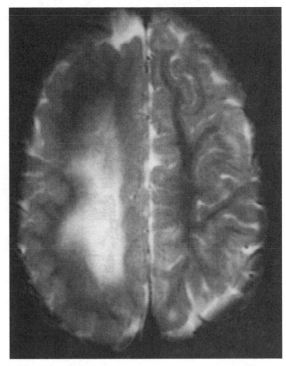

Figure 22-1. Hemimegalencephaly. Axial T2-weighted magnetic resonance image shows abnormally enlarged hemisphere with smooth cortex and abnormal white-matter signal changes.

pathologic appearance is identical to FCD with balloon cells.[1]

FCD probably is the most common form of focal developmental disorder diagnosed in patients with intractable focal epilepsy. The characteristic pathologic abnormalities of these lesions consist of disruption of cortical lamination with poorly differentiated glial cell elements. FCD can encompass a spectrum of changes. These changes range from mild cortical disruption without apparent giant neurons to the most severe forms in which cortical dyslamination, large bizarre cells, and astrocytosis are present.[13,14] The presence of balloon cells differentiates FCD type I (without balloon cells) from FCD type II (with balloon cells).

The clinical manifestations of patients with FCD vary.[15] Seizures begin in the first decade of life, usually after age 2 or 3 but sometimes shortly after birth. In some patients, seizures present in the second decade. The seizures may be of the partial sim-

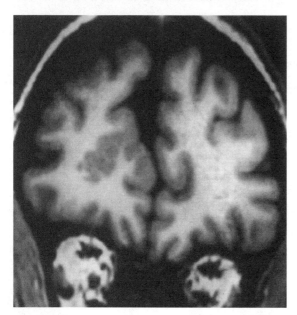

Figure 22-2. Focal cortical dysplasia. Coronal T1-weighted magnetic resonance image shows abnormal gray-matter area with underlying thickening of cortex.

ple motor, partial complex, or secondary generalized type. The location of the lesion will correlate with the clinical presentation.[16] The majority of patients have extratemporal cortical dysplasia involving the frontal lobes, in particular the pre- and postcentral gyrus. MRI findings include abnormal gyral thickening with underlying T2-weighted white-matter changes (Figure 22-2). These abnormalities can be rather circumscribed in nature. Interictal EEG scans may show very frequent spikes or even localized subclinical ictal EEG discharges.

FCD involving the temporal lobes also has been reported.[13,14] Both mesial and lateral neocortical structures can be affected. The seizures and clinical course in these patients appear to be similar to those in patients who have temporal lobe epilepsy due to hippocampal sclerosis, but EEG abnormalities usually are less circumscribed. MRI shows cortical thickening of temporal convolutions associated with poor differentiation of the gray-white junction. Focal dysplasia associated with hippocampal sclerosis also has been reported as "dual pathology."

Malformations Due to Neuronal Migration

Most true malformations of neuronal migration can be identified on imaging studies by the pres-ence of abnormal white and gray matter in the subependymal or subcortical regions. These findings vary in extent and severity from lissencephaly to focal subcortical or subependymal heterotopia. Some of these entities are seen primarily in neonates and infants with severe developmental delay, such as the lissencephalies, and are succinctly described.

Classic Lissencephaly and Subcortical Band Heterotopia

Classic lissencephaly (agyria) is a severe brain malformation manifested by a smooth cerebral surface, an abnormally thick four-layered cortex, diffuse neuronal heterotopia, and enlarged and dysplastic ventricles with preservation of the corpus callosum.[3,17] Subcortical band heterotopia (SBH) consist of symmetric and circumferential bands of gray matter found just beneath the cortex and separated from it by a thin band of white matter (Figure 22-3).[18] The overlying cortical surface appears normal, although this cortex can have more pyramidal cells than usual (B. Harding, personal communication, 2000). SBH sometimes is called *double cortex*, although this is a misnomer, as the underlying band does not have the normal six-layered cortical structure. Most bands are diffuse, but both partial frontal and partial posterior bands have been observed. In lissencephaly and SBH, the brainstem and cerebellum usually appear normal on imaging studies, although a few patients have mild vermis hypoplasia, and a very few have moderate vermis hypoplasia.

Lissencephaly and SBH compose a single malformation spectrum that is referred to as the *agyria-pachygyria-band spectrum*. This nomenclature is based on observation of patients with areas of classic lissencephaly, which merge into pachygyria,[19,20] and of multiple families with X-linked lissencephaly in male members and SBH in female members and the presence of similar mutations in both malformations. What distinguishes the gene defect is the anteroposterior (AP) morphologic pattern, which creates a characteristic gradient. Most patients with lissencephaly have a predominance of the posteroanterior (PA) gradient. The same AP and PA gradients are seen in patients with SBH, although the AP gradient is more common among SBH patients.

Children with classic lissencephaly or other diffuse malformations of the cortex often appear normal as newborns but sometimes exhibit apnea, poor feeding, or hypotonia. Seizures are uncommon during the first few days of life, but most have onset of seizures before 6 months. The epileptic spectrum in patients with the various lissencephalies is homogenous. Approximately 80% of children present with infantile spasms in the first year of life. Hypsarrhythmia and the typical EEG fast spike pattern often is seen at first. The infantile spasms respond initially to therapy with adrenocorticotropic hormone or other anticonvulsants in more than one-half of affected children, but the long-term response to treatment often is poor, and most children continue to have frequent seizures and severe developmental delay. Typical seizure types include myoclonic, tonic, and tonic-clonic seizures; many meet criteria for Lennox-Gastaut syndrome. Other neurologic manifestations include profound mental retardation and hypotonia followed by spasticity.

In contrast, most patients with SBH are female, have mild to moderate mental retardation (although both normal intelligence and severe mental retardation occur), minimal pyramidal signs, and dysarthria.[21] Seizures usually begin in childhood, although they may not begin until later, and controlling multiple seizure types that occur may be difficult. However, seizure frequency and severity vary. Cognitive development may slow after onset of the seizures.[18] EEG investigations usually demonstrate generalized spike and wave discharges or multifocal EEG abnormalities.[22] The neurologic outcome depends on the thickness of the heterotopic band as seen on MRI.[18]

Recent studies have identified two genes associated with the isolated lissencephaly sequence, including the *LIS1* gene on chromosome 17p13.3 and the *XLIS* (DCX) gene on chromosome Xq22.3-q23. Both appear to produce microtubule-associated proteins. Mutations of these two genes are the major cause of classic lissencephaly. Recent genotype-phenotype correlation has shown that patients with *LIS1* mutations have a PA gradient, whereas patients with *XLIS* mutations have the reverse (AP) gradient.[23] The same

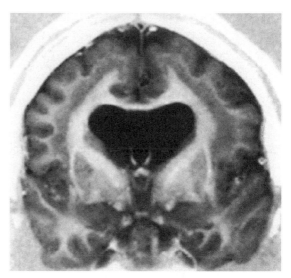

Figure 22-3. Band heterotopia. Coronal T1-weighted magnetic resonance image shows abnormal rim of gray matter underneath a white-matter rim. The overlying cortex appears normal.

gradients are seen in patients with SBH. Thus, molecular testing can be prioritized on the basis of the appearance of the scan.

Other syndromes with lissencephalies include the Miller-Dieker syndrome, which consists of classic lissencephaly, typical facial abnormalities, and sometimes other birth defects. The facial changes include a prominent forehead, bitemporal hollowing, a short nose with upturned nares, a protuberant upper lip, a thin vermilion border of the upper lip, and a small jaw.[24] Chromosome and fluorescent in situ hybridization analyses show visible deletions of chromosome 17p13.3 in all patients, with the *LIS1* gene being the primary cause of the lissencephaly in this syndrome. Lissencephaly occurs in several other rare syndromes. The clinical manifestations with intractable epilepsy are similar to those in children with classic lissencephaly. Examples include several types of lissencephaly with agenesis of the corpus callosum, cerebellar hypoplasia, or both.

Heterotopia

Heterotopia are defined as nodular gray-matter masses that can be diffuse, bilateral, or unilateral.

They may be isolated or may develop in conjunction with other central nervous system malformations (e.g., Chiari II malformations, basilar cephaloceles, or agenesis of the corpus callosum) or metabolic disorders (e.g., Zellweger syndrome and neonatal adrenoleukodystrophy). Patients (approximately 80%) with heterotopia are likely to develop epilepsy, their first seizures developing most commonly during the second decade of life. However, some patients with subependymal heterotopia are neurologically and developmentally normal, with the heterotopia being detected incidentally during imaging evaluation for unrelated conditions.[25] Disorders of cognition are less common in the unilateral focal group (<20%) and most common in the bilateral diffuse group, albeit with a clear male skew of severe mental retardation. The incidence of impaired cognition seems to parallel the incidence of associated malformations (of both brain and other viscera).[25] Subependymal heterotopia can be diagnosed readily on MRI. Its appearance is fairly characteristic: The nodules are round to ovoid, isointense to mature gray matter, and pro-

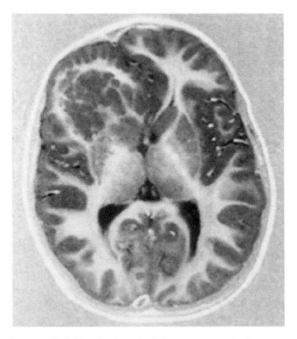

Figure 22-4. Focal subcortical heterotopia with abnormal cortex (cortical dysplasia). Axial T1-weighted magnetic resonance image shows large mass of heterotopic gray matter in the frontal lobe. Note involvement of basal ganglia and frontal lobe cortex.

truding slightly into the ventricular lumen, resulting in an irregular ventricular outline.

Several syndromes occur in conjunction with heterotopia. The best-defined syndrome is bilateral diffuse heterotopia or periventricular nodular heterotopia secondary to mutation of chromosome Xq28.[20] Filamin 1 is the gene defect. Filamin is an actin filament cross-linking protein and also links membrane proteins to actin. Because this disorder is X-linked, it is observed primarily in women. The disorder is rare in men, and those affected have an incidence of neurodevelopmental abnormalities much higher than that in female subjects. Other reported anomalies are seen in male persons, including cerebellar hypoplasia and syndactyly,[26] short-gut syndrome,[27] congenital nephrosis,[28] and frontonasal dysplasia.

Most patients with periventricular nodular heterotopia come to medical attention because of epilepsy. Seizures may be generalized or may appear localization-related, suggesting mesial temporal, neocortical temporal, or parieto-occipital onset.[29] Seizures usually begin during the second decade (mean age, 17 years), relatively later than in other MCDs. Scalp EEG scans show generalized or multifocal abnormalities, but pseudotemporal lobe localization has been described.

Subcortical heterotopia (SCH) are considerably less common than are subependymal heterotopia and have a different etiology. Patients with focal SCH have variable motor and intellectual disturbances, depending on the extent and localization of the lesions. Patients with bilateral, thick SCH present with moderate to severe developmental delay and motor dysfunction, whereas those with unilateral heterotopia have less severe deficits. Almost all affected patients eventually develop localization-related epilepsy, usually during the first or second decades.[30] EEG studies demonstrate regional rather than focal areas of epileptogenesis. Diagnosis is made on MRI, on which nodules of gray-matter intensity extend in a curvilinear course through the white matter from the ventricular surface to the cerebral cortex (Figure 22-4). The overlying cortex is thin, with small gyri and shallow sulci, and the white matter is thin. The corpus callosum is agenetic or hypogenetic in ~70% of affected brains. SCH often is sporadic, which suggests that somatic rather than germline mutations may be involved. The observation of discordant occurrence of SCH in monozygotic twins underscores the somatic origin of this malformation, at least in most patients.

Malformations of Cortical Organization

Malformations of cortical organization include those in which neurons reach the cortex but do not form normal cortical layers or intracortical connections. They are characterized by an abnormal gyral pattern with histologically normal thickness of the cortex and with no heterotopia in the subcortical or subependymal regions. The classic malformations in this category are polymicrogyria and schizencephaly. However, the observation that schizencephaly is layered by polymicrogyria supports the concept of a single entity currently known as the *schizencephaly-polymicrogyria complex.*

Polymicrogyria

Polymicrogyria is characterized by many small microgyri separated by shallow sulci, neuronal heterotopia and, often, enlarged ventricles. Frequently, polymicrogyria is superimposed on areas of apparent pachygyria that represent areas of fused gyri rather than true pachygyria. Multiple causes explain polymicrogyria, including environmental and genetic causes. The best-known cause is intrauterine cytomegalovirus infection, which usually is associated with diffuse or patchy white-matter changes and often diffuse or multifocal periventricular calcifications.[31]

Studies over the last 5–10 years have reported at least five distinct syndromes associated with polymicrogyria.[32–34] On the basis of experience with several families having affected relatives, diffuse polymicrogyria with no associated abnormalities appears to be X-linked in some families. Similarly, several families with bilateral perisylvian polymicrogyria appear to exhibit X-linked inheritance as well.

The clinical presentation in these conditions varies, except for the congenital bilateral perisylvian syndrome, or Kuzniecky syndrome.[32] Patients with the congenital bilateral perisylvian syndrome have prominent pseudobulbar paresis, severe but variable dysarthria, and minimal to severe developmental delay. Seizures occur in 60–80% of patients. Of those with seizures,

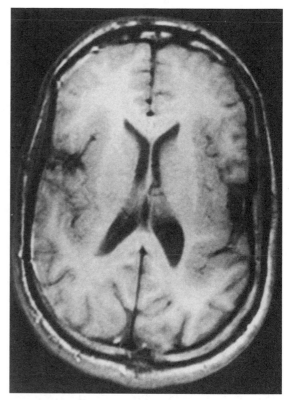

Figure 22-5. Congenital bilateral perisylvian syndrome. Axial T1-weighted magnetic resonance image shows bilateral opercular abnormalities with thick cortex representing (fused) polymicrogyria. The abnormalities are asymmetric in location and extent.

more than one-half experience frequent epilepsy. Seizures consist of atypical absence seizures, tonic-atonic attacks, and generalized tonic-clonic seizures. A unique seizure type consists of perioral seizures with bilateral facial involvement. EEG abnormalities include generalized spike and wave or multifocal abnormalities. The diagnosis can be made on the basis of the clinical features and can be confirmed on cranial MRI (Figure 22-5).

Another syndrome is unilateral polymicrogyria with transient, continuous, nonconvulsive status epilepticus during sleep. Affected patients have unilateral perirolandic lesions with mild to moderate hemiparesis from birth. Seizures often are localization-related at first but, eventually, a generalized epileptic encephalopathy develops. The transition usually occurs in childhood (age 5–8 years) but can occur in puberty. During this period, patients develop atypical absence seizures, generalized tonic-clonic seizures, and other clinical manifestations of generalized EEG discharges. EEG scans during slow-wave sleep will demonstrate continuous epileptiform discharges. Treatment often is required during that period, but spontaneous improvement has been reported.

Schizencephaly-Polymicrogyria Complex

The schizencephaly-polymicrogyria complex is included in the same category with polymicrogyria because the cortex around the lips of the cleft is polymicrogyric. The schizencephaly-polymicrogyria complex can be seen in patients with septo-optic dysplasia[35,36] or in isolation. These disorders generally are considered sporadic, but a recent report supports a genetic basis for some forms of the schizencephaly-polymicrogyria complex.[37]

The clinical manifestations of the schizencephaly-polymicrogyria complex often are related to the type of defect, with open or type II clefts often associated with contralateral pyramidal signs, developmental delay, and seizures. Callosal agenesis also is a marker for poor outcome. Seizures usually are focal and often intractable, but clinical variability is observed. EEG localization despite gross structural lesions often is regional rather than focal. Surgery is not often possible, owing to the central localization of the lesions and the presence of widespread areas of epileptogenic activity.

References

1. Barkovich A, Kuzniecky R, Dobbyns W, et al. A classification scheme for malformations of cortical development. Neuropediatrics 1996;27:59–63.
2. Barkovich AJ, Ferriero DM, Barr RM, et al. Microlissencephaly: a heterogeneous malformation of cortical development. Neuropediatrics 1998;29:113–119.
3. Dobyns WB, Truwit CL, Ross ME, et al. Differences in the gyral pattern distinguish chromosome 17–linked and X-linked lissencephaly. Neurology 1999;53:270–277.
4. Barkovich AJ, Gressens P, Evrard P. Formation, maturation, and disorders of brain neocortex. AJNR Am J Neuroradiol 1992;13:423–446.
5. Warkany J, Lemire RJ, Cohen MM Jr. Mental Retardation and Congenital Malformations of the Central Nervous System. Chicago: Yearbook Medical, 1981.
6. Dobyns WB, Barkovich AJ. Microcephaly with simplified gyral pattern (oligogyric microcephaly) and microlissencephaly: reply. Neuropediatrics 1999;30:104–106.
7. Norman RM. Cerebellar hypoplasia in Werdnig-Hoffmann disease. Arch Dis Child 1961;36:96–101.
8. Barth PG, Mullaart R, Stam FC, Slooff JL. Familial lissencephaly with extreme neopallial hypoplasia. Brain Dev 1982;4:145–151.
9. Pavone L, Curatolo P, Rizzo R, et al. Epidermal nevus syndrome: a neurological variant with hemimegalencephaly, gyral malformation, mental retardation, seizures and facial hemihypertrophy. Neurology 1991;41:266–271.
10. Dodge NN, Dobyns WB. Agenesis of the corpus callosum and Dandy-Walker malformation associated with hemimegalencephaly in the sebaceous nevus syndrome. Am J Med Genet 1995;56:147–150.
11. Vigevano F, Bertini E, Boldrini R, et al. Hemimegalencephaly and intractable epilepsy: benefits of hemispherectomy. Epilepsia 1989;30:833–843.
12. Taylor DC, Falconer MA, Bruton CJ, Corsellis JAN. Focal dysplasia of the cerebral cortex in epilepsy. J Neurol Neurosurg Psychiatry 1971;34:369–387.
13. Hardiman O, Burke T, Phillips J, et al. Microdysgenesis in resected temporal neocortex: incidence and clinical significance in focal epilepsy. Neurology 1988;38:1041–1047.
14. Kuzniecky R, Garcia J, Faught E, Morawetz R. Cortical dysplasia in TLE: MRI correlations. Ann Neurol 1991;29:293–298.
15. Wyllie E, Baumgartner C, Prayson R, et al. The clinical spectrum of focal cortical dysplasia and epilepsy. J Epilepsy 1994;7:303–317.
16. Kuzniecky RI, Jackson GD. Neuroimaging in Epilepsy. In RI Kuzniecky, GD Jackson (eds), Magnetic Resonance in Epilepsy. New York: Raven Press, 1995;27–48.
17. Barkovich A. Non-lissencephalic cortical dysplasias: correlation of imaging findings with clinical deficits. AJNR Am J Neuroradiol 1992;13:95–103.
18. Barkovich AJ, Guerrini R, Battaglia G, et al. Band heterotopia: correlation of outcome with magnetic resonance imaging parameters. Ann Neurol 1994;36:609–617.
19. Dobyns WB, Truwit CL. Lissencephaly and other malformations of cortical development: 1995 update. Neuropediatrics 1995;26:132–147.
20. Pilz DT, Kuc J, Matsumoto N, et al. Subcortical band heterotopia in rare affected males can be caused by missense mutations in DCX (XLIS) or LIS1. Hum Mol Genet 1999;8:1757–1760.
21. Dobyns WB, Andermann E, Andermann F, et al. X-linked malformations of neuronal migration. Neurology 1996;47:331–339.
22. Palmini A, Andermann F, Aicardi J, et al. Diffuse cortical dysplasia, or the "double cortex" syndrome: the clinical and epileptic spectrum in 10 patients. Neurology 1991;41:1656–1662.
23. Pilz DT, Matsumoto N, Minnerath S, et al. LIS1 and XLIS (DCX) mutations cause most classical lissen-

cephaly, but different patterns of malformation. Hum Mol Genet 1998;7:2029–2037.

24. Dobyns WB, Curry CJR, Hoyme HE, et al. Clinical and molecular diagnosis of Miller-Dieker syndrome. Am J Hum Genet 1991;48:584–594.

25. Eksioglu Y, Scheffer I, Cardenas P, et al. Periventricular heterotopia: an X-linked dominant epilepsy locus causing aberrant cerebral cortical development. Neuron 1996;16:77–87.

26. Nezelof C, Jaubert F, Lyon G. Syndrome familial associant grele court, malrotation intestinale, hypertrophie du pylore et malformation cerebrale: etude anatomoclinique de trois observations. Ann Anat Pathol (Paris) 1976;21:401–412.

27. Palm L, Hagerstrand I, Kristoffersson U, et al. Nephrosis and disturbances of neuronal migration in male siblings—a new hereditary disorder? Arch Dis Child 1986;61:545–548.

28. Guerrini R, Dobyns WB. Bilateral periventricular nodular heterotopia with mental retardation and frontonasal malformation. Neurology 1998;51:499–503.

29. Dubeau F, Tampieri D, Lee N, et al. Periventricular and subcortical nodular heterotopia: a study of 33 patients. Brain 1995;118:1273–1287.

30. Barkovich AJ. Pediatric Neuroimaging. New York: Raven Press, 1995;668.

31. Barkovich AJ, Lindan CE. Congenital cytomegalovirus infection of the brain: imaging analysis and embryologic considerations. AJNR Am J Neuroradiol 1994; 15:703–715.

32. Kuzniecky RI, Andermann F, Guerrini R. The congenital bilateral perisylvian syndrome: study of 31 patients. The Congenital Bilateral Perisylvian Syndrome Multicenter Collaborative Study. Lancet 1993;341:608–612.

33. Guerrini R, Dubeau F, Dulac O, et al. Bilateral parasagittal parietooccipital polymicrogyria and epilepsy. Ann Neurol 1997,41.65–73.

34. Guerrini R, Dobyns WB, Dulac O, et al. Genetically Determined Forms of Partial Symptomatic Epilepsies: Clinical Phenotype, Neuropathology and Neurogenetic Basis of Seizures. In SF Berkovic, P Genton, E Hirsch, F Picard (eds), Genetics of Focal Epilepsies: Clinical Aspects and Molecular Biology. London: John Libbey, 1999;125–147.

35. Aicardi J, Goutieres F. The syndrome of absence of the septum pellucidum with porencephalies and other developmental defects. Neuropediatrics 1981;12:319–329.

36. Kuban KCK, Teele RL, Wallman J. Septo-optic-dysplasia-schizencephaly: radiographic and clinical features. Pediatr Radiol 1989;19:145–150.

37. Brunelli S, Faiella A, Capra V, et al. Germline mutations in the homeobox gene EMX2 in patients with severe schizencephaly. Nat Genet 1996;12:94–96.

Chapter 23

Controlling Seizures in Children with Developmental Disabilities: An Overview

Blaise F. D. Bourgeois

Although the treatment of seizures in children with developmental disabilities follows the same basic principles as those that guide the treatment of all children with seizures, several distinguishing features characterize the therapeutic management of epilepsy in this subgroup of children. As a group, these patients have a different spectrum of seizure types and epilepsy syndromes. In general, controlling their seizures is more difficult, and alternative treatments are more likely to be tried, such as the ketogenic diet, epilepsy surgery, a vagal nerve stimulator implant, and experimental new antiepileptic drugs (AEDs). Because their seizures tend to be more refractory, such patients are more likely to receive AED polytherapy. As a group, children with developmental disabilities and seizures have a higher risk of experiencing status epilepticus or acute repetitive seizures. Also, children with developmental disabilities may be more susceptible to experiencing certain adverse effects from AEDs, including the phenomenon of seizure exacerbation that occurs with certain AEDs. Finally, even if their seizures are brought under control for a longer period, such children have a higher risk of seizure relapse when an attempt is made to take them off their medications.

Difference in Seizure Types and Epilepsy Syndromes

Children with developmental disabilities and seizures are much more likely to have a symptomatic or cryptogenic epilepsy than an idiopathic epilepsy.

They also are more likely to have generalized or multifocal epilepsies than strictly focal epilepsies, because isolated single lesions are less likely to cause developmental disabilities. Therefore, conditions characterized by a combination of epilepsy and developmental disabilities usually are associated with generalized encephalopathies, such as diffuse congenital anomalies, tuberous sclerosis, chromosomal disorders (e.g., Angelman's syndrome), postinfectious or postanoxic encephalopathies, and neurometabolic disorders (e.g., ceroid lipofuscinosis), among many others.

As can be seen in Table 23-1, symptomatic and cryptogenic epilepsies include epilepsy syndromes that differ notably from those that are considered to be idiopathic epilepsies. Most of these syndromes are known to be associated often or even invariably with developmental disabilities. The best-known examples are West's syndrome and the Lennox-Gastaut syndrome. These specific epilepsies have their own seizure types and treatment modalities. Affected patients now are involved in their own set of drug trials.[1–6] Practitioners involved in the treatment of such patients must be familiar with the therapeutic aspects of these syndromes. Choices of treatments and drug sequences for various syndromes are discussed briefly at the end of this chapter.

Likelihood of Refractory Seizures

As a group, children with developmental disabilities and epilepsy are less likely to experience freedom

Table 23-1. Generalized Epilepsy: Epileptic Syndromes

Idiopathic
   Childhood absence epilepsy
   Juvenile absence epilepsy
   Juvenile myoclonic epilepsy
   Myoclonic-astatic epilepsy
   Benign neonatal convulsions
   Benign myoclonic seizures in infancy
   Generalized tonic-clonic seizures on awakening
   Other generalized idiopathic epilepsy
Symptomatic or cryptogenic
   West's syndrome
   Lennox-Gastaut syndrome
   Early myoclonic encephalopathy
   Myoclonic absence epilepsy
   Specific etiologies
   Early infantile epileptic encephalopathy with
      suppression-burst

from seizures in response to therapy.[7,8] This limitation is due largely to the underlying cerebral pathology responsible for both the seizures and the developmental disability. In a review of intractable epilepsy, Aicardi and Shorvon[9] stated that "intractability is not evenly distributed among patients with

Table 23-2. Clinical Factors Associated with Chronic Active Epilepsy

Certain epilepsy syndromes	West's syndrome, Lennox-Gastaut syndrome, severe or progressive myoclonic epilepsy
Certain etiologies	Tuberous sclerosis, Sturge-Weber syndrome, metabolic disorders, tumor, hamartoma, gross malformation, arteriovenous malformation, damage following cerebral infection or trauma
Certain seizure types	Tonic seizures, atonic seizures, atypical absence seizures
Associated clinical features	Mental retardation, neurologic handicap, neuropsychiatric handicap, long duration of epilepsy without remission

Source: Modified from J Aicardi, SD Shorvon. Intractable Epilepsy. In JJ Engel, TA Pedley (eds), Epilepsy: A Comprehensive Textbook. Philadelphia: Lippincott–Raven, 1997;1325–1331. Courtesy of Lippincott–Raven Publishers.

epilepsy. It is more common in those with mental retardation, neurologic deficits, or both, and generally in patients with detectable structural brain damage." They identified a group of clinical factors associated with chronic active epilepsy. As can be seen from Table 23-2, most of these factors are relevant for the population of children with developmental disabilities. Delgado et al.[10] followed 531 patients with both diagnosed cerebral palsy and epilepsy. Over a period of approximately 10 years, only 69 (13%) of these patients had experienced freedom from seizures for 2 years or more.

Because their seizures are not controlled easily, patients with developmental disabilities are more likely to undergo trials of many different medications and to be enrolled in trials with new, nonmarketed AEDs. Such patients may have to be considered for treatment with drugs that are judged to be less safe, such as felbamate[11] or vigabatrin for infantile spasms.[4] They also are more likely to be considered for other therapeutic modalities, such as the ketogenic diet, epilepsy surgery, and the vagal nerve stimulator. At present, treatment of the Lennox-Gastaut syndrome and similar syndromes remains the main indication for the ketogenic diet[12] and for the use of felbamate.[11]

Antiepileptic Drug Polytherapy

Because they tend to have refractory seizures, children with developmental disabilities and epilepsy commonly receive AED polytherapy. Although polytherapy in such patients is the rule rather than the exception, little scientific evidence demonstrates the benefit of this practice. On the basis of several independent observations that reducing the number of AEDs can lessen the number or severity of side effects with little or no loss in seizure control, monotherapy has been strongly advocated.[13–19] In addition, adding a second drug after failure of the first was found to be associated with only modest benefit.[20] However, AED combinations can be expected to be used for as long as single-drug therapy fails to control every patient's seizures.

Combination drug therapy has several disadvantages. With few exceptions among the newer drugs, the majority of AEDs display pharmacokinetic interactions. These interactions not only create a need for more frequent drug level monitoring and dosage readjustments but increase the likelihood of subtherapeutic drug levels or clinical toxicity. A good example is seen in the inhibition of lamotrigine elimination by valproate, which increases the level-dose ratio of lamotrigine. This interaction is considered to be responsible for the higher incidence of rashes when lamotrigine is added to valproate than when it is added to another drug.[21]

It has been demonstrated also that AED combination therapy can result in cumulative toxicity. As a result, two drugs combined are more likely to cause side effects, despite levels in the therapeutic range, than would each drug alone at the same concentration. This concept is supported by a series of clinical studies in which reduction of AED polypharmacy resulted in fewer side effects.[13–18] Several of these studies were carried out in institutionalized patients with mental retardation. More recently, Pellock and Hunt[19] carried out an open, 10-year study of 244 epileptic, mentally retarded patients. The percentage of patients receiving monotherapy could be increased from 36.5% to 58.1% with no evidence of loss in seizure control.

Finally, the interpretation of drug effect often is more difficult with AED polytherapy. Determining which drug is responsible for a reduction in seizure frequency and which drug has caused dose-related or idiosyncratic side effects may become very difficult, especially when several changes in the drug regimen occur within a short time.

Combination drug therapy does have potential advantages, including (1) better seizure control with similar or fewer side effects, (2) same seizure control but with fewer side effects, and (3) reduction in the frequency of two or more different seizure types that respond only to different drugs. Only very few systematic clinical comparisons have been carried out between the effect of two drugs each given sequentially in monotherapy and their effect when they were administered in combination. A group of five patients with absence seizures became seizure-free when ethosuximide and valproate were combined, although their absence seizures had remained refractory to ethosuximide or to valproate in monotherapy.[22] A more recent crossover trial provided evidence supporting the combination of lamotrigine with valproate.[23] Among 13 patients who failed to experience a seizure reduction when valproate and

lamotrigine were added individually and sequentially to their pre-existing regimen, four became seizure-free when valproate and lamotrigine were added together.

Based on the paucity of clinical studies documenting the superiority of specific AED combinations, the selection of a combination often has to be based on careful clinical observation in individual patients.[24] Rational drug combinations rarely can be predicted. A rational AED combination for any given patient will have been identified if a patient does better in terms of seizure control versus side effects while taking drugs A and B together (at any doses) than while taking drug A alone or drug B alone at their respective optimal doses.

Risk of Status Epilepticus

In children who have developmental disabilities and epilepsy, the occurrence of episodes of status epilepticus is relatively common. Although they do not necessarily experience generalized tonic-clonic status epilepticus more frequently than do other patients with epilepsy, they are particularly prone to clusters of acute repetitive seizures and to nonconvulsive status epilepticus. For instance, patients with the Lennox-Gastaut syndrome are prone to develop atypical absence status that can last hours to days and has been described also as *spike-wave stupor*. Status epilepticus has been reported in more than two-thirds of patients with the Lennox-Gastaut syndrome.[25] The occurrence of status epilepticus has been well described also in patients with Angelman's syndrome (partial monosomy 15q). A high percentage of these patients experience nonconvulsive status epilepticus characterized by hypotonia and decreased alertness that can last days or weeks.[26] These episodes often relapse and may become intractable. In addition to nonconvulsive status epilepticus, patients with Angelman's syndrome also may experience episodes of myoclonic status.[27,28] Overall, a high percentage of patients with developmental disabilities and seizures require intermittent administration of oral, intravenous, or rectal benzodiazepines for status epilepticus or acute repetitive seizures.[29] For the same reason, these patients have a relatively high risk of emergency room visits.

Adverse Effects of Medications

A fairly large body of literature indicates that among children with epilepsy, those with developmental disabilities are more susceptible to experiencing more frequent or specific adverse effects of AEDs. In the most recent review of valproate hepatic fatalities in the United States, Bryant and Dreifuss[30] identified four risk factors for this complication: young age, polytherapy, developmental delay, and coincidental metabolic disorders. Of these four risk factors, three may be present in the population under discussion. For children who are younger than 2 years or who are developmentally delayed, metabolic testing has been recommended before treatment with valproate, and children should not receive valproate if they have a known or suspected metabolic disorder.[31]

Some independent reports have cited behavioral side effects of gabapentin in children,[32–35] consisting mainly of aggressive and oppositional behavior. Every patient in these series had either a baseline learning disability or attention-deficit hyperactivity disorder and developmental delay, or mental retardation. Similarly, agitation or hyperkinesia was found to be a frequent adverse effect of vigabatrin in children and seems to occur mostly in mentally retarded patients.[36,37] A group of three patients was reported to have experienced incontinence after the introduction of gabapentin.[38] All three had urinary incontinence, and two also had fecal incontinence, which was reversible after discontinuation of gabapentin. Two of these patients were mentally retarded, and one had attention-deficit hyperactivity disorder.

More than 30 years ago, enzyme-inducing AEDs were demonstrated to inactivate vitamin D and thereby cause clinical osteomalacia or rickets.[39–47] The overwhelming majority of reported patients were institutionalized and mentally retarded. Although contributing factors, such as low vitamin D intake and inactivity, had been cited, the main cause has been suggested to be lack of exposure to sun in these institutionalized handicapped children.[44]

These findings of increased susceptibility to adverse effects of medications have significant implications for the management of children with developmental disabilities and epilepsy. What also should be emphasized is that, as a group, these children are less likely to speak about adverse effects from their medication. Therefore, those involved in their care should have a higher index of suspicion and should look more actively for evidence of drug side effects.

Seizure Exacerbation by Antiepileptic Drugs

Well recognized is that certain AEDs can exacerbate the seizure frequency or cause de novo seizures in certain patients.[48] This phenomenon of seizure exacerbation has also been called *acute aberrant reaction* or *paradoxical intoxication*.[49] This response seems to be more prevalent in generalized epilepsies, particularly symptomatic generalized epilepsies, which are common in patients with developmental disabilities. In the earliest reports, primarily phenytoin was incriminated.[49,50] A more specific reaction has been observed repeatedly in patients with the Lennox-Gastaut syndrome. As mentioned, these patients have a tendency to experience nonconvulsive status epilepticus. When they receive intravenous benzodiazepines in an attempt to interrupt this nonconvulsive status, they may experience generalized tonic status epilepticus.[51–54]

Seizure exacerbation in patients with the Lennox-Gastaut syndrome seems to be caused by several different AEDs. Gabapentin was noted to cause a dramatic and reversible exacerbation of absence and myoclonic seizures in a 14-year-old boy with the Lennox-Gastaut syndrome.[55] In addition, hemi–tonic-clonic seizures became stronger and longer. More recently, Guerrini et al.[56] reported the case of an 8-year-old who had Lennox-Gastaut syndrome and experienced myoclonic status epilepticus after her dose of lamotrigine was increased to 20 mg/kg per day. Rapid disappearance of clinical and electrophysiologic manifestations of her myoclonic status epilepticus followed discontinuation of lamotrigine.

Carbamazepine also has been reported repeatedly and independently to cause seizure exacerbation in children. Five children (ages 3–11) experienced the onset of myoclonic atypical absence or atonic seizures (or both) within a few days of the addition of carbamazepine to their drug regimen.[57] Three of these five children had underlying central nervous system pathology. In another series of 15 children, carbamazepine was found to exacerbate generalized atypical absence seizures in 11 and generalized convulsive seizures in 4 children.[58] Fourteen had generalized seizures at baseline, and the patients were considered to have "intractable mixed seizure disorders." In this series, bilaterally synchronous spike and wave discharges of 2.5–3.0 Hz appeared to be predictive of exacerbation of atypical absence seizures by carbamazepine, whereas exacerbation of generalized convulsive seizures appeared more likely in patients with 1- to 2-Hz spike and wave discharges. On the basis of observations in six children with AED-induced seizures, Lerman[59] also found the presence of generalized spike and wave discharges to be a common denominator. He concluded that drug-induced seizure exacerbation is particularly likely to occur in children with conditions refractory to therapy and with slow spike and wave discharges in their electroencephalogram, such as children with the Lennox-Gastaut syndrome. Talwar et al.[60] found a high correlation between the new appearance of generalized spike, polyspike, and wave discharges and the occurrence of clinical seizure exacerbation by carbamazepine.

Vigabatrin has been reported to aggravate seizures in some patients with nonprogressive myoclonic epilepsies[36,61] and infantile spasms[62] and in patients with Angelman's syndrome.[63]

In conclusion, little doubt remains that patients with developmental disabilities are more susceptible to experiencing episodes of seizure exacerbation in response to certain AEDs. What is important is for those involved in their care to anticipate and recognize this possibility.

Seizure Relapse after Antiepileptic Drug Discontinuation

In addition to having more refractory epilepsies, patients with developmental disabilities also are more likely to experience seizure recurrences after discontinuation of their AEDs, even if their seizures had been controlled previously for an adequate period. Some of the factors identified by Holowach et al.[64] as being associated with seizure relapse after drug withdrawal included long duration of epilepsy before control, neurologic dysfunction, and combination of seizure types. More recently, Shinnar et al.[65] also identified risk factors

for recurrence after AED discontinuation. These factors included remote symptomatic epilepsy and slowing on the electroencephalogram. In both these studies, the risk factors identified are those associated more commonly with neurologic impairment.

A group of 531 children with diagnosed cerebral palsy and epilepsy were studied for approximately 10 years.[10] Of these, as quoted earlier, only 69 (13%) had been seizure-free for 2 years or more. Sixty-five were followed up during and after drug withdrawal, until seizure relapse or until 2 years without recurrence. Their seizure relapse rate was 41%.

Similar results were found in an open 10-year study of AED reduction in 244 institutionalized, mentally retarded patients.[19] Criteria for complete drug discontinuation were met in 12.7% of these patients. After an attempt at discontinuing their medications, nearly one-half required reinitiation of therapy.

Dooley et al.[66] followed 97 children who were weaned from their AED therapy after 1 year without seizure. The overall probability of seizure recurrence 2 years after drug discontinuation was 39% for the entire group. However, analysis of subgroups revealed that seizures recurred at 2 years in 51% of those who were neurologically handicapped, as opposed to 32% of those without a neurologic handicap.

In conclusion, several independent observations provide similar numbers, indicating that children with developmental disabilities have a 40–50% risk of seizure recurrence after elective discontinuation of AED therapy, even after 1 year or more without seizure before drug withdrawal.

Drug Selection by Seizure Type or Epilepsy Syndrome

Proper seizure or epilepsy syndrome diagnosis is the most important initial step in the process of managing seizures in children with developmental disabilities. The next step is to select the most appropriate medication of first choice. If an affected patient's seizures remain uncontrolled, the most appropriate sequence of drugs to use then represents the next challenge. The place of drugs in the treatment

Table 23-3. Role of Newer Antiepileptic Drugs in the Treatment Sequence of Seizures and Epileptic Syndromes in Children

Partial seizures with or without secondary generalization	
First choice	Carbamazepine, oxcarbazepine
Second choice	Gabapentin, lamotrigine, topiramate, valproate, levetiracetam
Third choice	Tiagabine, phenobarbital, primidone, phenytoin, zonisamide
Generalized tonic-clonic seizures	
First choice	Valproate, carbamazepine, phenytoin
Second choice	Topiramate, lamotrigine
Third choice	Phenobarbital, primidone
Absence seizures	
Before age 10 years	
First choice	Ethosuximide, valproate
Second choice	Lamotrigine
Consider	Methsuximide, acetazolamide, benzodiazepine, topiramate, zonisamide
After age 10 years	
First choice	Valproate
Second choice	Lamotrigine
Third choice	Ethosuximide, methsuximide, acetazolamide, benzodiazepine, topiramate, zonisamide
Juvenile myoclonic epilepsy	
First choice	Valproate
Second choice	Lamotrigine, clonazepam, topiramate
Third choice	Phenobarbital, primidone, zonisamide
Lennox-Gastaut and related syndromes	
First choice	Valproate
Second choice	Topiramate, lamotrigine
Third choice	Ketogenic diet, zonisamide, felbamate, benzodiazepine, phenobarbital
Consider	Ethosuximide, methsuximide, ACTH or steroids, pyridoxine, vigabatrin
Infantile spasms	
First choice	ACTH, vigabatrin
Second choice	Valproate
Third choice	Topiramate, lamotrigine, benzodiazepine, zonisamide
Consider	Pyridoxine, felbamate, tiagabine
Benign epilepsy with centrotemporal spikes	
First choice	Gabapentin, valproate, sulthiame
Second choice	Carbamazepine, phenytoin
Third choice	Phenobarbital, primidone, benzodiazepine
Consider	Lamotrigine, topiramate

ACTH = adrenocorticotropic hormone.

sequence of seizures or epilepsy syndromes is not established firmly and is not scientifically determined. Any attempt at assigning a place to the available drugs will have to be reassessed periodically as newer drugs are released or as new information becomes available regarding previously released drugs. The decision to assign a certain place to any drug in the treatment sequence of a seizure type or epilepsy syndrome will be influenced by various considerations. These factors include available efficacy data, available adverse effects data, pharmacokinetics and interactions, titration rate, personal experience, familiarity with different AEDs, and personal prescribing habits. Among these considerations, efficacy against seizures to be treated and adverse effects should have the highest priority in guiding the choice.

With this concept in mind, an attempt is made in Table 23-3 to assign places to various AEDs in the treatment sequence of several seizure types and epilepsy syndromes. Drugs are divided into drugs of first, second, and third choice, regardless of whether they are approved formally for a particular seizure type, epilepsy syndrome, or age group or for monotherapy. When two or more drugs are listed in the same category, the actual choice of a single drug may have to be made individually in any given patient on the basis of side effect profile, age, gender, and preference.

References

1. The Felbamate Study Group in Lennox-Gastaut Syndrome. Efficacy of felbamate in childhood epileptic encephalopathy (Lennox-Gastaut syndrome). N Engl J Med 1993;328:29–33.
2. Motte J, Trevathan E, Arvidsson JF, et al. Lamotrigine for generalized seizures associated with the Lennox-Gastaut syndrome. N Engl J Med 1997;337:1807–1812.
3. Sachdeo R, Glauser T, Ritter F, et al. A double-blind, randomized trial of topiramate in Lennox-Gastaut syndrome. Neurology 1999;52:1882–1887.
4. Vigevano F, Cilio M. Vigabatrin versus ACTH as first-line treatment for infantile spasms: a randomized, prospective study. Epilepsia 1997;38:1270–1274.
5. Granström M, Gaily E, Liukkonen E. Treatment of infantile spasms: results of a population-based study with vigabatrin as the first drug for spasms. Epilepsia 1999;40:950–957.
6. Åberg L, Kirveskari E, Santavuori P. Lamotrigine therapy in juvenile neuronal ceroid lipofuscinosis. Epilepsia 1999;40:796–799.
7. Huttenlocher PR, Hapke RJ. A follow-up study of intractable seizures in childhood. Ann Neurol 1990;28:699–705.
8. Juul-Jensen P. Epidemiology of Intractable Epilepsy. In D Schmidt, Morselli P (eds), Intractable Epilepsy. New York: Raven Press, 1986;5–11.
9. Aicardi J, Shorvon SD. Intractable Epilepsy. In JJ Engel, TA Pedley (eds), Epilepsy: A Comprehensive Textbook. Philadelphia: Lippincott-Raven, 1997;1325–1331.
10. Delgado MR, Riela AR, Mills J, et al. Discontinuation of antiepileptic drug treatment after two seizure-free years in children with cerebral palsy. Pediatrics 1996;97:192–197.
11. French J, Smith M, Faught E, Brown L. Practice advisory: the use of felbamate in the treatment of patients with intractable epilepsy. Neurology 1999;52:1540–1545.
12. Nordli DRJ, DeVivo DC. The ketogenic diet revisited: back to the future. Epilepsia 1997;38:743–749.
13. Reynolds EH, Shorvon SD. Single drug or combination therapy for epilepsy? Drugs 1981;21:374–382.
14. Fischbacher E. Effect of reduction of anticonvulsants on well-being. BMJ 1982;285:423–424.
15. Bennett HS, Dunlop T, Ziring P. Reduction of polypharmacy for epilepsy in an institution for the retarded. Dev Med Child Neurol 1983;25:735–737.
16. Schmidt D. Reduction of two-drug therapy in intractable epilepsy. Epilepsia 1983;24:368–376.
17. Theodore WH, Porter RJ. Removal of sedative-hypnotic antiepileptic drugs from the regimen of patients with intractable epilepsy. Ann Neurol 1983;13:320–324.
18. Albright P, Bruni J. Reduction of polytherapy in epileptic patients. Arch Neurol 1985;42:797–799.
19. Pellock JM, Hunt PA. A decade of modern epilepsy therapy in institutionalized mentally retarded patients. Epilepsy Res 1996;25:263–268.
20. Schmidt D. Two antiepileptic drugs for intractable epilepsy with complex-partial seizures. J Neurol Psychiatry 1982;45:1119–1124.
21. Besag FMC, Wallace SJ, Dulac O, et al. Lamotrigine for the treatment of epilepsy in childhood. J Pediatr 1995;127:991–997.
22. Rowan AJ, Binnie CD, Warfield CA, et al. The delayed effect of sodium valproate on the photoconvulsive response in man. Epilepsia 1979;20:61–68.
23. Pisani F, Oteri G, Russo M, et al. The efficacy of valproate-lamotrigine comedication in refractory complex partial seizures: evidence for a pharmacodynamic interaction. Epilepsia 1999;40:1141–1146.
24. Meinardi H. Use of Combined Antiepileptic Drug Therapy. In RH Levy, RH Mattson, BS Meldrum (eds), Antiepileptic Drugs (4th ed). New York: Raven Press, 1995;91–97.
25. Beaumanoir A, Foletti G, Magistris M, Volanschi D. Status Epilepticus in the Lennox-Gastaut Syndrome. In E Niedermeyer, R Degen (eds), The Lennox-Gastaut Syndrome. New York: Alan R Liss, 1988;283–299.
26. Matsumoto A, Kumagai T, Miura K, et al. Epilepsy in Angelman syndrome associated with chromosome 15q deletion. Epilepsia 1992;33:1083–1090.
27. Guerrini R, DeLorey TM, Bonanni P, et al. Cortical myoclonus in Angelman syndrome. Ann Neurol 1996;40:39–48.
28. Viani F, Romeo A, Viri M, et al. Seizure and EEG patterns in Angelman's syndrome. J Child Neurol 1995;10:467–471.
29. Dreifuss FD, Rosman NP, Cloyd JC, et al. A comparison of rectal diazepam gel and placebo for acute repetitive seizures. N Engl J Med 1998;338(26):1869–1975.
30. Bryant A, Dreifuss FE. Valproic acid hepatic fatalities: III. U.S. experience since 1986. Neurology 1996;46:465–469.
31. König SA, Siemes H, Bläker F, et al. Severe hepatotoxicity during valproate therapy: an update and report of eight new fatalities. Epilepsia 1994;35:1005–1015.
32. Wolf S, Shinnar S, Kang H, et al. Gabapentin toxicity in children, manifesting as behavioral changes. Epilepsia 1995;36:1203–1205.

33. Lee D, Steingard R, Cesena M, et al. Behavioral side effects of gabapentin in children. Epilepsia 1996;37:87–90.

34. Tallian K, Nahata M, Lo W, Tsao C-Y. Gabapentin associated with aggressive behavior in pediatric patients with seizures. Epilepsia 1996;37:501–502.

35. Khurana D, Riviello J, Helmers S, et al. Efficacy of gabapentin in children with refractory partial seizures. J Pediatr 1996;128:829–833.

36. Luna D, Dulac O, Pajot N, Beaumont D. Vigabatrin in the treatment of childhood epilepsies: a single-blind placebo-controlled study. Epilepsia 1989;30:430–437.

37. Dulac O, Chiron C, Luna D, et al. Vigabatrin in childhood epilepsy. J Child Neurol 1991:S30–S37.

38. Gil-Nagel A, Gapany S, Blesi K, et al. Incontinence during treatment with gabapentin. Neurology 1997;48:1467–1468.

39. Kruse R. Osteopathien bei antiepileptischer Langzeittherapie. Monatsschr Kinderheilk 1968;116:378.

40. Dent CE, Richens A, Rowe DJF, Stamp TCB. Osteomalacia with long-term anticonvulsant therapy in epilepsy. BMJ 1970;6:69.

41. Baud L, Paunier L, Preece MA, et al. Concentrations plasmatiques de 25-hydroxycholécalciférol et traitement anticonvulsivant. Schweiz Med Wochenschr 1974;104:1908–1910.

42. Liakakos D, Papadopoulos Z, Vlachos P, et al. Serum alkaline phosphatase and urinary hydroxyproline values in children receiving phenobarbital with and without vitamin D. J Pediatr 1975;87:291–296.

43. Tolman KG, Jubiz W, Sannella JJ, et al. Osteomalacia associated with anticonvulsant drug therapy in mentally retarded children. Pediatrics 1975;56:45–50.

44. Morijiri Y, Sato T. Factors causing rickets in institutionalised handicapped children on anticonvulsant therapy. Arch Dis Child 1981;56:446–449.

45. Hoikka V, Savolainen K, Karjalainen P, et al. Treatment of osteomalacia in institutionalized epileptic patients on long-term anticonvulsant therapy. Ann Clin Res 1982;14:72–75.

46. Davie MWJ, Emberson CE, Lawson DEM, et al. Low plasma 25-hydroxyvitamin D and serum calcium levels in institutionalized epileptic subjects: associated risk factors, consequences and response to treatment with vitamin D. Q J Med 1983;52:79–91.

47. David HP, Woloszczuk W, Kovarik J. Antiepileptikainduzierte osteomalazie und vitamin D therapie. Nervenarzt 1983;54:647–650.

48. Perucca E, Gram L, Avanzini G, Dulac O. Antiepileptic drugs as a cause of worsening seizures. Epilepsia 1998;39:5–17.

49. Troupin AS, Ojemann LM. Paradoxical intoxication—a complication of anticonvulsant administration. Epilepsia 1975;16:753–758.

50. Levy LL, Fenichel GM. Diphenylhydantoin activated seizures. Neurology 1965;15:716–722.

51. Tassinari CA, Gastaut H, Dravet C, Roger J. A paradoxical effect: status epilepticus induced by benzodiazepines (Valium and Mogadon). Electroencephalogr Clin Neurophysiol 1971;31:182.

52. Tassinari CA, Dravet C, Roger J, et al. Tonic status epilepticus precipitated by intravenous benzodiazepine in five patients with Lennox-Gastaut syndrome. Epilepsia 1972;13:421–435.

53. Prior PF, Maclaine GN, Scott DF, Laurance BM. Tonic status epilepticus precipitated by intravenous diazepam in a child with petit mal status. Epilepsia 1972;13:467–472.

54. Bittencourt PRM, Richens A. Anticonvulsant-induced status epilepticus in Lennox-Gastaut syndrome. Epilepsia 1981;22:129–134.

55. Vossler D. Exacerbation of seizures in Lennox-Gastaut syndrome by gabapentin. Neurology 1996;46:852–853.

56. Guerrini R, Belmonte A, Parmeggiani L, Perucca E. Myoclonic status epilepticus following high-dosage lamotrigine therapy. Brain Dev 1999;21:420–424.

57. Shields WD, Saslow E. Myoclonic, atonic, and absence seizures following institution of carbamazepine therapy in children. Neurology 1983;33:1487–1489.

58. Snead OC, Hosey LC. Exacerbation of seizures in children by carbamazepine. N Engl J Med 1985;313:916–921.

59. Lerman P. Seizures induced or aggravated by anticonvulsants. Epilepsia 1986;27:706–710.

60. Talwar D, Arora MS, Sher PK. EEG changes and seizure exacerbation in young children treated with carbamazepine. Epilepsia 1994;35:1154–1159.

61. Lortie A, Chiron C, Mumford J, Dulac O. The potential for increasing seizure frequency, relapse, and appearance of new seizure types with vigabatrin. Neurology 1993;43:S24–S27.

62. Buti D, Rota M, Marvulli I, et al. Myoclonus induced by gamma-vinyl GABA (vigabatrin, GVG) in 3 children with infantile spasms (abstract). Epilepsia 1993;34[Suppl 2]:118–119.

63. Kuenzle C, Steinlin J, Wohlrab G, et al. Adverse effects of vigabatrin in Angelman syndrome. Epilepsia 1998;39:1213–1215.

64. Holowach Thurston J, Thurston DL, Hixon BB, Keller AJ. Prognosis in childhood epilepsy: additional follow-up of 148 children 15 to 23 years after withdrawal of anticonvulsant therapy. N Engl J Med 1982;306:831–836.

65. Shinnar S, Berg AT, Moshé SL, et al. Discontinuing antiepileptic drugs in children with epilepsy: a prospective study. Ann Neurol 1994;35:534–545.

66. Dooley J, Gordon K, Camfield P, et al. Discontinuation of anticonvulsant therapy in children free of seizures for 1 year: a prospective study. Neurology 1996;46:969–974.

Chapter 24

Initiating and Discontinuing Antiepileptic Drugs in Children with Neurologic Handicaps and Epilepsy

Peter Camfield and Carol S. Camfield

Many children with epilepsy have concurrent neurologic or mental handicaps. In the Nova Scotia population–based cohort of 504 children with partial or generalized epilepsies (excluding absence and most secondary generalized epilepsies), approximately 40% of children had a concurrent neurologic handicap.[1] Twenty percent had a significant learning disorder, and 4% had an isolated mental handicap. Approximately 9% were of normal intelligence but had other neurologic disability sufficient to impair function, and 7.4% had a combination of mental handicap and neurologic disability. Children with secondary generalized epilepsy have an even higher rate of neurologic handicap. For this chapter, *handicapped* is defined as mental handicap or neurologic handicap (or both) sufficient to impair function.

Handicapped children who develop epilepsy have a poor epilepsy prognosis at every stage of disease. The chance of recurrence after a first seizure is higher[2]; the chance of becoming seizure-free on medication is reduced[1]; the chance of intractable epilepsy is increased[1]; and the chance of successfully stopping medication after a seizure-free period is reduced.[3] However, none of these concerns is absolute, and exceptions occur. This chapter makes use of information about treatment response in handicapped children to suggest an approach to the decisions of initiating and terminating antiepileptic drugs (AEDs).

Reasons for Initiating Antiepileptic Drugs

Reasons for starting AEDs in any child with seizures are not always straightforward. At least six considerations are involved: (1) prevention of injury from a seizure, (2) prevention of brain damage, (3) prevention of discomfort from seizures, (4) prevention of death, (5) reduction of social stigma, and (6) hope for improving the long-term outcome. Each of these issues should be reviewed carefully before AED use is begun.

Prevention of Injury

No studies indicate whether those with handicap are more or less likely to be injured during a seizure. In our experience, the rate of injury in all children with epilepsy is relatively small; however, there are specific epilepsy syndromes associated with neurologic handicaps that seem to increase the risk of injury. The most striking are epilepsies with akinetic-atonic seizures, mainly the Lennox-Gastaut syndrome. Children who fall forward with akinetic-atonic seizures have a very high rate of facial lacerations and dental injuries. Protective headgear (i.e., a helmet) often is ineffective unless a full-face mask is attached. The social stigma and disturbance of vision that accompany use of a helmet render this approach difficult.

Prevention of Brain Damage

The debate about brain injury from seizures is lively.[4,5] Few or no data regarding humans are available to prove that seizures damage the brain, and a fair amount of data show that they do not. The number of seizures before treatment does not alter the prognosis.[6] In animals, severe and repetitive seizures can be shown to damage the brain,[4,7] but the relevance of these data to humans remains controversial.

In clinical practice, encountering children who have developmental stagnation with the onset of severe frequent seizures (catastrophic epilepsy) is not uncommon. Is the brain actually damaged, is development simply slowed, or is the real potential of an affected child's nervous system just becoming apparent, irrespective of seizures? Many of the catastrophic epilepsies begin at the time of blossoming of an infant's or toddler's cognitive function, which creates difficulty in knowing whether intellectual function would have been better if seizures had not occurred. However, it is difficult to ignore the remarkable dulling of interest and affect that occurs with the onset of such disorders as infantile spasms.[8]

Status epilepticus can injure the brain. A predominance of children with status epilepticus are neurologically abnormal.[9] Of 193 children with status epilepticus seen at a single center, 38% had pre-existing neurologic handicaps. Suspicion that a child with newly diagnosed epilepsy is at especially increased risk of status epilepticus may influence decisions regarding the use of AEDs.

Therefore, the decision to start treatment should be influenced by fear of brain damage if the epilepsy syndrome is catastrophic. If an affected child has a small number of partial or generalized tonic-clonic seizures, fear of brain damage apparently is not a sufficient concern to justify treatment.

Prevention of Discomfort from a Seizure

Postictally, many children and adults may have nausea, vomiting, headache, and somnolence. These symptoms may be more prominent than the seizures and be sufficiently incapacitating to warrant treatment. No evidence suggests that this concern is less or more frequent in handicapped people.

Prevention of Death

Sudden, unexpected death is rare in children with epilepsy. The death rate in epileptic children with neurologic handicap is considerably higher than in the general population, but the epilepsy does not contribute much to this risk. In Finland, a 9.4% population sample was ascertained in 1962.[10] Overall, 2,677 people had mental handicap, and 243 also had epilepsy. Follow-up 35 years later through the national death registry documented that the rate of death for those with mental handicap and epilepsy was increased only marginally over the death rate of those with mental handicap alone. Death appeared to be the result of complications of neurologic dysfunction, not epilepsy. Therefore, fear of death normally should not influence the decision to prescribe AEDs.

Reduction of Social Stigma

Children with neurologic handicap typically are socially isolated. Not known is whether the addition of epilepsy increases the social stigma. Also unknown is whether AED treatment alters the social isolation. If seizures are very frequent and severe, a reasonable expectation is that social isolation would increase; therefore, even in the absence of data, this issue may help to justify AED treatment.

Long-Term Remission

A growing consensus maintains that our current medications are not antiepileptic. AEDs control seizures but do not influence the chance of remission.[11,12] No studies compare treatment with absence of treatment in any epileptic syndrome associated with handicap. Early vigorous treatment has not been proven or disproven to have an effect on the long-term outcome of epilepsy.

Reasons to Delay Treatment

Side effects from medication constitute the major reason not to treat. Some special issues influence this decision in neurologically impaired children. In nonverbal children, recognizing cognitive side effects may be more difficult. Nitrazepam and other benzodiazepines may interfere with swallowing, especially in children with existing bulbar problems, which could result in recurrent aspiration.[13] Increased drooling caused by the same mechanism is a personal care concern and very socially disabling. Drugs that interact with the P450 system in the liver may have an effect on vitamin D metabolism, which contributes to osteoporosis.[14] Handicapped children have additional risk factors for osteoporosis, including marginal nutrition, decreased sun exposure, and decreased mobility. Toxic hepatitis from valproic acid may be more common in children who are younger than 2 and have serious neurologic handicap.[15]

When to Initiate Therapy

Prescription of an AED for a child with a few seizures should not be a reflex. An individual decision for an individual child is appropriate. After a first partial or generalized tonic-clonic seizure, the chance of recurrence is very high for handicapped children, although not 100%. In our series of 168 children assessed after a first seizure, 73% of children with significant abnormalities on neurologic examination had a recurrent seizure, as compared with 47% of those who were normal.[16] In the meta-analysis by Berg and Shinnar,[2] the relative risk for recurrence after a first seizure in children with neurologic abnormalities in eight studies varied between 1.2 and 2.9.[2] If medication is started after a first seizure, it appears to be equally effective in the presence or absence of neurologic abnormality.[17]

The recurrence risk after two unprovoked seizures is very high, in the range of 80%.[16,18] The influence of neurologic handicap on this risk is still unclear. The hazards of waiting for a second seizure seem low, with little absolute need to start treatment before two seizures have occurred. Delaying treatment for more than two seizures may be entirely reasonable provided an affected child's activities are not overly restricted. For children with catastrophic epilepsy or at high risk of injury, the decision to start treatment is more straightforward.

When to Discontinue Therapy

For some children, epilepsy is a short-lived disorder. After 6–24 months of AED treatment of such children, drugs may be withdrawn and seizures do not recur.[3,11,12,18] Is there a downside to treating handicapped children any differently from others? In our population-based study, children with handicap had a lower chance of becoming seizure-free for a sufficient time to justify discontinuing medication, as compared to those without handicap: 293 of 383 (76.5%) versus 41 of 99 (41%; $p < .0001$).[1] For those who did become seizure-free, the length of seizure-free time before consideration of stopping treatment was the same in both groups (average for handicap group, 50.0 ± 25.7 months; no-handicap group, 44.2 ± 24.7 months).

The handicapped who were fortunate enough to be seizure-free long enough to stop medication had the same success rate as those without handicap (70.0% vs. 72.4%). This result is different from that seen in most publications. Berg and Shinnar's[3] meta-analysis of discontinuing medication found a relative risk for recurrence of 1.66 (95% confidence interval, 1.30–2.12) in those with epilepsy and mental handicap as compared with those with idiopathic epilepsy.[3] These authors also found a relative risk of recurrence of 1.79 (1.13–2.83) in children with epilepsy and motor deficits as compared with those with idiopathic epilepsy. From a practical point of view, this finding means that stopping medication in a child with epilepsy and handicap forecasts a decent chance of success, although probably less so than in an otherwise normal child.

Only a few publications address the long-term outcome of children who have recurrent seizures after medication is stopped. In our series, many normal children who discontinued medication a first time had recurrent seizures, started back on medication, and eventually discontinued medication successfully a second time. The number of cases was insufficient to examine the same sequence in handicapped children. However, we do note that of 41 handicapped children who stopped medication a first time, only 2 (4.5%) went on to have intractable epilepsy, as compared with 4 of 293 (1.3%) of those without handicap. In other words, if a child with handicap becomes seizure-free, stops medication, and has recurrent seizures, the epilepsy nearly always will be controlled again.

Therefore, withdrawing medication seems reasonable if a handicapped child becomes seizure-free for a suitable time. A pertinent issue is the length of seizure-free time before terminating medication. In the meta-analysis of Berg and Shinnar,[3] that issue was not addressed clearly; however, the standard of practice at the time of their writing varied from 2 to 5 seizure-free years, and individual publications all found a similar rate of recurrence of approximately 30%.

A 1-year study by Dooley et al.[19] of seizure-free patients found an overall recurrence rate of 39%. If affected children had a significant neurologic abnormality, the risk of recurrence was increased to 51%, as compared with 32% for those without neurologic abnormality. In the Netherlands, Peters et al.[11] reported a randomized study of AED withdrawal after 6 months versus 12 seizure-free months in children whose epilepsy was brought quickly under control. The recurrence risk after 6 months' treatment was increased to approximately 55%; however, after 2 years, the rate of remission was the same in both groups. Neither of these studies included children with secondary generalized epilepsies.

Overall, little would seem to be gained by AED treatment beyond 2 seizure-free years. If treatment is stopped before that, a somewhat higher rate of recurrence can be anticipated.

Infantile Spasms

The evolution of West's syndrome is so different from that of most other epilepsies that it warrants separate discussion. Treatment of infantile spasms nearly always is indicated, but the treatment duration may be very short. The majority of children with spasms have neurologic problems prior to the time of diagnosis,[20] and only rarely do such children turn out to be cognitively normal in the long term. The onset of spasms often is associated with developmental regression, and some authorities suggest that early treatment is associated with a quicker response to medication, although no randomized trials have addressed this issue. Therefore, treatment nearly always seems justified as soon as the diagnosis is confirmed. Evidence suggests that treatment with vigabatrin is effective in more than 50%, with response within a few days.[21] Unclear is how long treatment with vigabatrin should be continued once spasms have stopped. In contrast, the more traditional treatment has been with intramuscular adrenocorticotropic hormone. Treatment is continued for a few weeks only, with a high percentage of children experiencing a permanent or long-lasting remission.[22]

References

1. Camfield C, Camfield P, Gordon K, et al. Outcome of childhood epilepsy: a population-based study with a simple predictive scoring system for those treated with medication. J Pediatr 1993;122:861–868.
2. Berg AT, Shinnar S. The risk of seizure recurrence following a first unprovoked seizure: a meta-analysis. Neurology 1991;41:965–972.
3. Berg AT, Shinnar S. Relapse following discontinuation of anti-epileptic drugs: meta-analysis. Neurology 1994;44:601–608.
4. Wasterlain CG. Recurrent seizures in the developing brain are harmful. Epilepsia 1997;38:728–734.
5. Camfield PR. Recurrent seizures in the developing brain are not harmful. Epilepsia 1997;38:735–737.
6. Camfield C, Camfield P, Gordon K, Dooley J. Does the number of seizures before treatment influence ease of control or remission of childhood epilepsy? Not if the number is 10 or less. Neurology 1996;46:41–44.
7. Holmes GL, Gairsa JL, Chevassus-Au-Louis N, Yekezkel BA. Consequences of neonatal seizures in the rat: morphological and behavioural effects. Ann Neurol 1998;44:845–857.
8. Dulac O, Chiron C, Robain O, et al. Infantile spasms: a pathophysiological hypothesis. Semin Pediatr Neurol 1994;1:83–89.

9. Maytal J, Shinnar S, Moshé SL, Alvarez LA. Low morbidity and mortality of status epilepticus in children. Pediatrics 1989;83:323–331.
10. Iivanainen M, Patja K. Lifespan and mortality of epileptic persons with intellectual disability. Poster 3.150. Presented at the Twenty-Third International Epilepsy Congress, Prague, September 15, 1999.
11. Peters AC, Brouwer OF, Gerts AT, et al. Randomized prospective study of early discontinuation of AEDs in children with epilepsy. Neurology 1998;50:724–730.
12. Braathen G, Anderson T, Gylie H, et al. Comparison between one and three years of treatment in uncomplicated childhood epilepsy—a prospective study: 1. Outcome in different seizure types. Epilepsia 1996;37:822–832.
13. Wyllie E, Wyllie R, Cruse RP, et al. Mechanism of nitrazepam drooling and aspiration. N Engl J Med 1986;314:35–38.
14. Sheth RD, Wesolowski CA, Jacob JC, et al. Effect of carbamazepine and valproate on bone mineral density. J Pediatr 1995;127:256–262.
15. Dreifuss FE, Santilli N, Langer DH, et al. Valproic acid fatalities: a retrospective review. Neurology 1987;37:379–385.
16. Camfield PR, Camfield CS, Dooley JM, et al. Epilepsy after a first unprovoked seizure in childhood. Neurology 1985;35:1657–1660.
17. First Seizure Trial Group. Randomised clinical trial on the efficacy of antiepileptic drugs in reducing the risk of relapse after a first unprovoked tonic-clonic seizure. Neurology 1993;43:478–482.
18. Hauser WA, Rich SS, Lee JR, et al. Risk of recurrent seizures after two unprovoked seizures. N Engl J Med 1998;338:429–434.
19. Dooley JM, Gordon K, Camfield PR, et al. Discontinuation of anticonvulsant therapy in children free of seizures for 1 year. Neurology 1996;46:969–974.
20. Dulac O, Plouin P, Schlumberger E. Infantile Spasms. In E Wyllie (ed), The Treatment of Epilepsy: Principles and Practice (2nd ed). Baltimore: Williams & Wilkins, 1997;540–572.
21. Aicardi J, Mumford JP, Dumas C, Wood S. Vigabatrin as initial therapy for infantile spasms: a European retrospective survey. Epilepsia 1996;37:638–642.
22. Vigevano F, Cilio MR. Vigabatrin versus ACTH as first-line treatment for infantile spasms: a randomized, prospective study. Epilepsia 1997;38:1270–1274.

Chapter 25

Community-Based Antiepilepsy Treatment in the Developmentally Disabled

Ross B. FineSmith

This chapter reviews the unique factors associated with the management of epilepsy and antiepileptic drugs (AEDs) in the community-based population of individuals with developmental disabilities (DD). Many of the same principles that are established for AED therapy in the nonhandicapped population can be applied to individuals with DD. These principles can be used as guidelines in making decisions about initiating drug therapy or determining the most appropriate AED.[1] The guidelines are as listed in Table 25-1. Additional specific challenges confront the community physician treating patients with epilepsy and moderate to profound DD. These factors include a higher incidence of medically refractory epilepsy, cognitive disabilities that can limit feasibility of neurodiagnostic testing, and inability to describe or report symptoms in those with limited communicative ability. Also, DD patients are more likely to experience adverse effects from AEDs.[2]

Relocation of Persons with Disabilities

In the past, most patients with severe childhood disabilities and epilepsy were treated by pediatricians or pediatric neurologists. Often, such patients were admitted in late childhood or as young adults to long-term care facilities at which staff physicians provided their medical and neurologic care. The current trend of deinstitutionalization of individuals with moderate to profound DD has "relo-

cated" this group to a variety of community settings, including group homes, sponsored living, supported-living arrangements, and supervised apartment living. Their medical and neurologic care now is the responsibility of physicians located in these communities. Unlike the staff physicians in the developmental centers, most physicians in the community have limited experience or exposure to persons with significant DD. This is not a result of discrimination but one simply of demographics. These patients were institutionalized and typically did not receive treatment from outside physicians. The relocating process has resulted in a marked increase in medical consumers who have DD and require medical care in our communities.

In New Jersey, 5,841 people were living in developmental centers in 1986; as of March 1999, the number was 3,623. These 2,000 persons have been relocated and now are living in many communities throughout New Jersey. The number of individuals residing in group homes has tripled in the last 8 years; in addition, 2,900 persons are on the urgent waiting list, with 1,000 names on a nonurgent waiting list.[3,4] This trend is national and is not specific to one state.[5]

The relocation has been especially challenging to those physicians treating patients with epilepsy. A 30–50% incidence of epilepsy exists in individuals with DD,[6] and as many as 45% of those have medically refractory epilepsy.[7–9] Patients with this type of epilepsy require significantly more of physicians' practice time than do other patients with

Table 25-1. Principles of Antiepileptic Drug Therapy

Assess the risk-benefit ratio of initiating medication.
Choose an appropriate medication based on the seizure type.
If seizures persist, consider adding or substituting a second antiepileptic drug.
Diligently monitor for medication side effects and quality of life.

epilepsy in the community. Patients in this group often need more aggressive management and treatment and often require the use of more novel therapies, such as the vagal nerve stimulator and the ketogenic diet and, when appropriate, a referral for evaluation for epilepsy surgery.

The remainder of this chapter is designed to familiarize the reader with and aid in the development of a community-based program to treat more effectively patients with epilepsy and moderate to profound DD. The state of New Jersey serves as a model.

Legal Guardians and Family Members

Approximately 50% of individuals approved and eligible for services from the division of developmental disabilities (DDD) are residing with parents or family members.[3] Many of these persons are on waiting lists for group home placement. These individuals frequently will be seen by the same family physician who has cared for them most of their lives. Referral to a neurologist may occur in the event of an initial seizure or a change in seizure status in those with pre-existing epilepsy.

Complicated neurologic histories are frequently incomplete when the patient is accompanied by an unfamiliar group home staff member. Family members have a greater personal interest in the care of a relative, and concern may be reflected in the accuracy of the interval history, management of medication, and vigilance in reporting undesirable side effects. Many disabled children continue to live at home well into adulthood, and aging parents may have difficulty remembering to administer medications, count seizures accurately, and recognize side effects. Parents may have difficulty physically in transporting their child to the office or

hospital. This is especially problematic if an affected child has a physically handicapping condition, such as cerebral palsy.

Most adults with moderate to profound DD and cognitive impairment are evaluated and assessed not to be competent to make decisions for their own well-being. A legal guardian, therefore, must be appointed. Parents and other family members may live nearby and be involved with affected DD persons' care and yet elect not to be their legal guardian. However, many individuals have no close family members involved, and legal guardianship is assigned to a legal representative within the DDD. For those providing medical care to this population, it is good practice to routinely obtain the name and address of the legal guardian and to contact that person by phone to establish a relationship. Such calls are necessary in the event of any questions regarding the need for written consent for a given procedure. Changing medications, laboratory blood work, and noninvasive radiologic and electrophysiologic studies usually do not require consent. However, conscious sedation and general anesthesia occasionally are necessary to perform a routine test or procedure, and because there is additional medical risk, written consent should be obtained in advance. The risks and benefits of any invasive procedure should be discussed with the legal guardian. Some individuals with moderate DD are their own guardian. Regardless of whether affected persons have a legal guardian, attempts should be made to explain all medical information at a level that is appropriate for that individual. Some states strictly regulate the enrollment of persons with DD into research protocols. A research protocol must be approved by a regional institutional review board, and additional review may require a state's department of DD research committee. This precaution ensures that such patients are not enrolled unnecessarily in higher-risk protocols.

The primary caregivers for adults with DD often are group home staff, a situation that frequently can cause the family to be overlooked in the medical treatment process. Family members may participate in medical decisions, but, owing to parental age, health, and living arrangements, some parents are unable to be present for visits. Health care providers should contact the next of kin to introduce themselves and to obtain additional medical information. Relatives usually are happy to hear from a medical provider and can provide valuable medical background. If family members express interest in the treatment plan, they should be encouraged to be present at office visits. This arrangement can provide invaluable information, as the following account illustrates. The following vignette exemplifies the necessity of family involvement, because the patients frequently are nonverbal or cognitively impaired.

An individual with autism and epilepsy was evaluated by a neurologist, who was requested to provide ongoing neurologic care. The patient was accompanied by a residential home staff member who had known him for 2 months. A previous discharge summary from the developmental center reported that no seizures were observed in the last 4 years the patient had lived there. Electroencephalographic (EEG) and magnetic resonance imaging (MRI) findings were unremarkable; based on the recent history and these reports, the patient was considered a relatively low risk for seizure relapse if the AED was discontinued. His legal guardian was a DDD representative, and the next of kin was an aunt living in the next state. She was contacted by phone at the time of the office visit and reported that over the last 9 years, three separate neurologists had attempted to wean her nephew off carbamazepine because he had been seizure-free for up to 4 years at a time. All three occasions resulted in status epilepticus and, during one hospitalization, the patient developed severe pneumonia. The neurologist elected not to pursue this option. The patient has been followed for 3 years since and continues to be seizure-free on carbamazepine.

Group Home Structure and Staff

Group home staff, sponsors, and personal aides are of great importance in the execution of the medical treatment plan for persons with DD. Staff members accompany patients to the office and often are the only source of information at that time. Persons relocating from developmental centers should have a brief medical discharge summary. The level of experience, motivation, and competence of the staff varies significantly. Staff names always should be noted in the margins of the chart adjacent to the medical note. This allows for tracking and resolving communication problems. The health care providers should educate the accompanying staff and tell them what is needed during each visit to assess the patient's response to therapy. Community or agency presentations and "in-services" can be helpful in educating care providers.

Group home managers oversee the care and treatment of each of the residents and typically are reliable and dedicated. Unfortunately, many of the support staff are unfamiliar with the patient's medication and seizure pattern. It may be necessary to communicate directly with the manager regarding the more difficult to control or fragile epilepsy patients.

Physicians can develop a seizure record form that the group home staff must complete after each seizure. The form can be tailored by physicians to obtain pertinent information describing the event and allows for more accurate documentation of the number and characterization of seizures. This form is especially helpful when the staff member who witnessed the seizure does not accompany the patient to the office visit. The seizure record form can be reviewed quickly at each visit. It also allows for a more accurate assessment of the current treatment; from it, more effective medication adjustments can be made. The seizure logs should remain in the medical chart for quick reference. Group homes often have a folder that accompanies a patient to each visit.

Most group homes keep accurate medication records and log books. In addition, many now have prescriptions filled at pharmacies that offer "bubble packs." Each dose is individually encased in a small air bubble on a sheet with multiple rows of individual doses. After the dose is given, a mark is made at the corresponding time in a patient's medication log. This system provides a much lower likelihood of missed doses. Because it is easy to tell if an individual "bubble" was not opened, not all group home staff members are allowed to administer and dispense medications. Those staff members allowed to perform this duty must have some formal training about dispensing medication.

Working within the regulations to which the group homes are mandated to follow can be tedious and frustrating to those unfamiliar with the requirements. The regulations are not established by the group homes but are state mandated in an attempt to ensure safety. For example, on prescriptions, the physician must write the specific times at which medications are to be administered (e.g., "8 a.m. and 8 p.m. daily," instead of "b.i.d."). Staff members cannot administer any medication without these times, and the prescription must be rewritten. If doses are adjusted by phone, the adjustment must be followed by a written prescription that is mailed or faxed, ensuring appropriate documentation at the group home. This procedure is problematic when these changes are made during on-call hours because the physicians are not in the office.

Neurodiagnostic Testing

Persons with significant disabilities and cognitive impairment often do not understand why they are having a test performed and may respond in a similar fashion to that of a child who is the same mental age. In addition, a higher incidence of psychological and psychiatric conditions compounds the difficulty in obtaining these studies. Therefore, conscious sedation often is required. An MRI of the brain requires a patient to lie very still for approximately 40 minutes, and several different forms of sedation can be administered. This may simply include oral benzodiazepines or may require intravenous conscious sedation provided by an anesthesiologist. Because an electroencephalogram can be altered significantly and may suppress eleptogenic potentials with many of the sedating medications, the utility of EEG study is limited in some cases. The determination of the seizure type then would have to be based on the clinical description of the event, patient history, and the MRI. Neurodiagnostic studies of DD patients can be very time consuming and often frustrating for busy MRI facilities and EEG laboratories.

Antiepileptic Medications

After the diagnosis of epilepsy and seizure type has been established, the AED that is believed to be most effective and to present the least chance of side effects is determined. This is based on whether the seizures are primary generalized, partial, atonic, or myoclonic. A careful review of the history is necessary to ensure that an AED that was used previously with adverse effects is not reinstituted. This may be difficult to avoid in some cases because medical records from institutions and previous treating physicians are not available.

Comorbid conditions and mode of drug delivery are prominent issues in treating DD patients. A higher incidence of behavioral and psychiatric conditions exists in the DD population, and AEDs may exacerbate an underlying or comorbid condition. Psychiatric comorbidities have been reported to occur in 25% and severe maladaptive behavior in up to 55% of those meeting criteria for mental retardation.[10] Valproate and carbamazepine are AEDs used most commonly in the treatment of bipolar disorder, mania, intermittent explosive disorder, and aggressive behavior. Therefore, in choosing a medication to treat seizures, the psychiatric history must be obtained. If a patient was treated previously with valproate or carbamazepine as a mood stabilizer and the agent was tolerated and effective, the same medication should be considered for an initial anticonvulsant. This choice lowers the risk of adverse events, because it was previously tolerated and also may influence behaviors. Conversely, a previously documented adverse effect, such as agitation, would preclude selection of that medication.

Carbamazepine

Carbamazepine (Tegretol, Carbatrol) is a first-line AED for partial-onset and some forms of generalized epilepsy. This agent is an excellent choice in the treatment of individuals with DD because it has minimal adverse effects on cognition and behavior. Carbamazepine is indicated also in the treatment of bipolar disorder and trigeminal neuralgia. It can be used as a single agent to treat the relatively common comorbidity of mood disorder and epilepsy,[11] although carbamazepine is not an effective antidepressant. Adverse behavioral reactions occur infrequently and may be due to the tricyclic ring structure in carbamazepine. This outcome may result in mild mood-elevating properties that would be problematic in a patient having hypomania that has not been detected or diagnosed. Such patients may become agitated, irritable, and hyperactive.

Hyponatremia is a known side effect and can be exacerbated by patients who drink free water habitually or due to dryness as a side effect of antidepressants or antipsychotic medication.

An additional advantage of carbamazepine is the multiple formulations available. Tegretol is available in chewable tablets and an elixir that is ideal for patients unable to swallow tablets. Tegretol extended-release tablets allow for less frequent dosing; Carbatrol, a newer form of extended-release carbamazepine, is produced in a capsule that can be opened and sprinkled on food. This has allowed for the use of an extended-release form in young children.

Valproate

Valproate is a major AED that has a broad spectrum of antiepileptic effects and is effective against primary generalized, partial, and myoclonic seizures. Valproate is also indicated in the treatment of mania and migraine headaches. Migraine is significantly more common in patients with epilepsy; however, the frequency of migraine in patients with DD has not been well defined. Mania and agitated behavior are observed more frequently in epilepsy patients with DD than in the general population. Valproate can be effective in treating both conditions. Additional uses of valproate in the DD population include behavioral cycling,[12] aggressive behaviors,[13,14] and hyperactivity-agitation in autism.[15] This medication should be used in a very limited fashion or not at all in children younger than age 2 because this group of patients has a significant risk of hepatotoxicity. These patients are at even greater risk if they have a severe developmental delay, are on additional AEDs, or have a neurometabolic disorder.[16] Thrombocytopenia is another known side effect, although it is rarely serious. However, if an individual's DD includes ataxia with frequent falls, caution should be used. Valproate is also available in liquid and sprinkle formulation. A recent extended-release formulation allows for once-a-day dosing. Depacon is an intravenous preparation of valproate that may be used in the hospital for rapid bolusing during breakthrough seizures.

Phenytoin

Phenytoin (Dilantin) has a very safe profile and is effective in the treatment of partial and generalized seizures. The agent does not appear to affect mood or behavior. An advantage of phenytoin is that it has a long half-life and may be given once daily. This is helpful in patients with compliance problems, and phenytoin is available in liquid, chewable, and intravenous formulations. Phenytoin is not a first-choice AED in persons with DD because a selected side effect profile is especially problematic in this population. Oral hygiene commonly is deficient in individuals with DD, and this is complicated by the gingival hyperplasia caused by phenytoin. In addition, individuals with DD often are susceptible to balance disturbances, which can be exacerbated by phenytoin.[17]

Phenobarbital

Phenobarbital is the oldest and among the most effective AEDs in current use. Although life-threatening safety concerns are very rare, systemic and neurologic adverse effects limit its general use. Phenobarbital is the drug of choice for treating children younger than age 2 and is effective against a wide range of seizure types. It is not used commonly in older patients because it has been shown to slow cognition and learning and has adverse effects on mood, including irritability in children and depression in adults.[18] Phenobarbital can cause soft-tissue changes, such as frozen shoulder, soft-tissue growths, and Dupuytren's contractures. However, it is a very effective anticonvulsant, and some patients respond exceptionally well and may experience increased seizure activity when change is attempted.

Felbamate

Felbamate (Felbatol) was the first "new-generation" AED after a 15-year gap (1978–1993), and it was used widely and accepted until postmarketing experience revealed a high incidence of hepatic failure and aplastic anemia.[19] The agent is very effective against multiple seizure types and has a favorable side effect profile for many patients with DD. There is rarely sedation at higher doses, and it appears to have a mild stimulant effect. Therefore, it can be beneficial for psychomotor slowing and appetite reduction. This same effect may be more prominent in a subgroup and result in insomnia and anorexia. Felbatol has a wide spectrum of anticonvulsant activity and is especially effective in the Lennox-Gastaut syndrome. This medication should be used only when the risk-benefit ratio has been evaluated carefully by all those involved in an affected person's care. However, the combined risk of bone marrow or liver failure with felbamate is estimated at 1 in 2,000 individuals and likely would be reduced significantly by frequent blood monitoring (every 2–4 weeks for the first year of therapy). This level of monitoring surpasses that of other commonly used AEDs, but, in cases of severe epilepsy or adverse effects that severely impair quality of life, felbamate may be a reasonable alternative.

Gabapentin

Gabapentin (Neurontin) is effective as an adjunctive therapy in partial seizures. It is used widely for neuropathic pain syndromes and refractory bipolar disorder but is indicated only for partial seizures. Neurontin is available as a capsule only and has no serious medical side effects. In some children, particularly those with DD, gabapentin may cause behavioral exacerbations. It has minimal protein binding and hepatic metabolism, so it has limited interactions with other medications and can be used safely in other medical conditions.

Lamotrigine

Lamotrigine (Lamictal) also has a wide spectrum of anticonvulsant activity and is effective against the Lennox-Gastaut syndrome and in monotherapy. Lamictal also appears to have a mild mood-elevating quality and is rarely sedating. It also has mood-stabilizing qualities and is being used off-label in bipolar disorder. This combination of effects gives Lamictal a very favorable profile for use in individuals with DD.[20,21] However, some reports have cited adverse behavioral effects, including marked elevation of mood and agitation in this population of patients.[22,23]

Initially, lamotrigine was found to cause a concerning number of allergic skin reactions, with subsequent development of Stevens-Johnson syndrome. However, the etiology of this reaction has since been established to be directly related to the rate of titration. The slower the rate of titration, the less likely it is that a reaction will occur. The chance of complications is minimized if the agent is increased by 2.5–5.0 mg per week for children and 12.5 mg per week for adults. Lamictal is also available in 2- and 5-mg chewable tablets.

Topiramate

Topiramate (Topamax) is indicated for partial seizures and the Lennox-Gastaut syndrome. It has been very effective in refractory seizure disorders, is typically well tolerated, and is effective in monotherapy. Several studies have shown cognitive and behavioral side effects, including problems with concentration and attention, slowing of thought processes, word-finding difficulties, and memory problems. Cognitive and behavioral side effects can be minimized by gradual dose escalation. Notably, in the author's experience, cognitive and behavioral problems have not been a problem in the DD population. Topamax is available in 25-, 100-, and 200-mg tablets and is available also in 15- and 25-mg sprinkle formulation.

Tiagabine

Tiagabine (Gabitril) is approved for adjunctive treatment of partial seizures. Behavioral side effects are infrequent but may include tiredness, nervousness, difficulty in concentrating, irritability, or confusion. It is available only in tablet forms (4, 12, 16, and 20 mg).

Vigabatrin

Vigabatrin (Sabril) is not approved in this country and most likely will not gain U.S. Food and Drug Administration approval due to possible retinal dysfunction that can cause visual field deficits in up to 25% of treated patients. It can be obtained from other countries and is effective and well tolerated in persons with DD.[24] Sabril has been most useful in the treatment of infantile spasms and remains a treatment of choice for this disorder in many countries.

Oxcarbazepine

Oxcarbazepine (Trileptal) recently has become available. It is a variant of carbamazepine but metabolically bypasses the problematic epoxide intermediate that is responsible for many of the side effects of carbamazepine, including sedation. Therefore, patients are able to tolerate higher doses of oxcarbazepine, which will result in a greater chance of successful monotherapy. The agent should be very beneficial for use in individuals with DD.[25]

Adverse Effects Attributed to Antiepileptic Drugs

The abundance of conflicting reports concerning the adverse behavioral effects of AEDs on people with DD may be due to the fact that we are frequently unable to recognize pre-existing psychiatric disorders in handicapped individuals. This sometimes results in an AED choice that may aggravate a psychiatric condition. In addition, DD persons often are unable to communicate side effects they are experiencing and may act out only when the side effects are intolerable. Finally, DD patients are less likely to be able to compensate mentally for drug-induced side effects; therefore, the behavioral variability may be even greater among those with DD, given their altered neurologic baseline. Therefore, the effects of a specific AED on a specific individual with a DD probably is less predictable than in a patient with epilepsy without neurologic impairment.

Managing Developmentally Disabled Patients with Epilepsy in the Community Setting

Individuals recently discharged from developmental centers may have received appropriate AED management. Epileptologists may have

been contracted to aid in the management of patients with epilepsy residing in developmental centers. In other settings, physicians may continue AEDs indefinitely.[26] Re-evaluation of a patient's epilepsy and need for AEDs is frequently necessary on initial consultation. Monotherapy should be attempted, because it has been shown to be effective in up to 90% of institutionalized persons with epilepsy.[27,28] Withdrawing AEDs, especially phenobarbital and benzodiazepines, can result in a marked improvement in alertness and mood. An increase in muscle tone can be seen in some individuals with cerebral palsy or acquired hemiplegia after phenobarbital or a benzodiazepine is withdrawn. Baclofen may be added for the treatment of spasticity. Occasionally, an underlying personality or mood disorder is unmasked when the AED is withdrawn. Mania can appear as carbamazepine or valproate is withdrawn.[29] If there were no signs of side effects with medication that was withdrawn, that medication can simply be restarted to treat the unmasked psychiatric disorder.

Conclusion

The field of developmental neurology is in an early stage of evolution. It includes understanding both the unique medical needs of those with DD and the constraints involved in their medical care. Our ability to incorporate these unique provisions successfully into current clinical practice depends on the initiative, motivation, and cooperation we have as a medical community. Further collaborative studies are required to determine the efficacy of alternative therapies such as vagal nerve stimulation[30,31] and epilepsy surgery[28] in individuals with DD. Cooperating with diagnostic testing centers and educating our communities are essential to the successful ongoing implementation of appropriate neurologic care of those with moderate to profound DD.

References

1. Coulter DL. Comprehensive management of epilepsy in persons with mental retardation. Epilepsia 1997;38[Suppl 4]:S24–S31.

2. Alvarez N, Besag F, Iivanainen M. Use of antiepileptic drugs in the treatment of epilepsy in people with intellectual disability. J Intellect Disabil Res 1998;42(1):1–15.
3. New Jersey Department of Human Services: Division of Developmental Disabilities. Annual Report to the Constituency. August 21, 1998.
4. The Association for Retarded Citizens. Matrix of Program Services. July 15, 1998.
5. Braddock D, Hemp R, Bachelder L, Fujiura G. The State of States in Developmental Disabilities (4th ed). Washington, DC: American Association of Mental Retardation, 1995.
6. Sunder TR. Meeting the challenge of epilepsy in persons with multiple handicaps. J Child Neurol 1997;12(1):S38–S43.
7. Steffenberg U, Hedstrom A, Lindroth A, et al. Intractable epilepsy in a population-based series of mentally retarded children. Epilepsia 1998;39(7):767–775.
8. Marcus JC. Control of epilepsy in a population with mental retardation: lack of correlation with IQ, neurologic status, and the electroencephalogram. Am J Ment Retard 1993;[Suppl 98]:47–51.
9. Singh BK, Towle PO. Antiepileptic drug status in adult outpatients with mental retardation. Am J Ment Retard 1993;[Suppl 98]:41–46.
10. Deb S. Mental disorder in adults with mental retardation and epilepsy. Comp Psychol 1997;3:179–184.
11. Waisburg H, Alvarez N. Carbamazepine in the treatment of epilepsy in people with intellectual disability. J Intellect Disabil Res 1998;42(1):36–40.
12. Kastner T, FineSmith R, Walsh K. Long-term administration of valproic acid in the treatment of affective symptoms in people with mental retardation. J Psychopharmacol (Oxf) 1993;13(6):448–451.
13. Mattes JA. Valproic acid for nonaffective aggression in the mentally retarded. J Nerv Ment Dis 1992;9:601–602.
14. Wilcox J. Divalproex sodium in the treatment of aggressive behavior. Ann Clin Psychiatry 1994;6(1):17–20.
15. Pioplys AV. Autism: electroencephalogram abnormalities and clinical improvement with valproic acid. Arch Pediatr Adolesc Med 1994;148:220–222.
16. Friis ML. Valproate in the treatment of epilepsy in people with intellectual disability. J Intellect Disabil Res 1998;42[Suppl 1]:32–35.
17. Iivanainen M. Phenytoin: effective but insidious therapy for epilepsy in people with intellectual disability. J Intellect Disabil Res 1998;42(1):24–31.
18. Alvarez N. Barbiturates in the treatment of epilepsy in people with intellectual disability. J Intellect Disabil Res 1998;1:16–23.
19. Pellock JM, Brodie MJ. Felbamate: an update. Epilepsia 1997;38(12):1261–1264.
20. Besag FM. Lamotrigine in the treatment of epilepsy in people with intellectual disability. J Intellect Disabil Res 1998;42(1):50–56.
21. Davanzo PA, King BH. Open trial lamotrigine in the treatment of self-injurious behavior in an adolescent with profound mental retardation. J Child Adolesc Psychopharmacol 1996;6(4):273–279.
22. Ettinger AB, Weisbrot DM, Saracco J, et al. Positive and negative psychotropic effects of lamotrigine in patients with epilepsy and mental retardation. Epilepsia 1998;39(8):874–877.
23. Beran RG, Gibson RJ. Aggressive behavior in intellectually challenged patients with epilepsy treated with lamotrigine. Epilepsia 1998;39(9):1018–1019.
24. Ylinen A. Antiepileptic efficacy of vigabatrin in people with severe epilepsy and intellectual disability. J Intellect Disabil Res 1998;1:46–49.
25. Gaily E, Granstrom ML, Liukkonen E. Oxcarbazepine in the treatment of epilepsy in children and adolescents with intellectual disability. J Intellect Disabil Res 1998;1:41–45.
26. Baribeault JJ. Clinical advocacy for persons with epilepsy and mental retardation living in community-based programs. J Neurosci Nurs 1996;28(6):359–372.
27. Pellock JM, Hunt PA. A decade of modern epilepsy therapy in institutionalized mentally retarded patients. Epilepsy Res 1996;25(3):263–268.
28. Beckung E, Uvebrant P. Impairments, disabilities and handicaps in children and adolescents with epilepsy. Acta Paediatr 1997;86(3):254–260.
29. Ketter TA, Malow BA, Flamini R, et al. Anticonvulsant withdrawal-emergent psychopathology. Neurology 1994;44:55–61.
30. Parker AP, Polkey PE, Binnie CD, et al. Vagal nerve stimulation in epileptic encephalopathies. Pediatrics 1999;103(4):778–782.
31. Uthman BM, Wilder BJ, Hammond EJ, Reid SA. Efficacy and safety of vagus nerve stimulation in patients with complex partial seizures. Epilepsia 1990;3[Suppl 2]:S44–S50.

Chapter 26

The Role of New Antiepileptic Therapies

Steven C. Schachter

Epilepsy, one of the most common neurologic disorders encountered in the general population, affects between 2 and 4 million people in the United States, including 1 of 50 children and 1 of 100 adults.[1] The overall prevalence of epilepsy is approximately 14–24% among people with mental retardation[2–5] and may be as high as 82% in association with profound mental retardation.[6]

The annual costs for epilepsy diagnosed in the United States in 1990 were estimated at $3 billion.[7] Indirect costs, including lost income and costs of home care or institutionalization, account for up to two-thirds of the costs of epilepsy[8] and are disproportionately greater among patients with cognitive and neurologic deficits.

In fewer than one-half of all patients with epilepsy, the disorder has an identifiable cause. The causes of epileptic seizures include congenital brain malformations, inborn errors of metabolism, high fevers, head trauma, brain tumors, stroke, intracranial infection, cerebral degeneration, withdrawal states, and iatrogenic drug reaction.[9] Because the cerebral pathology underlying developmental disabilities (DD) is associated with epilepsy, a higher proportion of epilepsy in patients with DD has an identifiable cause, especially cortical malformations.

This chapter first briefly reviews the clinical evaluation of seizures in patients with DD. Then the epilepsy treatments that have been approved in the United States over the last 10 years are presented, including antiepileptic drugs (AEDs) and

vagus nerve stimulation (VNS); thus, vigabatrin is not included. Finally, the principles of epilepsy therapy for patients with DD are discussed.

Clinical Evaluation of Seizures in Patients with Developmental Disabilities

Prior to the choice of therapy, an affected patient's seizure type must be established. Usually this determination is based on a thorough history from the patient and firsthand descriptions of seizures from observers, such as family members. However, this process may be problematic when such patients are unable to describe their seizure experiences or the observations of witnesses to the seizures are unreliable. Therefore, obtaining an accurate medical history and seizure description may be difficult in dealing with some DD patients or their caregivers, especially when caregivers are not knowledgeable about epilepsy. Second, distinguishing epileptic seizures from recurrent behaviors that are nonepileptic, such as self-stimulatory behaviors and tics, may be difficult without prolonged electroencephalographic monitoring and, therefore, may be identified mistakenly as seizures.[10] Nevertheless, a concerted effort should be made to discern the seizure precipitants, ictal symptoms and signs, and postictal features of each identifiable seizure type that a patient may have, with the assistance of electroencephalographic monitoring when necessary. Elucidation of seizure types will facilitate treatment selection and monitoring of the effects of treatment, which may vary as a function of seizure type.

Each seizure type may occur among patients with DD, and patients often have multiple seizure types, including combinations of partial, tonic, atonic, myoclonic, and atypical absence seizures.

Similarly, making a diagnosis of an epilepsy syndrome may be difficult. Epilepsy syndromes are characterized by particular patterns of clinical features, including age at onset of seizures, family history of epilepsy, seizure type, and associated neurologic signs and symptoms.[11] Establishing a syndrome may allow clinicians to offer a prognosis, provide genetic counseling, and choose AED therapy. Although many patients with DD and seizures do not fit into a well-described syndrome, others clearly do, including childhood epileptic encephalopathy (Lennox-Gastaut syndrome) and infantile spasms (West's syndrome).

Recent Advances in Seizure Therapy

The usual objective of treating epilepsy is to enable the patient to lead a lifestyle as free from the medical and psychosocial complications of seizures as possible. The medical goals, thus, are to prevent seizures without causing disabling side effects. In 1985, a study of otherwise healthy adults with partial-onset seizures found that these goals of therapy were not met for nearly one-half of the enrolled patients with the standard AEDs available at that time.[12] As a result, a number of new AEDs and a device were developed for adults with partial-onset seizures and were cleared for marketing in the United States by the U.S. Food and Drug Administration, including felbamate (1993), gabapentin (1993), lamotrigine (1994), topiramate (1996), tiagabine (1997), VNS (1997), levetiracetam (1999), oxcarbazepine (2000), and zonisamide (2000). Subsequent to their initial approval, topiramate (TPM) was approved as adjunctive therapy for partial seizures in children as young as 2 years old and for primary generalized tonic-clonic seizures in adults and children 2 years of age and older, and lamotrigine (LTG) was approved as monotherapy in adults who had partial seizures and already were receiving therapy with a single enzyme-inducing AED and as adjunctive therapy

in the generalized seizures of Lennox-Gastaut syndrome in children and adults.

The goal of treating epilepsy in patients with DD is similar: to achieve the combination of seizure control and tolerability that results in the best possible quality of life, particularly with regard to alertness, behavior, and temperament. However, compared to other patients, those with DD are less likely to attain complete seizure control. Nonetheless, significant reduction of injury-producing seizures, such as atonic seizures, should be sought, both to protect the patient and to lessen the need for close supervision. With regard to tolerability, side effects (particularly behavioral) may be atypical and dose-limiting. Therefore, close attention to individualizing treatment regimens offers the best chance of achieving therapeutic success.

Pharmacotherapy

Felbamate

Felbamate (FBM) was the first new AED approved in the United States in nearly 15 years[13] and the first AED to be proven effective in Lennox-Gastaut syndrome in children.[14] Absorption of FBM from the gastrointestinal tract is nearly complete, and approximately 25% is protein-bound. FBM is metabolized by the hepatic cytochrome P450 system and is excreted in the urine (40–50% as the unchanged drug). The half-life of FBM is 15–24 hours. Drug-drug interactions are common: FBM increases serum concentrations of phenytoin (PHT), valproate (VPA), and carbamazepine-epoxide; consequently, dosage adjustments of concomitant AEDs usually are necessary.[15]

The mechanism of action of FBM is not completely known. In vitro, FBM potentiates γ-aminobutyric acid (GABA) function, and blocks voltage-dependent sodium channels and the ionic channel at the N-methyl-D-aspartate excitatory amino acid receptor.[16]

FBM is effective as monotherapy and add-on therapy for partial-onset seizures and tonic-clonic seizures in patients 14 years of age and older.[17] Studies have demonstrated also the effectiveness of FBM as an add-on for the atonic seizures associated with the Lennox-Gastaut syndrome in children aged 2–14 years.[13]

Typical side effects are insomnia, headache, nausea, anorexia, somnolence, vomiting, weight loss, and dizziness. Rare but potentially fatal side effects are aplastic anemia and liver failure.[18] Risk factors appear to be age older than 14, female gender, a history of autoimmune disorders, and previous hematologic reactions to medications. As a result, the use of FBM now is restricted largely to Lennox-Gastaut syndrome patients, for whom the possible benefits of treatment outweigh the risks.[19]

Doses should be titrated slowly over several weeks to months to minimize side effects. Starting doses in adults and children are 600 mg per day and 15 mg/kg per day, respectively. Daily dosages between 1,800 mg and 4,800 mg in adults and 45–60 mg/kg per day in children often are required for seizure control. Physicians should obtain signed informed consent from affected patients or legal representatives prior to starting treatment. Although routine monitoring of liver and bone marrow function is recommended, it does not predict the occurrence of potentially fatal liver and bone marrow failure. Studies are under way to determine whether a metabolite excreted in the urine may be predictive of idiosyncratic reactions.

Gabapentin

Gabapentin (GBP), which consists of a cyclohexyl group fused to GABA,[13] has a very favorable pharmacokinetic profile.[20] It does not undergo metabolism and does not affect the metabolism of other drugs. No protein binding occurs. Because of these pharmacokinetic attributes, drug-drug interactions are not a problem with GBP. However, its absorption depends on amino acid transporters in the gastrointestinal tract and, therefore, is saturable, typically at single doses of 1,200 mg or greater, which results in decreased bioavailability at higher doses. The half-life of GBP in patients with normal renal function is 4–9 hours; those with renal insufficiency usually need lower dosages at less frequent intervals. The mechanism of action of GBP is unknown. Despite its structural similarity to GABA, GBP does not bind to GABA receptors in

the central nervous system (CNS), although it may enhance GABA synthesis.

GBP is approved as adjunctive therapy for partial seizures in patients 12 years of age and older.[21] Side effects generally are mild to moderate and transient.[22] The side effects reported most commonly are drowsiness, ataxia, dizziness, and nystagmus. Children, particularly those with learning disabilities, may have behavioral side effects, such as explosive outbursts, aggression, and uncooperative behavior.[23–25] Weight gain occurs in up to 5% of patients. No idiosyncratic reactions or effects on bone marrow or hepatic function have been described.

GBP should be started in older children and adults at 300 mg per day and increased by 300 mg every 3–7 days to the maximum tolerated dose. The recommended dosage range is 900–1,800 mg per day; however, many patients need higher dosages for efficacy.[26,27] In younger children, the starting dose is 10 mg/kg per day, and the target dose is 30–60 mg/kg per day in three or four divided doses. A therapeutic serum concentration range has not been established.

Lamotrigine

LTG has good bioavailability, and plasma concentrations are linearly related to dose.[13] LTG is 55% protein-bound and is metabolized hepatically to inactive glucuronide conjugates that are excreted renally. Because VPA inhibits glucuronidation, comedication with VPA increases the half-life of LTG to 70 hours as compared to 14 hours when the concomitant AEDs are enzyme-inducing, as is carbamazepine (CBZ). The mechanism of action of LTG appears to be on voltage-sensitive sodium channels,[16,28] particularly on neurons that synthesize the excitatory neurotransmitters glutamate and aspartate.[29]

LTG is effective as adjunctive therapy and as a monotherapy AED for the treatment of partial seizures when concomitant AEDs are tapered.[30,31] Data suggest that the agent is effective also for the partial and generalized seizures associated with the Lennox-Gastaut syndrome in children.[32–34]

Common CNS-related side effects of LTG include insomnia, drowsiness, dizziness, headache, somnolence, diplopia, and ataxia. Rash and nausea are the primary systemic side effects of LTG. Up to 10% of patients develop a benign rash during the initial 1–2 months of therapy. Based on clinical trials and postmarketing reports, the risk of severe dermatologic reaction (erythema multiforme, Stevens-Johnson syndrome, or toxic epidermal necrolysis) in adults is 0.3% and approximately 1% in children aged 16 and younger.[35] Hence, the prompt evaluation of any rash is appropriate, and discontinuation of LTG, unless the rash is clearly not drug-related, is prudent. The risk factors for severe dermatologic reactions are young age, comedication with VPA, a rapid rate of LTG titration, and a high LTG starting dose.[36] Aggressive behavior in children with mental retardation has been reported in association with LTG.[37]

LTG is available in a variety of tablet strengths, from 25 to 200 mg, and as 5-mg, rapidly dispersible tablets. For adult patients not receiving VPA and taking an AED that induces hepatic enzymes, the initial dose is 25 mg twice daily, titrated upward by 5-mg increments every 1–2 weeks as needed. For adult patients taking VPA, the initial dose is 12.5–25.0 mg every other day, with increases of 12.5–25.0 mg every 2 weeks as needed and tolerated. The starting dose for children taking VPA is 0.2 mg/kg per day, and the dosage is increased every 2 weeks to a target dose of 1–5 mg/kg per day. For children not taking VPA, the starting dose is 2 mg/kg per day, and the dosage is increased every 2 weeks to a target dose of 5–15 mg/kg per day. Therapeutic serum concentrations of LTG have not been established.

Topiramate

TPM, a sulphamate-substituted monosaccharide,[13] is metabolized by the hepatic P450 microsomal enzymes. Therefore, the clearance of TPM˙ is accelerated by enzyme-inducing AEDs, resulting in decreased TPM concentrations.[38] Conversely, TPM may increase PHT plasma concentrations when PHT metabolism is near saturation. Nearly 70–80% of TPM is excreted unchanged in the urine. In patients with normal renal function, the half-life of TPM is approximately 21 hours, and the time to steady state is 4–5 days. TPM has multiple mechanisms of action.[28] It blocks voltage-dependent sodium channels, enhances the activity

of GABA at a nonbenzodiazepine site on GABA(A) receptors, antagonizes an N-methyl-D-aspartate-glutamate receptor, and weakly inhibits carbonic anhydrase.

TPM is effective as adjunctive therapy for the treatment of adults with partial seizures, children with the Lennox-Gastaut syndrome, atonic seizures in cognitively disabled patients, and primary generalized seizures.[39–44] A pilot study showed encouraging results for infantile spasms.[45] Side effects include psychomotor slowing, difficulty with concentration, speech and language problems, somnolence, or fatigue.[46] Side effects are more likely to occur with higher initial starting doses, rapid titration, and polytherapy. Additional side effects include decreased appetite, weight loss, and kidney stones. No idiosyncratic side effects (other than allergic dermatitis) have been noted.

TPM is available as tablets and as 15- and 25-mg sprinkle capsules that can be opened and sprinkled onto food. The initial and target adult doses are 25–50 mg per day and 200–400 mg per day divided in two doses, respectively. The initial and target doses for children are 0.5–1.0 mg/kg per day and 3–9 mg/kg per day, respectively, with weekly increases of 0.5–1.0 mg/kg. Therapeutic levels have not been established.

Tiagabine

Tiagabine (TGB) is absorbed quickly and nearly completely and is metabolized extensively by the P450 isozyme CYP3A.[47] Because TGB does not induce or inhibit hepatic enzymatic function and does not displace tightly protein-bound drugs, serum concentrations of concomitant AEDs, such as CBZ, PHT, theophylline, warfarin, and digoxin, are unaffected by TGB. VPA concentrations may be reduced slightly.

The half-life of TGB is 5–8 hours in patients who are not taking enzyme-inducing AEDs and is reduced by approximately 50% when hepatic metabolism is induced. TGB concentrations are increased in association with hepatic dysfunction but not renal failure. Therefore, dosage adjustments may be necessary in patients with hepatic disease but not in those with renal impairment.[48,49] TGB has linear, predictable pharmacokinetics, and children eliminate TGB slightly more rapidly than do adults. The mechanism of action is quite specific: TGB inhibits the neuronal and glial reuptake of GABA and, therefore, enhances GABA-mediated inhibition.[13]

TGB is effective as add-on therapy for partial seizures in dosages ranging from 32 mg to 56 mg daily.[50,51] Suggestive evidence indicated that TGB may be effective for infantile spasms.[52] Despite its short half-life, TGB is effective when dosed two to four times daily.

The initial and target adult doses are 4–8 mg per day and 32–56 mg per day in two to four divided doses, respectively, although some patients may require higher dosages. The initial and target doses for children are 0.1 mg/kg per day and 1.0 mg/kg per day, respectively, with weekly increases of 0.1 mg/kg.

Side effects include dizziness, fatigue, asthenia, nervousness, tremor, trouble in concentrating, depression, difficulty in speaking, and abdominal pain.[53] No clinically important laboratory abnormalities were noted in clinical studies, and therapeutic ranges have not been established.

Levetiracetam

Levetiracetam (LEV), the S enantiomer of the ethyl analog of piracetam,[54] is absorbed rapidly and nearly completely after oral administration. Peak serum concentrations are achieved within 2 hours, and daily doses and plasma concentrations are linearly related.[55] LEV is not protein-bound (<10%), and the major metabolic pathway is hydrolysis,[56,57] which is independent of the hepatic cytochrome P450 system. Consequently, the half-life of LEV is unaffected by concomitant AEDs.[55] In addition, LEV does not induce or inhibit the hepatic P450 system, so little potential exists for pharmacokinetic interactions with other drugs.[56] In children and adults, steady state is achieved after 2 days of twice-daily dosing. The mechanism of action of LEV is unknown and clearly different from all other AEDs.

The effectiveness of LEV in treating patients with refractory partial-onset seizures was demonstrated in three multicenter, randomized, double-blind, placebo-controlled, add-on studies in the United States and Europe.[58] Suggestive evidence indicates that LEV is effective for photosensitive epilepsy and for a variety of generalized seizure types.[59]

Side effects include fatigue, tiredness, somnolence, and dizziness. In clinical trials, minor but statistically significant decreases in total mean red blood cell count ($0.03 \times 10^6/mm^3$), mean hemoglobin (0.09 g/dl), and mean hematocrit (0.38%) occurred in LEV-treated patients as compared to placebo-treated patients.[58]

Treatment in adults is initiated with 500 mg twice daily. The dosage can be titrated by 1,000 mg every 2 weeks to 4,000 mg daily as needed for seizure control. The initial and target doses for children are 20 mg/kg per day and 40–60 mg/kg per day, respectively. A therapeutic range has not been established.

Oxcarbazepine

Oxcarbazepine (OXC) is chemically and structurally similar to CBZ but is metabolized differently. Whereas CBZ is oxidized to the 10,11 epoxide by an inducible enzyme, OXC is reduced to a monohydroxy derivative (MHD) by a noninducible ketoreductase. MHD is the active metabolite of OXC and accounts for the antiseizure activity of OXC.

The metabolism of OXC is unaffected by induction or inhibition of the hepatic P450 system, which reduces the potential for interactions with AEDs and drugs that inhibit the metabolism of CBZ, such as erythromycin, cimetidine, and propoxyphene.[60–63] However, OXC may elevate PHT concentrations when PHT metabolism is near saturation and also may reduce the potency of oral contraceptives.[64,65]

The half-life of MHD is 8–10 hours,[66,67] and steady state is achieved after three to four OXC doses in a twice-daily regimen.[67] MHD is approximately 40% protein-bound. OXC and its metabolites are excreted renally,[68] so hepatic impairment does not affect OXC or MHD pharmacokinetics.[67] The mechanism of action of OXC is similar to that of CBZ.[69,70]

The efficacy and tolerability of OXC are comparable to those of VPA and PHT in patients with newly diagnosed or previously untreated partial-onset or primary generalized seizures.[71–73] Other monotherapy studies confirm its effectiveness in patients with chronic medically refractory seizures.[74,75] Effectiveness in patients with cognitive disability has been reported,[76] and exacerbation of generalized seizure subtypes, such as myoclonic, absence, and atonic seizures, appears to occur less often than with CBZ.

Elevations of liver function tests[77] and skin reactions occur less frequently with OXC than with CBZ, but patients who have skin allergies to CBZ have approximately a 15–25% chance of a similar reaction to OXC.[78,79] Conversely, hyponatremia occurs more commonly with OXC than with CBZ. Although isolated cases of hyponatremic coma have been reported,[80] OXC-induced hyponatremia rarely is of clinical significance.[81–83] No clinically significant fluctuations of white blood cells have been observed in clinical studies.

The recommended dosage as monotherapy in adults is 600–1,200 mg per day; higher dosages may be necessary when the agent is used as polytherapy in patients with refractory seizures. The initial and target doses for children are 10 mg/kg per day and 30–60 mg/kg per day, respectively. The therapeutic range of MHD has not been established.

Zonisamide

Zonisamide (ZNS), a sulfonamide derivative that is unrelated chemically and structurally to other AEDs, is absorbed rapidly and nearly completely. ZNS is 40–60% protein-bound[84–86] and does not induce[87] or inhibit the hepatic P450 system. Dosages and plasma concentrations are related linearly in adults[88,89] and in children.[90] The plasma half-life in healthy volunteers after a single oral dose ranges from 50 to 68 hours.[84,85,91] In the presence of enzyme-inducing AEDs, ZNS half-life decreases by approximately 50%, and plasma concentration at steady state decreases.[85,92,93] ZNS blocks voltage-dependent sodium[94] and T-type (but not L-type) calcium channels.[95,96] ZNS also inhibits carbonic anhydrase.[85]

ZNS is effective for patients with refractory partial-onset seizures.[97,98] Suggestive evidence indicates that ZNS is effective also against generalized seizures,[85] infantile spasms,[99] seizures associated with the Lennox-Gastaut syndrome,[100] and myoclonic and generalized tonic-clonic seizures in patients with progressive myoclonic epilepsy of the Unverricht-Lundberg type or associated with ragged red fibers.[90,101–103]

Side effects include somnolence, ataxia, anorexia, confusion, difficulty in thinking, nervousness, fatigue, and dizziness.[97,98] Kidney stones occurred in 2.6% of ZNS-exposed subjects in the U.S. and European studies,[100] as compared to 0.2% of patients in Japanese studies.[103]

The recommended initial daily dose is 100–200 mg for adults in two divided doses. Because steady state is reached in 7–10 days, dosages should be increased at 2-week intervals to a target maintenance dose of 400–600 mg per day in adults.[100] Higher dosages may be tolerable and necessary in selected patients. Therapeutic drug monitoring will be useful, particularly to establish a therapeutic range for individual patients. The initial and target doses for children are 1–2 mg/kg per day and 5–8 mg/kg per day, respectively, with increases of 0.5–1.0 mg/kg every 2 weeks.

Principles of Pharmacotherapy in Patients with Developmental Disabilities

Monotherapy versus Polytherapy

The advantages of monotherapy over polytherapy in patients with DD are a wider therapeutic window, enhanced seizure control, less potential for drug interactions, and improved behavior.[104,105] Considering the greater likelihood of mixed seizures in patients with DD, reasonable AEDs to select as initial monotherapy are those with a broad spectrum of activity and minimal potential for sedation,[106] such as VPA and LTG.[107,108]

Although monotherapy does not provide adequate seizure relief for a substantial number of patients,[109] clinicians should consider why a patient's seizures have not responded to monotherapy treatment before considering combination AED therapy. Possible reasons include incorrect classification of seizure type (and, therefore, incorrect choice of AED), failure to titrate the dose high enough, and continued exposure to seizure precipitants, such as sleep deprivation and stress. Sources of stress for patients with DD may be subtle; therefore, recognizing them (e.g., a minor change in daily routine) may be difficult. Finally, comedication with psychoactive medications that may cause iatrogenic seizures should be avoided.

Some patients occasionally do experience abatement of seizure frequency or severity with a combination of AEDs. Considering the large number of available AEDs, emphasis has been placed on rationally selecting combinations of AEDs. Drugs with different side effect profiles and combinations that do not have a significant potential for drug-drug interactions are advisable. This caution is particularly important because patients often are taking non-AEDs that have actions on the CNS for control of moods, troublesome behaviors, or diminished attention spans. Further, AEDs that have different mechanisms of action have been suggested. However, the mechanisms of action of AEDs are not understood fully, and drugs with similar mechanisms may be effective when used in combination.

Monitoring Antiepileptic Drug Serum Concentrations

In the DD population, AED serum concentrations are helpful to evaluate whether a patient's reports or observations by a caregiver of adverse events are likely to be the result of medication side effects, and to establish the therapeutic concentration for a patient whose seizures are brought under control. Serum concentrations associated with neurotoxicity or cognitive-behavioral effects vary from one patient to another and often occur within the "therapeutic range," particularly in patients with significant cerebral pathology. Free (rather than total) concentrations are useful in managing AED dosages (particularly PHT and VPA) when patients have low albumin levels or take other tightly protein-bound medications.

Vagus Nerve Stimulation

The introduction of left VNS in 1997 opened up a new, nonpharmacologic approach to epilepsy treatment.[110] VNS is approved in the United States

for use as adjunctive therapy for adults and adolescents who are older than age 12 and have partial-onset seizures refractory to AEDs. The mechanism of action of VNS is uncertain.[111]

Within the first 2 postoperative weeks, ramping up the output current is initiated by the physician and is adjusted to patient tolerance. A typical treatment regimen consists of adjusting the current output to a 30-Hz signal frequency with a 500-msec pulse width for 30 seconds of on-time and 5 minutes of off-time. Once programmed, the generator will deliver intermittent stimulation at the desired settings until any additional programming instructions are received or until the battery life is expended, which typically occurs after 4 or more years of operation. In addition, the patient or a companion may activate the generator by placing the supplied magnet over the generator for several seconds; in some patients, this may interrupt a seizure or reduce its severity if administered at the onset of the seizure.

VNS is effective as adjunctive therapy for partial seizures. Several reports suggest efficacy in treating the Lennox-Gastaut syndrome,[112–114] and many centers have used VNS instead of performing corpus callosotomies for atonic seizures. The side effects of the implantation surgery are transient and include incisional pain, coughing, voice alteration, chest pain, and nausea. Adverse effects related to stimulation therapy usually are mild to moderate in severity, are temporally related to stimulation, and almost always resolve with adjustment in stimulation settings. Common treatment-related side effects are hoarseness, throat pain, coughing, dyspnea, and paresthesia. No cognitive, sedative, visual, affective, or coordination side effects have been reported; hence, conspicuously absent with VNS therapy are the typical CNS side effects of AEDs, which can be particularly difficult in patients with DD.

Summary

The successful management of epilepsy in patients with DD requires a thorough and individualized approach that accurately establishes affected patients' seizure types and, when possible, epilepsy syndromes. Selection of therapy should be rational and tailored to each patient. In this manner, clinicians will be able to take advantage of the new treatments for seizures to minimize the impact of the seizures and treatment side effects on their patients, thereby enabling them—and their caregivers—to ensure the best possible quality of life.

References

1. Hauser WA, Hesdorffer DC. Epilepsy: Frequency, Causes and Consequences. New York: Demos, 1990;378.
2. Deb S. Epilepsy and mental retardation. Epilepsie Bull 1997;25:91–94.
3. McGrother CW, Hauck A, Bhaumik S, et al. Community care for adults with learning disability and their careers: needs and outcomes from the Leicestershire register. J Intellect Disabil Res 1996;40:183–190.
4. Goulden KJ, Shinnar S, Koller H, et al. Epilepsy in children with mental retardation: a cohort study. Epilepsia 1991;32(5):690–697.
5. Forsgen I, Edvinsson SO, Blomquist HK, et al. Epilepsy in a population of mentally retarded children and adults. Epilepsy Res 1990;6(3):234–248.
6. Suzuki H, Aihara M, Sugai K. Severely retarded children in a defined area of Japan: prevalence rate, associated disabilities and causes. Brain Dev 1991;23(1):4–8.
7. Pachlatko C. The cost of epilepsy care to the community. Seizure 1997;6(6):415–417.
8. Jacoby A, Buck D, Baker G, et al. Uptake and costs of care for epilepsy: findings from a U.K. regional study. Epilepsia 1998;39(7):776–786.
9. Schachter SC. Iatrogenic seizures. Neurol Clin North Am 1998;16(1):157–170.
10. Coulter DL. Epilepsy and mental retardation: an overview. J Ment Retard 1993;98(5):1–11.
11. International League Against Epilepsy. Proposal for revised classification of epilepsies and epileptic syndromes. Commission on Classification and Terminology of the International League Against Epilepsy. Epilepsia 1989;30(4):389–399.
12. Mattson RH, Cramer JA, Collins JF, et al. Comparison of carbamazepine, phenobarbital, phenytoin, and primidone in partial and secondarily generalized tonic-clonic seizures. N Engl J Med 1985;313(3):145–151.
13. Bialer M, Johannessen SI, Kupferberg HJ, et al. Progress report on new antiepileptic drugs: a summary of the fourth EILAT conference (EILAT IV). Epilepsy Res 1999;34(1):1–41.
14. Felbamate Study Group in the Lennox-Gastaut Syndrome. Efficacy of felbamate in childhood epileptic encephalopathy. N Engl J Med 1993;328:29–33.
15. Walker MC, Patsalos PN. Clinical pharmacokinetics of new antiepileptic drugs. Pharmacol Ther 1995;67(3):351–384.
16. Macdonald RL, Kelly KM. Mechanisms of action of currently prescribed and newly developed antiepileptic drugs. Epilepsia 1994;35[Suppl 4]:S41–S50.
17. Bourgeois BF. Felbamate in the treatment of partial-onset seizures. Epilepsia 1994;35[Suppl 5]:S58–S61.
18. Kaufman DW, Kelly JP, Anderson T, et al. Evaluation of case reports of aplastic anemia among patients treated with felbamate. Epilepsia 1997;38(12):1265–1269.
19. Pellock JM, Brodie MJ. Felbamate: 1997 update. Epilepsia 1997;38(12):1261–1264.
20. Gram L. Pharmacokinetics of new antiepileptic drugs. Epilepsia 1996;37[Suppl 6]:S12–S16.
21. Mattson RH Managing epilepsy: the role of gabapentin. Neurology 1994;44[Suppl 5]:S3.
22. Morris GL 3rd. Efficacy and tolerability of gabapentin in clinical practice. Clin Ther 1995;17(5):891–900.
23. Tallian KB, Nahata MC, Lo W, Tsao CY. Gabapentin associated with aggressive behavior in pediatric patients with seizures. Epilepsia 1996;37(5):501–502.
24. Wolf SM, Shinnar S, Kang H, et al. Gabapentin toxicity in children manifesting as behavioral changes. Epilepsia 1995;36(12):1203–1205.
25. Mikati MA, Choueri R, Khurana DS, et al. Gabapentin in the treatment of refractory partial epilepsy in children with intellectual disability. J Intellect Disabil Res 1998;42[Suppl 1]:57–62.
26. Bruni J. Titration of gabapentin dose for optimal control of epileptic seizures. Adv Ther 1996;13(6):324–334.
27. Bruni J. Outcome evaluation of gabapentin as add-on therapy for partial seizures. "NEON" Study Investigators Group. Neurontin Evaluation of Outcomes in Neurological Practice. Can J Neurol Sci 1998;25(2):134–140.
28. Meldrum BS. Update on the mechanism of action of antiepileptic drugs. Epilepsia 1996;37[Suppl 6]:S4–S11.
29. Leach MJ, Marden CM, Miller AA. Pharmacological studies on lamotrigine, a novel potential antiepileptic drug: II. Neurochemical studies on the mechanism of action. Epilepsia 1986;27(5):490–497.
30. Schachter SC. Efficacy and safety of lamotrigine, a new anticonvulsant. Todays Ther Trend 1995;12(4):135–143.
31. Gilliam F, Vazquez B, Sackellares JC, et al. An active-control trial of lamotrigine monotherapy for partial seizures [see comments]. Neurology 1998;51(4):1018–1025.
32. Schlumberger E, Chavez F, Palacios L, et al. Lamotrigine in treatment of 120 children with epilepsy. Epilepsia 1994;35(2):359–367.

33. Motte J, Trevathan E, Arvidsson JF, et al. Lamotrigine for generalized seizures associated with the Lennox-Gastaut syndrome. Lamictal Lennox-Gastaut Study Group. N Engl J Med 1997;337(25):1807–1812.

34. Dulac O, Kaminska A. Use of lamotrigine in Lennox-Gastaut and related epilepsy syndromes. J Child Neurol 1997;12[Suppl 1]:S23–S28.

35. Dooley J, Camfield P, Gordon K, et al. Lamotrigine-induced rash in children. Neurology 1996;46(1):240–242.

36. Besag FM, Dulac O, Alving J, Mullens EL. Long-term safety and efficacy of lamotrigine (Lamictal) in paediatric patients with epilepsy. Seizure 1997;6(1):51–56.

37. Beran RG, Gibson RJ. Aggressive behaviour in intellectually challenged patients with epilepsy treated with lamotrigine. Epilepsia 1998;39(3):280–282.

38. Johannessen SI. Pharmacokinetics and interaction profile of topiramate: review and comparison with other newer antiepileptic drugs. Epilepsia 1997;38[Suppl 1]:S18–S23.

39. Sachdeo RC, Glauser TA, Ritter F, et al. A double-blind, randomized trial of topiramate in Lennox-Gastaut syndrome. Topiramate YL Study Group. Neurology 1999;52(9):1882–1887.

40. Elterman RD, Glauser TA, Wyllie E, et al. A double-blind, randomized trial of topiramate as adjunctive therapy for partial-onset seizures in children. Topiramate YP Study Group. Neurology 1999;52(7):1338–1344.

41. Kerr MP. Topiramate: uses in people with an intellectual disability who have epilepsy. J Intellect Disabil Res 1998;42[Suppl 1]:74–79.

42. Ben-Menachem E. Clinical efficacy of topiramate as add-on therapy in refractory partial epilepsy: the European experience. Epilepsia 1997;38[Suppl 1]:S28–S30.

43. Reife RA, Pledger GW. Topiramate as adjunctive therapy in refractory partial epilepsy: pooled analysis of data from five double-blind, placebo-controlled trials. Epilepsia 1997;38[Suppl 1]:S31–S33.

44. Biton V, Montouris GD, Ritter F, et al. A randomized, placebo-controlled study of topiramate in primary generalized tonic-clonic seizures. Topiramate YTC Study Group. Neurology 1999;52(7):1330–1337.

45. Glauser TA, Clark PO, Strawsburg RH. A pilot study of topiramate in the treatment of infantile spasms. Epilepsia 1998;39:1324–1328.

46. Sander JW. Practical aspects of the use of topiramate in patients with epilepsy. Epilepsia 1997;38[Suppl 1]:S56–S58.

47. Bopp B, Gustavson L, Johnson M. Pharmacokinetics and metabolism of [14C tiagabine] after oral administration to human subjects. Epilepsia 1995;36[Suppl 2]:S158.

48. Cato A, Qian JX, Gustavson LE. Pharmacokinetics and safety of tiagabine in subjects with various degrees of renal function. Epilepsia 1995;36[Suppl 3]:S159.

49. Cato A III, Gustavson LE, Qian J, et al. Effect of renal impairment on the pharmacokinetics and tolerability of tiagabine. Epilepsia 1998;39(1):43–47.

50. Lassen LC, Sommerville K, Mengel HB. Summary of five controlled trials with tiagabine as adjunctive treatment of patients with partial seizures. Epilepsia 1995;36[Suppl 3]:S148.

51. Schachter SC. Tiagabine: current status and potential clinical applications. Exp Opin Invest Drugs 1996;5(10):1377–1387.

52. Kugler S. Efficacy and tolerability of tiagabine in infantile spasms. Epilepsia 1999;40[Suppl 7]:134.

53. Schachter SC, Deaton R, Sommerville K. Long-term use of tiagabine for partial seizures. Epilepsia 1997;38[Suppl 8]:S105–S106.

54. Loscher W, Schmidt D. New drugs for the treatment of epilepsy. Curr Opin Invest Drugs 1993;2:1067–1095.

55. Patsalos PN, Walker MC, Ratnaraj N. The pharmacokinetics of levetiracetam (UCB L059) in patients with intractable epilepsy. Epilepsia 1995;36[Suppl 4]:52.

56. Nicolas J-M, Collart P, Gerin B, et al. In vitro evaluation of potential drug interactions with levetiracetam, a new antiepileptic agent. Drug Metab Dispos 1999;27:250–254.

57. Klitgaard H, Matagne A, Govert J, Wulfert E. Evidence for a unique profile of levetiracetam in rodent models of seizures and epilepsy. Eur J Pharmacol 1998;353(2–3):191–206.

58. Shorvon SD, van Rijckevorsel K, Verdru P. Pooled efficacy and safety data of levetiracetam (LEV) used as adjunctive therapy in patients with partial onset seizures. Epilepsia 1999;40[Suppl 7]:76.

59. Kasteleijn-Nolst Trenite DG, Marescaux C, Stodieck S, et al. Photosensitive epilepsy: a model to study the effects of antiepileptic drugs. Evaluation of the piracetam analogue, levetiracetam. Epilepsy Res 1996;25(3):225–230.

60. Baruzzi A, Albani F, Riva R. Oxcarbazepine: pharmacokinetic interactions and their clinical relevance. Epilepsia 1994;35[Suppl 3]:S14–S19.

61. Keränen T, Jolkkonen J, Klosterskov Jensen P, Menge GP. Oxcarbazepine does not interact with cimetidine in healthy volunteers. Acta Neurol Scand 1992;85(4):239–242.

62. Mogensen PH, Jorgensen L, Boas J, et al. Effects of dextropropoxyphene on the steady-state kinetics of oxcarbazepine and its metabolites. Acta Neurol Scand 1992;85(1):14–17.

63. Keränen T, Jolkkonen J, Klosterskov Jensen PK, et al. Absence of interaction between oxcarbazepine and erythromycin. Acta Neurol Scand 1992;86(2):120–123.

64. Klosterskov Jensen P, Saano V, Haring P, et al. Possible interaction between oxcarbazepine and an oral contraceptive. Epilepsia 1992;33(6):1149–1152.

65. Fattore C, Cipolla G, Gatti G, et al. Induction of ethinylestradiol and levonorgestrel metabolism by oxcarbazepine in healthy women. Epilepsia 1999;40(6):783–787.

66. Dickinson RG, Hooper WD, Dunstan PR, Eadie MJ. First dose and steady-state pharmacokinetics of oxcarbazepine and its 10-hydroxy metabolite. Eur J Clin Pharmacol 1989;37(1):69–74.

67. Lloyd P, Flesch G, Dieterle W. Clinical pharmacology and pharmacokinetics of oxcarbazepine. Epilepsia 1994;35[Suppl 3]:S10–S13.

68. Schutz H, Feldmann KF, Faigle JW, et al. The metabolism of 14C-oxcarbazepine in man. Xenobiotica 1986;16(8):769–778.

69. Schmutz M, Brugger F, Gentsch C. Oxcarbazepine: preclinical anticonvulsant profile and putative mechanisms of action. Epilepsia 1994;35[Suppl 5]:S47–S50.

70. Wamil AW, Portet C, Jensen PK, et al. Oxcarbazepine and its monohydroxy metabolite limit action potential firing by mouse central neurons in cell culture. Epilepsia 1999;32[Suppl 3]:65–66.

71. Christe W, Kramer G, Vigonius U, et al. A double-blind controlled clinical trial: oxcarbazepine versus sodium valproate in adults with newly diagnosed epilepsy. Epilepsy Res 1997;26:451–460.

72. Bill PA, Vigonius U, Pohlmann H, et al. A double-blind controlled clinical trial of oxcarbazepine versus phenytoin in adults with previously untreated epilepsy. Epilepsy Res 1997;27:195–204.

73. Guerreiro MM, Vigonius U, Pohlmann H, et al. A double-blind controlled clinical trial of oxcarbazepine versus phenytoin in children and adolescents with epilepsy. Epilepsy Res 1997;27:205–213.

74. Schachter SC, Vazquez B, Fisher RS, et al. Oxcarbazepine: double-blind, randomized, placebo-control monotherapy trial for partial seizures. Neurology 1999;52:732–737.

75. Sachdeo R, Beydoun A, Schachter S. Safety and efficacy of oxcarbazepine monotherapy. Neurology 1998;50:A200.

76. Gaily E, Granstrom M-L, Lliukkonen E. Oxcarbazepine in the treatment of epilepsy in children and adolescents with intellectual disability. J Intellect Disabil Res 1998;42[Suppl 1]:41–45.

77. Friis ML, Kristensen O, Boas J, et al. Therapeutic experiences with 947 epileptic out-patients in oxcarbazepine treatment. Acta Neurol Scand 1993;87(3):224–227.

78. Van Parys JAP, Meinardi H. Survey of 260 epileptic patients treated with oxcarbazepine (Trileptal) on a named-patient basis. Epilepsy Res 1994;19:79–85.

79. Jensen NO. Oxcarbazepine in patients hypersensitive to carbamazepine. Presented at the Sixteenth International Epilepsy Congress, Hamburg, Germany, 1983.

80. Steinhoff BJ, Stoll KD, Stodieck SR, et al. Hyponatremic coma under oxcarbazepine therapy. Epilepsy Res 1992;11:67–70.

81. Dam M. Practical aspects of oxcarbazepine treatment. Epilepsia 1994;35[Suppl 3]:S23–S25.

82. Van Amelsvoort T, Bakshi R, Devaux CB, Schwabe S. Hyponatremia associated with carbamazepine and oxcarbazepine therapy: a review. Epilepsia 1994;35(1):181–188.

83. Sachdeo RC, Wassertein AG, D'Souza J. Oxcarbazepine (Trileptal) effect on serum sodium. Epilepsia 1999;40[Suppl 7]:103.

84. Matsumoto K, Miyazaki H, Fujii T, et al. Absorption, distribution and excretion of 3-(sulfamoyl(14C)-methyl)-1,2-benzisoxazole (AD-810) in rats, dogs, monkeys and of AD-810 in man. Arzneimittelforschung 1983;33:961–968.

85. Seino M, Naruto S, Ito T, et al. Other Antiepileptic Drugs: Zonisamide. In RH Levy, RH Mattson, BS Meldrum (eds), Antiepileptic Drugs (4th ed). New York: Raven Press, 1995;1011–1023.

86. Matsumoto K, Miyazaki H, Fujii T, et al. Binding of sulfonamides to erythrocyte proteins and possible drug-drug interaction. Chem Pharm Bull (Tokyo) 1989;37:2807–2810.

87. Kochak GM, Page JG, Buchanan RA, et al. Steady-state pharmacokinetics of zonisamide, an antiepileptic agent for treatment of refractory complex partial seizures. J Clin Pharmacol 1998;38(2):166–171.

88. Wilensky AJ, Friel PN, Ojemann LM, et al. Zonisamide in epilepsy: a pilot study. Epilepsia 1985;26:212–220.

89. Ono T, Yagi K, Seino M. Clinical efficacy and safety of a new antiepileptic drug, zonisamide: a multi-institutional phase III study. Seishin Iyaku 1988;30:471–482.

90. Yagi K, Seino M. Open clinical trial of new antiepileptic drug, zonisamide (ZNA) on 49 patients with refractory epileptic seizures. Clin Psychiatry 1987;29:111–119.

91. Ito T, Yamaguchi T, Miyazaki H, et al. Pharmacokinetic studies of AD-810, a new antiepileptic compound. Phase 1 trials. Arzneimittelforschung 1982;32:1581–1586.

92. Ojemann LM, McLean JR, Buchanan RA. Comparative pharmacokinetics of zonisamide (CI-912) in epileptic patients on carbamazepine or phenytoin monotherapy. Ther Drug Monit 1986;8:293–296.

93. Sackellares JC, Donofrio PD, Wagner JG, et al. Pilot study of zonisamide (1,2-benzisoxazole-3-methanesulfonamide) in patients with refractory partial seizures. Epilepsia 1985;26:206–211.

94. Schauf CL. Zonisamide enhances slow sodium inactivation in Myxicola. Brain Res 1987;413:185–188.

95. Suzuki S, Kawakami K, Nishimura S, et al. Zonisamide blocks T-type calcium channel in cultured neurons of rat cerebral cortex. Epilepsy Res 1992;12:21–27.

96. Kito M, Maehara M, Watanabe K. Mechanisms of T-type calcium channel blockade by zonisamide. Seizure 1996;5(2):115–119.

97. Wilder BJ, Ramsay RE, Guterman A. A Double-Blind Multicenter Placebo-Controlled Study of the Efficacy and Safety of Zonisamide in the Treatment of Complex Partial Seizures in Medically Refractory Patients (internal report). Osaka, Japan: Dainippon Pharmaceutical Co., 1986.

98. Schmidt D, Jacob R, Loiseau P, et al. Zonisamide for add-on treatment of refractory partial epilepsy: a European double-blind trial. Epilepsy Res 1993;15:67–73.

99. Yanai S, Hanai T, Narazaki O. Treatment of infantile spasms with zonisamide. Brain Dev 1999;21(3):157–161.

100. Leppik IE. Zonisamide. Epilepsia 1999;40[Suppl 5]:S23–S29.

101. Henry T, Henry TR, Leppik IE, et al. Progressive myoclonus epilepsy treated with zonisamide. Neurology 1998;38:928–931.

102. Kyllerman M, Ben-Menachem E. Zonisamide for progressive myoclonus epilepsy: long-term observations in seven patients. Epilepsy Res 1998;29(2):109–114.

103. Yagi K, Seino M. Methodological requirements for clinical trials in refractory epilepsies—our experience with zonisamide. Prog Neuropsychopharmacol Biol Psychiatry 1992;16:79–85.

104. Collacott RA, Dignon A, Hauck A, Ward JW. Clinical and therapeutic monitoring of epilepsy in a mental handicap unit. Br J Psychiatry 1989;155:522–525.

105. Pellock JM, Hunt PA. A decade of modern epilepsy therapy in institutionalized mentally retarded patients. Epilepsy Res 1996;25:263–268.

106. Alvarez N. Barbiturates in the treatment of epilepsy in people with intellectual disability. J Intellect Disabil Res 1998;42[Suppl 1]:16–23.

107. Alvarez N, Besag F, Iivanainen M. Use of antiepileptic drugs in the treatment of epilepsy in people with intellectual disability. J Intellect Disabil Res 1998;42[Suppl 1]:1–15.

108. Besag FMC. Lamotrigine in the treatment of epilepsy in people with intellectual disability. J Intellect Disabil Res 1998;42[Suppl 1]:50–56.

109. Deb S, Joyce J. The use of antiepileptic medication in a population based cohort of adults with learning disability and epilepsy. Int J Psychiatry Clin Pract 1999;3:129–133.

110. Schachter SC, Saper CB. Progress in epilepsy research: vagus nerve stimulation. Epilepsia 1998;39:677–686.

111. Rutecki P. Anatomical, physiological, and theoretical basis for the antiepileptic effect of vagus nerve stimulation. Epilepsia 1990;31[Suppl 2]:S1–S6.

112. Helmers SL, Al-Jayyousi M, Madsen J. Adjunctive treatment in Lennox-Gastaut syndrome using vagal nerve stimulation. Epilepsia 1998;39[Suppl 6]:169.

113. Ben-Menachem E, Hellstrom K, Waldton C, Augustinsson LE. Evaluation of refractory epilepsy treated with vagus nerve stimulation for up to 5 years. Neurology 1999;52(6):1265–1267.

114. Lundgren J, Amark P, Blennow G, et al. Vagus nerve stimulation in 16 children with refractory epilepsy. Epilepsia 1998;39(8):809–813.

Chapter 27

The Titanic Impact of Partial Compliance on Medication Effectiveness

Joyce A. Cramer

The impact of poor medication compliance on treatment outcome is mirrored in the story of *Titanic*. Neither the patient who misses many doses nor the doctor who attributes continued seizures to lack of drug efficacy sees the iceberg ahead. Although the orders have been given to reverse the engines and turn hard to port (the doctor's prescription given with instructions to take the medication), *Titanic* (the patient) remains on her fatal collision course. Why did the ship not turn in time? Why does the doctor change to an alternative medication or add a second drug?

Inherent in the answers to these questions is a message for all clinicians who prescribe medications: Look under the surface. They should not assume that they know which patients take their medications regularly. They should not assume that a seizure exacerbation signals cellular deterioration or a tumor. Rather, clinicians must develop skills to improve communication about what they prescribe, to teach patients skills to follow a dosing plan, and to reinforce the message.

A definition of *compliance* in the medical setting is yielding to a request or following a physician's instructions closely. Patients who are partially compliant differ from those who are noncompliant, in that noncompliant patients do not return for treatment. Another definition is treatment persistence, with a focus on long-term continuation of dosing. Both definitions include the concept of partial compliance, ranging from the occasional missed dose to the occasional extra dose. The pattern for partial compliance may be erratic, or it may be consistent but different from what a physician prescribed. Patients who are partially compliant are making an effort to participate in their treatment but neither achieve their intention nor receive the full effect of their treatment. Common reasons are forgetfulness, a dosage change that is not understood fully, or lack of efficacy.[1] Persistence is an issue when patients feel that they no longer need medication. Some people test themselves by purposely omitting doses, and others simply become lax about daily dosing. If seizures do not recur, they may feel that the medication no longer is necessary.

Measuring Compliance

Although for thousands of years doctors have been asking patients about compliance, measurement techniques provide varied results. Asking patients about their compliance is the easiest method, but it is not always an accurate measure of compliance. Patients tend to tell physicians what they think the physician wants to hear.[2,3] Patients' assessments of failure to take medication tend to be accurate, whereas denials of noncompliance are not.[3] Drug levels do not measure overall compliance because most drugs are absorbed rapidly and reach detectable levels in the blood quickly after a few doses.[4] One clear indication of noncompliance is a blood level of zero, because it indicates unarguably that no drug has been ingested for some time.[5]

The newest technology available for assessing dosing is continuous electronic monitoring using a variety of devices.[6] Widely used units are the medication event monitor and the electronic drug exposure monitor (APREX, a division of AARDEX Ltd., Union City, California). These units use a standard prescription bottle equipped with a microprocessor in the cap to record the date and time the bottle is opened.[6,7] Each opening of the cap is counted as a presumptive dose. Data from the units can be downloaded to a personal computer to show a calendar plot of the number of openings for each day. The system also displays the exact time and date of every bottle opening, which provides a very good understanding of drug usage and the dosing interval or the number of hours between doses. The patient's pattern of usage can be compared with the prescribed regimen to determine how many doses were taken on schedule, too late, too early, or not at all.[7,8] In other devices are boxes equipped with compartments for dosing of several medications. Data are transmitted to a central computer for reports.

Predicting Compliance

In electronic monitoring studies of people taking antiepileptic drugs, we have determined that most epilepsy patients take approximately 50–90%, although the overall range is 0–100%.[3,7] On average, patients take approximately 75% of medication as prescribed.[7] Detailed neuropsychological studies showed that compliance does not correlate with intelligence, memory, personality disorder, age, or education.[7] The number of drugs taken by a patient also does not correlate with compliance. Patients who are prescribed several medications tend to take all types of drugs together (e.g., three medications, six pills with breakfast) or forget all of them when they miss that dose.[7] The conclusion is that the number of medications is not as important as the number of times daily at which doses must be remembered.[7] A linear decline in compliance rates has been demonstrated with an increasing number of doses per day, with the greatest decline occurring when dosing increased from three to four times daily. Compliance rates with

one-, two-, three-, and four-times-daily dosing of antiepileptic drugs were 87%, 81%, 77%, and 39%, respectively.[7] Even once-daily dosing does not lead to perfect compliance.[9]

The effect of medication compliance on drug effectiveness is based on the following question: Did the drug fail, or did the patient fail to take the drug?[7,8,10] We have shown that medication dosing habits vary over time. Dosing was good (86%) in the 5 days before and after a visit, but declined significantly to approximately 70% 1 month after the visit.[8] These data suggest that higher compliance rates just before may be related to anticipation of the visit. However, the message lasts only for a brief period after the visit; no good methods are available for predicting which patients will follow prescribed medication regimens or when patterns will change.[7] Establishing the minimum number of dosing times per day and teaching patients how to remember dose times should help to improve compliance. Table 27-1, a calendar plot, reveals erratic compliance on weekdays with a three-times-daily regimen and neglect on weekends.

Strategies for Improving Compliance with Medication

A patient reporting good compliance with a prescribed regimen rarely intends to deceive. If such a person has forgotten to take doses, the lapse also is forgotten. Thus, reporting good compliance signifies lack of awareness of a problem. Electronic monitoring dispelled the myth of deception by demonstrating daily dosing events to individuals. Most patients were surprised to see how many doses they had omitted inadvertently. Until we can give every patient an electronic unit, we can supplement good intentions with structured compliance education.

Compliance Education

The key to compliance education is to facilitate dosing by rendering the schedule easy and relevant to the patient's individual needs.[1] The four principal strategies for improving compliance are education, planning of dosing regimens, clinical scheduling, and communication.[1] These

Table 27-1. Electronic Dosing Record for a Patient Prescribed a Medication to Be Taken Three Times Daily*

Sunday	Monday	Tuesday	Wednesday	Thursday	Friday	Saturday
—	3	3	2	3	2	1
1	3	3	3	2	2	0
0	0	3	2	2	2	1
0	2	2	2	2	1	0
0	0	1	2	0	—	—

*Digits indicate numbers of doses taken per day.

strategies and the practical suggestions listed later can be applied to all patient groups regardless of underlying medical illness. Physicians who use these strategies clarify to patients that they want to help and are interested in how medication is taken.

Planning Number of Medications, Dosing Schedules, and Cues

Some of the essential aspects of prescribing that will enhance patient compliance are selecting the fewest number of doses to be taken daily, with consideration of other medications patients must take; scheduling the times at which doses are to be taken; and helping patients to select a reminder or "cue." A simple system is to help patients to develop their own reminder cues.[11] A cue can be any regularly performed activity to which a patient can tie a medication regimen. Basic cues are clock times, meal times, or daily rituals. For example, if patients are aware of certain times during the day or wear a watch, and if they are on a simple medication regimen (i.e., once or twice daily), specific clock times can be selected as medicine times (e.g., 7 a.m. and 7 p.m.). Other good cues are meal times, shaving, fixing one's hair, or inserting contact lenses. Most patients will be able to establish a patterned behavior that will work for them. The cue training can be accomplished by health care staff trained in the technique. Clinicians should ask patients regularly about their cues and how well they are reminded to take their medication. Consistent queries not only help patients to develop a personalized cueing system but reinforce the interest of physicians in their well-being. Follow-up visits should reinforce the compliance message after the

initial dosing regimen and reminder cue are established with the patient.

Repetitive Follow-Up Questioning

Treatment persistence requires development of a long-term strategy that considers the patient's inability and reluctance to modify behavior and the likelihood that compliance will be less than perfect. The message will be reinforced if the same questions are asked at each visit. Many people stop taking medication after being seizure-free for a long period. Abrupt discontinuation occurs when a prescription is not refilled. Most patients begin to taper dosing to test whether they really need the medication or when they simply realize that they have missed many doses with no consequence. Some patients need a reminder that good seizure control is related to good compliance. If the medication is not taken regularly, the seizure threshold could change.[2,12] Anxiety often is related to concern about adverse effects or fear of "becoming addicted" to the medication. Clear answers that address these real concerns should help the patient. Health care providers develop individual styles for counseling about development of a compliance program. A good provider-patient relationship that engages affected patients in dosing decisions could have an impact on compliance.[12,13]

Feedback about Dosing

Physicians cannot predict who will be a good complier when first prescribing a medication or who has been a good complier in long-term treatment. The availability of electronic monitoring at reduced cost has extended its use into physicians' offices. Electronic monitors can be used to detect occult noncompliance and to teach affected patients how to improve dosing. The Medication Usage Skills for Effectiveness Program (MUSE-P) was developed as a rapid, simple teaching program that can be initiated by nonmedical personnel spending a few minutes with affected patients.[6,13] The first step is to teach the patient how to select a dosing cue and to take all doses from the special bottle. During return visits, the unit is "read" using proprietary software. On a computer screen in a calendar format, patients see a record of all doses taken (see Table 27-1). The simple, two-dimensional format provides a clear message in the style of a report card. A zero indicates that no doses were taken that day; 2 indicates that two doses were taken. The nonprofessional staff person then asks whether the cues have been helpful and, if they were not, the cues are changed. Questions about special problems on days when doses were missed engage the patient in a review of dosing habits. The visual and verbal lesson is that doses were missed by the patient and that improvement can be achieved with better attention. The MUSE-P has been effective in a population with severe schizophrenia (with cognitive deficits) and mood disorders (lack of interest in helping themselves). We found significant differences between patients receiving MUSE-P as compared to controls receiving usual medication education.[13] This technique takes up only minutes of a staff person's time in teaching skills that might be useful for a lifetime.

Conclusion

Even patients with poorly controlled seizures take only approximately three-fourths of medication as prescribed.[7] However, we do not know which patients will be erratic, or when, or to what degree in complying with prescribed regimens. Addressing compliance issues is important because of the direct and indirect costs of seizures that affect the health care system.[10] Clinicians who routinely discuss compliance and dose schedules and who help patients to select a personal cue reminder engage patients in their own care. In an environment in which patient satisfaction is a measure of successful medical care, attention to compliance is a simple way to demonstrate special attention and to improve medical success.

References

1. Cramer JA. Identifying and Improving Compliance Patterns: A Composite Plan for Health Care Providers. In JA Cramer, B Spilker (eds), Patient Compliance in Medical Practice and Clinical Trials. New York: Raven Press, 1991;387–392.
2. Cramer JA. Overview of Methods to Measure and Enhance Patient Compliance. In JA Cramer, B Spilker (eds), Patient Compliance in Medical Practice and Clinical Trials. New York: Raven Press, 1991;3–10.
3. Cramer JA, Mattson RH. Monitoring Compliance with Antiepileptic Drug Therapy. In JA Cramer, B Spilker (eds), Patient Compliance in Medical Practice and Clinical Trials. New York: Raven Press, 1991;123–137.
4. Pullar T, Kumar S, Tindall H, Feely M. Time to stop counting the tablets? Clin Pharmacol Ther 1989;46:163–168.
5. Norell SE. Methods in assessing drug compliance. Acta Med Scand 1983;683:35–40.
6. Cramer JA. Microelectronic systems for monitoring and enhancing patient compliance with medication regimens. Drugs 1995;49:321–327.
7. Cramer JA, Mattson RH, Prevey ML, et al. How often is medication taken as prescribed? A novel assessment technique. JAMA 1989;261:3273–3277.
8. Cramer JA, Scheyer RD, Mattson RH. Compliance declines between clinic visits. Arch Intern Med 1990;150:1509–1510.
9. Cramer JA. Consequences of intermittent treatment for hypertension: the case for medication compliance and persistence. Am J Manag Care 1999;4:1563–1568.
10. Cramer JA. Partial medication compliance: the enigma in poor medical outcomes. Am J Manag Care 1995;1:45–52.
11. Cramer JA. Medication use by the elderly: enhancing patient compliance in the elderly. Role of packaging aids and monitoring. Drugs Aging 1998;12:7–15.
12. Lima J, Nazarian L, Charney E, Lahti C. Compliance with short-term antimicrobial therapy: some techniques that help. Pediatrics 1976;57:383–386.
13. Cramer JA, Rosenheck R. Enhancing medication compliance for people with serious mental illness. J Nerv Ment Dis 1999;187:52–54.

Chapter 28

Cognitive Toxicity of Antiepileptic Drugs

Daniel L. Drane and Kimford J. Meador

The use of antiepileptic drugs (AEDs) can significantly improve the quality of life (QOL) of epilepsy patients by preventing the striking disruption of function resulting from a seizure episode as well as the untoward cumulative effects of uncontrolled seizure activity on cerebral integrity and subsequent cognitive functioning. Despite the obvious benefits of AEDs in controlling neuronal irritability, these medications can contribute to compromised cognitive processing by dampening normal neuronal excitability. Effective clinicians will seek not only to minimize seizure activity but to help their patients maintain a normal level of arousal and optimal cognitive functioning through the appropriate use of AEDs.

The purpose of this chapter is twofold: to equip the clinician with the available knowledge necessary to make the most effective treatment decisions in the use of AEDs and to identify areas in which additional research is required to maximize optimal treatment delivery. Topics discussed include the general intellectual functioning of epilepsy patients and a review of what is known about the effects on cognition of both the older, well-established AEDs and some of the newer medications. Methodologic issues involved in AED research, which have often resulted in conflicting conclusions, are reviewed. The effects of AEDs on the cognition of patients at the extremes of age and patients with developmental delay or intellectual disability also are discussed, as is the possible impact of in utero exposure to these agents. Throughout this review, attention is devoted to the improvement in QOL that can be achieved by striking a balance between seizure control and the maintenance of optimal cognitive functioning.

Cognitive Functioning in Epilepsy

To assess accurately the possible adverse effects of AEDs on cognition, clinicians must know the baseline intellectual capacity of their epilepsy patients and should be acquainted with the multiple factors that have shaped the patients' cognitive development. Otherwise, clinicians may mistakenly attribute preexisting cognitive deficits, which could have resulted from a variety of psychosocial or disease-related variables, to the AEDs being used for seizure control. Premorbid influences on cognition include the usual mix of environmental, psychosocial, and hereditary concerns that typically enter into any discussion of intelligence (e.g., socioeconomic status, other medical conditions, parental intelligence quotient [IQ]).[1] In addition, numerous variables specific to the disorder of epilepsy must be considered.[2,3] These include age of patient at seizure onset; duration, severity, and frequency of epileptogenic episodes; etiology of seizure disorder (idiopathic versus known pathology); seizure type; and both intraictal and interictal physiologic dysfunction resulting from the seizures themselves. Patients with earlier seizure onset tend to exhibit greater intellectual impairment owing to the effects of these noxious variables on early cerebral development and consequent impairment of formative learning. Furthermore, some patients will have undergone surgical interventions that can radically alter and shape their subsequent development and intellectual capacity. Careful review of a patient's medical and psychosocial history, along with a clinical evaluation of mental status, will help to establish that patient's baseline functioning, against which change can be measured. In some situations, a thorough neuropsychological evaluation may be indicated. These could include cases in which subtle deficits could have a significant impact on vocational or educational functioning or in which patients are complaining of cognitive dysfunction resulting from current AEDs.

In general, an increased incidence of cognitive deficits is noted among patients with epilepsy. However, the majority of epilepsy patients have normal cognitive function,[3] as shown in the seminal work of William Lennox,[4] one of the first investigators to study the effects of AEDs on cognition. The increased incidence of cognitive dysfunction among this group seems to be explained in part by the high incidence of epilepsy in patients with mental retardation, focal brain damage, or other underlying cerebral diseases.

General Effects of Polypharmacy and Dosage

In general, optimal cognitive functioning is more likely to be achieved by avoiding polypharmacy and by not exceeding the recommended standard therapeutic ranges for AED blood levels. Studies in which the number of AEDs used in the treatment of epilepsy patients was reduced have consistently shown decreased drowsiness, improved attention or concentration and mood, heightened drive, and enhanced psychomotor performance.[5–7] Furthermore, adverse effects of polypharmacy are present even when all employed AEDs are kept within standard therapeutic ranges.[8,9] Some studies have linked a reduction in polypharmacy to improvements on measures of general intellectual functioning and higher cognitive processing.[10,11]

When standard therapeutic AED blood levels are exceeded, the risk of cognitive impairment by AEDs is increased.[3,12] Even patients receiving multiple AEDs perform better on a variety of neuropsychological measures when maintained at lower AED blood levels. Improvement has been observed on measures of vigilance and reaction time,[13,14] general intellectual functioning,[15] cognitive processing speed,[9] visual scanning and tracking,[9,14] and immediate and recent memory.[9,14] Similarly, several monotherapy studies demonstrate a strong relationship between higher AED dosages and increasing cognitive impairment.[16–18]

Despite clear evidence of the detrimental effects of these practices, polypharmacy and AED dosages that exceed standard therapeutic levels may be required in some cases to manage seizure occurrence effectively. Clinicians must evaluate the risk-benefit ratio on a case-by-case basis while keeping in mind these general principles.

Established Antiepileptic Drugs and Cognition

A plethora of research studies exist that examine the cognitive effects of the older, established AEDs. However, many of these studies, plagued by poor experimental designs, have tended to create only a morass of antithetical results and conclusions.[19] Such contradictory information renders difficult a clinician's effective decision making regarding medication selection. Several recent review articles have highlighted the methodological flaws that have confounded the design of most AED studies, and an attempt has been made to clarify this confusion objectively by considering only those studies that meet minimal research standards.[2,20] Frequent problems include subject selection bias, nonequivalence on clinical and dependent variables, insufficient statistical power, and inadequate statistical control for multiple comparisons.[12,20]

Although all the major AEDs can produce cognitive side effects, the magnitude of these effects tends to be modest, for the most part, when monotherapy is practiced within the standard therapeutic range.[3,21] When such effects are observed, they usually tend to involve attentional processing, psychomotor speed, and response accuracy.[3,22] Clinical drug studies have shown that the greatest deleterious effects on cognition result from the use of barbiturates and benzodiazepines.

The cognitive effects produced by carbamazepine, phenytoin, and valproate seem modest and similar between drugs.[12] Although some controversy remains regarding the differential effects of these well-established AEDs, recent studies attempting to control carefully for confounding variables have failed to find any significant differences between these medications in either patients or healthy volunteers.[12,23,24] Dodrill and Troupin,[25] using a well-designed, double-blind, randomized crossover study to compare the cognitive effects of carbamazepine and phenytoin, had originally concluded that phenytoin contributed to more adverse effects on cognition than did carbamazepine. However, after these researchers later reanalyzed their data to control for differing AED blood levels, the differences between the agents' effects evaporated.[26] In addition, the well-known VA Cooperative Study,[27] which examined the cognitive effects of carbamazepine, phenytoin, phenobarbital, and primidone in a parallel study of new-onset epilepsy patients, found no "consistent patterns" of impairment attributable to AED type. Furthermore, variations between the cognitive effects of these AEDs were small, despite a very large sample size. Similarly, Meador et al.[28,29] found no clinically significant differential cognitive effects among carbamazepine, phenytoin, and valproate using randomized, double-blind crossover designs in healthy volunteers. However, performance was worse overall for subjects receiving phenobarbital.

Given that most studies have examined the effects of AEDs only for short treatment durations, one might wonder about the possible long-term, cumulative effects of AED treatment. However, the work of Dodrill and Wilensky[30] helps to address this issue by examining the neuropsychological performance in patients with epilepsy over a longer span of time. Three treatment groups—treated with phenytoin alone, phenytoin in combination with other AEDs, or an alternative AED regimen apart from phenytoin—were examined over 5 years. No differences were observed among these groups for the duration of the study.

Even though the AED effects on cognition are modest, such cognitive effects could have an impact on the performance of epilepsy patients engaged in complex tasks involving sustained attention, motor speed, or learning. With little apparent differential variation between the common AEDs, the clinician is free to base AED choice on other clinical factors. However, the differences we have discussed are based on group performance; therefore, the clinician should remain aware that individual patients may react uniquely to any administered medication.

New Antiepileptic Drugs

As new AEDs are being introduced, comparisons to the older AEDs and to one another are necessary. A number of studies have already been completed, and many more are currently under way. Although initial results for several of these new AEDs as compared to placebo have been promising, few direct comparisons to the older, established AEDs have been made.[12]

Clobazam

Clobazam was introduced initially as an anxiolytic drug during the mid-1970s, although its antiepileptic effects were recognized soon thereafter.[31,32] Its chemical structure differs slightly from that of clonazepam and diazepam, and it is less likely to cause psychomotor impairment or sedation.[33] Although its mechanism of action remains somewhat unclear, it is believed to potentiate the inhibitory actions of γ-aminobutyric acid (GABA).[34] Studies have demonstrated the antiepileptic properties of clobazam and have suggested that it may be useful in adults and children with many types of epilepsy.[35,36] Notable behavioral side effects have included sedation, changes in mood, aggression, and disinhibition.[37] However, only one recent study has attempted to examine the cognitive and behavioral impact of this medication in a systematic fashion. This study, using a randomized, double-blind prospective design, found no significant differences between clobazam and standard monotherapy (i.e., either carbamazepine or phenytoin) on a variety of neurocognitive and mood measures in children.[38]

Felbamate

Given that felbamate has been plagued with restrictions due to its toxicity to bone marrow and liver, well-controlled, systematic studies are unlikely. Felbamate may be hyperarousing, in contrast to the older AEDs, and can cause insomnia in some patients.

Gabapentin

Gabapentin is a relatively new AED, the exact mechanism of action of which remains uncertain, but it appears to have a good cognitive profile in initial studies. Most studies have not found a significant effect of gabapentin on cognitive functioning.[39–42] Further, improved ratings have often been observed on measures of mood and QOL.[40,43] In contrast, some authors have reported adverse effects on the behavior of children treated with gabapentin, which have ceased following dose reduction or discontinuation of gabapentin treatment.[44,45]

One of the first studies completed with gabapentin, involving a comparison of low-dose gabapentin and placebo, observed subtle improvement on several psychometric tests, including measures of concentration, numeric memory, and complex reaction time.[39] Several positive effects also were reported on both neuropsychological and QOL measures after conversion to gabapentin monotherapy among a group of patients with refractory partial seizures.[46] However, this study was limited by its lack of a placebo group to control for test-retest effects. More recently, the same researchers found no differences on any measures of cognitive function between a large sample of patients treated with gabapentin and a reference group of patients treated with placebo.[40]

One small study (n = 21) comparing gabapentin to placebo in patients with partial epilepsy used a double-blind, dose-ranging (1,200–2,400 mg per day), add-on, crossover design, which produced differences on only 1 of 11 cognitive measures (i.e., a positive effect of gabapentin on one variable).[47] No differences were observed on QOL measures between patients treated with gabapentin versus placebo in this study. However, gabapentin produced significantly more drowsiness and side effects.

Another recent study, using a double-blind, randomized crossover design with two 5-week treatment periods, compared the cognitive effects of gabapentin and carbamazepine in 35 healthy subjects. Although both AEDs produced some effects, gabapentin produced significantly fewer untoward cognitive effects as compared to carbamazepine (i.e., subjects performed better on 26% of all cognitive variables when treated with gabapentin versus carbamazepine).[48]

As regards QOL and behavioral issues, subjective improvements in mood were reported in a double-blind clinical trial using gabapentin as add-on therapy in patients with epilepsy.[43] In this study, a greater number of gabapentin-treated patients (46%) reported improvements in general well-being as compared to control patients receiving placebo medications (29%). Similarly, in an open-label, add-on study of 114 patients, QOL ratings improved after addition of this AED.[49] In the recent study by Dodrill et al.,[40] patients treated with gabapentin exhibited better scores on QOL measures than did the placebo-treated comparison group. Patients treated with gabapentin tended to report better moods and less anxiety and discouragement than did members of the reference group. Of note, the reference group was not a true control group as it had served as a comparison group during a prior AED study. Finally, although gabapentin appears generally to be well tolerated in children, behavioral side effects include irritability, hyperactivity, and agitation.[44,45,50] The children in these studies had preexisting problems with attention-deficit hyperactivity disorder, developmental delay, or learning disability, and behavioral disruption ceased with dose reduction or discontinuation of treatment with gabapentin.

Lamotrigine

The main mechanism of action for lamotrigine is blockade of voltage-dependent sodium channels, which results in the stabilization of neuronal membranes and reduction of excitatory neurotransmitter release.[51,52] Lamotrigine is effective in the management of both partial and generalized seizures and is well tolerated in studies involving patients and healthy volunteers.[53,54] Smith et al.[55] found no cognitive effects attributable to lamotrigine when compared to placebo as an add-on treatment in patients with partial epilepsy. However, the neuropsychological battery employed was limited in nature. A study comparing several new AEDs in healthy volunteers found no significant cognitive effects for either lamotrigine or gabapentin.[42] However, this study was limited by a small sample size and a parallel group design. Two studies examining the impact of AEDs on healthy volunteers suggested that lamotrigine may produce fewer adverse central nervous system effects than do diazepam, carbamazepine, and phenytoin.[56,57] Preliminary results were presented recently from a study that used a double-blind, randomized, crossover design to compare the neuropsychological effects of lamotrigine and carbamazepine in healthy adult volunteers.[58] Performance was statistically superior on lamotrigine as compared to carbamazepine for 17 of the 40 variables.

Several studies suggest that lamotrigine can improve perception of psychological well-being.[53,55,59] Higher QOL ratings have also been attributed to lamotrigine in comparison to carbamazepine and phenytoin.[60] Lamotrigine can be beneficial in bipolar disorder[61–63] and may improve behavior in children with epilepsy who have severe cognitive deficits or autism.[64,65] Among patients with Lennox-Gastaut syndrome, the addition of lamotrigine can improve the behavior of some individuals (e.g., reduced irritability and hyperactivity, decreased lethargy, contribution to improved social engagement and cooperation) while leading to heightened problems in others (e.g., hyperactivity, irritability, and stereotypy).[66] These conflicting results may reflect both diversity of the psychosocial and behavioral problems experienced by persons with developmental delay and the possible interaction of other AEDs or psychotropic medications. Taken together, these studies suggest that lamotrigine has psychotropic properties, although future studies are required to determine the interplay of other medications and patient variables.

Levetiracetam

Recently approved by the U.S. Food and Drug Administration, levetiracetam appears to work via a novel mechanism of action, and it has a favorable efficacy-toxicity ratio.[67] However, no formal studies on its cognitive effects have yet been published.

Oxcarbazepine

Cognitive or behavioral effects of oxcarbazepine, a derivative of carbamazepine, have been examined in only a handful of studies, although initial clinical trials suggest that it is better tolerated than carbamazepine or phenytoin. No differential cognitive effects were observed when this AED was compared with phenytoin in a small, randomized, double-blind, parallel group study in patients with new-onset epilepsy.[68] A small crossover study employing healthy adults produced mixed results. Performance on reaction time measures appeared slowed by oxcarbazepine, whereas improvement was observed in subjective alertness and performance on a visual cancellation task.[69] Although no other published cognitive studies with oxcarbazepine are available, a preliminary report noted few cognitive effects in patients treated with oxcarbazepine, carbamazepine, or valproate.[70]

Rufinamide

Rufinamide remains in the early stages of development but appears to have a good efficacy-toxicity ratio. Nevertheless, no published studies regarding the effects of this medication on cognition have yet been published.

Tiagabine

Initial studies with tiagabine, which inhibits the reuptake of GABA,[71] have not shown any adverse cognitive effects. Three independent studies using an add-on design found no effect on cognition, mood, or QOL in epileptic patients.[70,72–74] The first of these investigations found no significant cognitive changes in a double-blind crossover study of patients with partial epilepsy treated with low-dose add-on therapy.[73] Similarly, no adverse neuropsychological effects were observed in a relatively small, randomized, placebo-controlled, parallel group–design study of patients either during the double-blind phase at low dosages or in the open-label phase at higher dosages.[72] Finally, Dodrill et al.[74] found no clinically significant changes on either neurocognitive or QOL measures in a large, double-blind, add-on, placebo-controlled, parallel, multicenter, dose-response efficacy study in patients with focal seizures.

Dodrill et al.[75] have recently contributed the first report of the effects of tiagabine monotherapy on mental abilities, adjustment, and mood. Multiple measures of cognition, mood, and QOL were administered to patients with complex partial seizures who were randomly switched to low-dose (6 mg per day) or high-dose (36 mg per day) tiagabine monotherapy. Patients who achieved tiagabine monotherapy tended to experience positive changes in mood that were greatest among the group receiving the lower dosage of tiagabine. Cognitive improvements, which were greatest among the patients treated with the higher tiagabine dosage, were observed in the areas of motor speed, concentration, and generative fluency. In the 25% of patients who did not achieve tiagabine monotherapy, negative changes in mood were observed among the patients receiving the higher dosage. These researchers attributed the negative change in mood to a rapid titration to high-dose tiagabine therapy. This study lacked a control group for direct comparison. However, these researchers used the same battery of tests for which they have established a reference group during earlier investigations with the same clinical population. Comparison of tiagabine to other AEDs and at varying dosage levels are needed to clarify its effects.

Topiramate

Topiramate is believed to act on the GABA neurotransmitter system and to block voltage-sensitive sodium channels and the kainate/AMPA species of glutamate receptor.[76] Although few studies directly investigated the cognitive effects of topiramate, observations during clinical trials showed a tendency to produce somnolence, psychomotor slowing, language problems, and difficulty with memory.[77,78] A preliminary report with formal cognitive testing noted modest but significant effects in epilepsy patients receiving topiramate as add-on therapy.[79] However, effect size appeared similar to test-retest effects. A recent study compared the cognitive effects of topiramate, gabapentin, and lamotrigine in 17 healthy adults using a single-blind, randomized, parallel group study.[42] Patients receiving topiramate performed worse than the other groups on generative fluency and visual attention tasks during the acute dosing phase. They also scored worse on measures of verbal memory and psychomotor speed at 1 month of treatment. Limitations of this study included the use of a parallel group design and the use of a titration rate for topiramate that was faster than recommended guidelines. Preliminary results recently were presented comparing the cognitive effects of topiramate to valproate in a randomized add-on parallel group study of adult epilepsy patients. The researchers reported only minor differences.[80] Overall, initial evidence suggests that topiramate has some impact on cognition, although its absolute effects in epilepsy patients relative to other AEDs remains to be determined.

Vigabatrin

One of the most frequently examined novel AEDs, vigabatrin was the first AED developed for a targeted mechanism of action.[32] Vigabatrin inhibits the breakdown of the enzyme γ-aminobutyric acid transaminase, thereby leaving greater amounts of GABA present in the brain.[81] Although vigabatrin has been tolerated well in clinical trials, some concern was expressed initially that it might produce adverse cognitive side effects. Such concerns arose because vigabatrin inhibits the breakdown of GABA (the major inhibitory neurotransmitter) and causes intramyelinic edema in laboratory animals.[82] However, intramyelinic edema has not been demonstrated in primates or humans,[83,84] and multiple comparisons to placebo have shown few untoward effects on cognition or QOL.[17,85–87]

Most of the comparisons of vigabatrin to placebo have employed a double-blind, randomized, add-on design in patients with epilepsy. Although one of these studies reported improvement on some cognitive measures,[88] most simply showed no change after the addition of vigabatrin to the current medication regimen.[85,86] Kälviainen et al.[89] compared the effects of vigabatrin and carbamazepine in epilepsy patients. They reported fewer adverse effects for vigabatrin on cognition, but limitations in sample size and the experimental design employed in this study preclude any firm conclusions. One study also has attempted to examine the impact of vigabatrin versus lorazepam on the cognitive function of healthy adults.[90] Vigabatrin produced less impairment than lorazepam in this group. However, this study used only a single dose of vigabatrin that was insufficient to produce a maximal effect on the inhibitory neurotransmitter GABA. Taken together, these studies suggest that vigabatrin has few adverse effects on cognition. However, systematic, well-controlled studies are required to support any improvement in cognitive function. Moreover, direct comparisons with both the old and new AEDs would be helpful.

Finally, depression and psychotic reactions have sometimes been reported to occur in some patients treated with vigabatrin in controlled clinical trials.[81,91,92] However, results of studies examining mood and QOL ratings have not demonstrated these adverse behavioral effects.[85,86] In fact, some studies have found positive changes in mood and QOL ratings.[93] A recent pilot study, examining the use of vigabatrin in a sample of epilepsy patients with mental retardation and psychiatric or behavioral comorbidity, found the drug to be well tolerated and reported that it reduced stereotypies and aggressiveness in some patients.[94] Currently, no evidence exists to show that this medication leads to a greater risk for adverse behavior than does any other AED.[95]

Zonisamide

Zonisamide is a sulfonamide derivative that appears fairly comparable to the established AEDs in its ability to control seizure activity.[96] The exact mechanism of action for this AED is unknown, although it can block sodium and calcium channels. Only one study examined the impact of zonisamide on cognitive functioning. Berent et al.,[97] conducting a small, preliminary evaluation of zonisamide in patients with refractory partial seizures, found that patients experienced deficits in

the learning and acquisition of novel verbal information. Learning impairment was material-specific and appeared to resolve after a couple of months as tolerance developed.

Promise of the New Antiepileptic Drugs

Drawing any firm conclusions regarding the cognitive effects of the new AEDs is difficult on the basis of the limited number of studies completed to date. However, initial trends suggest that several of these new medications produce minimal cognitive dysfunction. Ultimately, direct comparison with the established AEDs is required. Recognizing the limitations in the state of current AED research, the clinician may use these new antiepileptic medications with cautious optimism while carefully examining future studies as they appear in the literature.

Antiepileptic Drugs and Age Extremes

Despite the sensitivity of persons at the extremes of age to the cognitive side effects of medications, few AED studies focus on these vulnerable groups. The elderly are more susceptible to medication side effects, owing to both pharmacokinetic and pharmacodynamic reasons.[98] Children are at higher risk owing to the impact that medications can have on their physical and cognitive development.[99] When administering AEDs among these age groups, the clinician should carefully monitor cognitive performance in some manner. This might involve neuropsychological assessment, obtaining feedback from family members regarding daily functioning and, in the case of children, monitoring school performance.

Further research involving the elderly is needed.[100] Only two studies have been published to date that examine the use of AEDs in the aged. The first study found only minimal differences when comparing phenytoin to valproate and when comparing both AEDs to nondrug baselines in an elderly population.[101] Another recent study demonstrated that making modest increases (within the standard therapeutic range) in the dosage levels of standard AEDs (i.e., carbamazepine, sodium valproate, or phenytoin) used in monotherapy did not contribute to any alteration in the neurocognitive performance of an elderly sample of patients when compared to a group of placebo controls.[102]

Discriminating between the relative contribution of AEDs and other factors affecting cognitive and behavioral problems among children can be especially complex. Few studies currently exist, and these have generally been limited to the standard AEDs. Vining et al.,[103] using a double-blind, randomized, crossover design, found that performance of 21 children with epilepsy on phenobarbital was worse than performance on valproate for several cognitive and behavioral measures. These children performed better on a learning task and on several nonverbal performance measures while on valproate. While on phenobarbital, their behavior was rated as significantly worse by their parents in a few areas, and they were also described as more hyperactive. In an open-label, parallel study of phenobarbital and valproate using a control group of nonepileptic children,[104] the group treated with phenobarbital failed to show any test-retest improvement in either performance or full-scale IQ obtained from the Wechsler Intelligence Scale for Children–Revised. However, drawing any firm conclusions about this AED's long-term impact on learning ability is difficult owing to significant baseline differences in intellectual functioning between the control group and the children treated with phenobarbital. Adverse cognitive effects for phenobarbital have also been found in placebo-controlled parallel group studies of children with febrile convulsions on measures of memory and general intellectual functioning.[104–106] A recent follow-up to one of these studies, which had originally examined infants who had experienced febrile seizures, found that those who had been treated with phenobarbital rather than placebo had significantly lower scores on a measure of reading recognition and a slightly lower but nonsignificant mean IQ when tested 3–5 years later.[107] Researchers suggested that treatment with phenobarbital may have interfered with developing verbal skills.

Aldenkamp et al.,[108] using a controlled, parallel group design to compare cognitive performance in children being withdrawn from standard AED monotherapy (groups included patients treated with carbamazepine, phenytoin, or valproic acid), found significant improvement on only one vari-able after complete discontinuation of therapy. These researchers concluded that these standard AEDs had little impact on higher cognitive functions, although they believed that phenytoin might produce mild impairment of psychomotor speed. Similarly, other AED withdrawal studies in children have shown little alteration in cognitive functioning after discontinuation of the standard AEDs.[109,110]

Forsythe et al.,[111] comparing children with new-onset epilepsy who were randomly assigned to treatment with carbamazepine, phenytoin, or sodium valproate, reported that recent memory functioning was worse for the group treated with carbamazepine. Williams et al.,[112] also comparing children with new-onset epilepsy, found no significant differences on a number of neurocognitive measures between children treated with a variety of AEDs in monotherapy and a group of control patients with diabetes mellitus. Most of the children in this study were treated with carbamazepine or valproate, although a small number were receiving ethosuximide, lamotrigine, gabapentin, or phenytoin. Combining different treatment groups made it impossible to examine any differential effects of the employed AEDs. Although researchers were careful to control for AED blood levels, baseline differences, and ongoing seizure activity, this study lacked random assignment of subjects.

Mandelbaum and Burack[113] examined the cognitive and behavioral performance in children ages 4–16 years with new-onset, idiopathic seizures both at baseline and at 6- and 12-month intervals after the initiation of AED therapy. They found that seizure type accounted for differences between subjects at baseline and found no significant effects of AED treatment (carbamazepine, sodium valproate, or ethosuximide) at follow-up. Limitations in sample size at follow-up, apparently resulting from participant attrition, restrict the conclusions that can be drawn from this study about the overall effect of AEDs. Nevertheless, this study did highlight the impact of seizure type on cognition.[113]

Overall, one is left with only tentative conclusions regarding the impact of AEDs on the age extremes, owing to the paucity of studies completed with children or the elderly. However, initial studies suggest that although the standard AEDs can affect both cognition and behavior, these drugs' effects tend to be modest in the short term. Nevertheless, even subtle AED effects could be harmful during critical periods of learning and childhood development. As with studies involving adults, phenobarbital seems to have a more adverse profile with children than does carbamazepine, valproate, or phenytoin. Additional studies are needed that involve larger sample sizes and more rigorous methodologic designs among these extreme age groups. Moreover, no studies examining cognitive impact of the novel AEDs at the age extremes are currently available; these, too, are needed.

Antiepileptic Drugs in Patients with Developmental Delay

Epilepsy patients experiencing developmental delay or intellectual disability may be more adversely affected by the potential side effects of AEDs than patients without such limitations. These patients may have fewer cognitive and emotional resources with which to cope with even mild restrictions in intellectual functioning. Also, increased behavioral problems and irritability may occur in such patients because they sometimes are less able to report adverse effects from AEDs when they occur (e.g., oversedation, diplopia, dizziness).[114] This could be particularly problematic for those patients with limitations in communication, such as those who have autism or profound mental retardation.

Studies examining the impact of AEDs on the cognitive and behavioral functioning of patients with intellectual and developmental disabilities and epilepsy have been limited. Moreover, given that patients with developmental disorders often have a higher base rate of behavioral and psychiatric problems, determining the unique contribution of administered AEDs can be difficult.[115] Few AED studies specifically target such patient groups. More typically, the impact of AEDs on these populations has been reported in anecdotal fashion or as a secondary finding of a larger study. Existing studies, although small in number, suggest that AEDs can intensify baseline behavior and cognitive problems in these groups and also can contribute to new-onset behavioral issues and cognitive dysfunction.[44,45,66] Therefore, great care

is needed in choosing an appropriate AED for such patients.

Initial studies with lamotrigine suggested that it may be well tolerated by patients with intellectual limitations or developmental delay.[64,66,116,117] Several open-label studies reported positive findings, including decreased autistic symptoms[64]; enhanced alertness and attention span; and improved mobility, speech, and independence.[117] In addition, two blinded, placebo-controlled studies suggest that lamotrigine has a positive impact on behavior, mood, and communication in patients with Lennox-Gastaut syndrome.[118,119] The first study reported improvement in behavior, speech, nonverbal communication, and gross and fine motor coordination in patients treated with lamotrigine versus placebo. In the second study, parents of 130 patients with Lennox-Gastaut syndrome completed QOL questionnaires after a single-blind, placebo phase and again after 16 weeks of add-on therapy. Parents of the children included in the lamotrigine group reported significant improvements in the mood and sociability of their children. Despite these positive reports, not all results have been favorable. Some individuals developed heightened problems, including increased hyperactivity and irritability.[66] Beran and Gibson[120] reported that 5 of 19 intellectually handicapped patients with epilepsy exhibited aggressive behaviors during lamotrigine treatment. These conflicting results may reflect both the diversity of the psychosocial and behavioral problems experienced by persons with developmental delay and the possible interaction of other AEDs or psychotropic medications.[66,116]

Gabapentin may produce behavioral side effects, including irritability, hyperactivity, and agitation, in children with attention-deficit hyperactivity disorder, developmental delay, or learning disability, despite being generally well tolerated by children.[44,45,50] All behavioral changes ceased in these children with dose reduction or discontinuation of treatment with this AED. One recent study suggested that children younger than 10 years who have intellectual disabilities were at greater risk of adverse behavior as a result of gabapentin therapy than were older children.[121] The severity of intellectual disability did not appear to affect the occurrence of side effects significantly.

Kälviainen[122] has suggested that tiagabine might represent a good choice for persons who are intellectually disabled, as it tends to have a low side effect profile in the cognitive area.

However, controlled trials examining its impact in a clinical population with intellectual disability or developmental delay are not available. Carbamazepine and valproate often are used in these special populations, as adverse cognitive impact has tended to be minimal and positive psychotropic effects may be helpful.[114,123]

Topiramate is effective in treating the atonic seizures associated with Lennox-Gastaut syndrome[124] and has broad-based efficacy across a range of both generalized and partial seizures. Side effects such as sedation, confusion, and word-finding difficulty may limit its usefulness, but patients with developmental delay and intellectual disability usually tolerate this AED without problems. Thus, topiramate should be one of the AEDs considered for use in such populations, given that control of seizures frequently is difficult in these patients.

Overall, the appropriate management of seizures can maximize the intellectual functioning of those with developmental delay by improving their capacity to learn and by offsetting potentially permanent cerebral changes resulting from prolonged seizure activity or frequent epileptiform discharges. Nevertheless, many more studies are required to understand the impact of both the old and new AEDs on persons with developmental and intellectual disabilities, as well as the interactions of these agents with other potential psychotropic medications used in these populations.

Neurodevelopmental Effects of In Utero Antiepileptic Drug Exposure

From a theoretic perspective, the greatest risk of adverse effects of AED treatment might result from in utero exposure. In animal models, such exposure causes permanent alterations in anatomic structures and behavioral functions.[125] Likewise, negative developmental outcomes have been seen in children whose mothers were treated with AEDs during pregnancy.[126] However, controversy exists as to the differential effects, because a well-designed study controlling for variables such as maternal age, IQ, socioeconomic background, and seizure type and frequency during pregnancy has not been conducted.

Animal Studies

Animal studies suggest that somatic and developmental abnormalities can result from in utero exposure to AEDs.[127] Many of these malformations and delays appear to have clinical counterparts.[128,129] Although the AED dosage required to produce somatic anomalies in animals is usually several times higher than the standard therapeutic dosage used in humans, developmental and behavioral effects in animal offspring appear to occur at much lower dosages, with blood levels comparable to those in humans.[130–132] Nevertheless, differences involving interspecies and intraspecies susceptibility to AED-induced malformations make difficult the extrapolation from these studies of effects of AEDs on humans. Research examining the specific effects of AEDs are lacking, and no current data are available on the newer antiepileptic medications.

In utero phenobarbital produces neuronal deficits and reduced brain weight in mice at maternal levels of 40–200 μg/ml. Prenatal phenobarbital also impairs the development of several reflexes, open-field activity, schedule-controlled behavior, and brain levels of catecholamines in mice.[126,132] Early exposure to phenobarbital in mice may alter postsynaptic components of the hippocampal cholinergic system, impairing hippocampus-related behavior.[133]

Exposure to phenytoin in utero leads to a variety of behavioral abnormalities in rats, including abnormal circling behavior, decreased learning ability, hyperactivity, impaired motor coordination, and delayed reflex development.[134–141] These studies have established a dose-effect relationship, using maternal plasma levels (10–25 mg/kg) that overlap the standard human therapeutic range.[130,135,136] The behavioral effects observed in these studies are chronic, do not resolve with advancing age of the animals, and are not explained by malnutrition, the impact of seizures, or patterns of maternal rearing.[137–139] Among newborn mice exposed to phenytoin doses ranging from 10 to 35 mg/kg, total brain weight, cerebral weight, and cerebellar weight were reduced significantly in mice receiving doses of either 25 or 35 mg/kg as compared to untreated controls.[140] Phenytoin also alters neuronal membranes in the hippocampus.[141]

Vorhees[142,143] found similar but less striking neurobehavioral effects in the offspring of rats after intrauterine exposure to valproate (150–200 mg/kg) and trimethadione (250 mg/kg) at relevant maternal blood concentrations and nonmalforming doses. Phenobarbital resulted in only minor behavioral effects, although higher doses (400–600 mg/kg) were maternally toxic or resulted in a high rate of embryonic deaths or the occurrence of major somatic abnormality.[144] Finally, valproic acid has also been shown to alter neuronal membranes in the hippocampus.[145]

Overall, animal studies suggest that a number of developmental and behavioral problems, as well as structural cerebral defects, can result from intrauterine exposure to AEDs. In addition, such deficits can occur at maternal plasma levels that are both concordant with those used in humans and below those levels necessary to produce significant physical malformations or embryotoxicity. Deficits appear to be most noticeable as task complexity increases[135] and can emerge at developmental stages subsequent to initial exposure.[130] However, interspecies differences and the lack of comparative information on pharmacokinetics and developmental outcome make difficult direct extrapolation from animal studies to AED use in humans.

Human Studies

Although AEDs are potential teratogenic agents and can cause developmental and behavioral dysfunction in animals, the effects of intrauterine exposure in humans remains unclear and somewhat controversial. Many variables, including paternal IQ and socioeconomic status, maternal seizure type and frequency during pregnancy, and maternal age, can contribute to the intellectual capacity, cognitive functioning, and developmental achievement of a patient's offspring. Infants of mothers with epilepsy tend to have higher rates of malformations than do those whose mothers are

without epilepsy, even when the infants of mothers with epilepsy are not being exposed to medications.[146] Studies controlling for these variables in a careful fashion are lacking.

Perhaps this confusion is best captured by the recent consensus guidelines to manage pregnant women with epilepsy.[147] The participants who developed these guidelines could not delineate, based on available data, which of the four major AEDs—carbamazepine, phenobarbital, phenytoin, or valproate—is the most teratogenic. "Each of the four major AEDs has been considered more teratogenic than the other three AEDs, depending on the author cited."[147] The guideline authors noted that mixed findings resulted from a variety of study confounders, including polypharmacy, different dosage levels, various combinations of AEDs, different patient populations, and different genotypes that were exposed to the AEDs. This panel concluded that the present consensus opinion is that "the AED that stops seizures in a given patient should be used."[147] They added that this is often the drug of choice for a given seizure type and epilepsy syndrome. The panel also endorsed monotherapy rather than polytherapy. Unfortunately, although further studies have been released over the last few years, little has changed to resolve the confusion surrounding the differential teratogenic effects of the major AEDs, and even less is known about their newer counterparts.

Most investigators found an increased risk of developmental delay in children of mothers with epilepsy,[148–158] although a few studies found no greater risk than in the general public.[159,160] Children of mothers with epilepsy have an increased risk of mental retardation as compared to children of mothers without epilepsy, but this risk is not observed in children of fathers with epilepsy. Multiple factors could contribute to the observed differences, but animal studies suggest that AEDs play at least a partial role.

Although children of mothers with epilepsy are at greater risk of experiencing cognitive problems as compared to the normal population, the specific causes remain uncertain. The risk of mental retardation in children of mothers with epilepsy, for example, has been associated with intrauterine growth retardation, major malformations, numerous (≥9) minor malformations, and in utero AED exposure.[161] Gailey et al.[151] compared performance on neuropsychological tests of 104 children exposed in utero to AEDs (primarily phenytoin) and a comparable number of control children at the age of 5.5 years. Although children of the mothers with epilepsy performed worse on some measures, results suggested that these differences were related to seizures during pregnancy, maternal partial seizure disorder, and low paternal education rather than the effects of AED exposure. Fujioka et al.[162] suggested complex interrelationships, the risk being increased with increased dose and numbers of AEDs, decreased maternal education, impaired maternal-child relation, and maternal partial seizure disorder.

Scolnik et al.[163] attempted to control for many of the confounding variables in assessing the possible cognitive effects of in utero exposure to AEDs (phenytoin and carbamazepine) by conducting a case-controlled, prospective, blinded observational investigation. Each mother exposed to either phenytoin or carbamazepine was paired with the next woman attending the clinic who matched the index mother on a number of variables, including age and socioeconomic class. Nonepileptic mothers were attending this clinic to receive counseling after gestational exposure to nonteratogens (e.g., penicillin). The offspring of these mothers, as well as the mothers themselves, were examined by a team of physicians and psychologists between 18 and 36 months after the infants' delivery. The practitioners' evaluation included neurocognitive and intellectual assessment. On the basis of their results, these practitioners concluded that phenytoin adversely affected neurobehavioral development, whereas carbamazepine did not. However, a significantly greater proportion of the group treated with carbamazepine included nonepileptic mothers who were treated with this medication for other reasons (e.g., bipolar disorder). Likewise, the mean maternal AED dose was less in the carbamazepine group (534 mg per day of the 800- to 1,200-mg per day range for carbamazepine vs. 354 mg per day of the 300- to 400-mg per day range for phenytoin). Further, the maternal groups were matched a priori by education rather than IQ. Although the carbamazepine group turned out to be well matched to its control group on IQ, the phenytoin group was not. Between-group differences on these variables tend to confound the results of this study. This point is driven home by the fact that the resulting IQ differences between the maternal and child groups for carbamazepine and phenytoin turned out to be of the same order of magnitude as one another. Finally, the data analysis did not directly compare the case-control difference scores for the two AED treatment groups. When the appropriate statistical analysis was performed comparing the difference scores of the two paired groups of children, no significant difference was found.[164] Although the reported difference may be real, a study with a larger sample size and tighter control of confounding variables will be required to demonstrate it conclusively.

Renisch et al.[165] reported the results of two double-blind studies involving independent samples of adult men and examining the effects of in utero phenobarbital exposure on general intellectual functioning. Men exposed prenatally to phenobarbital had significantly lower verbal IQ scores than predicted using regression models based on control subjects (approximately 7 IQ points, or 0.5 standard deviation [SD]). Lower economic status, late gestational exposure to phenobarbital, and being the offspring of an "unwanted" pregnancy increased the magnitude of the negative effects. One weakness of the study is that phenobarbital was prescribed primarily for hypertension, but the researchers did not control for the effects of hypertension and preeclampsia in the analyses. Nevertheless, these findings suggest that behavioral teratologic sequelae of prenatal phenobarbital exposure in humans can continue into adulthood. They also suggest that socioeconomic and psychological factors may interact with drug exposure to exacerbate cognitive and developmental deficits.

Overall, both animal and human studies suggest that in utero AED exposure has some negative impact on the development of exposed offspring. Also, polytherapy can have greater adverse effects on outcome than monotherapy. Nevertheless, the differential effects of AEDs remain uncertain owing to methodological difficulties involved in this area of research. Larger studies are needed that attempt to control for a variety of confounding variables, including parental IQ, socioeconomic status, secondary health problems during pregnancy, and maternal seizure activity.

Possible Mechanisms Underlying Antiepileptic Drug Effects on Neurodevelopment

Teratogens are environmental agents that cause a structural abnormality after fetal exposure. A teratogen operates on a susceptible genotype, and its effects may be mediated by an interaction of multiple liability genes.[166] This interaction of environment and genetics can lead to discordant outcomes in offspring exposed to the same teratogen. For example, differing outcomes have been observed for dizygotic twin fetuses exposed to phenytoin.[167] Functional deficits can occur at dosages lower than those required to produce somatic abnormalities, and whether the same mechanisms are involved in both functional and anatomic defects remains unclear. Proposed possible mechanisms underlying functional teratogenicity of AEDs include epoxides,[167,168] free radicals,[169] ischemia,[170] folate,[171,172] and neuronal suppression.[173]

Ecological Validity and Quality-of-Life Issues in Clinical Antiepileptic Drug Trials

Another potential limitation in studying cognitive effects of AEDs involves the assessment procedures that are commonly employed. Adams et al.,[174] in reviewing the available human and animal studies on the developmental effects of phenytoin, suggested that the behavioral end point of human studies has tended to lag behind that of animal paradigms. For example, most human studies have examined the rate of occurrence of morphologic abnormalities rather than attempting to assess the effects of AEDs on cognition and behavioral measures. In contrast, animal paradigms often involve complex behavioral tasks. In animal studies that found adverse effects after in utero exposure to AEDs, behavioral abnormalities often were observed only in the most complex behavioral activities (e.g., complex maze learning).[174,175] Therefore, researchers should try to employ test batteries and behavioral paradigms that tap a range of relevant cognitive domains, including executive functioning and complex learning and memory; likewise, they should include measures that assess QOL.

Many studies have used measures of general intellectual functioning (e.g., Wechsler Adult Intelligence Scale, Revised; Wechsler Adult Intelligence Scale, third edition) to assess cognition. However, subtle cognitive dysfunction can be obscured if only global scores are examined.[176] Further, such tests do not adequately assess sustained attention, memory, and learning, all areas that could potentially suffer from the impact of neuronal dampening. Executive functioning could include measures of planning and organization, response inhibition, self-monitoring (metacognition), and complex problem solving. Assessment procedures in the area of executive functioning have tended to lag behind other areas of cognitive evaluation.[176,177] Because AEDs can affect mood and aggression,[178–180] likely through their effect on limbic structures and related neurotransmitters, the impact of emotional processing on decision making and cognitive processing may be a valuable measure to assess. Damasio's somatic marker hypothesis[181] and behavioral paradigms for exploring such issues in humans suggests that we often underestimate the impact of emotional functioning on cognition. Assessing motor planning and initiation of both simple and complex behavioral sequences might also be helpful, given that many of the animal studies resulted in abnormal patterns of movement (e.g., aberrant circling behavior). Also, increasing the use of measures with greater ecological validity might help us to avoid overestimating the real-world impact of effects that might be functionally inconsequential despite their having reached the level of statistical significance.

Finally, assessing QOL issues in epilepsy might help to demonstrate the more global response of a patient to AED therapy. QOL research involves a movement to examine the patient's perception of illness, treatment, and impairment of daily functioning.[182] Such an endeavor, which has its roots in oncology research,[183] can provide the clinician with useful information regarding the impact of treatment on the patient's psychosocial, emotional, spiritual, and vocational functioning. To date, QOL in epilepsy has not been very thoroughly investigated, although initial scale development has been undertaken. The Quality of Life in Epilepsy–89 (QOLIE-89) scale appears particularly promising and is being employed more frequently in recent studies. Self-perceptions derived from the QOLIE-89 have been shown to correlate with measures of cognitive and emotional functioning.[184] A version of this measure specifically for use with adolescents also was developed recently (QOLIE-AD-48).[185] Such instruments may help clinicians to understand better the needs of their epilepsy patients and may help to justify various treatment decisions in this current age of managed care.

AEDs are only one treatment component that may exert influence on QOL. Other treatment factors include surgical interventions and clinical programs designed to equip patients with the skills necessary for everyday functioning (e.g., social skills training, vocational counseling, cognitive remediation). Many epilepsy patients, particularly those experiencing intractable seizures, have missed significant opportunities for training and development. Lacking functional competence in social or vocational settings may create or compound negative perceptions regarding self-esteem and competence. Effective management of seizures through the use of AEDs plays a fundamental part in assisting patients with epilepsy to maximize their functional capacity in all spheres of life. Generally, QOL perceptions are improved in epilepsy patients on AEDs, especially if seizure freedom is obtained. Further, as mentioned earlier, initial studies with gabapentin and lamotrigine suggest that these agents may affect QOL, perhaps through psychotropic effects.[46,55]

Studies that determine both the general and differential effects of the major and novel AEDs—particularly in the case of in utero exposure—represent elaborate and time-consuming undertakings. Controlling for the many familial, environmental, and disease-related variables poses a daunting task. Designing an assessment battery that is comprehensive, valid, and efficient represents a worthwhile endeavor necessary to optimize the results of a careful, rigorous, methodologic design. Improved psychometric batteries and procedures are being used more frequently, although many studies are still lacking in this regard.

Conclusion

All AEDs can affect cognition adversely if standard therapeutic dosages are exceeded or if these medications are employed in polypharmacy. The older, established AEDs produce only modest effects when used in monotherapy within the standard therapeutic ranges. Barbiturates, bromides, and benzodiazepines have been shown to produce greater levels of sedation and impaired cognition, as compared to the established AEDs. Differential effects appear slight among phenytoin, carbamazepine, and valproate. Initial studies with some of the newer AEDs suggest few adverse cognitive effects. Research investigating the impact of these newer AEDs on cognition remains scant and currently includes few direct comparisons with the older AEDs.

Although the effects of AEDs on cognition appear modest when they are used in monotherapy and at standard dosages, even slight effects can have clinical importance for some patient groups. Such groups might include children participating in school or adults whose jobs depend on vigilance or response speed. In such cases, the use of monotherapy at the lowest possible dosage may be indicated. In general, the magnitude of AED effects on cognition is commonly much less than the impact of other factors in epilepsy. Further, modest cognitive effects of AEDs may be offset in part by reduced seizure frequency.

Future research studies are needed to compare the new AEDs directly with the established AEDs. The possible effects of AED exposure in utero and on groups at the extremes of age must be more thoroughly evaluated as well. Adverse consequences would be expected to be most severe among these more vulnerable groups. Initial studies examining the impact of AEDs on children and older adults, although limited in nature, suggest that the patterns of drug effect among these groups are similar to those observed in studies of adults. Animal research and initial human studies examining in utero AED exposure suggest that these medications have some negative effect on the developmental outcome of children. Nevertheless, differential AED effects remain unclear.

Future research needs to continue examining the impact of AEDs on factors affecting the epilepsy patient's QOL and to employ test batteries that are sensitive to both gross disruption of cognitive processes (e.g., attention) and the complexities of real-world behaviors. The effective clinician will attempt to control seizure activity while minimizing cognitive impairment. Each patient must be viewed on a case-by-case basis. Our suggestions represent general guidelines and may not apply to the individual patient, although careful, ongoing monitoring of cognitive status is essential to maximize patient potential.

References

1. Anastasi A. Psychological Testing. New York: Macmillan, 1988;336–370.
2. Meador KJ, Loring DW. Cognitive Effects of Antiepileptic Drugs. In O Devinsky, WH Theodore (eds), Epilepsy and Behavior. New York: Wiley-Liss, 1991;151–170.
3. Smith DB. Cognitive effects of antiepileptic drugs. Adv Neurol 1991;55:197–212.
4. Lennox WG. Brain injury, drugs and environment: a cause of mental decay in epilepsy. Am J Psychiatry 1942;99:174–180.
5. Milano Collaborative Group of Studies on Epilepsy. Long-term intensive monitoring in the difficult patient: preliminary results of 16 months of observations—usefulness and limitations. In C Gardner-Thorpe (ed), Antiepileptic Drug Monitoring. Tunbridge Wells, UK: Pitman Medical, 1977;197–213.
6. Shorvon SD, Reynolds EH. Reduction in polypharmacy for epilepsy. BMJ 1979;2:1023–1025.
7. Reynolds EH, Shorvon SD. Monotherapy or polytherapy for epilepsy? Epilepsia 1981;22:1–10.
8. Schain RJ, Ward JW, Guthrie D. Carbamazepine as an anticonvulsant in children. Neurology 1977;27:476–480.
9. Thompson PJ, Trimble MR. Anticonvulsant drugs and cognitive functions. Epilepsia 1982;23:531–544.
10. Ludgate J, Keating J, O'Dwyer R, Callaghan N. An improvement in cognitive function following polypharmacy reduction in a group of epileptic patients. Acta Neurol Scand 1985;71:448–452.
11. Prevey ML, Mattson RH, Cramer JA. Improvement in cognitive functioning and mood state after conversion to valproate monotherapy. Neurology 1989;39:1640–1641.
12. Meador KJ. Cognitive Effects of Epilepsy and of Antiepileptic Medications. In E Wyllie (ed), The Treatment of Epilepsy: Principles and Practice (2nd ed). Baltimore: Williams & Wilkins, 1996;1–33.
13. Dekaban AS, Lehman EJB. Effects of different dosages of anticonvulsant drugs on mental performances in patients with chronic epilepsy. Acta Neurol Scand 1975;52:319–330.
14. Trimble MR, Thompson PJ. Anticonvulsant drugs, cognitive function, and behavior. Epilepsia 1983;24[Suppl 1]:S55–S63.
15. Tchicaloff M, Gaillard F. Quelques effets indesirables des medicaments anti-epiletiques, sur le rendements intellectuels. Rev Neuropsychol Infant 1970;18:599–602.
16. Dodrill CB. Diphenylhydantoin serum levels, toxicity, and neuropsychological performance in patients with epilepsy. Epilepsia 1975;16:593–600.
17. Gillham RA, Blacklaw J, McKee PJW, Brodie MJ. Effect of vigabatrin on sedation and cognitive function in patients with refractory epilepsy. J Neurol Neurosurg Psychiatry 1993;56:1271–1275.
18. O'Dougherty M, Wright FS, Cox S, Walson P. Carbamazepine plasma concentration relationship to cognitive impairment. Arch Neurol 1987;44:863–867.
19. Dodrill CB. Behavioral effects of antiepileptic drugs. Adv Neurol 1991;55:213–224.
20. Vermeulen J, Aldenkamp AP. Cognitive side-effects of chronic antiepileptic drug treatment: a review of 25 years of research. Epilepsy Res 1995;22:65–95.
21. Meador KJ. Cognitive side effects of antiepileptic drugs. Can J Neurol Sci 1994;21[Suppl 3]:S12–S16.
22. Dodrill CB, Temkin NR. Motor speed is a contaminating factor in evaluating the "cognitive" effects of phenytoin. Epilepsia 1989;30:453–457.
23. Pullianen V, Jokelainen M. Effects of phenytoin and carbamazepine on cognitive functions in newly diagnosed epileptic patients. Acta Neurol Scand 1994;89:81–86.
24. Smith KR, Goulding PM, Wilderman D, et al. Neurobehavioral effects of phenytoin and carbamazepine in patients recovering from brain trauma: a comparative study. Arch Neurol 1994;51:653–660.
25. Dodrill CB, Troupin AS. Psychotropic effects of carbamazepine in epilepsy: a double-blind comparison with phenytoin. Neurology 1977;27:1023–1028.
26. Dodrill CB, Troupin AS. Neuropsychological effects of carbamazepine and phenytoin: a reanalysis. Neurology 1991;41:141–143.
27. Smith DB, Mattson RH, Cramer JA, et al. Results of a nationwide veterans administration cooperative study comparing the efficacy and toxicity of carbamazepine, phenobarbital, phenytoin, and primidone. Epilepsia 1987;28[Suppl 3]:S50–S58.
28. Meador KJ, Loring DW, Allen ME, et al. Comparative cognitive effects of carbamazepine and phenytoin in healthy adults. Neurology 1991;41:1537–1540.

29. Meador KJ, Loring DW, Moore EE, et al. Comparative cognitive effects of phenobarbital, phenytoin, and valproate in healthy adults. Neurology 1995;45:1494–1499.

30. Dodrill CB, Wilensky AJ. Neuropsychological abilities before and after 5 years of stable antiepileptic drug therapy. Epilepsia 1992;33:327–334.

31. Gastaut H. Essai préliminaire d'une benzodiazépine en epileptologie. Nouv Presse Méd 1978;7:2400.

32. Dichter MA, Brodie MJ. Drug therapy: new antiepileptic drugs. N Engl J Med 1996;334:1583–1590.

33. Hindmarch I, Haller J, Sherwood N, Kerr JS. Comparison of five anxiolytic benzodiazepines on measures of psychomotor performance and sleep. Neuropsychobiology 1991;24:84–89.

34. Haefely W, Kulcsar A, Mohler H, et al. Possible involvement of GABA in the central actions of benzodiazepines. Adv Biochem Psychopharmacol 1975;14:131–151.

35. Hentschel B, Froscher W. Clobazam in the treatment of epilepsy. Drugs Today 1992;28:567–572.

36. Canadian Clobazam Cooperative Group. Clobazam in treatment of refractory epilepsy: the Canadian experience. A retrospective study. Epilepsia 1991;32:407–416.

37. Robertson MM. Current status of the 1,4- and 1,5-benzodiazepines in the treatment of epilepsy: the place of Clobazam. Epilepsia 1986;27[Suppl 1]:S27–S41.

38. Canadian Study Group for Childhood Epilepsy, Bawden HN, Camfield CS, et al. The cognitive and behavioural effects of clobazam and standard monotherapy are comparable. Epilepsy Res 1999;33:133–143.

39. Saletu B, Gunberger J, Linzmayer L. Evaluation of encephalotrophic and psychotropic properties of gabapentin in man by pharmaco-EEG and psychometry. Int J Clin Pharmacol Ther Toxicol 1986;24:362–373.

40. Dodrill CB, Arnett JL, Hayes AG, et al. Cognitive abilities and adjustment with gabapentin: results of a multisite study. Epilepsy Res 1999;35:109–121.

41. Mortimore C, Trimble M, Emmers E. Effects of gabapentin on cognition and quality of life in patients with epilepsy. Seizure 1998;7:359–364.

42. Martin R, Kuzniecky R, Ho S, et al. Cognitive effects of topiramate, gabapentin, and lamotrigine in healthy young adults. Neurology 1999;52:321–327.

43. Dimond KR, Pande AC, Lamoreaux L, Pierce MW. Effect of gabapentin (Neurontin) on mood and well-being in patients with epilepsy. Prog Neuropsychopharmacol Biol Psychiatry 1996;20:407–417.

44. Lee DO, Steingard RJ, Cesena M, et al. Behavioral side effects of gabapentin in children. Epilepsia 1996;37:87–90.

45. Wolf SM, Shinnar S, Kang H, et al. Gabapentin toxicity in children manifesting as behavioral changes. Epilepsia 1995;36:1203–1205.

46. Dodrill CB, Arnett JL, Hayes AG, et al. Evaluation of quality of life during a double-blind multicenter study of gabapentin (GBP; Neurontin) monotherapy in patients with medically refractory partial seizures. Epilepsia 1995;36[Suppl 4]:S88.

47. Leach JP, Girvan J, Paul A, Brodie MJ. Gabapentin and cognition: a double-blind, dose-ranging placebo-controlled study in refractory epilepsy. J Neurol Neurosurg Psychiatry 1997;62:372–376.

48. Meador KJ, Loring DW, Ray PG, et al. Differential cognitive effects of carbamazepine and gabapentin. Epilepsia 1999;40(9):1279–1285.

49. Bruni J. Outcome evaluation of gabapentin as add-on therapy for partial seizures. Can J Neurol Sci 1998;25:134–140.

50. Tallian KB, Nahata MC, Lo W, Tsao C-Y. Gabapentin associated with aggressive behavior in pediatric patients with seizures. Epilepsia 1996;37:501–502.

51. Lees G, Leach MJ. Studies on the mechanism of action of the novel anti-convulsant lamotrigine (Lamictal) using primary neuroglia: cultures from rat cortex. Brain Res 1993;612:190–199.

52. Leach MJ, Marden CM, Miller AA. Pharmacological studies on lamotrigine, a novel potential antiepileptic drug: 2. Neurochemical studies on the mechanism of action. Epilepsia 1986;27:490–497.

53. Brodie M, Richens A, Yuen AWC, UK Lamotrigine/Carbamazepine Monotherapy Trial Group. Double-blind comparison of lamotrigine and carbamazepine in newly diagnosed epilepsy. Lancet 1995;345:476–479.

54. Cohen AF, Land GS, Breimer D, et al. Lamotrigine, a new anticonvulsant. Pharmacol Ther 1987;42:535–541.

55. Smith D, Baker G, Davies G, et al. Outcomes of add-on treatment with lamotrigine in partial epilepsy. Epilepsia 1993;34:312–322.

56. Cohen AF, Ashby L, Crowley D, et al. Lamotrigine (BW430C) potential anticonvulsant. Effects on the central nervous system in comparison with phenytoin and diazepam. Br J Clin Pharmacol 1985;29:619–629.

57. Hamilton MJ, Cohen AF, Yuen AWC, et al. Carbamazepine and lamotrigine in healthy volunteers: relevance to early tolerance and clinical trial dosages. Epilepsia 1993;34:166–173.

58. Meador KJ, Loring DW, Ray PG, et al. Differential cognitive effects of carbamazepine and lamotrigine. Neurology 2000;54[Suppl 3]:A84.

59. Gillham R, Baker G, Thompson R, et al. Standardization of a self-report questionnaire for use in evaluating cognitive, affective and behavioral side-effects of antiepileptic drug treatments. Epilepsy Res 1996;24:47–55.

60. Binnie CD. Lamotrigine. Epilepsia 1995;36[Suppl 3]:S32.

61. Sporn J, Sachs G. The anticonvulsant lamotrigine in treatment-resistant manic-depressive illness. J Clin Psychopharmacol 1997;17:185–189.

62. Walden J, Hesslinger B, van Calker D, Berger M. Addition of lamotrigine to valproate may enhance effi-

cacy in the treatment of bipolar affective disorder. Pharmacopsychiatry 1996;29:193–195.

63. Calabrese JR, Bowden CL, Sachs GS, et al. A double-blind placebo-controlled study of lamotrigine monotherapy in outpatients with bipolar I depression. J Clin Psychiatry 1999;60(2):79–88.

64. Uvebrant P, Bauziene R. Intractable epilepsy in children. The efficacy of lamotrigine treatment, including non-seizure-related benefits. Neuropediatrics 1994;25:284–289.

65. Meador KJ, Baker GA. Behavioral and cognitive effects of lamotrigine. J Child Neurol 1997,12[Suppl 1]:S44–S47.

66. Ettinger AB, Weisbrot DM, Saracco J, et al. Positive and negative psychotropic effects of lamotrigine in patients with epilepsy and mental retardation. Epilepsia 1998;39:874–877.

67. Bialer M, Johannessen SI, Kupferberg HJ, et al. Progress report on new antiepileptic drugs: a summary of the fourth Eliat conference (EILAT IV). Epilepsy Res 1999;34(1):1–41.

68. Äikiä M, Kälviainen R, Sivenius J, et al. Cognitive effects of oxcarbazepine and phenytoin monotherapy in newly diagnosed epilepsy: one-year follow-up. Epilepsy Res 1992;11:199–203.

69. Curran HV, Java R. Memory and psychomotor effects of oxcarbazepine in healthy human volunteers. Eur J Clin Pharmacol 1993;44:529–533.

70. Kälviainen R, Äikiä M, Riekkinen PJ. Cognitive adverse effects of antiepileptic drugs. CNS Drugs 1996;6:358–368.

71. Braestrup C, Nielsen EB, Sonnewald U, et al. (R)-N-[4,4-Bis(3-methyl-2-thienyl)but-3-3n-1-yl] nipecotic acid binds with high affinity to the brain gamma-aminobutyric acid uptake carrier. J Neurochem 1990;54:639–647.

72. Sveinbjornsdottir S, Sander J, Patsalos P, et al. Neuropsychological effects of tiagabine, a potential new antiepileptic drug. Seizure 1994;3:29–35.

73. Riekkinen PJ, Kälviainen R, Äikiä M, et al. Cognitive and electrophysiological effects of tiagabine add-on therapy: a randomized double-blind placebo-controlled study. Neurology 1994;44[Suppl 2]:A321.

74. Dodrill CB, Arnett JL, Sommerville KW, Shu V. Cognitive and quality of life effects of differing dosages of tiagabine in epilepsy. Neurology 1997;48:1025–1031.

75. Dodrill CB, Arnett JL, Shu V, et al. Effects of tiagabine monotherapy on abilities, adjustment, and mood. Epilepsia 1998;39:33–42.

76. White HS, Brown SD, Woodead JH, et al. Topiramate enhances GABA-mediated chloride flux and GABA-evoked chloride currents in murine brain neurons and increases seizure threshold. Epilepsy Res 1997;28:167–179.

77. Faught E, Wilder BJ, Ramsey RE, et al. Topiramate placebo-controlled dose-ranging trial in refractory partial epilepsy using 200-, 400-, and 600-mg daily dosages. Neurology 1996;46:1684–1690.

78. Privitera M, Fincham R, Penry J, et al. Topiramate placebo-controlled dose-ranging trial in refractory partial epilepsy using 600-, 800-, and 1000-mg daily dosages. Neurology 1996;46:1678–1683.

79. Meador KJ, Kamin M, Topiramate TPS-TR Study Team. Assessing cognitive effects of a new AED without the bias of practice effects. Epilepsia 1997;38[Suppl 3]:60.

80. Aldenkamp AP, Baker G, Mulder OG, et al. A randomized clinical study comparing the cognitive effects of topiramate versus valproate in a first-line add-on design. Epilepsia 1999;40[Suppl 40]:83.

81. Petroff OA, Rothman DL, Behar KL, Mattson RH. Initial observations on effect of vigabatrin on in vivo 1H spectroscopic measurements of gamma-aminobutyric acid, glutamate, and glutamine in human brain. Epilepsia 1995;36:457–464.

82. Grant SM, Heel RC. Vigabatrin: a review of its pharmacodynamic and pharmacokinetic properties, and therapeutic potential in epilepsy and disorders of motor control. Drugs 1991;6:889–926.

83. Cocito L, Maffini M, Loeb C. MRI findings in epileptic patients on vigabatrin for more than 5 years. Seizure 1992;1:163–165.

84. Hammond EJ, Ballinger WE Jr, Lu L, et al. Absence of cortical white matter changes in three patients undergoing long-term vigabatrin therapy. Epilepsy Res 1992;12:261–265.

85. Dodrill CB, Arnett JL, Sommerville KW, Sussmann NM. Evaluation of the effects of vigabatrin on cognitive abilities and quality of life in epilepsy. Neurology 1993;43:2501–2507.

86. Dodrill CB, Arnett JL, Sommerville KW, Sussmann NM. Effects of differing dosages of vigabatrin (Sabril) on cognitive abilities and quality of life in epilepsy.Epilepsy 1995;36:164–173.

87. Grunewald RA, Thompson PJ, Corcoran R, et al. Effects of vigabatrin on partial seizures and cognitive function. J Neurol Neurosurg Psychiatry 1994;57:1057–1063.

88. McGuire AM, Duncan JS, Trimble MR. Effects of vigabatrin on cognitive function and mood when used as add-on therapy in patients with intractable epilepsy. Epilepsia 1992;33:128–134.

89. Kälviainen R, Äikiä M, Saukkone AM, et al. Vigabatrin versus carbamazepine monotherapy in newly diagnosed patients with epilepsy: a randomized controlled study. Arch Neurol 1995;52:989–996.

90. Saletu B, Grunberger J, Linzmayer L, et al. Psychophysiological and psychometric studies after manipulating the GABA system by vigabatrin, a GABA-transaminase inhibitor. Int J Psychophysiol 1986;4:63–80.

91. Brodie MJ, McKee PJW. Vigabatrin and psychosis. Lancet 1990;335:1279.

92. Sander JW, Hart YM, Trimble MR, Shorvon SD. Vigabatrin and psychosis. J Neurol Neurosurg Psychiatry 1991;54:435–439.

93. Lee BI, Huh K, Kim JS, et al. Vigabatrin open trial in patients with medically intractable seizures under carbamazepine monotherapy (abstract). Epilepsia 1991;32[Suppl 1]:S103.

94. Veggiotti P, De Agostini G, Muzio C, et al. Vigabatrin use in psychotic epileptic patients: report of a prospective pilot study. Acta Neurol Scand 1999;99: 142–146.

95. Ferrie CD, Robinson RO, Panayiotopoulous CP. Psychotic and severe behavioral reactions with vigabatrin: a review. Acta Neurol Scand 1996;93:1–8.

96. Wilensky AJ, Friel PN, Ojeman LM, et al. Zonisamide in epilepsy: a pilot study. Epilepsia 1985;26:212–220.

97. Berent S, Sackellares JC, Giordani B, et al. Zonisamide (CI-912) and cognition: results from preliminary study. Epilepsia 1987;28:61–67.

98. Leppik IE. Metabolism of antiepileptic medication: newborn to elderly. Epilepsia 1992;33[Suppl 4]:S32–S40.

99. Morselli PL. Pharmacokinetics in Infancy, Childhood and Adolescence. In E Wyllie (ed), The Treatment of Epilepsy. Philadelphia: Lea & Febiger, 1993;752–768.

100. Dodrill CB. Cognitive and Adjustmental Consequences of Seizures and Antiepileptic Drugs in the Elderly. In AJ Rowan, RE Ramsawy, M Miller (eds), Seizures and Epilepsy in the Elderly. Newton, MA: Butterworth–Heinemann, 1997;179–190.

101. Craig I, Tallis R. The impact of sodium valproate and phenytoin on cognitive function in elderly patients: results of a single-blind randomized comparative study. Epilepsia 1994:35:381–390.

102. Read CL, Stephen LJ, Stolarek IH, et al. Cognitive effects of anticonvulsant monotherapy in elderly patients: a placebo-controlled study. Seizure 1998;7:159–162.

103. Vining EP, Mellits ED, Dorsen MM, et al. Psychologic and behavioral effects of antiepileptic drugs in children: a double-blind comparison between phenobarbital and valproic acid. Pediatrics 1987;80:165–174.

104. Calandre EP, Dominguez-Granados R, Gomez-Rubio M, Molina-Font JA. Cognitive effects of long-term treatment with phenobarbital and valproic acid in school children. Acta Neurol Scand 1990;81:504–506.

105. Camfield CS, Chaplin S, Doyle AB, et al. Side effects of phenobarbital in toddlers: behavioral and cognitive aspects. J Pediatr 1979;95:361–365.

106. Farwell JR, Lee YJ, Hirtz DG, et al. Phenobarbital for febrile seizures—effects on intelligence and on seizure recurrence. N Engl J Med 1990;322:364–369.

107. Sulzbacher S, Farwell JR, Temkin N, et al. Late cognitive effects of early treatment with phenobarbital. Clin Pediatr 1999;38:387–394.

108. Aldenkamp AP, Alpherts WC, Blennow G, et al. Withdrawal of antiepileptic medication in children—effects on cognitive function: the Multicenter Holmfrid Study. Neurology 1993;43:41–50.

109. Toonby B, Nilsson HL, Aldenkamp AP, et al. Withdrawal of antiepileptic medication in children. Correlation of cognitive function and plasma concentration—the multicentre "Holmfrid" study. Epilepsy Res 1994;19:141–152.

110. Riva D, Devoti M. Carbamazepine withdrawal in children with previous symptomatic partial epilepsy: effects on neuropsychologic function. J Child Neurol 1999;14:357–362.

111. Forsythe I, Butler R, Berg I, McGuire R. Cognitive impairment in new case of epilepsy randomly assigned to carbamazepine, phenytoin, and sodium valproate. Dev Med Child Neurol 1991;33:524–534.

112. Williams J, Bates S, Griebel ML, et al. Does short-term antiepileptic drug treatment in children result in cognitive or behavioral changes? Epilepsia 1998;39:1064–1069.

113. Mandelbaum DE, Burack GD. The effect of seizure type and medication on cognitive and behavioral functioning in children with idiopathic epilepsy. Dev Med Child Neurol 1997;39:731–735.

114. Alvarez N, Besag F, Iivanainen M. Use of antiepileptic drugs in the treatment of epilepsy in people with intellectual disability. J Intellect Disabil Res 1998;42[Suppl 1]:1–15.

115. Schaal DW, Hackenberg T. Toward functional analysis of drug treatment for behavior problems of people with developmental disabilities. Am J Ment Retard 1994;99:123–140.

116. Besag FM. Lamotrigine in the treatment of epilepsy in people with intellectual disability. J Intellect Disabil Res 1998;42[Suppl 1]:50–56.

117. Buchanan N. The efficacy of lamotrigine on seizure control in 34 children, adolescents and young adults with intellectual and physical disability. Seizure 1995;4:233–236.

118. Mullens L, Gallagher J, Manasco P. Improved neurological function accompanies effective control of the Lennox-Gastaut syndrome with Lamictal: results of a multinational, placebo-controlled trial. Epilepsia 1996;37[Suppl 5]:163.

119. Jacoby A, Baker G, Bryant-Constock L. Lamotrigine add-on therapy is associated with improvement in mood in patients with severe epilepsy. Epilepsia 1996;37[Suppl 5]:202.

120. Beran RG, Gibson RJ. Aggressive behavior in intellectually challenged patients with epilepsy treated with lamotrigine. Epilepsia 1998;39:280–282.

121. Mikati MA, Choueri R, Khurana DS, et al. Gabapentin in the treatment of refractory partial epilepsy in children with intellectual disability. J Intellect Disabil Res 1998;42[Suppl 1]:57–62.

122. Kalviainen R. Tiagabine: a new therapeutic option for people with intellectual disability and partial epilepsy. J Intellect Disabil Res 1998;42[Suppl 1]:63–67.

123. Waisburg H, Alvarez N. Carbamazepine in the treatment of epilepsy in people with intellectual disability. J Intellect Disabil Res 1998;42[Suppl 1]:36–40.

124. Kerr MP. Topiramate: uses in people with an intellectual disability who have epilepsy. J Intellect Disabil Res 1998;42[Suppl 1]:74–79.

125. Reinisch JM, Sanders SA. Early barbiturate exposure: the brain, sexually dimorphic behavior, and learning. Neurosci Biobehav Rev 1982;6:311–319.

126. Fishman RHB, Yanai J. Long-lasting effects of early barbiturates on central nervous system and behavior. Neurosci Biobehav Rev 1983;7:19–28.

127. Finnell RH, Dansky LV. Parental epilepsy, anticonvulsant drugs and reproductive outcome—epidemiologic and experimental findings spanning three decades: 1. Animal studies. Reprod Toxicol Rev 1991;5:281–299.

128. Dansky LV, Finnell RH. Parental epilepsy, anticonvulsant drugs, and reproductive outcome—epidemiologic and experimental findings spanning three decades: 2. Human studies. Reprod Toxicol Rev 1991;5:301–335.

129. Fisher JE, Vorhees C. Developmental toxicity of antiepileptic drugs: relationship to postnatal dysfunction. Pharm Res 1992;26:207–221.

130. Vorhees CV. Developmental effects of anticonvulsants. Neurotoxicology 1986;7:235–244.

131. Vorhees CV. Fetal hydantoin syndrome in rats: dose-effect relationships of prenatal phenytoin on postnatal development and behavior. Teratology 1987;35:287–303.

132. Yanai J, Sze PY, Iser C, Melamed E. Studies on brain monoamine neurotransmitters in mice after prenatal exposure to barbiturate. Pharmacol Biochem Behav 1985;23:215–219.

133. Rogel-Fuchs Y, Newman ME, Trombka D, et al. Hippocampal cholinergic alterations and related behavioral deficits after early exposure to phenobarbital. Brain Res Bull 1992;29:1–6.

134. Mullenix P, Tassinari MS, Keith DA. Behavioral outcome after prenatal exposure to phenytoin in rats. Teratology 1983;27:149–157.

135. Vorhees CV. Maze learning in rats: a comparison of performance in two water mazes in progeny prenatally exposed to different doses of phenytoin. Neurotoxicol Teratol 1987;9:235–241.

136. Weisenburger WP, Minck DR, Acuff KD, Vorhees CV. Dose-response effects of prenatal phenytoin exposure in rats: effects on early locomotion, maze learning, and memory as a function of phenytoin-induced circling behavior. Neurotoxicol Teratol 1990;12:145–152.

137. Schilling MA, Inman SL, Morford LL, et al. Prenatal phenytoin exposure and spatial navigation in offspring: effects on reference and working memory and on discrimination learning. Neurotoxicol Teratol 1999;21:567–578.

138. Vorhees CV, Minck DR. Long-term effects of prenatal phenytoin exposure on offspring behavior in rats. Neurotoxicol Teratol 1989;11:295–305.

139. Vorhees CV, Rindler JM, Minck DR. Effects of exposure period and nutrition on the developmental neurotoxicity of anticonvulsants in rats: short and long-term effects. Neurotoxicology 1990;11:273–283.

140. Hatta T, Ohmori H, Murakami T, et al. Neurotoxic effects of phenytoin on postnatal mouse brain development following neonatal administration. Neurotoxicol Teratol 1999;21:21–28.

141. Vorhees CV, Rauch SL, Hitzemann RJ. Prenatal phenytoin exposure decreases neuronal membrane order in rat offspring hippocampus. Int J Dev Neurosci 1990;8:283–288.

142. Vorhees CV. Fetal anticonvulsant syndrome in rats: dose- and period-response relationships of prenatal diphenylhydantoin, trimethadione, and phenobarbital exposure on the structural and functional development of the offspring. J Pharmacol Exp Ther 1983;227:274–287.

143. Vorhees CV. Behavioral teratogenicity of valproic acid: selective effects on behavior after prenatal exposure to rats. Psychopharmacology (Berl) 1987;92:173–179.

144. Vorhees CV. Teratogenicity and developmental toxicity of valproic acid in rats. Teratology 1987;35:195–202.

145. Vorhees CV, Rauch SL, Hitzemann RJ. Prenatal valproic acid exposure decreases neuronal membrane order in rat offspring hippocampus cortex. Neurotoxicol Teratol 1991;13:471–474.

146. Kaneko S. Antiepileptic drug therapy and reproductive consequences: functional and morphologic effects. Reprod Toxicol 1991;5:179–198.

147. Delgado-Escueta AV, Janz D. Consensus guidelines: preconception counseling, management, and care of the pregnant woman with epilepsy. Neurology 1992;42[Suppl 5]:149–160.

148. Hanson JW, Myrianthopoulos NC, Harvey MAS, Smith DW. Risks to the offspring of women treated with hydantoin anticonvulsants, with emphasis on the fetal hydantoin syndrome. J Pediatr 1976;89:662–668.

149. Janz D. On Major Malformations and Minor Anomalies in the Offspring of Parents with Epilepsy: Review of the Literature. In D Janz, M Dam, A Richens, et al. (eds), Epilepsy, Pregnancy, and the Child. New York: Raven Press, 1982;211–222.

150. Kallen B. A register study of maternal epilepsy and delivery outcome with special reference to drug use. Acta Neurol Scand 1986;73:253–259.

151. Gaily E, Kantola-Sorsa E, Granström ML. Specific cognitive dysfunction in children with epileptic mothers. Dev Med Child Neurol 1990;32:403–414.

152. Lander CM, Eadie MJ. Antiepileptic drug intake during infancy and malformed offspring. Epilepsy Res 1990;7:77–82.

153. Granström ML, Gaily E. Psychomotor development in children of mothers with epilepsy. Neurology 1992;42:144–148.

154. Koch S, Lösche G, Jäger-Roman E, et al. Major birth malformations and antiepileptic drugs. Neurology 1992;42[Suppl 5]:83–88.

155. Lindhout D, Meinardi, H, Meijer JWA, Nau H. Antiepileptic drugs and teratogenesis in two consecutive cohorts: changes in prescription policy paralleled by changes in pattern of malformations. Neurology 1992;42[Suppl 5]:94–110.

156. Vanoverloop D, Schnell RR, Harvey EA, Holmes LB. The effects of prenatal exposure to phenytoin and other anticonvulsants on intellectual function at 4 to 8 years of age. Neurotoxicol Teratol 1992;14:329–335.

157. Losche G, Steinhausen H-C, Koch S, Helge H. The psychological development of children of epileptic parents: II. The differential impact of intrauterine exposure to anticonvulsant drugs and further influential factors. Acta Paediatr 1994;83:961–966.

158. Steinhausen HC, Losche G, Koch S, Helge H. The psychological development of children of epileptic parents: I. Study design and comparative findings. Acta Paediatr 1994;83:955–960.

159. Dieterich E, Steveling A, Lukas A, et al. Congenital anomalies in children of epileptic mothers and fathers. Neuropediatrics 1980;11:274–283.

160. Granström ML, Hiilesmaa VK. Physical Growth of the Children of Epileptic Mothers: Preliminary Results from the Prospective Helsinki Study. In D Janz, M Dam, A Richens, et al (eds), Epilepsy, Pregnancy, and the Child. New York: Raven Press, 1982;397–401.

161. Hill RM, Tennyson LM. Maternal drug therapy: effect on fetal and neonatal growth and neurobehavior. Neurotoxicology 1986;7:121–140.

162. Fujioka K, Kaneko S, Hirano T, et al. A Study of the Psychomotor Development of the Offspring of Epileptic Mothers. In T Sato, S Shinagawa (eds), Antiepileptic Drugs and Pregnancy. Amsterdam: Excerpta Medica, 1984;415–424.

163. Scolnik D, Nulman I, Rovet J, et al. Neurodevelopment of children exposed in utero to phenytoin and carbamazepine monotherapy. JAMA 1994;271:767–770.

164. Loring DW, Meador KJ, Thompson WO. Neurodevelopment effects of phenytoin and carbamazepine (letter). JAMA 1994;272:850–857.

165. Renisch JM, Sanders SA, Mortensen EL, Rubin DB. In utero exposure to phenobarbital and intelligence deficits in adult men. JAMA 1995;274:1518–1525.

166. Finnell RH, Chernoff GF. Gene-Teratogen Interactions. An Approach to Understanding the Metabolic Basis of Birth Defects. In H Nau, WJ Scott (eds), Pharmacokinetics in Teratogenesis. Boca Raton, FL: CRC Press, 1987;97–109.

167. Phelan MC, Pellock JM, Nance WE. Discordant expression of fetal hydantoin syndrome in heteropaternal dizygotic twins. Med Intell 1982;307:99–101.

168. Juchau MR. Chemical Teratogenesis. In E Jucker (ed), Progress in Drug Research. Basel: Birkhauser Verlag, 1993;9–50.

169. Wells PG, Kim PM, Laposa RR, et al. Oxidative damage in chemical teratogenesis. Mutat Res 1997;396:65–78.

170. Juchau MR. Chemical Teratogenesis in Humans: Biochemical and Molecular Mechanisms. In E Jucker (ed), Progress in Drug Research. Basel: Birkhauser Verlag, 1997;25–92.

171. Dansky LV, Andermann E, Rosenblatt D, et al. Anticonvulsants, folate levels and pregnancy outcome: a prospective study. Ann Neurol 1987;21:176–182.

172. Zhu M, Zhou S. Reduction of the teratogenic effects of phenytoin by folic acid and a mixture of folic acid, vitamins, and amino acids: a preliminary trial. Epilepsia 1989;30:246–251.

173. Bennett GD, Lau F, Calvin JA, Finnell RH. Phenytoin-induced teratogenesis: a molecular basis for the observed developmental delay during neurulation. Epilepsia 1997;38:415–423.

174. Adams J, Vorhees CV, Middaugh LD. Developmental neurotoxicity of anticonvulsants: human and animal evidence on phenytoin. Neurotoxicol Teratol 1990;12:203–214.

175. Conde CA, Costa V, Tomaz C. Measuring emotional memory in the elevated T-maze using a training-to-criterion procedure. Pharmacol Biochem Behav 1999;63:63–69.

176. Lezak MD. Neuropsychological Assessment (3rd ed). New York: Oxford University Press, 1995.

177. Dugbartey AT, Rosenbaum JG, Sanchez PN, Townes BD. Neuropsychological assessment of executive functions. Semin Clin Neuropsychiatry 1999;4:5–12.

178. Post RM, Denicoff KD, Frye MA, et al. A history of the use of anticonvulsants as mood stabilizers in the last two decades of the 20th century. Neuropsychobiology 1998;38:152–166.

179. Fava M. Psychopharmacologic treatment of pathologic aggression. Psychiatr Clin North Am 1997;20:427–451.

180. Letterman L, Markowitz JS. Gabapentin: a review of published experience in the treatment of bipolar disorder and other psychiatric conditions. Pharmacotherapy 1999;19:565–572.

181. Damasio AR. The somatic marker hypothesis and the possible functions of the prefrontal cortex. Philos Trans R Soc Lond B Biol Sci 1996;35:1413–1420.

182. Meador KJ. Research use of the new Quality-of-Life in Epilepsy Inventory. Epilepsia 1993;34[Suppl 4]:S34–S38.

183. Karnofsky DA, Burchenal J. The Clinical Evaluation of Chemotherapeutic Agents in Cancer. In C MacLeod (ed), Evaluation of Chemotherapeutic Agents. New York: Columbia University Press, 1949;191–205.

184. Perrine K, Hermann BP, Meador KJ, et al. The relationship of neuropsychological functioning to quality of life in epilepsy. Arch Neurol 1995;52:997–1003.

185. Cramer JA, Westbrook LE, Devinsky O, et al. Development of the Quality of Life in Epilepsy Inventory for Adolescents: the QOLIE-AD-48. Epilepsia 1999;40:1114–1121.

Chapter 29

Adverse Effects of Antiepileptic Drugs

Daniel J. Luciano

As many as 50% of patients treated with antiepileptic drugs (AEDs) will experience adverse effects (AEs) at some point. Simply put, AEs are undesirable responses caused by drugs. Such effects usually are mild and reversible and occur predominantly during the initial phases of therapy. AEs may be acute and clinically obvious or may arise more insidiously, at times only in the form of subclinical laboratory abnormalities. This chapter presents an overview of AEs of AEDs and highlights the relatively small body of data specific to the developmentally disabled (DD) and of particular relevance to this population.

Adverse Effects of Antiepileptic Drugs in the Developmentally Disabled

The appropriate use of AEDs and management of associated AEs can be extremely challenging, even in a normal patient population. Certain characteristics of the DD population and their epilepsy puts these AED users at even greater risk of developing AEs. In addition, management of DD patients is more difficult than management of other persons with epilepsy and requires greater awareness and anticipation of AEs on the part of caregivers and physicians. DD patients often have trouble communicating their symptoms, so, aside from direct behavioral effects of AEDs, physical symptoms may be expressed as behavioral changes such as withdrawal, irritability, or temper tantrums.

DD patients are inherently more sensitive to many of the AEs of AEDs, but information regarding AED use in these individuals is relatively limited, as they usually are excluded from preliminary drug studies. Owing to the presence of baseline brain dysfunction, the DD epileptic population is at particular risk for neurotoxic and behavioral AEs. The DD population is also more sensitive to the negative motor effects of AEDs, as they already frequently experience motor instability. In addition, DD patients are much more likely to have epilepsy that is difficult to control and to experience multiple seizure types. As a result, they are much more likely to require prolonged high levels of medication and AED polytherapy—both of which increase the incidence of AEs. The likely chronicity of treatment in this population further increases the chances that long-term AEs of AEDs eventually will develop. Finally, monitoring AEs in this population can be extremely challenging owing to communication difficulties and requires great acumen and anticipation on the part of caregivers.

Many of the new AEDs have fewer central nervous system and systemic toxicities than do older agents. In addition, several (lamotrigine, topiramate, felbamate) are broad-spectrum AEDs, allowing the use of AED monotherapy in many patients with disabilities and multiple seizure types, thus decreasing AE incidence.

Types of Adverse Effects of Antiepileptic Drugs

The different types of AEs that occur as a result of AED use are local, dose-related neurotoxic or systemic, idiosyncratic, and chronic. Table 29-1 lists

Table 29-1. Common Adverse Effects of Antiepileptic Drugs

Antiepileptic Drug	Dose-Related Neurotoxic Adverse Effects	Dose-Related Systemic Adverse Effects	Idiosyncratic Adverse Effects	Chronic Adverse Effects
Phenobarbital	Lethargy	Impotence	Rash, hypersensitivity syndrome,[a] agranulocytosis,[a] aplastic anemia,[a] hepatitis[a]	Contractures, frozen shoulder, short-term memory problem, deficiencies of folate and vitamins D and K
Primidone (Mysoline)	Lethargy, dizziness, ataxia	Impotence	Rash, leukopenia,[a] thrombocytopenia,[a] agranulocytosis,[a] aplastic anemia,[a] adenopathy,[a] hepatitis,[a] SLE[a]	Deficiencies of folate and vitamins D and K
Clonazepam (Klonopin)	Lethargy, ataxia, drooling	—	Rash, hair loss, anemia,[a] thrombocytopenia,[a] leukopenia[a]	—
Ethosuximide (Zarontin)	Lethargy, dizziness, headache	—	Rash, anemia, leukopenia, pancytopenia,[a] agranulocytosis,[a] aplastic anemia,[a] SLE[a]	—
Phenytoin (Dilantin)	Lethargy, nystagmus, ataxia, diplopia, chorea,[b] increased seizures[b]	—	Rash, agranulocytosis,[a] aplastic anemia,[a] Stevens-Johnson syndrome,[a] hepatitis,[a] pseudolymphoma,[a] SLE[a]	Gingival hyperplasia, hirsutism, acne, facial dysmorphism, osteopenia, cerebellar degeneration, neuropathy, deficiencies of folate and vitamins D and K
Carbamazepine (Tegretol, Carbatrol)	Lethargy, headache, diplopia, dizziness, ataxia	Cardiac arrhythmias, conduction block, hyponatremia	Rash, leukopenia, aplastic anemia,[a] agranulocytosis,[a] hypersensitivity syndrome, hepatitis	Spina bifida (0.5–1.0%), decreased vitamin D, weight gain, hypercholesterolemia
Valproate (Depakote)	Lethargy, tremor	Thrombocytopenia, elevated LFTs, hyperammonemia	Hepatic necrosis, pancreatitis, stupor or coma	Weight gain, polycystic ovaries, hair loss, decreased vitamin D, hearing loss, dementia or Parkinson's disease,[a] spina bifida (1%)
Felbamate (Felbatol)	Headache, lethargy, insomnia, dizziness	Anorexia	Aplastic anemia, hepatic failure, Stevens-Johnson syndrome, hypersensitivity syndrome	Weight loss
Gabapentin (Neurontin)	Lethargy, dizziness, ataxia, diplopia, worsened seizures	Leukopenia,[a] thrombocytopenia,[a] anemia[a]	—	Weight gain
Lamotrigine (Lamictal)	Dizziness, headache, diplopia, ataxia, insomnia, lethargy, tremor	—	Rash, Stevens-Johnson syndrome, hypersensitivity syndrome, renal failure	—

Topiramate (Topamax)	Dizziness, lethargy, trouble concentrating, speech problems, confusion, paresthesias	Nephrolithiasis	—	Weight loss
Tiagabine (Gabitril)	Dizziness, lethargy, impaired concentration, confusion, tremor	Hypertension	Rash	—
Oxcarbazepine (Trileptal)	Lethargy, headache, dizziness, ataxia	Hyponatremia	Rash	—
Levetiracetam (Keppra)	Lethargy, ataxia, dizziness	Minor decrease in hemoglobin and hematocrit,[a] leukopenia[a]	—	—
Zonisamide (Zonegran)	Lethargy, ataxia, trouble concentrating, speech problems	Anorexia, anhidrosis, nephrolithiasis, elevated blood urea nitrogen and creatinine levels	—	Rash[a]
Vigabatrin (Sabril)	Lethargy	Anemia,[a] leukopenia[a]	—	Weight gain, visual field defect

LFT = liver function test; SLE = systemic lupus erythematosus.

[a]Occurs rarely.

[b]Occurs with toxic levels. Topiramate may cause paresthesias that, akin to the adverse effects of acetazolamide, appear to be related to carbonic anhydrase inhibition and that may be ameliorated by the administration of citrate (Bicitra).

various AEDs and the most common or notable AEs in these drug classes.

Local Effects

Virtually all AEDs can cause some degree of gastrointestinal (GI) upset, a local irritative effect. This AE is seen most commonly with carbamazepine (CBZ; Tegretol, Carbatrol), valproic acid (VPA; Depekene, Depakote), felbamate (FBM; Felbatol) and lamotrigine (LTG; Lamictal). GI toxicity usually is seen at drug initiation but abates with continued therapy. It can be alleviated by the initial use of small frequent doses and by coadministration of the drug with food or an antacid. However, these measures may affect the degree of absorption of some of the older AEDs, such as phenytoin (PHT; Dilantin) or CBZ. The absorption of most newer AEDs is not similarly affected. The time to achieve a maximal serum level may be prolonged, but the value of the maximal level is, for the most part, unchanged.

When administered intramuscularly, PHT can cause local tissue necrosis due to crystallization. Administered intravenously, it can cause venous irritation, phlebitis, and cording. Extravasation from a vein also can cause severe tissue necrosis, rarely necessitating amputation. These problems occur because the drug is dissolved in a basic solvent. Such problems are not seen with fosphenytoin (Cerebyx), which is dissolved in a neutral vehicle.

Dose-Related Neurotoxic Effects

Dose-related neurotoxic effects are the most common AEs and are seen with virtually all AEDs, particularly at the time of initiation or dosage change, with high levels, and in polytherapy. In these situations, most AEDs can cause lethargy, dizziness, diplopia, and ataxia. However, the incidence of such AEs often is significantly lower in monotherapeutic trials. In most instances, dose-related neurotoxic effects abate with time or a reduction in cotherapy. Aside from these ubiquitous AEs, Table 29-1 lists more specific neurotoxic AEs of AEDs.

In the DD population, excessive sedation should be avoided, as it may lead to further impairment of limited intellectual capacity. Such sedation may also paradoxically increase seizure frequency in some DD patients whose seizures are more frequent in states of drowsiness or sleep, such as those with the Lennox-Gastaut syndrome. FBM and LTG, which have been reported to cause lethargy, appear to be more stimulant in monotherapy, at times resulting in insomnia. Although a stimulant effect is preferable to sedation, in some cases the result may be a worsening of seizures secondary to sleep-deprivation. In this case, the long half-life of these agents may allow a single administration of the medication early in the day, or twice-daily administration at breakfast and lunch.

Although much less common, many AEDs can cause an exacerbation of seizures, usually at high blood levels.[1] Clonazepam (Klonopin) can cause an increase in tonic seizures, and coadministration with other agents has rarely been reported to precipitate tonic status epilepticus.[2] Gabapentin (GBP; Neurontin) has also been reported to increase seizures by as much as 27%.[3] In some instances, specific AEDs worsen certain seizure types. For example, CBZ and PHT, drugs primarily used in partial epilepsy, can worsen the myoclonic and absence seizures of generalized epilepsy.[4] In addition, at toxic levels, PHT can worsen seizures that it effectively controls at therapeutic levels.[5]

Abnormal movements can occur as an AE of most AEDs, particularly with high serum levels of these agents. In many cases, patients experiencing such AEs have developmental disabilities and baseline motor dysfunction. Tremor due to VPA is perhaps the most common example[6] and may be improved with propranolol or acetazolamide.[7] Hyperammonemia due to VPA may also incite asterixis.[6] PHT is notable in causing choreoathetosis and orofacial dyskinesias at toxic levels.[5] Similar abnormal movements have been reported with VPA and FBM.[8,9] Myoclonus sometimes is seen as an AE of CBZ and has also been reported recently in conjunction with GBP use.[10]

Dose-Related Systemic Effects

Many AEDs, particularly the older agents, are associated with systemic AEs that often are dose-related (see Table 29-1). The most common involve alterations in liver function tests (LFTs) and complete blood cell count, (CBC), although these are rarely of clinical significance and often normalize despite continued therapy.

LFTs are elevated in many patients taking AEDs, particularly with the use of VPA, but also with phenobarbital (PB), PRM, PHT, and CBZ. Gamma-glutamyl transferase is particularly sensitive and is elevated in as many as 50% of patients treated with AEDs.[11] For appropriate management, the practitioner must realize that most elevations in LFTs represent hepatic activation as opposed to cellular damage. As a result, LFT values as high as three times the laboratories' upper limit of normal may be tolerated as long as they are clinically asymptomatic.

Abnormalities in the CBC are also very common. Most of the aromatic AEDs cause macrocytosis, sometimes accompanied by mild anemia due to a deficiency of folate caused by these agents. CBZ often causes mild leukopenia and neutropenia, but no concern is warranted unless the absolute neutrophil count falls to fewer than 1,500.[12] This effect generally is not seen with oxcarbazepine (OXC; Trileptal), despite the fact that it is chemically related to CBZ.

CBZ is well-known to cause hyponatremia, which is usually mild and asymptomatic. Hyponatremia also may occur during treatment with OXC. The effect may be due to altered sensitivity of hypothalamic osmoreceptors. In a population of 40 children and adolescents with intellectual disabilities treated with OXC, asymptomatic hyponatremia was seen in 24%.[13] As long as the sodium level is stable and the patient remains asymptomatic, sodium levels as low as 125 mg/dl can be tolerated chronically. If clinically significant, such hyponatremia can usually be eliminated with fluid restriction. If fluid restriction is not successful, doxycycline or demeclocycline may be effective.[14]

CBZ use has resulted rarely in atrioventricular conduction delays and bradyarrhythmias, primarily in elderly patients with underlying cardiac disease.[15] However, heart block has been reported—again rarely—in normal children, and patients with tuberous sclerosis and cardiac rhabdomyoma may be at risk.[15] Caution should be exercised using this AED in those with pre-existing conduction abnormalities such as a prolonged QT interval and atrioventricular blocks.

VPA often causes dose-related thrombocytopenia, particularly at a serum level exceeding 110 μg/ml.[16] However, clinical hemorrhage does not usually occur unless the platelet count drops below 20,000. VPA may also cause an idiosyncratic platelet adhesion defect akin to that of aspirin, as well as a deficiency of clotting factors such as fibrinogen. Such effects may express clinically as easy bruising or prolonged bleeding. Although most surgical series have not demonstrated increased hemorrhagic complications in patients treated with VPA,[17] a study of 114 patients with cerebral palsy undergoing spinal surgery demonstrated a significant difference in bleeding times, blood loss, and postoperative blood product administration in those receiving VPA monotherapy.[18] As a result, in patients on VPA who are scheduled to undergo surgery, bleeding times should be assessed in addition to a platelet count and coagulation studies.

VPA also causes hyperammonemia in as many as 50% of patients.[19] This may be due to altered renal production or elimination, induced carnitine deficiency, or the unmasking of underlying metabolic defects, such as ornithine transcarbamylase deficiency, and may be compounded in polytherapy.[6] TPM can compound VPA-induced hyperammonemia, possibly via its inhibition of carbonic anhydrase and cerebral glutamine synthetase.[20] Hyperammonemia occurs without associated elevations in hepatic enzymes and may be associated with lethargy, confusion, irritability, and a worsening of seizures. In the DD and elderly populations, the problem may be further compounded by constipation, which may lead to an even greater degree of hyperammonemia via the overgrowth of urea-splitting bacteria. Symptoms may sometimes be eliminated by supplementation with L-carnitine (Carnitor; 50 mg/kg per day) and, if necessary, lactulose (15–30 ml per day).

TPM is associated with a 1.5% risk of developing renal stones, which is more common in men.[21] Risk is increased with a personal or family history of renal stones. This appears to be related to the carbonic anhydrase inhibitor activity of TPM, with decreased urinary citrate excretion and subsequent alkalinization of urine. Acetazolamide causes renal stones via the same mechanism, and renal calculi may also occur during treatment with zonisamide (ZNS) and the ketogenic diet. When using TPM, good hydration must be maintained and, particularly in a nonverbal patient, urine must be examined for evidence of crystal formation or blood; likewise, the practitioner must be alert for the possibility of renal colic if there is evi-

Table 29-2. Cognitive and Behavioral Adverse Effects of Antiepileptic Drugs

Antiepileptic Drug	Adverse Effects
Phenobarbital	Depression, irritability, hyperactivity, memory loss
Clonazepam	Irritability, depression, psychosis
Ethosuximide	Psychosis, parkinsonian changes, aggression
Phenytoin	Delirium,[a] psychosis[a]
Carbamazepine	Depression, irritability, agitation, aggression, psychosis[b]
Valproate	Depression, irritability, hallucinosis, delirium, pseudodementia, or parkinsonism
Felbamate	Insomnia, anxiety, depression, agitation
Gabapentin	Aggression (children), dysphoria
Lamotrigine	Insomnia, agitation
Topiramate	Confusion, trouble concentrating, word-finding problems, psychosis
Tiagabine	Nervousness, irritability, trouble concentrating, depression
Oxcarbazepine	Trouble concentrating, speech problems
Levetiracetam	Psychosis, depression
Zonisamide	Psychosis, depression, irritability, insomnia
Vigabatrin	Depression, psychosis, anxiety, irritability, confusion, hyperactivity (children)

[a]With toxic level.
[b]Primarily in combination therapy.

dence of distress. In one patient who developed renal stones, the author prevented recurrence with the administration of vitamin C (500 mg twice daily) for urinary acidification.

The use of benzodiazepines such as clonazepam may cause increased salivation and bronchial secretions that can be particularly problematic in children and in DD patients.[2]

The newly approved AED ZNS has rarely been reported to cause oligohidrosis or anhidrosis associated with hyperpyrexia in children, including one DD child.[22]

Cognitive and Behavioral Effects

Virtually all AEDs may cause cognitive and behavioral AEs, and the DD population is at greater risk for these effects due to underlying cerebral dysfunction and a significant incidence of such problems at baseline. Table 29-2 lists common or notable cognitive and behavioral AEs of AEDs. (For a more detailed review of this subject, the reader is referred to Chapters 18 and 28 in this book.) With some of the newer AEDs, these AEs were reported in preliminary studies but have not yet been subjected to systematic neuropsychological study.

Most AEDs, particularly older agents, are capable of producing cognitive AEs such as trouble with attention and memory, although such effects are usually minimal when AEDs are used at therapeutic levels.[23,24] Cognitive AEs are more commonly seen with high AED levels and in polytherapy.[23,24] In addition, such effects are modest as compared to the cognitive difficulties produced by factors such as underlying cerebral lesions and uncontrolled seizures.[23,24]

The cognitive effects of PHT, CBZ, and VPA appear to be very similar.[24] Barbiturates and benzodiazepines generally cause the greatest cognitive difficulties.[23,24] Of the new AEDs, GBP appears to have minimal unwanted cognitive effects and, in this respect, was found superior to CBZ in a population of healthy volunteers.[25] In patients with epilepsy, no cognitive AEs were found associated with the use of LTG or tiagabine (TGB).[24] No cognitive differences were noted between PHT and OXC in a small randomized study.[26]

Some concern has been expressed among clinicians about the possible cognitive AEs of the drug TPM, including problems with word finding, concentration, and memory. Kerr[27] reported that in a DD population with Lennox-Gastaut syndrome, somnolence, anorexia, and behavioral changes were seen twice as frequently as in a placebo group. However, AEs of this drug were minimal in monotherapy as opposed to polytherapy.[27] The author has had the experience of treating multiple DD patients with TPM, initially with concern about potential cognitive AEs. However, in the majority of such patients, cognition and behavior improved along with improvements in seizure control.

In the DD population, the barbiturates and benzodiazepines have been primarily implicated in behavioral deterioration. Although usually sedative in nature, these agents used in this setting (particularly in children) may induce paradoxic irritability, hyperactivity, and aggression.[2] Worsening of behavior in the DD population may occur with vigabatrin (VGB),[28] although others have not found this to be so.[29] This agent also is capable of producing psychosis, with risk factors being a past history of psychosis and the abrupt cessation of seizures.[30,31] VGB may cause depression,[30] as can the new AEDs ZNS and levetiracetam (LEV). CBZ can cause a deterioration in behavior in the DD population, primarily in those with brain damage and pre-existing abnormal behavior.[4] In the DD population, GBP can be associated with hyperactivity, irritability, and aggression, particularly in those younger than 10 years with developmental disabilities and baseline attention-deficit disorder.[32] LTG, particularly in monotherapy, may be a good AED in the DD population because it is broad-spectrum, more stimulating in monotherapy, and has been reported to have positive cognitive and behavioral effects in DD patients.[33] Aggressive behavior with this agent has rarely been reported in the DD population,[34] but one must wonder whether this perhaps represents a "release" phenomenon, which may occur with the elimination of sedative AEs of AEDs or improvement in seizure control.[33] In such situations, the apparent AE actually represents clinical improvement, and social learning is required to establish more adaptive behavior.[35]

Idiosyncratic Effects

Idiosyncratic AEs of AEDs are the most worrisome, as they are relatively unpredictable and are potentially life-threatening. In one form or another, they may occur in 5–10% of patients treated with AEDs.[28] These AEs are unrelated to dosage and may be a consequence of allergic drug hypersensitivity, which may involve an active metabolite of the AED. These effects tend to occur within the first few months of treatment and can range from mild rashes (most common) to a severe AED hypersensitivity syndrome that is potentially life-threatening. Such effects are most common with the aromatic AEDs (e.g., PB, PHT, CBZ) but have also been seen with the new agents FBM and LTG.

Rash is the most common idiosyncratic AE and occurs in 5–10% of patients treated with aromatic AEDs and LTG.[36,37] The rash is usually mild, morbilliform, located primarily on the head and trunk, and appears within the first 2 months of therapy. It occurs more commonly with rapid AED titration.[38] Rash often is transient and usually resolves with dose reduction, drug discontinuation or, in many cases, even with continued therapy. Symptomatic treatment can be provided with antihistamines and, if the rash is severe, corticosteroids. At least in the case of CBZ, such treatment may hasten resolution of the rash and allow continued therapy.[39] When patients do experience a rash, assessment is crucial for associated symptoms that suggest a full-blown hypersensitivity reaction, such as fever, adenopathy, and intraoral lesions (vide infra).

Practitioners should be aware that many patients will tolerate a drug rechallenge without recurrent rash. For example, Besag et al.[40] found that all seven patients who experienced a mild rash from LTG tolerated slow reintroduction of this agent without rash recurrence. In some instances (such as with CBZ use), the rash may be due to coloring agents or other additives rather than the drug itself, and the rash can be eliminated by changing drug preparations.[41] Although chemically related to CBZ, OXC has only a 27% chance of causing cross-reactivity in patients with rash due to CBZ.[42]

Antiepileptic Drug Hypersensitivity Syndrome

AED hypersensitivity syndrome is a severe systemic reaction that occurs in 1 in every 3,000 AED exposures, usually within the first 2–8 weeks.[43] It is most common with the aromatic AEDs (i.e., PB, PHT, CBZ) but has also been seen with FBM and LTG.[44] The syndrome is characterized by fever, rash, facial swelling, adenopathy, eosinophilia, and organ involvement (e.g., hepatitis, nephritis). In most instances, symptoms resolve within a few weeks of drug discontinuation, although flares may occur after a few weeks.[43] Progression to Stevens-Johnson syndrome and toxic epidermal necrolysis may occur in 9–13% of hypersensitive patients.[43] Identification and appropriate treatment of the syndrome is crucial, as mortality may be as high as 20% when hepatic failure is associated. In severe cases, systemic corticosteroids and antihistamines are administered.[44] When the syndrome occurs, cross-reactivity among AEDs can be as high as 70–80%.[43] Therefore, it is suggested that benzodiazepines, GBP, VPA, or, possibly, TPM be at least temporarily substituted if an AED is required, as these agents exhibit a very low incidence of hypersensitivity reactions and can usually be added fairly rapidly.[44] LEV may also prove useful in this situation owing to its lack of significant hypersensitivity reactions.

Stevens-Johnson Syndrome and Toxic Epidermal Necrolysis

Stevens-Johnson syndrome (SJS) and toxic epidermal necrolysis (TEN) are severe, idiosyncratic, dermatologic reactions associated with use of the aromatic AEDs (i.e., PB, PHT, CBZ), FBM, LTG, and ZNS. They usually appear within the first few weeks of therapy and often are preceded by fever and malaise. As opposed to AED hypersensitivity syndrome, SJS is associated with oral mucosal blisters, and GI and respiratory mucosa may also be involved. Target lesions are seen, and less than 10% detachment of the body surface occurs, as opposed to greater than 30% in TEN. Corneal scarring also is common with SJS. Mortality is approximately 5% in SJS and 30% in TEN.[45]

LTG has provoked severe dermatologic reactions, including SJS and TEN, in as many as 1 of 50 children and 1 of 1,000 adults.[45] Several fatalities have occurred. Such reactions appear to be related to rapid titration and coadministration of VPA, which doubles the half-life of LTG.[37,45] This is an important consideration, as many DD patients take VPA for their mixed seizure disorders. With slow initial titration, the incidence of such severe reactions dropped dramatically.[46] Subsequently, when LTG is added to VPA, initial dosage should not be more than 25 mg every other day, and increases should not be more than 25 mg every 2 weeks.

Aplastic Anemia

Aplastic anemia is a severe idiosyncratic reaction to AEDs that is characterized by bone marrow suppression and having a fatality rate as high as 30%. CBZ has classically been associated with this complication, with an incidence of approximately 5.1 per million; CBZ also is associated with agranulocytosis, with an incidence of 1.4 per million.[15] However, in recent history, aplastic anemia has most closely been associated with the use of FBM. FBM initially appeared to be an extremely safe medication and was the first AED to be approved in monotherapy for partial epilepsy and for treating patients with the Lennox-Gastaut syndrome.[47] Unfortunately, after FBM's release, 33 patients developed aplastic anemia, and 7 deaths occurred in association with this drug's use. This represents an incidence of 300 cases of aplastic anemia per million, whereas the incidence in the general population is 2 per million. A relationship to FBM dose was not evident, and all cases occurred within the first year of treatment. Interestingly, no cases occurred in patients younger than 13 years. In all but three cases, confounding factors were present, such as cotherapy with other AEDs. A risk profile emerged, with patients having the following characteristics being more likely to develop aplastic anemia with FBM use: adult, female, white, receiving polytherapy, having a history of allergy to other AEDs (especially rash), having experienced cytopenia with other AEDs (especially thrombocytopenia), and having overt or serologic evidence of immune disease.[47] No new cases have been reported since 1994, although 10,000–12,000 patients still are taking FBM. The aplastic anemia may be due to the creation of an active intermediate, phenylpropenal (atropaldehyde).[47,48] The ratio of urinary metabolites of this agent can now be assessed and may predict risk.[48] Studies to evaluate the reliability of this testing are ongoing.

Hepatic Failure

Aside from dose-related, asymptomatic elevation of LFTs, VPA is associated with idiosyncratic fatal hepatic necrosis, with an overall incidence of 1 in 10,000–45,000 exposures.[6] This appears to be due to an active 4-ene-valproate metabolite and occurs within the first 6 months of therapy. The lowest risk is in patients older than 20 years who are on monotherapy. The greatest risk is in those younger than 2 years who are receiving polytherapy.[49] In this group, the incidence can be as high as 1 in 500–800 exposures.[49] Greater risk is present when a patient's family history includes severe hepatic disease, metabolic disorders (e.g., carnitine or ornithine carbamoyl transferase deficiency), and severe seizure disorders accompanied by mental retardation or organic brain disease.[6] Thus, DD children may be particularly at risk.

After release of FBM, 18 cases of hepatic failure and 5 deaths occurred in patients on the drug.[47]

Both adults and children were affected. Confounding factors were identified in nine patients but, in seven patients, hepatic failure was believed most likely to be attributable to FBM. Time from drug initiation to hepatic failure onset varied, with a mean of 217 days. The cause remains unknown, although one must wonder whether the atropaldehyde metabolite is responsible for this severe AE in addition to aplastic anemia.

Other Idiosyncratic Effects

VPA has rarely been associated with an idiopathic encephalopathy. This condition may be expressed as stupor or coma, which, in some cases, has been associated with carnitine deficiency, hyperammonemia, elevated PB levels, and polytherapy.[6] VPA also may cause idiosyncratic pancreatitis, usually within the first year, and is more common in young people.[6] In a DD population taking VPA, the incidence of pancreatitis was 7%, which is considered rare.[50] Mortality is as high as 20%, and an inability of DD patients to communicate symptoms may place them at greater risk for delayed diagnosis and possible fatality.[51] The pancreatitis usually is reversed by VPA discontinuation.[6]

Pancreatitis and other severe AEs of VPA (e.g., hepatic dysfunction) may be related to a VPA-induced deficiency in glutathione peroxidase and the elemental cofactors zinc and selenium.[52,53] Supplementation with these minerals may reverse or prevent a recurrence of such problems. For example, the author has had the experience of successfully rechallenging a young girl with major VPA-induced LFT elevations and a young boy with several bouts of VPA-induced acute pancreatitis by prescribing for these patients daily 50-mg zinc and 20-μg selenium supplements.

Routine monitoring of amylase generally is not recommended, as VPA may cause asymptomatic elevations of amylase, which may be salivary in origin; in addition, in rare instances, pancreatitis occurs with normal amylase levels but elevation of other pancreatic enzymes.[54] Practitioners should reserve a high index of suspicion for possible pancreatitis in DD patients on VPA, given the associated mortality of this condition and this population's difficulties in communicating symptoms. If blood tests are to be performed, multiple pancreatic enzymes should be assayed.

Long-Term Effects

Some AEs of AEDs occur only with chronic therapy and may appear after months, years, or even decades of treatment (see Table 29-1). Such AEs are more common with higher doses, polypharmacy, and prolonged treatment, all characteristics of AED use in the DD population. Thus, DD patients are at particular risk of developing such AEs. Most of the newer AEDs do not appear to provoke long-term effects similar to those brought on by older agents, although experience to date with the new AEDs is fairly limited.

Several metabolic and hormonal effects are seen with long-term AED treatment. Many of these effects are due to hepatic microsomal enzyme induction by AEDs, with resultant hypermetabolism of other substances, such as hormones. Metabolic and hormonal effects are most prominent with older AEDs and are not seen at all with benzodiazepines, VPA, or GBP. Given their limited hepatic metabolism and inductive effects, the new AEDs LTG, TPM, TGB, LEV, and ZNS would also not be expected to have significant effects.

Metabolic Effects

PB, PHT, CBZ, and VPA cause a lowering of vitamin D and calcium levels, least prominent with CBZ. Such reductions can be associated with osteomalacia, and the DD population is at increased risk due to dietary factors, limited sunlight exposure, and immobility. The problem may present clinically as repeated fractures or an apparent painful proximal myopathy. If these AEDs are used chronically, the practitioner should consider performing bone densitometry and supplementing with vitamin D (vitamin D_2, 1,000 IU per day) and calcium.

Enzyme-inducing AEDs also cause a deficiency of vitamin K, which may result in hemorrhagic complications in newborns of women with epilepsy, particularly if they are premature. Supplementation with oral vitamin K (10–20 mg per day) should be given for the month prior to delivery and should also be given intravenously during labor. Vitamin K and fresh-frozen plasma may also be necessary for the newborn.[55]

PB, PHT, CBZ, and VPA also are associated with folate deficiency, due in part to impaired absorption and to hypermetabolism,[56] which commonly expresses itself as macrocytosis, although usually without associated anemia. Folate deficiency may be a crucial factor in the occurrence of fetal malformations associated with AED use (*vide infra*).

Enzyme-inducing AEDs lead to a hypermetabolism of thyroid hormones, with PHT and CBZ causing 60% and 74% decreases in total thyroxine, respectively.[57] However, these AEDs displace triiodothyronine and thyroxine from binding proteins, resulting in normal free levels of these hormones.[57] When abnormalities are found, the thyroid-stimulating hormone level should be checked to confirm the euthyroid state of the patient.[57]

VPA interferes with mitochondrial intermediate metabolism, thereby causing decreases in carnitine and increases in ammonia and glycine.[6] The risk of such problems may be increased by genetic enzymatic defects. An increased risk of hyperammonemia is present in patients with hepatic disease or urea cycle defects, the most common being a partial deficiency of ornithine transcarbamylase.[6]

Weight changes are seen with the chronic use of several AEDs. VPA causes weight gain that has been associated with polycystic ovaries and hyperandrogenism.[58] Weight gain also is seen with GBP and VGB.[59] Conversely, ethosuximide, TPM, and, particularly, FBM may cause weight loss, which can be problematic when patients are already severely underweight. In such cases, the use of high-calorie supplements (e.g., Ensure) is indicated. In addition, the administration of cyproheptadine hydrochloride (Periactin) in selected patients may effectively increase appetite.

Sexual and Reproductive Effects

Although perhaps not of primary importance in the DD population, epilepsy and chronic AED treatment may negatively affect sexual and reproductive function. Most commonly, epilepsy is associated with hyposexuality, which, in many cases, may be directly related to the effects of epilepsy itself on hypothalamic function. However, AEDs may also contribute to this problem, and barbiturates, such as primidone, have most commonly been associated with decreased libido and impotence.

Enzyme-inducing AEDs cause an increase in hepatic synthesis of sex hormone–binding globulin and increase the metabolism of hormones, including contraceptives, leading to an increase in the required dosage of contraceptive hormones. PHT and CBZ may directly block testosterone synthesis[60] and may elevate estradiol levels.[61] Decreased free testosterone due to higher protein binding may be a cause of hyposexuality in men.[4,62] Menstrual disorders also are seen with such AEDs as CBZ and VPA and correlate with sex hormone changes.[4] In women, exposure to VPA has been associated with hyperandrogenism, polycystic ovarian disease, obesity, and menstrual irregularities.[63]

The approximately twofold increased risk of fetal malformations in women with epilepsy may be multifactorial, although AED exposure is a major risk. The risk appears greater with polytherapy and higher AED levels.[64] Malformations are most likely to occur with AED exposure during the period of organogenesis, in the first trimester, and cardiac defects, orofacial clefts, genitourinary malformations, and neural tube defects are most common.[65] PHT initially had been associated with fetal malformations subsumed under the name *fetal hydantoin syndrome*. This syndrome is characterized by growth deficiency, microcephaly, a broad and depressed nasal ridge, distal digital hypoplasia, and intellectual disability. However, all of the older AEDs also have been associated with such effects, and the syndrome is more appropriately called the *fetal AED syndrome*. CBZ and VPA are specifically known to cause fetal spina bifida, which may be an idiosyncratic effect due to the presence of active intermediates. Although genetics may play a part in teratogenicity, folate deficiency caused by older AEDs appears crucial, and supplementation has been shown to lower the incidence of malformations, particularly neural tube defects.[66] A folate dosage of at least 0.4 mg per day is recommended.

The safety of new AEDs in pregnancy is not yet known owing to the small number of pregnant women receiving these agents, but no definite significant problems have been associated with the use of the new drugs.

Long-Term Adverse Effects of Specific Antiepileptic Drugs

Although chronic PB therapy causes fewer systemic AEs than do other AEDs, long-term use is associated with a number of rheumatologic effects, including Dupuytren's contractures and frozen shoulder syndrome.[28] Similar problems may be seen with chronic PHT use. Chronic exposure to PHT can cause a number of cosmetic AEs (see Table 29-1). For this reason, PHT often is avoided in the pediatric population, if at all possible. It also generally is not recommended as a first-choice AED in DD patients, particularly if ataxia or cognitive problems are present at baseline, owing to the potential for exacerbation of these problems with long-term treatment.[5] Although toxic serum PHT levels generally are implicated in the genesis of these AEs, patients with severe brain damage who are receiving AED polytherapy may be especially susceptible to the chronic neurotoxic effects of PHT, even with low serum levels.[5]

PHT is associated with cerebellar degeneration, which appears to be related to duration of therapy and toxic serum levels. In the DD population, the end result may be permanent immobility.[5] Iivanainen et al.[67] retrospectively studied 131 patients with mental retardation receiving PHT. PHT intoxication was found in 73 subjects (56%), and 18 of these had a persistent loss of locomotion after experiencing a clinical PHT toxicity syndrome for a mean of 22.8 months. In some, permanent loss was seen after only 1 month of intoxication. In the same study, a positive correlation was noted between PHT levels and brain damage but not between toxic PHT levels and frequent seizures. It was found that more rapid motor deterioration occurred in the presence of higher PHT levels and larger fourth ventricles.

Chronic PHT exposure also causes a peripheral neuropathy with associated areflexia.[5,28] In addition, lymphadenopathy (pseudolymphoma) and a lupus-like syndrome can occur. Chronic exposure to VPA rarely causes reversible syndromes of dementia with parkinsonian features, as well as mental deterioration associated with cortical pseudoatrophy.[68] VPA sometimes (although rarely) causes a reversible sensorineural hearing loss.[6] In the DD population, this problem might manifest as apparent unresponsiveness or, possibly, agitation as a result of auditory illusory phenomena secondary to sensory deprivation.

VGB can cause retinal toxicity with peripheral visual field defects in 10% or more of patients treated chronically.[69] As a result, whether VGB will ever gain U.S. Food and Drug Administration approval remains unclear.

Laboratory Testing

Physicians are accustomed to monitoring regularly those patients receiving AEDs by assessing drug levels, CBC, and chemistries (especially sodium and LFTs). Many of the newer AEDs are much safer systemically, so routine blood monitoring is not required. However, a majority of patients on AEDs demonstrate some abnormalities on testing, which are rarely of clinical significance. Common examples include mild leukopenia with CBZ and thrombocytopenia and elevated LFTs with VPA. Such findings often lead to unnecessary additional testing, as well as the possible unnecessary discontinuation of medications that were otherwise useful.[47] The presumed value of routine blood monitoring is based on the assumption that severe AEs (e.g., aplastic anemia and hepatic failure) can be detected before the appearance of clinical signs and symptoms. However, the necessity, value, and cost-effectiveness of such testing has been questioned.[47] For example, in the case of VPA, clinical signs including nausea, vomiting, anorexia, edema, lethargy, and a worsening of seizures often precede an elevation of LFTs and are more reliable predictors of clinically significant liver toxicity than the laboratory measures.[49]

Particularly when older AEDs are being initiated, blood should be drawn for a CBC and chemistries before commencing therapy, to establish a baseline for future comparison. Blood tests, including AED levels (if appropriate), should then be repeated once or twice in the first 3–6 months, while the dose is being titrated upward. It is during this period that most abnormalities arise. After the first 3–6 months, the necessity of continued regular testing is questionable, particularly after a patient has been on an AED for longer than 1 year. Rather, patients and caregivers should be instructed to report signs and symptoms suggestive of problems, such as unexplained fever, easy bruising, and petechiae.

The use of FBM warrants special mention. When FBM is being used, a CBC and LFTs should be performed at baseline and then every 1–2 weeks for the first year.[70] However, the value of such testing in predicting aplastic anemia or hepatic failure is unclear. At the time these problems arose, routine blood testing was not being performed owing to the perceived safety of FBM; therefore, data on the possible predictive value of laboratory testing was not collected. Hence, patients or caregivers should be advised of the early clinical signs of hepatic and hematologic toxicity. When this agent is being prescribed, testing of the patient's urine after each dosage change for the atropaldehyde metabolites of FBM is worthwhile; such testing is conducted with kits provided by Carter-Wallace Laboratories (Cranbury, New Jersey) in the hope of averting aplastic anemia.

Knowledge of therapeutic drug levels can be valuable, but such information should not be used to direct most clinical decisions regarding medication dosage. Although they tend to maintain drug levels within the therapeutic range, physicians should be aware that this range applies to a majority but not the entire population. Some patients will be well controlled with "subtherapeutic" levels, whereas others require levels in the "toxic" range and will not experience AEs from such apparent overdosing. Many new AEDs have much wider therapeutic windows than earlier agents, and their levels are currently less well defined and clinically useful. The guiding principle should always be to treat the patient, not the blood level. Therapeutic changes should, for the most part, be based on the occurrence of seizures and clinical AEs, much as was done in the past. AED levels should generally be tested only when there is questionable compliance or absorption, poor seizure control, a dosage change, the addition of other medication with possible interactions, clinical intoxication, pregnancy, or new disease states.

Managing and Preventing Adverse Effects of Antiepileptic Drugs in the Developmentally Disabled

The management of AEs of AEDs in the DD population can be extremely challenging and requires first that caregivers know which AEs are most likely to be encountered with the use of a particular AED. Given that communication problems are common in such patients, practitioners and caregivers should be aware of the clinical signs that might be exhibited. One must remember that in a nonverbal patient, multiple symptoms (e.g., nausea, dizziness, and diplopia) might all be expressed similarly as agitation.

In selecting an AED, broad-spectrum agents should be used whenever possible, and polytherapy should be avoided. If possible, in treatment of the DD population, drugs should be used that are the least likely to cause negative behavioral effects. Barbiturates and benzodiazepines should generally

be avoided. Seizure control and behavior can be improved in the DD population with monotherapy and particularly with the avoidance or elimination of PB.[71] In some instances, agitation or other apparent negative behavioral effects of AEDs may not truly represent a negative AE but, rather, a positive release phenomenon as a result of eliminating sedative AEs. In such instances, the appropriate course of action is to teach adaptive responses as opposed to eliminating the drug.

The drug preparation used will affect the incidence of AEs. Liquid formulations are more rapidly absorbed, resulting in the more rapid attainment of higher peak serum levels and a greater chance of neurotoxic AEs. If at all possible, timed-release preparations of AEDs are preferable, as peaks and troughs are minimized, resulting in better seizure control and a lesser incidence of AEs.

In adding AEDs, upward titration should be as slow as possible, and the lowest effective dosage should be used. The physician should be aware that many AEs—particularly those that are neurotoxic—tend to occur at initiation or shortly after a change in dosage, while blood levels are rising. The majority of such AEs resolve by the time a new equilibrium has been reached, approximately five half-lives after the change. Only intolerable AEs that persist after equilibrium is established should prompt reduction or discontinuation of a drug. Otherwise, the patient may not receive a fair trial of a medication that may have proven effective.

Individualization of AED regimens can also diminish the risk of AEs. Although a particular AED might usually be given on a three-times-daily regimen, a patient experiencing only nocturnal seizures may be effectively dosed only at bedtime with a drug having a relatively short half-life, thereby controlling seizures while simultaneously minimizing the chance of diurnal AEs. If AEs occur at peak dose levels, AEDs may be given in smaller, more frequent doses than usual, which will serve to lower peak levels and associated AEs. In addition, such a strategy may help to minimize GI symptoms associated with certain AEDs. Particularly with the new AEDs, such GI symptoms may also be diminished via coadministration with food or antacids, which do not significantly affect their absorption.

At times, determining whether a clinical sign or symptom represents an AE or an ictal phenomenon may be difficult. Careful observation should reveal whether the episode is temporally related to medication administration, in which case the former is more likely. In addition, drug AEs are, in general, much more prolonged than seizures, which usually last for only a few minutes. One might consider a temporary reduction in medication as a diagnostic or therapeutic trial if a drug effect appears more likely and the risk of major seizures is not great. If questions remain, consideration should be given to evaluating the patient at a comprehensive epilepsy center where continuous video-electroencephalographic monitoring can be performed in order to answer these questions.

Finally, total seizure control, particularly if seizure events are minor, may not be worth achieving if, in the process, a patient's quality of life is sacrificed to AEs of medication. This is particularly true if seizure control itself would not significantly improve a given patient's quality of life.

References

1. Genton P, McMenamin J (eds). Can antiepileptic drugs aggravate epilepsy? Epilepsia 1998;39:S1–S29.
2. Isojarvi JIT, Tokola RA. Benzodiazepines in the treatment of epilepsy in people with intellectual disability. J Intellect Disabil Res 1998;42[Suppl 1]:80–92.
3. US Gabapentin Study Group No. 5. Gabapentin as add-on therapy in refractory partial epilepsy: a double-blind, placebo-controlled, parallel-group study. Neurology 1993;43:2292–2298.
4. Waisburg H, Alvarez N. Carbamazepine in the treatment of epilepsy in people with intellectual disability. J Intellect Disabil Res 1998;42[Suppl 1]:36–40.
5. Iivanainen M. Phenytoin: effective but insidious therapy for epilepsy in people with intellectual disability. J Intellect Disabil Res 1998;42[Suppl 1]:24–31.
6. Dreifuss FE. Valproic Acid: Toxicity. In RH Levy, RH Mattson, BS Meldrum (eds), Antiepileptic Drugs (4th ed). New York: Raven Press, 1995;641–648.
7. Lancman ME, Asconape JJ, Walker F. Acetazolamide appears effective in the management of valproate induced tremor. Mov Disord 1994;9:369.
8. Lancman ME, Asconape JJ, Penry JK. Choreiform movements associated with the use of valproate. Arch Neurol 1994;51(7):702–704.
9. Luciano D, Devinsky O, Raguthu S, et al. Movement disorders during felbamate therapy. Epilepsia 1994;35[Suppl 8]:159.
10. Asconape J, Diedrich A, DellaBadia J. Myoclonus associated with the use of gabapentin. Epilepsia 2000;41:479–481.
11. Sano J, Kawada H, Yamaguchi N, et al. Effects of phenytoin on serum gamma-glutamyl transpeptidase activity. Epilepsia 1981;22:331–338.
12. Silverstein FS, Boxer L, Johnston MV. Hematological monitoring during therapy with carbamazepine in children (letter). Ann Neurol 1983;13:685–686.
13. Gaily E, Granstrom ML, Liukkonen E. Oxcarbazepine in the treatment of epilepsy in children and adolescents with intellectual disability. J Intellect Disabil Res 1998;42[Suppl 1]:41–45.
14. Brewerton TD, Jackson CW. Prophylaxis of carbamazepine-induced hyponatremia by demeclocycline in six patients. J Clin Psychiatry 1994;55:249–251.
15. Holmes GL. Carbamazepine: Toxicity. In RH Levy, RH Mattson, BS Meldrum (eds), Antiepileptic Drugs (4th ed). New York: Raven Press, 1995;567–579.
16. Beydoun A, Sackellares JC, Shu V. Safety and efficacy of divalproex sodium monotherapy in partial epilepsy: a double-blind, concentration-response design clinical trial. Depakote Monotherapy for Partial Seizures Study Group. Neurology 1997;48:182–188.
17. Anderson GD, Lin YX, Berge C, Ojemann GA. Absence of bleeding complications in patients undergoing cortical surgery while receiving valproate treatment. J Neurosurg 1997;87(2):252–256.
18. Chambers HG, Weinstein CH, Mubarak SJ, et al. The effect of valproic acid on blood loss in patients with cerebral palsy. J Pediatr Orthop 1999;19(6):792–795.
19. Kugoh T, Yamamoto M, Hosokawa K. Blood ammonia level during valproic acid therapy. Jpn J Psychiatry Neurol 1986;40:663–668.
20. Hamer HM, Knake S, Schomburg U, Rosenow F. Valproate-induced hyperammonemic encephalopathy in the presence of topiramate. Neurology 2000;54(1):230–232.
21. Shorvon SD. Safety of topiramate: adverse events and relationships to dosing. Epilepsia 1996;37:S18–S22.
22. Iinuma K, Minami T, Cho K, et al. Long-term effects of zonisamide in the treatment of epilepsy in children with intellectual disability. J Intellect Disabil Res 1998;42[Suppl 1]:68–73.
23. Devinsky O. Cognitive and behavioral effects of antiepileptic drugs. Epilepsia 1995;36[Suppl 2]:S46–S65.
24. Meador KJ. Current discoveries on the cognitive effects of antiepileptic drugs. Pharmacotherapy 2000;20(8):185S–190S.
25. Meador KJ, Loring DW, Ray PG, et al. Differential cognitive effects of carbamazepine and gabapentin. Epilepsia 1999;40(9):1279–1285.
26. Aikis M, Kalviainen R, Sivenius J, et al. Cognitive effects of oxcarbazepine and phenytoin monother-

apy in newly diagnosed epilepsy: one-year follow-up. Epilepsy Res 1992;11:199–203.

27. Kerr MP. Topiramate: uses in people with an intellectual disability who have epilepsy. J Intellect Disabil Res 1998;42[Suppl 1]:74–79.

28. Mattson RH. The role of the old and the new antiepileptic drugs in special populations: mental and multiple handicaps. Epilepsia 1996;37[Suppl 6]:S45–S53.

29. Ylinen A. Antiepileptic efficacy of vigabatrin in people with severe epilepsy and intellectual disability. J Intellect Disabil Res 1998;42[Suppl 1]:46–49.

30. Levinson DF, Devinsky O. Psychiatric adverse events during vigabatrin therapy. Neurology 1999;53(7):1503–1511.

31. Thomas L, Trimble M, Schmitz B, Ring H. Vigabatrin and behavior disorders: a retrospective survey. Epilepsy Res 1996;25:21–27.

32. Mikati MA, Choueri, R, Khurana DS, et al. Gabapentin in the treatment of refractory partial epilepsy in children with intellectual disability. J Intellect Disabil Res 1998;42[Suppl 1]:57–62.

33. Besag FMC. Lamotrigine in the treatment of epilepsy in people with intellectual disability. J Intellect Disabil Res 1998;42[Suppl 1]:50–56.

34. Beran RG, Gibson RJ. Aggressive behaviour in intellectually challenged patients with epilepsy treated with lamotrigine. Epilepsia 1998;39:280–282.

35. Alvarez N, Besag F, Iivanainen M. Use of antiepileptic drugs in the treatment of epilepsy in people with intellectual disability. J Intellect Disabil Res 1998;42[Suppl 1]:1–15.

36. Chadwick D, Shaw MD, Foy P, et al. Serum anticonvulsant concentrations and the risk of drug induced skin eruptions. J Neurol Neurosurg Psychiatry 1984;47:642–644.

37. Messenheimer JA. Lamotrigine. Epilepsia 1995;36[Suppl 2]:S87–S94.

38. Rapp RP, Norton JA, Young B, Tibbs PA. Cutaneous reactions in head-injured patients receiving phenytoin for seizure prophylaxis. Neurosurgery 1983;13:272–275.

39. Murphy JM, Mashman J, Miller JD, Bell JB. Suppression of carbamazepine-induced rash with prednisone. Neurology 1991;41:144–145.

40. Besag FM, Ng GY, Pool F. Successful re-introduction of lamotrigine after initial rash. Seizure 2000;9(4):282–286.

41. Koppel BS, Harden CL, Daras M. Tegretol excipient-induced allergy. Arch Neurol 1991;48(8):789.

42. Dam M, Ostergaard LH. Oxcarbazepine. In RH Levy, RH Mattson, BS Meldrum (eds), Antiepileptic Drugs (4th ed). New York: Raven Press, 1995;987–995.

43. Schlienger RG, Shear NH. Antiepileptic drug hypersensitivity syndrome. Epilepsia 1998;39[Suppl 7]:S3–S7.

44. Hamer HM, Morris HH. Hypersensitivity syndrome to antiepileptic drugs: a review including new anticonvulsants. Cleve Clin J Med 1999;66:239–245.

45. Pellock JM. Overview of lamotrigine and the new anti-epileptic drugs: the challenge. J Child Neurol 1997;12[Suppl 1]:S48–S52.

46. Wong IC, Mawer GE, Sander JW. Factors influencing the incidence of lamotrigine-related skin rash. Ann Pharmacother 1999;33:1037–1042.

47. Pellock JM. Felbamate in epilepsy therapy. Evaluating the risks. Drug Saf 1999;21:225–239.

48. Thompson CD, Barthen MT, Hopper DW, et al. Quantification in patient urine samples of felbamate and three metabolites: acid carbamate and two mercapturic acids. Epilepsia 1999;40(6):769–776.

49. Dreifuss FE, Langer DH, Moline KA, Maxwell JE. Valproic acid hepatic fatalities: II. U.S. experience since 1984. Neurology 1989;39:201–207.

50. Buzan RD, Firestone D, Thomas M, Dubovsky SL. Valproate-associated pancreatitis and cholecystitis in six mentally retarded adults. J Clin Psychiatry 1995;56(11):529–532.

51. Evans RJ, Miranda RN, Jordan J, Krolikowski FJ. Fatal acute pancreatitis caused by valproic acid. Am J Forensic Med Pathol 1995;16(1):62–65.

52. Pippenger CE, Meng X, van Lente F, Rothner AD. Valproate therapy depresses free radical scavenging activity: a probable mechanism for induction of acute pancreatitis or hepatotoxicity. Neurology 1989;39[Suppl 1]:214.

53. Graf WD, Oleinik OE, Glauser TA, et al. Altered antioxidant enzyme activities in children with a serious adverse experience related to valproic acid therapy. Neuropediatrics 1998;29(4):195–201.

54. Otusbo S, Huruzono T, Kobae H, et al. Pancreatitis with normal serum amylase associated with sodium valproate: a case report. Brain Dev 1995;17:219–221.

55. Moslet U, Hansen ES. A review of vitamin K, epilepsy and pregnancy. Acta Neurol Scand 1992;85:39–43.

56. Kishi T, Fujita N, Eguchi T, Ueda K. Mechanism for reduction of serum folate by antiepileptic drugs during prolonged therapy. J Neurol Sci 1997;145:109–112.

57. Surks MI, DeFesi CR. Normal serum free thyroid hormone concentrations in patients treated with phenytoin or carbamazepine. A paradox resolved. JAMA 1996;275(19):1495–1498.

58. Isojarvi JIT, Laatikainen TJ, Pakarinen AJ, et al. Polycystic ovaries and hyperandrogenism in women taking valproate for epilepsy. N Engl J Med 1993;329:1383–1388.

59. Shorvon S, Stefan H. Overview of the safety of newer antiepileptic drugs. Epilepsia 1997;38[Suppl 1]:S45–S51.

60. Kuhn-Velten WN, Herzog AG, Muller MR. Acute effects of anticonvulsant drugs on gonadotropin-stimulated and precursor-supported androgen production in the rat testis. Eur J Pharmacol 1990;181:151–155.

61. Herzog AG, Levesque LA, Drislane FW, et al. Phenytoin-induced elevation of serum estradiol and reproductive dysfunction in men with epilepsy. Epilepsia 1989;32:550–553.

62. Barragry JM, Makin HL, Trafford DJ, Scott DF. Effect of anticonvulsants on plasma testosterone and sex hor-

mone binding globulin levels. J Neurol Neurosurg Psychiatry 1978;41:913–914.

63. Vainionpaa LK, Rattya J, Kinp M, et al. Valproate-induced hyperandrogenism during pubertal maturation in girls with epilepsy. Ann Neurol 1999;45:444–450.

64. Kaneko S, Otani K, Fukushima J, et al. Teratogenicity of antiepileptic drugs: analysis of possible risk factors. Epilepsia 1988;29:459–467.

65. Nulman I, Laslo D, Koren G. Treatment of epilepsy in pregnancy. Drugs 1999;57(4):535–544.

66. Czeizel AE, Dudas I. Prevention of the first occurrence of neural-tube defects by periconceptional vitamin supplementation. N Engl J Med 1992;327:1832–1835.

67. Iivanainen M, Viukari M, Helle EP. Cerebellar atrophy in phenytoin-treated mentally retarded epileptics. Epilepsia 1977;18:375–386.

68. Guerrini R, Belmonte A, Canapicchi R, et al. Reversible pseudoatrophy of the brain and mental deterioration associated with valproate treatment. Epilepsia 1998;39(1):27–32.

69. Eke T, Talbot JF, Lawden MC. Severe persistent visual field constriction associated with vigabatrin. BMJ 1997;314:180–181.

70. French J, Smith M, Faught E, Brown L. Practice advisory: the use of felbamate in the treatment of patients with intractable epilepsy. Report of the Quality Standards Subcommittee of the American Academy of Neurology and the American Epilepsy Society. Neurology 1999;52:1540–1545.

71. Pellock JM, Hunt PA. A decade of modern epilepsy therapy in institutionalized mentally retarded patients. Epilepsy Res 1996;25:263–268.

Chapter 30

The Ketogenic Diet

Karen Ballaban-Gil

The ketogenic diet (KD) is a high-fat, low-carbohydrate, low-protein diet used in the treatment of pediatric epilepsy since the 1920s.[1] Currently, it is being used primarily for refractory childhood epilepsy.

The history of the KD dates back to biblical times when it was recognized that in patients with epilepsy, fasting often improved seizure control. In 1921, Dr. Wilder, a diabetologist at the Mayo Clinic, developed the KD, in which the high fat, low protein, and low carbohydrate intake mimicked the therapeutic effects of the fasting state.[1] Variations of the diet have been used successfully in the United States since the 1920s for the treatment of epilepsy. However, with the development of effective antiepileptic drugs (AEDs) in the 1940s and 1950s, the use of this rigorous diet was substantially decreased.

Since 1994, the KD has attracted renewed interest for managing intractable epilepsy. Numerous clinical trials have been reported, and animal studies have been conducted, to evaluate both the efficacy of the diet and its mechanism of action. This chapter reviews these data.

Dietary Content of the Classic Ketogenic Diet

The KD is calculated to be very high in fats and low in carbohydrates and protein. In the classic 4-to-1 ratio diet, each meal contains 4 g fat for each gram of protein and carbohydrate that is consumed. Typically, caloric intake is approximately 75% of normal recommended calorie intake, which is based on the child's age and ideal weight (50% weight for any given length), and a minimum of 1 g protein per kilogram of body weight per day is required. Some practitioners also restrict fluid intake to an average of 65 ml per kilogram of body weight per day, although the importance of fluid restriction to the efficacy of the diet has not been established. Each meal consists of a protein source (meat, fish, poultry, egg, or cheese), a carbohydrate (either fruit or vegetable), a fat source (butter, margarine, oil, or mayonnaise), and 36–40% heavy whipping cream, which contains protein, carbohydrate, and fat calories. Table 30-1 shows a typical day's meals for a 5-year-old, 18-kg child.

For youngsters with severe developmental disabilities who are unable to take food orally, the diet can be administered by liquid, tube feedings. Such feedings are most often composed of Ross Carbohydrate-Free Formula, Microlipid, and Polycose powder, combined with sterile water.

Efficacy of the Ketogenic Diet

Clinical Trials

In 1924, in the era before effective AEDs, Peterman[2] reported that 60% of patients were seizure-free and an additional 35% had greater than 50% improvement in seizure frequency on the KD. Barborka[3] reported that of 100 adults with epilepsy, 12 had complete seizure control on the diet, 44 had improved but incomplete seizure control, and 44 demonstrated no benefit. In 1963, in a 10-year follow-up study of patients treated at the Mayo Clinic, Keith[4] reported that 22.2% were seizure-free, 17.6% had improved seizure control, and 28.2% had no change or worsening of their seizure frequency. In his textbook, Livingston[5] reported his results in more than 1,000 patients treated with the

Table 30-1. Classic 4-to-1 Ketogenic Diet

Breakfast
    60 g 36% heavy cream
    20 g fruit
    39 g eggs
    22 g butter
Lunch
    60 g 36% heavy cream
    35 g vegetable
    19 g white tuna fish
    24 g butter or margarine
Dinner
    60 g 36% heavy cream
    24 g vegetable
    31 g beef hot dog
    14 g butter or margarine
    40 g sugar free gelatin

Note: One-day menu for 18-kg, 5-year-old youngster.

KD. Seizures were controlled in 52%, reduced in 27%, and unchanged in 21%.

One of the more widely quoted studies, at least in the lay literature, was reported by Kinsman et al.[6] in 1992. This retrospective review involved 58 children who were treated at the Johns Hopkins Hospital and who had a mean age of 60 months and a mean follow-up of 31 months. Kinsman's group[6] reported that 29% had "virtually complete" seizure control, 38% had a 50% or greater reduction in seizure frequency, and 29% experienced no improvement or worsening of seizure control.

Prior to recent renewed interest in the KD, the only prospective study of the efficacy of the diet was that of Schwartz et al.[7] These researchers compared the efficacy and tolerability of the classic 4-to-1 KD with the medium-chain triglyceride (MCT) diet and a modified MCT oil diet. At follow-up at 3 months, 40% of patients had at least a 90% reduction in seizures, approximately 40% had more than a 50% reduction in seizure frequency, and 19% noted less than a 50% seizure reduction. They found no difference in efficacy among the three diets, although a difference in side effects and tolerability was noted, with the MCT diet being less well tolerated.

After publication of *The Epilepsy Diet Treatment: An Introduction to the Ketogenic Diet*,[8] much publicity surrounding the diet appeared in the lay press, which provoked other prospective evaluations of the efficacy of the KD. Nigro et al.[9] reported their results

in 34 children, 45% of whom experienced at least a 75% reduction in seizures and 14% of whom demonstrated a 50–75% reduction in seizures. The diet was discontinued by 32% of the children, largely owing to their failure to respond.

Swink et al.[10] conducted a prospective study of 68 children having a mean age of 6.4 years. Their reported results were based on those subjects who remained on the diet for 12 months (n = 27). Of these 27 children, 22% were seizure-free, 22% had more than 90% seizure control, and 46% had 50–90% seizure control. However, when one calculates these data on an intent-to-treat (n = 68), only 9% were seizure-free, an additional 9% had greater than 90% seizure control, and 18% had 50–90% seizure control. Forty percent of patients discontinued the diet, 16 owing to poor seizure control and 10 because of poor tolerance.

Holt et al.[11] reported results of the diet in 22 children. Fifty-nine percent (n = 13) had "significant seizure improvement," which the authors defined as greater than a 90% decrease in seizures or a prolonged period of being seizure-free among children who previously experienced daily seizures. In nine children, the diet failed, in that no improvement in seizure frequency was noted in five cases and the family was unable to manage the diet in four cases.

Summ et al.[12] treated 44 children having a mean age of 4.5 years and average follow-up of 9 months (range, 1–16 months). During the follow-up period, 73% of patients (32) remained on the diet. Of these, 91% had at least a 50% seizure reduction (66% of original group) and 19% were seizure-free (14% of original group). Five patients (11% of original group) had initial seizure control but then experienced seizure recurrence.

Freeman et al.[13] treated 150 children having a mean age of 5.3 years. At 1-year follow-up, 27% had greater than a 90% reduction in seizure frequency, with a total of 50% having greater than a 50% decrease in seizures. Forty-five percent of their patients discontinued the diet within the first year.

Vining et al.[14] reported the results of a multicenter study performed to determine the efficacy of the KD at seven independent sites. Fifty-one children with a mean age of 4.7 years (range, 1.3–8.6 years) were enrolled. They had been treated with an average of seven AEDs and were experiencing an average of 230 seizures per month (range, 11–1,880 seizures) during the 1-month baseline period prior to diet initiation. Many children had multiple seizure types. KD efficacy was evaluated at 3, 6, and 12 months. At 6-month follow-up, 12% of patients were seizure-free, 29% had greater than a 90% reduction in seizure frequency, and 53% had greater than a 50% reduction in seizures. Twenty-seven percent of children had discontinued the diet by the 6-month follow-up. At 12-month follow-up, of the 47% of children still enrolled, 10% were seizure-free, 22% had greater than a 90% reduction in seizure frequency, and 40% had greater than a 50% reduction in seizure frequency. By the 12-month follow-up, 53% of the patients had discontinued the diet. Notably, no differences in outcome were obvious at 1 year based on age, gender, or electroencephalographic abnormalities.

At the Montefiore-Einstein Comprehensive Epilepsy Center from November 1994 through August 1996 (unpublished data), 47 children with refractory epilepsy were started on the classic KD, using the protocol of the Johns Hopkins Hospital[8] and were followed in a prospective manner. The mean age of the children was 6.63 years (range, 1.5–16.5 years). Eight of these children also were enrolled in the multicenter prospective study of the efficacy of the KD.[14] At least three conventional AEDs had failed to benefit all these patients prior to initiation of the diet. One child was lost to follow-up after diet initiation, and two others remained on the diet for less than 2 weeks. Of the remaining 44 children, at 1-year follow-up, 7% were seizure-free and an additional 7% had greater than a 90% reduction in seizure frequency. Fifty percent of children had less than a 50% reduction in seizure frequency. Within 1 year of initiation, 59% of children had discontinued the diet, most because of lack of efficacy. Interestingly, no difference in outcome was noted on the basis of intellect or associated disabilities.

Overall, the results of these prospective studies of the KD indicate that it is an effective modality in the treatment of intractable childhood epilepsy.

Effect of Seizure Type on Efficacy

It has often been stated that the KD is most effective in the treatment of myoclonic and atonic sei-

zures and least effective in the treatment of partial and absence seizures.[8] However, no data are available to support these assumptions, and most studies have not demonstrated any differences in efficacy based on seizure type. The possible exception to this may be partial seizures, as many studies exclude purely partial seizures. Kinsman et al.[6] reported that seizure type was not predictive of outcome. Schwartz et al.[7] similarly found no significant difference in KD efficacy based on seizure type. The multicenter trial conducted by Vining et al.[14] further substantiated this finding.

Animal Studies

Despite more than 75 years of clinical experience with the KD, the mechanism of action of the diet remains unknown. Relatively few animal studies of the effectiveness of this treatment have been undertaken, and even fewer were aimed at understanding the KD's mechanism of action. In addition, substantial differences in methodology characterize these studies, including differences in animal species and age, KD formulation, duration of treatment, methods of inducing seizures, and outcome measures.[15] An extensive review of these animal studies can be found in a recent article by Stafstrom.[15]

In 1933, in the first animal study of the efficacy of the KD, Keith[16] showed that rabbits treated with intravenous acetoacetate were protected against the development of thujone-induced convulsions.

Appleton and DeVivo[17] developed an animal model to study both the efficacy of the KD and its effects on cerebral metabolism. Adult rats were fed a KD for 5 weeks, and their responses to electroconvulsive shock were evaluated. These researchers showed that ketogenic rats had an increased threshold to seizure induction with electroconvulsive shock and that the onset of antiepileptic effect was gradual. The initial response of increased voltage threshold began approximately 10–12 days after initiation of the KD, and the maximal effect on convulsive threshold was not reached until approximately 20 days. Also, once ketosis was reversed by the introduction of a high-carbohydrate diet, seizure susceptibility returned quickly. Within 48 hours, rats needed only the lower electrical stimulus to produce maximal convulsion. Interestingly, this is similar to a clinical phenomenon that has been observed in children treated with the KD; a time lag between initiation of the KD and a reduction in seizures may be noted, and some youngsters quickly experience a recurrence of seizures when they lose ketosis (often because of ingesting carbohydrates).

Appleton and DeVivo found that ketogenic rats had significantly higher serum and brain concentrations of β-hydroxybutyrate than did control animals. However, although serum acetoacetate was elevated in ketogenic animals, no difference in brain acetoacetate concentration was noted. Similarly, no difference was found between the ketogenic animals and the controls in brain potassium, calcium, phosphate, water content, glutamic acid, glutamine, γ-aminobutyric acid (GABA), alanine, or aspartic acid levels. They suggested that the mechanism of action of the KD was that ketosis alters cerebral metabolism of glucose, leading to an elevation in electroconvulsive threshold.

In a study to evaluate the antiepileptic mechanism of the KD, Al-Mudallal et al.[18] measured cerebral intracellular pH, glucose, lactate, adenosine triphosphate, phosphocreatine, and GABA levels in adult rats fed a KD for 5–6 weeks. They found that although the ketogenic rats had a greater than 10-fold increase in their plasma ketones, no significant differences existed in cerebral pH or cerebral levels of glucose, lactate, adenosine triphosphate, phosphocreatine, or GABA between the ketogenic rats and controls. The researchers concluded that the antiepileptic effect of the KD was unlikely to be mediated by cerebral acidosis or by increased cerebral GABA.

Hori et al.[19] used a kindling model of seizures to evaluate the anticonvulsant effectiveness and behavioral consequences of the KD. This was the first study to evaluate the efficacy of the KD using an animal model of epilepsy. Adult rats were kindled and then placed on a KD for 5 weeks. They were compared to control rats that were kindled and then fed normal rat chow. Afterdischarge threshold and stage V seizure thresholds were compared between the two groups. The researchers found that the ketogenic rats had transiently increased afterdischarge and seizure thresholds during the first 3 weeks of treatment but that the protective effect was lost in the last 2 weeks of treatment. Notably, even during the first 3 weeks of treatment, ketogenic rats had no increased protection from seizure spread. Furthermore, ketogenic rats did not show improved learning on the water-maze or open-field tests. However, it is noteworthy that the level of ketosis in these animals was significantly lower than that seen in children or in other animal studies. In addition, the authors point out that more robust antiepileptic effects might have been seen if immature animals had been evaluated.

Bough and Eagles[20] used pentylenetetrazole-induced seizures in adult rats to evaluate the antiepileptic effect of the KD. After 35 days of treatment with the KD, the ketogenic rats had a significantly increased threshold for seizure induction as compared to controls. Of note, once the diet was initiated, no difference in seizure severity between the ketogenic rats and the controls was found.

Animal data about the efficacy of the KD in young animals is very limited. Rho et al.[21] studied the effects of the KD on flurothyl seizure susceptibility in juvenile mice treated with the KD for 3, 7, and 12 days and in adult mice treated for 15 days. Juvenile mice treated with the KD for 7 and 12 days had significantly increased latency to the first flurothyl-induced (clonic) seizure as compared to control animals. Juvenile mice fed the KD for only 3 days did not exhibit this seizure protection. Interestingly, the KD did not have an antiepileptic effect against the second (tonic extension) seizure induced by flurothyl in any of the juvenile groups, but it significantly delayed tonic extension in the adult group. Furthermore, the juvenile mice fed the KD had a lower mortality rate after flurothyl-induced seizures as compared to controls.

These data provide strong evidence in animal models for the anticonvulsant efficacy of the KD and suggest possible underlying mechanisms of the diet's antiepileptic effect. However, further studies, particularly in young, developing animals, are needed to help us to understand better the diet's mechanisms of action.

Adverse Effects of the Ketogenic Diet

Few serious complications caused by the classic or modified KD have been reported. Short-term complications during the initial hospital stay include dehydration, hypoglycemia, acidosis, vomiting, diarrhea, and refusal to eat.[2] Long-term complications (1 week–2 years) include kidney stones (3–5%), recurrent infections (2%), metabolic derangements (hyperuricemia [2%], decreased amino acid levels, acidosis [2%]), hypercholesterolemia (29–59%), irritability, lethargy, and refusal to eat.[6,12,22–25] Carnitine deficiency has also been demonstrated in some children on the KD.[26,27] Very long-term complications (greater than 2 years) have not been studied.

We reported results in five children who experienced serious adverse events after initiation of the KD.[28] Two of these developed severe hypoproteinemia within 1 month of diet initiation, and one also developed lipemia and hemolytic anemia. A third child developed Fanconi's tubular acidosis within 1 month of diet initiation, and the other two developed elevated liver function test results. The latter three children were being treated with valproate at the time of initiation of the KD, and we postulated that the diet may potentiate valproate toxicity.

Conclusion

Retrospective and prospective studies in children have demonstrated that the KD is an effective treatment for refractory childhood epilepsy. Animal studies have similarly confirmed the anticonvulsive efficacy of the KD and have suggested some possible underlying mechanisms of its antiepileptic effects. A better understanding of these mechanisms could help clinicians to optimize use of the diet and might lead to the development of novel antiepileptic therapies.

References

1. Wilder RM. The effect of ketonemia on the course of epilepsy. Mayo Clin Proc 1921;2:307–308.
2. Peterman MG. The ketogenic diet in epilepsy. JAMA 1925;84:1979–1983.
3. Barborka CJ. Epilepsy in adults: results of treatment by ketogenic diet in one hundred cases. Arch Neurol Psychiatry 1930;23:904–914.
4. Keith HM. Convulsive Disorders in Children: With Reference to Treatment with Ketogenic Diet. Boston: Little, Brown, 1963.
5. Livingston S. Dietary Management of Epilepsy. In S Livingston (ed), Comprehensive Management of Epilepsy in Infancy, Childhood and Adolescence. Springfield, IL: Charles C Thomas 1972;378–405.
6. Kinsman SL, Vining EPG, Quaskey SA, et al. Efficacy of the ketogenic diet for intractable seizure disorders: review of 58 cases. Epilepsia 1992;33:1132–1136.
7. Schwartz RH, Eaton J, Bower BD, Aynsley-Green A. Ketogenic diets in the treatment of epilepsy: short-term clinical effects. Dev Med Child Neurol 1989;31:145–151.
8. Freeman JM, Kelly MT, Freeman JB. The Epilepsy Diet Treatment: An Introduction to the Ketogenic Diet. New York: Demos, 1994.
9. Nigro MA, Ventimiglia J, Selcen D, Beierwaltes P. Seizure frequency, behavioral, and performance effects of the ketogenic diet. Ann Neurol 1995;38:549–550.
10. Swink TD, Vining EPG, Kelly MC, et al. Efficacy of the classical ketogenic diet in children with refractory epilepsy: a prospective study. Epilepsia 1996;37[Suppl 5]:108.
11. Holt PJ, Barry PM, O'Leary ED. Successes, failures and adverse events on the ketogenic diet. Epilepsia 1996;37[Suppl 5]:109.
12. Summ JM, Woch MA, McNeil T, et al. Success and complications of the ketogenic diet for intractable childhood epilepsy. Epilepsia 1996;37[Suppl 5]:109.
13. Freeman JM, Vining EPG, Pillas DJ, et al. The efficacy of the ketogenic diet–1998: a prospective evaluation of intervention in 150 children. Pediatrics 1998;102:1358–1363.
14. Vining EPG, Freeman JM, Ballaban-Gil K, et al. A multicenter study of the efficacy of the ketogenic diet. Arch Neurol 1998;55:1433–1437.
15. Stafstrom CE. Animal models of the ketogenic diet: what have we learned, what can we learn? Epilepsy Res 1999;37:241–259.
16. Keith HM. Factors influencing experimentally produced convulsions. Arch Neurol Psychiatry 1933;29:148–154.
17. Appleton DB, DeVivo DC. An animal model for the ketogenic diet. Epilepsia 1974;15:211–217.
18. Al-Mudallal AS, LaManna JC, Lust WD, Harik SI. Diet induced ketosis does not cause cerebral acidosis. Epilepsia 1996;37:258–261.
19. Hori A, Tandon P, Holmes GL, Stafstrom CE. Ketogenic diet: effects on expression of kindled seizures and behavior in adult rats. Epilepsia 1997;38:750–758.
20. Bough KJ, Eagles DA. A ketogenic diet increases the resistance to pentylenetetrazole-induced seizures in the rat. Epilepsia 1999;40:138–143.
21. Rho JM, Kim DW, Robbins CA, et al. Age-dependent differences in flurothyl seizure sensitivity in mice treated with a ketogenic diet. Epilepsy Res 1999;37:233–240.
22. Schwartz RH, Boyes S, Aynsley-Green A. Metabolic effects of three ketogenic diets in the treatment of severe epilepsy. J Dev Med Child Neurol 1989;31:152–160.

23. Vining EPG, Kwiterovich P, Hsieh S, et al. The effect of the ketogenic diet on plasma cholesterol. Epilepsia 1996;37[Suppl 5]:109.

24. Chesney D, Brouhard BH, Wyllie E, Powaski K. Biochemical abnormalities of the ketogenic diet in children. Clin Pediatr 1999;38:107–109.

25. Delgado MR, Mills J, Sparagana S. Hypercholesterolemia associated with the ketogenic diet. Epilepsia 1996;37[Suppl 5]:108.

26. Demeritte EL, Ventimiglia J, Coyne M, Nigro MA. Organic acid disorders and the ketogenic diet. Ann Neurol 1996;40:305.

27. Rutledge SL, Kinsman SL, Geraghry MT, et al. Hypocarnitinemia and the ketogenic diet. Ann Neurol 1989;26:472.

28. Ballaban-Gil K, Callahan C, O'Dell C, et al. Complications of the ketogenic diet. Epilepsia 1998;39:744–748.

Chapter 31

Vagus Nerve Stimulation for the Treatment of Medically Intractable Epilepsy

Eric B. Geller

Although the majority of people with epilepsy achieve good control of seizures with standard anti-epileptic drugs (AEDs), approximately 25–35% have medically refractory epilepsy.[1] Some of these patients are candidates for neurosurgical intervention, which can offer seizure-free rates of 70% or greater in properly selected cases.[2] However, a significant number of people remain who are not surgical candidates or for whom surgery has failed. Alternative treatment has typically involved trials of medication combinations or enrollment in experimental drug trials. It is in this context that vagus nerve stimulation (VNS) has emerged as a unique alternative therapy for such medically refractory patients. This chapter reviews the preclinical and clinical trial data leading up to U.S. Food and Drug Administration approval and commercial release of VNS in 1997, postmarketing data, and the growing evidence regarding the use of VNS in developmentally disabled (DD) patients.

Background

The idea that afferent stimulation might abort a seizure dates back to ancient Greece.[3] Many of my patients describe various personal techniques that they believe prevent their seizures, such as touching part of the body or employing mental concentration.

The vagus nerve is a mixed nerve containing parasympathetic efferent fibers, approximately 80% of which are sensory fibers that provide the brain with visceral sensory information from the head, neck, thorax, and abdomen.[4] The cell bodies of the vagus nerve fibers are located in the nodose ganglion near the jugular foramen. The first central synapse is in the nucleus tractus solitarius (NTS) of the medulla. The NTS has three main output pathways: feedback loops to the autonomic preganglionic and somatic motor neurons in the medulla and spinal cord; the reticular formation of the medulla; and ascending projections to the forebrain, relayed via the parabrachial nucleus in the dorsal pons. Major forebrain targets include the thalamus, hypothalamus, insula, anterior cingulate, amygdala, and basal forebrain.[4]

In 1938, Bailey and Bremer[5] described the cortical representation of the vagus nerve and noted alteration of the electroencephalogram owing to afferent vagal stimulation. Despite similar reports over the years, it was not until the mid-1980s that VNS was studied as a treatment for epileptic seizures.[6] Numerous animal studies demonstrate that acute vagal stimulation may abort a seizure and chronic, intermittent stimulation may prevent seizures. VNS shows efficacy in multiple animal seizure models, including seizures incited by pentylenetetrazol, maximal electroshock, strychnine, penicillin-induced foci, alumina-gel, and kindling.[6–12] In amygdaloid kindling, an experimental model of temporal lobe epilepsy, VNS retards the development of spontaneous seizures, suggesting an effect on epileptogenesis.[12]

Human Trials of Vagus Nerve Stimulation

The first VNS implants in humans occurred in 1988. The initial pilot studies, termed *E01* and *E02*, were single-blind studies in 14 patients with refractory partial epilepsy.[13] These studies suggested a reduction in seizures and established the safety of VNS. Safety evaluation included extensive testing with Holter monitoring,[14] electroencephalographic (EEG) scanning,[15] evoked potential testing,[16] and gastric pH monitoring[14] to assess possible adverse effects of VNS. These studies showed no significant effects of stimulation on cardiac or gastric function and no clear changes in EEG recordings or evoked potential results.

These studies led to two major clinical trials (termed *E03* and *E05*), which were multicenter, randomized, double-blind trials.[17–19] Because the patient can feel stimulation, a true inactive placebo arm could not be accomplished in these trials. The trials were designed to test the hypothesis that if stimulation is effective, more stimulation (i.e., relatively high settings) would be more effective than less stimulation (i.e., relatively low settings). Both trials were similar in their patient population and design. They included patients with medically refractory partial epilepsy who were as young as 12 years. High-stimulation parameters were as follows: 30 Hz, 30 seconds of on time, 5 minutes of off time, and a 500-microsecond pulse width. In contrast, low stimulation consisted of 1 Hz, 30 seconds of on time, 180 minutes of off time, and a 130-microsecond pulse width.[17–19] The strength of the electrical current was titrated to tolerance, in increments of 0.25 mA to a maximum of 3.5 mA. Patients and investigators were blinded to the stimulation protocol used, and an unblinded investigator who was not involved in clinical assessment programmed the stimulator. Similar to many AED studies, a 12-week baseline period was established for seizure counting; then, stimulation was initiated 2 weeks after stimulator implantation and a ramp-up period for the stimulation current, followed by a 14-week study period. After the initial study period, patients were entered into a long-term follow-up study. The E05 trial differed from the E03 trial in excluding nonmotor simple partial seizures from the analysis and excluding patients who had undergone prior epilepsy surgery.[15]

Efficacy was measured as the mean or median reduction in seizure frequency from the baseline period, as well as the percentage of the group experiencing 50% or greater reduction in seizures (the response rate [RR]). The RR has become a popular measure among AED trials, giving an estimate of the chance of significant response and allowing comparison of efficacy among different drugs. The median seizure reduction in the high- and low-stimulation groups was 24.5% versus 6.1% in E03 ($p = .01$)[18] and 28% versus 15% in E05 ($p = .039$).[19] The RR in the high- and low-stimulation groups was 31% versus 13% in E03[18] and 22% versus 16% in E05.[19] Although the low-stimulation group appears to have more than a minimal response, it was not a truly inactive placebo. These studies supported the hypothesis that within the ranges studied, a greater amount of stimulation is more efficacious.

Several studies have looked at the long-term effects of VNS. Efficacy in the extension phase to 12 months after implantation was not only maintained but even increased.[20] Salinsky et al.[20] reported on 100 of the 114 patients in the E03 study who had completed at least 12 months of stimulation. They found median seizure frequency to be reduced by 20% as compared to baseline in the first 3-month period and by 32% in the fourth 3-month period. Amar et al.[3] examined the 1-year follow-up data from 164 patients who completed the open-label, nonblinded extension phase of the E05 study. Median reduction in seizure frequency at 15 months was 45%, the RRs being 39% with greater than 50% reduction, 21% with greater than 75% reduction, and 2% seizure-free. The percentage of patients in the E05 extension phase who were seizure-free for the preceding 6 months increased from 0.5% at 9 months to 2.4% at 15 months, 5.3% at 21 months, and 11.8% at 27 months after implantation.[21] The entire cohort of E01–E05 study participants was examined by Morris et al.[22] A total of 440 patients were followed out to 3 years after stimulator implantation. RRs were 36.8% at 1 year, 43.2% at 2 years, and 42.7% at 3 years. The percentage of patients experiencing side effects decreased over the 3 years, indicating increasing tolerance. Thus, not only was the benefit maintained, but the effect seemed to increase over time. Such findings are extremely important when considering that patients are committing to a device implant with years of battery life.

The E04 study was a compassionate-use trial, which included patients excluded from the E03 and E05 trials, such as children (see later) and patients with generalized epilepsies. The generalized epilepsy group was analyzed by Labar et al.[23] This group of 24 patients had both idiopathic (seven patients) and symptomatic generalized epilepsies. For all seizure types, median seizure reduction was 46%, with an RR of 46%. No significant difference in response among seizure types or epilepsy syndromes was noted. These data demonstrate that patients with generalized epilepsies may experience benefits from VNS similar to the benefits enjoyed by patients with partial epilepsies.

These studies led to the 1997 U.S. approval of the Cyberonics Neurocybernetic Prosthesis system. On the basis of these studies, the official indication is for the treatment of medically refractory partial epilepsy in patients who are at least 12 years old. Since the release of the Neurocybernetic Prosthesis in 1997, several thousand patients have undergone implantation, and numerous postmarketing studies have been published or presented at scientific meetings. The most remarkable feature of the postmarketing experience has been the apparently greater efficacy than was noted in the clinical trials. RRs of 40–60% are routinely reported, with seizure-free rates of 5–10%.[3,21–27] The reasons for such an improvement in efficacy are unclear, although lack of blinding may contribute. Good results with VNS have been reported in patients with generalized epilepsy and children younger than 12 years, groups excluded from the original studies (see later). All seizure types and epilepsy syndromes reported have shown some improvement with VNS.

Although seizure reduction and quality of life are important issues for people with epilepsy, a more important issue is the potential for a foreshortened life span. Annegers et al.[28] studied mortality, particularly sudden unexpected death in epilepsy patients (SUDEP) having VNS for 2 years. Among the group of 1,819 patients, 25 deaths occurred over the 2-year period. The overall mortality in the group was lower than that in other populations with severe epilepsy, and SUDEP rates were lower after 2 years of follow-up. Although not definitive, these results suggest that VNS may protect against the adverse effects of seizures as well as against the seizures themselves.

Efficacy of Vagus Nerve Stimulation in Patients with Developmental Disabilities

People with developmental disabilities and epilepsy have a number of important issues that differ from those in the general epilepsy population. Brain injury or dysfunction of any type may be a risk factor for epilepsy.[1] Patients having such a condition, such as those with the Lennox-Gastaut syndrome, are more likely to have multiple seizure types and may be more prone to injuries from falls during seizures. Patients with baseline cognitive and motor impairments may have a greater sensitivity to the adverse effects of AEDs, especially as polypharmacy frequently is necessary. Compliance with complicated medical regimens puts an increased burden on caregivers and may be especially difficult for DD patients attempting some degree of independence in life skills. Medically refractory DD patients are less likely to be candidates for curative epilepsy surgery, making the use of alternative therapies imperative.

Although VNS has become a popular therapy among the DD population, published studies are few and include only small numbers of subjects. Several studies have looked specifically at patients with the Lennox-Gastaut syndrome.

Thirteen patients (ages 4–44 years) with the Lennox-Gastaut syndrome were treated with VNS and followed up for 6 months.[26] After 6 months, median seizure rate reduction was 52% (range, 0–93%). Three patients had a greater than 90% reduction, two had a greater than 75% reduction, and one had a greater than 50% reduction.

A group of seven patients (ages 4–33 years) with the Lennox-Gastaut syndrome received VNS for 6 months.[24] One became seizure-free, and five had a 60–90% reduction in seizure frequency. Both partial and generalized seizures responded to VNS. Four patients improved with rapid cycling parameters when standard settings were ineffective after 1 month.

Nine children with the Lennox-Gastaut syndrome were similarly studied; seven of nine had a greater than 50% seizure reduction, and one achieved seizure freedom with VNS monotherapy.[29] In yet another study, among five patients with the Lennox-Gastaut syndrome who were followed up for 9 months after VNS, a median seizure reduction of 41% was noted (range, 28–93%), with no patients' seizure frequency worsening.[23] In this group, there was no change in seizure frequency over time, but the benefit occurred early and was maintained for the study period.

An increasing number of studies target VNS in children with epilepsy. Murphy et al.[25,30] studied VNS in 19 children with refractory epilepsy. Mean age at stimulator implantation was 10.2 years (range, 4–19 years), and the mean duration of epilepsy was 8.7 years. All children in the study had severe epilepsy, with 10 experiencing more than one seizure daily and 4 having undergone previous neurosurgical procedures. Primary generalized seizures occurred in 8 patients, whereas 11 had partial seizures. Symptomatic causes of epilepsy included brain tumor, abnormal cortical organization, pachygyria, encephalitis, asphyxia, postpertussis encephalopathy, and Rett syndrome. All the patients had an intelligence quotient of less than 70. In this group, 53% had a greater than 50% reduction in seizures, and 32% had a 90% reduction in seizure frequency. Magnet activation was effective in aborting seizures in five patients, and a change to rapid cycling improved the outcome in four of five patients. The best responders appeared to be those in whom the Lennox-Gastaut syndrome had been diagnosed and children who had failed previous callosotomy. The total number of medications was reduced by 12% after VNS initiation, and monotherapy was achieved in five patients, but in no patients were AEDs eliminated completely. Side effects were similar to those found in adult studies and were well tolerated.

The results of VNS in children younger than 18 years who were enrolled in the E03, E04, and E05 trials have been analyzed separately.[31] Sixty children having a mean age of 13.5 years were enrolled, the youngest being 3.6 years old. The cause of epilepsy was known in 33.3% and was idiopathic in 66.7%. Five patients exited from the study: three owing to lack of efficacy, one because of erosion of the device through the skin, and one owing to death by aspiration pneumonia. Median percentage reduction in seizures was 23% at 3 months after implantation and showed steady improvement over 18 months to 43% reduction.

No significant differences in response on the basis of seizure type, etiology, or age were noted.

VNS may have positive effects on cognition in DD children. In a group of 15 children with epileptic encephalopathies who had VNS for at least 1 year, only a mild (17%) median seizure reduction was observed, but improvement in perceived treatment side effects and general behavior occurred; in six patients, verbal performance improved significantly.[32]

Progressive myoclonic epilepsies are rare conditions characterized by severe intractable seizures and progressive neurologic deterioration, sometimes worsened by certain AEDs. One 34-year-old patient with progressive myoclonic epilepsy of the Unverricht-Lundborg type, at 1-year follow-up after VNS, had a greater than 90% reduction in seizure frequency, and cerebellar ataxia had also improved.[33]

Practical Issues Regarding Vagus Nerve Stimulation in Developmentally Disabled Patients

A number of practical issues related to VNS are encountered in the DD population. Little information on this subject has been published. Consequently, the following are my personal observations from working with many patients with developmental disabilities and epilepsy and their families and caregivers.

A common concern is the assessment of VNS adverse effects in a nonverbal individual. Nonverbal patients cannot communicate pain or discomfort as easily as can verbal patients. The most common side effects related to VNS in the E03 study were hoarseness (37%), throat pain (11%), cough (7%), dyspnea (6%), paresthesia (6%), and muscle pain (6%).[4] Hoarseness is not relevant to nonverbal patients. Cough and alterations of breathing are easily observed. Assessment of more subjective sensations such as paresthesia and pain is more difficult. My experience has been that severely impaired nonverbal individuals will display a change in behavior (e.g., arrest of activity or looking around) when stimulation is initiated; this appears to be a reaction to a novel sensation and disappears quickly. Such patients have expressed discomfort by moaning or becoming agitated; the discomfort resolves rapidly with readjustment of VNS settings. Swallowing generally has not been a problem, but one of my patients had visibly increased drooling with higher VNS settings that resolved with lowering of the stimulation threshold. Because of the limited patient feedback in such individuals, I recommend increasing stimulation very gradually, usually using the lowest current (0.25 mA) initially and increasing only by 0.25 mA at each programming session. If visible side effects occur, the patient is allowed to go home, only if careful observation is possible and if the patient can return to the office on short notice for readjustment if tolerance does not develop adequately.

Some family members have told me that a given patient cannot communicate that pain is occurring. In such a situation, whether VNS is tolerated in the absence of visible side effects cannot be readily discerned. Reassurance can be difficult, and this concern has caused some families to defer VNS implantation. However, most families and caregivers can be reassured that pain, which is rare with VNS in any patient group, can be detected by observing for changes in facial expression (e.g., grimace) or in behavior. Such changes would be temporally linked to stimulation (e.g., once every 5 minutes), further facilitating their detection.

Swallowing may be impaired in patients with severe motor disabilities, and so some patients or their families or caregivers may express concern regarding the potential of VNS to cause aspiration or to increase swallowing difficulties. Schallert et al.[34] used barium swallow studies in eight children to compare swallowing when VNS was off, on, and at maximally tolerated settings. This study found that laryngeal penetration of barium occurred in three patients without stimulation and in one patient with stimulation. Aspiration did not occur in any patient at clinically relevant VNS settings.

Compliance with AED therapy can be difficult at the best of times; in the DD population, these problems may be magnified. Some patients are fully dependent on their families or on institutions for care and may receive medications multiple times per day without difficulty, although this increases the burden on the caregiver. Higher-functioning DD individuals may be attempting a greater degree of independence, either in a group home or in an independent living situation. These people may experience more difficulty managing a complicated medical regimen of two or more medications given two to four times daily. VNS offers a therapy that requires no active compliance by the patient or caregiver, making it an easy addition to the AED regimen.

The magnet activation function of the VNS can be very useful for patients in the DD population. Many such patients may not have an aura or may not be physically capable of using the magnet themselves. However, caregivers can use the magnet to try to abort or shorten seizures or to interrupt seizure clusters. This is particularly useful for patients in a school or workshop setting and may reduce the disruption in a patient's daily activities caused by the seizures. Using the magnet is easy and can be learned in minutes after a simple demonstration. Parents or other immediate caregivers should be instructed in magnet use before hospital discharge after the implant; at our center this is typically done by the epilepsy nurse practitioner. School or workshop personnel can be educated by the family or by outreach programs from an epilepsy center. Cyberonics also provides clinical specialists who can perform this training.

Assessment of efficacy can be challenging in the DD population. Likewise, keeping detailed seizure calendars, particularly if multiple seizure types are present, can be difficult. DD patients may have other paroxysmal behaviors, such as movement disorders or self-stimulatory behaviors, that can be mistaken for seizures. In such a situation, video-EEG monitoring can be extremely helpful in clarifying seizure types and setting appropriate goals for VNS therapy.

Identifying Candidates for Vagus Nerve Stimulation

Proper selection of patients is critical for any antiepileptic therapy. Although VNS appears to provide some benefit for a broad spectrum of epilepsies and seizure types, certain principles are critical in the evaluation.

First, the presence of epilepsy must be confirmed. Other physiologic conditions, such as syncope or movement disorders, may mimic epileptic seizures. Psychogenic nonepileptic seizures are reported to occur in 5–20% of outpatient epilepsy populations and in 10–40% of patients referred to specialty epilepsy centers.[35] If outpatient EEG and magnetic resonance imaging testing is not conclusive, inpatient video-EEG monitoring should be performed to characterize the seizure types and epilepsy syndrome definitively. Patients with surgically amenable lesions that cause partial epilepsy should be identified if possible, as surgical resection can lead to seizure freedom in 60–90% of well-selected patients with mesial temporal sclerosis or other structural lesions.[2] Many patients initially evaluated for epilepsy surgery turn out to be poor candidates, because of either multiple or nonlocalizable foci; these patients may be good candidates for VNS. Some patients may appear to be medically intractable because the wrong AED was used (e.g., carbamazepine for generalized absence epilepsy). In such cases, change of medication may lead to significant seizure improvement.

A reasonable trial of appropriate AED therapy should be attempted before VNS is considered. The definition of *reasonable trial* will vary from patient to patient, depending on seizure frequency, titration schedules, and adverse effects of medication.

Patient education is critical before VNS implantation is attempted. The patient and caregivers must be told of the potential benefits, based on prior experience, and be aware of potential adverse effects, both stimulation- and surgery-related. Cyberonics has produced a patient education videotape, which is useful in giving the patient an overview of VNS prior to the discussion with the physician or epilepsy nurse. Patient-to-patient contact is extremely useful, as it allows the patient considering VNS to ask questions of someone who has already undergone the implantation procedure, to see the actual scarring produced by the incisions, and to hear the effect on the voice.

Because the published data indicates continued improvement over time, I ask my patients to commit to VNS therapy for at least 1 year before considering an explant for lack of efficacy. I also advise them that prior to explantation, I recommend that the patient allow a several-month trial period, during which the device is shut off to determine whether the patient's condition worsens without use of VNS.

The patient and physician must jointly set goals for VNS therapy before implantation. Clear goals make assessment of efficacy easier and allow the patient to have realistic expectations prior to undergoing surgical implantation. Although reduction in seizure frequency is always an important goal, reduction in dose and number of AEDs often is desired as well and may be achieved without worsening of seizure frequency or severity.

Conclusion

VNS is a unique therapy for medically resistant epilepsy. Efficacy has been demonstrated in both partial and generalized epilepsies and in all age groups. The profile of adverse effects differs from that of AEDs, and VNS generally is well tolerated. VNS offers the opportunity to terminate seizures using magnet activation. DD patients may benefit from VNS, but specific issues among this patient population must be addressed prior to and after stimulator implantation.

References

1. Annegers JF. Epidemiology and genetics of epilepsy. Neurol Clin 1994;12:15–29.
2. Doyle WK, Spencer DD. Anterior Temporal Resections. In J Engel Jr, TA Pedley (eds), Epilepsy: A Comprehensive Textbook. Philadelphia: Lippincott–Raven, 1997;1807–1817.
3. Amar AP, DeGiorgio CM, Tarver WB, Apuzzo ML. Long-term multicenter experience with vagus nerve stimulation for intractable partial seizures. Results of the XE5 trial. Stereotact Funct Neurosurg 1999;73:104–108.
4. Schachter SC, Saper CB. Vagus nerve stimulation. Epilepsia 1998;39:677–686.
5. Bailey P, Bremer F. A sensory cortical representation of the vagus nerve. J Neurophysiol 1983;1:405–412.
6. Zabara J. Inhibition of experimental seizures in canines by repetitive vagal stimulation. Epilepsia 1992;33:1005–1012.
7. McLachlan RS. Suppression of interictal spikes and seizures by stimulation of the vagus nerve. Epilepsia 1993;34:918–923.
8. Woodbury JW, Woodbury DM. Effects of vagal stimulation on experimentally induced seizures in rats. Epilepsia 1990;31[Suppl 2]:S7–S19.
9. Woodbury JW, Woodbury DM. Vagal stimulation reduces the severity of maximal electroshock seizures in intact rats: use of a cuff electrode for stimulating and recording. Pacing Clin Electrophysiol 1991;14:94–107.

10. Lockard JS, Congdon WC, DuCharme LL. Feasibility and safety of vagal stimulation in monkey model. Epilepsia 1990;31[Suppl 2]:S20–S26.

11. Takaya M, Terry WJ, Naritoku DK. Vagus nerve stimulation induces a sustained anticonvulsant effect. Epilepsia 1996;37:1111–1116.

12. Fernandez-Guardiola A, Martinez A, Valdes-Cruz A, et al. Vagus nerve prolonged stimulation in cats: effects on epileptogenesis (amygdala electrical kindling). Behavioral and electrographic effects. Epilepsia 1999;40:822–829.

13. Uthman BM, Wilder BJ, Penry JK, et al. Treatment of epilepsy by stimulation of the vagus nerve. Neurology 1993;43:1338–1345.

14. Ramsay RE, Uthman BM, Augustinsson LE, et al. Vagus nerve stimulation for treatment of partial seizures: 2. Safety, side effects, and tolerability. Epilepsia 1994;35:627–636.

15. Hammond EJ, Uthman BM, Reid SA, Wilder BJ. Electrophysiological studies of cervical vagus nerve stimulation in humans: I. EEG effects. Epilepsia 1992;33:1013–1020.

16. Hammond EJ, Uthman BM, Reid SA, Wilder BJ. Electrophysiological studies of cervical vagus nerve stimulation in humans: II. Evoked potentials. Epilepsia 1992;33:1021–1028.

17. Ben-Menachem E, Manon-Espaillat R, Ristanovic R, et al. Vagus nerve stimulation for treatment of partial seizures: 1. A controlled study of effect on seizures. Epilepsia 1994;35:616–626.

18. The Vagus Nerve Stimulation Study Group. A randomized controlled trial of chronic vagus nerve stimulation for treatment of medically intractable seizures. Neurology 1995;45:224–230.

19. Handforth A, DeGiorgio CM, Schachter SC, et al. Vagus nerve stimulation therapy for partial-onset seizures. A randomized active-control trial. Neurology 1998;51:48–55.

20. Salinsky MC, Uthman BM, Ristanovic RK, et al. Vagus nerve stimulation for the treatment of medically intractable seizures: results of a 1-year open-extension trial. Arch Neurol 1996;53:1176–1180.

21. Morris GL, Pallagi J, Vagus Nerve Study Group. Seizure freedom analysis on 195 refractory epilepsy patients receiving vagus nerve stimulation therapy. Neurology 1999;52[Suppl 2]:A239.

22. Morris GL 3rd, Mueller WM. Long-term treatment with vagus nerve stimulation in patients with refractory epilepsy. The Vagus Nerve Stimulation Study Group E01–E05. Neurology 1999;53:1731–1735.

23. Labar D, Nikolov B, Tarver B, Fraser R. Vagus nerve stimulation for symptomatic generalized epilepsy: a pilot study. Epilepsia 1998;39:201–205.

24. Helmers SL, Al-Jayyousi M, Madsen J. Adjunctive treatment in Lennox-Gastaut syndrome using vagal nerve stimulation. Epilepsia 1998;39[Suppl 6]:169.

25. Hornig GW, Murphy JV, Schallert G, Tilton C. Left vagus nerve stimulation in children with refractory epilepsy: an update. South Med J 1997;90:484–488.

26. Hosain S, Nikalov B, Harden C, Fraser R. Vagus nerve stimulation treatment for Lennox-Gastaut syndrome. J Child Neurol 2000;15:509–512.

27. Labar D, Murphy J, Tecoma E, E04 VNS Study Group. Vagus nerve stimulation for medication-resistant generalized epilepsy. Neurology 1999;52:1510–1512.

28. Annegers JF, Coan SP, Hauser WA, Leestma J. Epilepsy, vagal nerve stimulation by the NCP system, all-cause mortality, and sudden, unexpected, unexplained death. Epilepsia 2000;41:549–553.

29. Murphy JV, Hornig G. Chronic intermittent stimulation of the left vagal nerve in nine children with Lennox-Gastaut syndrome. Epilepsia 1998;39[Suppl 6]:169.

30. Murphy JV, Hornig GW, Schallert G. Left vagal nerve stimulation in children with refractory epilepsy. Arch Neurol 1995;52:886–889.

31. Murphy JV. Left vagal nerve stimulation in children with medically refractory epilepsy. The Pediatric VNS Study Group. J Pediatr 1999;134:563–566.

32. Parker AP, Polkey CE, Binnie CD, Madigan C. Vagal nerve stimulation in epileptic encephalopathies. Pediatrics 1999;103:778–782.

33. Smith B, Shatz R, Elisevich K, et al. Effects of vagus nerve stimulation on progressive myoclonus epilepsy of Unverricht-Lundborg type. Epilepsia 2000;41:1046–1048.

34. Schallert G, Foster J, Lindquist N, Murphy JV. Chronic stimulation of the left vagus nerve in children: effect on swallowing. Epilepsia 1998;39:1113–1114.

35. Alper K. Nonepileptic seizures. Neurol Clin 1994;12:153–173.

Chapter 32

Developmental Disabilities and Epilepsy Surgery

Edwin Liu and Michael Duchowny

Developmental disabilities frequently complicate the management of chronic epilepsy in childhood. The impact of physical and mental disability on the medical management of epilepsy has been reviewed in several recent articles.[1,2] For several reasons, however, a bias has developed against surgical therapy for patients with intractable epilepsy and significant developmental disabilities. This bias is unfortunate, as early seizure freedom typically improves the overall quality of life for handicapped individuals and their families, particularly for infants with catastrophic epilepsy.

Although developmental disabilities often complicate surgical management, they are rarely an absolute barrier to surgery. In this chapter, we review the influence of developmental disabilities on the surgical management of patients with pharmacoresistant seizures, including the identification of potential surgical candidates, the presurgical workup, the surgical procedures, and the implications for developmental outcome.

Definitions and Epidemiology

The Developmental Disabilities Assistance and Bill of Rights Act defined a *developmental disability* as a severe, chronic disability that is found in an individual 5 years of age or older and is attributable to a mental or physical impairment or combination of mental and physical impairments. The disability must manifest before age 22 years, be permanent, and result in substantial functional limitation in three or more of the following areas of major life activity: (1) self-care, (2) receptive and expressive language, (3) learning, (4) mobility, (5) self-direction, (6) capacity for independent living, and (7) economic self-sufficiency. The disability also should reflect an affected individual's need for a combination and sequence of special, interdisciplinary, or generic services, supports, or other assistance that is lifelong or of extended duration. This definition, therefore, includes the broad categories of cerebral palsy, mental retardation, and pervasive developmental delay as well as selective severe impairments of sensory function or communication. Etiologies that commonly result in developmental disabilities and intractable epilepsy include prenatal, perinatal, or postnatal hypoxic-ischemic insults or vascular events, malformations of brain development, early traumatic brain injury, neonatal meningitis, and chromosomal or metabolic disorders.[3,4]

In addition, the catastrophic childhood epilepsies or epileptic encephalopathies—such as early infantile epileptic encephalopathy (Ohtahara's syndrome),[5] infantile spasms (West's syndrome), the Lennox-Gastaut syndrome, or the severe myoclonic epilepsies—typically cause very frequent and severe seizures associated with significant developmental delay or deterioration. Table 32-1 categorizes the various etiologies based on the time of occurrence and the potential for surgical treatment. For purposes of this review, we extend

Table 32-1. Common Etiologies of Epilepsy and Developmental Disabilities

Potentially surgically treatable
   Prenatal: malformations of cortical development
      Focal cortical dysplasia
      Focal pachygyria, polymicrogyria
      Focal schizencephaly
   Hemimegalencephaly: neurocutaneous syndromes
      Tuberous sclerosis
      Sturge-Weber syndrome
   Perinatal
      Periventricular leukomalacia
      Stroke
      Neonatal meningitis
   Postnatal
      Stroke
      Traumatic brain injury
      Viral or bacterial meningitis
      Catastrophic childhood epilepsies
         Ohtahara's syndrome
         Infantile spasms
         Lennox-Gastaut syndrome
Not surgically treatable (prenatal)
   Diffuse malformations of cortical development
      Lissencephaly
      Aicardi's syndrome
      Holoprosencephaly
   Chromosomal disorders
      Rett syndrome
      Angelman's syndrome
   Metabolic disorders
      Neuronal ceroid lipofuscinosis
      Peroxisomal disorders
      Pyridoxine deficiency
      Mitochondrial encephalomyopathies
      Alpers' disease
      Glucose transporter defects
Progressive myoclonic encephalopathies

our observations to include children younger than age 5 (see Table 32-1).

Developmental disabilities are present in 20–35% of all children with epilepsy[6–8] and in the majority (61%) of children with intractable epilepsy.[9] Numerous studies have shown that seizures are more likely to begin earlier, to be of greater severity, and to be refractory to medical treatment in individuals with disabilities.[10–17] For example, studies have found that 50–69% of disabled individuals have seizures that were refractory to medication after 5 years, whereas only 26–31% of patients who were free of disability still experienced refractory seizures after a similar period.[13,15] In a Swedish study of 195 children with active epilepsy who were followed up for 12 years, those without a neurologic deficit had an annual remission rate of 13%, whereas those with disabilities had a remission rate of 3%.[12] Similarly, in a study of 145 children with seizures refractory to therapy for at least 2 years, Huttenlocher and Hapke[9] found a remission rate of 4.0% in those with intelligence quotients greater than 70 and a rate of 1.5% in those with intelligence quotients of less than 70.[9] The discrepancy is even greater when seizures begin within the first year of life.[18] Finally, even when seizure control is achieved, a higher rate of relapse after discontinuation of antiepileptic medication occurs in children with disabilities (Figure 32-1).[19]

Conversely, developmental disabilities are more likely to be severe if seizures are present.[20–22] Among children with profound mental retardation, 59% have epilepsy, whereas only 8% with mild retardation are epileptic.[20] Furthermore, among individuals with epilepsy, handicaps are much more likely to be multiple.[20,23–26] Steffenburg et al.[23] found that 69% of children with epilepsy and mental retardation had at least one additional diagnosis of cerebral palsy, visual impairment, or autism. In the case of the catastrophic epilepsies, often pronounced deterioration of mental function is coincident to the onset of seizures and severe interictal electroencephalographic (EEG) abnormalities. Several studies of adrenocorticotropic hormone treatment for infantile spasms found a poorer developmental outcome in patients with a longer interval between the onset of spasms and initiation of treatment,[27,28] although some researchers found this only among cryptogenic cases.[29,30] Whether this supports the view that, under certain circumstances, seizure duration affects developmental outcome and whether subtler degrees of cognitive decline also may be seen in other chronic epilepsies remains controversial.[31]

Identification of Surgical Candidates

Several potential obstacles might hinder referral of patients with developmental disabilities for surgical evaluation. Clinicians may adopt a nihilistic attitude, harboring the belief that epilepsy surgery would be a "heroic effort" in these individuals because of their limited life expectancy or nursing a misperception that the impact of seizure freedom on the quality of life is minimal. In our opinion, this view is unjustified for a number of reasons. Predicting developmental outcome can be difficult in significantly handicapped individuals, particularly in infants and young children, the group for which surgery is most likely to have maximal benefit. Clinicians' perceptions of outcome in developmentally handicapped individuals often are unduly pessimistic and likely to bias treatment decisions negatively.[32] A 1977 survey found that more than one-half of pediatricians would not support high-risk surgery in children with Down syndrome,[33] yet our experience suggests that a reduction in the frequency of seizures in patients with epilepsy, even devastated individuals, often has a positive impact on the quality of life of the child and caregivers. In addition, as we discuss later, evidence suggests that early surgical intervention may improve long-term developmental outcome.[34–36] For this reason, the potential for poor developmental outcome should prompt more urgent consideration of surgical therapy.

The decision to perform surgery in developmentally disabled patients is influenced also by the assumption that global disability is a marker for generalized or multifocal pathology that is not amenable to surgery. For this reason, early advocates of epilepsy surgery argued that the presence of mental retardation was a strict contraindication.[37,38] More recently, the pendulum has swung back with the realization that such fears are unfounded. Although it is likely that, as a group, individuals with disabilities have more diffuse pathology, when a single epileptic focus can be identified, data from both adult and pediatric epilepsy surgery centers have failed to demonstrate a clinically significant correlation between overall intelligence quotient and seizure outcome.[39–42]

Furthermore, even when diffuse or multifocal abnormalities are documented, seizure control may be achieved after focal resection. Through functional imaging and surgical outcome, secondary generalized seizures arising from a single focus have been documented in some patients with infantile spasms[43] and Ohtahara's syn-

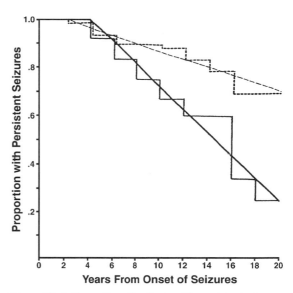

Figure 32-1. Proportion of patients with persistent seizures (>1/year) as a function of follow-up from onset of seizures (life-table method). Solid lines represent a group with intelligence quotient ≥70; stippled lines represent a group with intelligence quotient <70. (Reprinted from PR Huttenlocher, RJ Hapke. A follow-up study of intractable seizures in childhood [see comments]. Ann Neurol 1990;28[5]:699–705, with permission.)

drome.[44] Multifocal disorders, such as tuberous sclerosis[45,46] or periventricular leukomalacia[47] have also been linked to a single region of seizure onset. Finally, even multiple potential seizure foci may respond to palliative procedures, such as corpus callosotomy.[48]

The identification of surgical candidates with disabilities follows the same principles as those for other candidates, including documentation of medical intractability, evaluation of psychological preparedness of the individual and family, identification of the seizure focus, and overlap with eloquent cortical regions. For disabled patients, discussion of the goals and expected outcome of surgery is especially important so that clinicians and family may assess the risks and benefits. Can prolonged seizure freedom reasonably be expected, or is the procedure for palliative purposes? Is an improvement in developmental outcome expected? Are any functional deficits expected? Procedures that may be unacceptable in healthy individuals because of incomplete or transient seizure freedom or functional deficit might be worthwhile in the developmentally disabled population if developmental outcome might be improved.

Presurgical Workup

The presence of developmental disabilities adds complexity to the presurgical workup. The basic approach is similar to that for nondisabled patients and includes psychological and neuropsychological assessment, structural and functional imaging studies, noninvasive and invasive electrophysiologic investigations, and functional mapping studies. The presence of developmental disabilities also mandates that other factors be excluded. Metabolic and chromosomal disorders must be screened, as they contraindicate surgery or affect management decisions (e.g., the choice of surgical procedure, prognosis). One should not be deterred by a preexisting diagnosis of perinatal asphyxia or viral meningitis, as these terms often are applied when no other etiology is readily apparent. The presence of dysmorphic features, particularly if multiple, should prompt a thorough genetic evaluation. Clues to the presence of a metabolic disorder include progressive deterioration in development, microcephaly or macrocephaly, ophthalmic or cutaneous lesions, a family history of similarly affected individuals, and unusual magnetic resonance imaging abnormalities, including whitematter changes or progressive cerebral atrophy. Psychomotor regression also may accompany the severe or progressive myoclonic epilepsies. The genes for many of these disorders recently have been mapped, facilitating diagnosis and genetic counseling.[49]

Common metabolic or chromosomal causes of intractable epilepsy that should be considered include the neuronal ceroid lipofuscinoses (NCLs),[50] peroxisomal[51] and mitochondrial disorders,[52] Alpers' disease,[53] and Angelman's[54] and Rett syndromes.[55] Consideration should be given to screening for disorders that may lead to severe epilepsy and developmental delay but are not typically included in standard metabolic batteries: Examples are a urine dipstick for sulfite oxidase or molybdenum cofactor deficiency,[56] a trial of pyridoxine,[57] very long chain–fatty acid assessment, spinal fluid evaluation for hypoglycorrhachia due to a glucose transporter defect,[58] buffy coat evalua-

tion for NCL,[59] or muscle biopsy for mitochondrial disorders. The presence of cortical dysplasia does not a priori exclude an inborn error of metabolism, as developmental brain malformations may be seen in peroxisomal disorders and nonketotic hyperglycinemia, among others.

Issues surrounding maturation and plasticity render the neuropsychological evaluation of developmentally disabled individuals unreliable for purposes of localization. Nonetheless, a baseline evaluation of developmental, cognitive, and adaptive abilities is important. Accurate assessment of baseline deficits is required to aid in planning surgery that could result in further deficits, to assist clinicians in making a realistic prognosis for developmental outcome, and to provide a baseline for follow-up evaluations. Close attention must be paid to the proper choice of testing instruments in young, very low-functioning, or physically handicapped individuals.

Neuroradiologic studies provide important information for selecting candidates and planning surgery, particularly in the developmentally disabled who have a higher incidence of multifocal pathology. Searching for abnormalities outside the seizure focus is important, particularly in the contralateral hemisphere, as the demonstration of contralateral activation predicts poor long-term seizure outcome. However, multifocal abnormalities do not preclude the possibility of a single epileptic focus. In tuberous sclerosis, for example, although radiographic abnormalities often are multifocal, affected patients' habitual seizures often originate from a single tuber. In these cases, limited focal resections can result in a long-term seizure-free outcome.[45,46] Magnetic resonance imaging may aid in identifying the epileptogenic tuber, which usually is the largest and often is calcified.[60]

Nuclear medicine studies (e.g., single-photon emission computed tomography or positron emission tomography) are useful in the presurgical evaluation but must be interpreted cautiously in handicapped individuals, because metabolic or structural abnormalities of the brain may cause alterations in cerebral blood flow or metabolism unrelated to the seizure focus.[61] In addition, structural asymmetries may not allow for comparisons with the contralateral side. In certain instances, comparison of ictal and interictal studies may clarify confounding factors. Occasionally, however, very electrically active dysplastic lesions may be paradoxically hyperperfused interictally.[62] Obtaining true "ictal" single-photon emission computed tomographic studies may be difficult in the catastrophic childhood epilepsies characterized by brief seizures that preclude timely ictal injection of isotope. In infantile spasms, seizures may occur repetitively or in clusters for several minutes. Anecdotal experience suggests that injecting during a cluster still may be useful, although such a conclusion awaits further analysis.

Video-EEG monitoring of developmentally disabled individuals is especially challenging, because behavioral problems and cognitive deficits often lead to logistical problems in the monitoring. The pulling off of wires and electrodes by a patient can render recordings uninterpretable, and special precautions are required to prevent a patient's strangulation on cables or explantation of invasive electrodes. A parent or guardian should be in the room at all times. For ethical reasons, we do not employ physical restraints.

Deficits of communication may limit the ability of developmentally disabled individuals to describe experiential phenomena, such as auras; therefore, the video record must be reviewed closely for localizing behavioral correlates. These correlates might include running to the parent, a fearful facial expression, or crying in response to an aura; slow tracking movements of the eyes or head in response to a visual aura; grabbing or pointing to the ear in response to an auditory hallucination; or gagging and drooling due to insular involvement.

The interpretation of the ictal and interictal EEG recording is complicated by the diverse seizure symptomatology in developmentally disabled patients. Symptoms include polymorphous patterns of infantile or axial spasms, tonic or atonic seizures, and drop attacks. Although seizures may be generalized secondarily, their spread typically is rapid, and evidence of focalization often is subtle. Interictally, epileptiform features may exist multifocally or in a hypsarrhythmic or suppression-burst pattern. The focus may be inferred only by a consistent asymmetry of clinical or electrographic features or by the coexistence of partial seizures.[63–66]

In evaluating electrophysiologic data, the practitioner must bear in mind several points with regard to the developmentally disabled population. First, an EEG study may offer clues to etiology. Characteristic rhythmic epileptiform discharges or continuous epileptiform discharges occur in focal cortical dysplastic lesions.[67] Several genetic and metabolic disorders have distinctive interictal EEG patterns, such as notched rhythmic delta in Angelman's syndrome,[68] central spikes in Rett syndrome,[69] delta brushlike complexes in Alpers' disease,[70] progressive flattening of the EEG recording in infantile NCL,[71] or giant visual evoked potentials during low-frequency photic stimulation in late infantile NCL.[72] Attention to these possibilities, which may have been overlooked in the metabolic screen, is critical, as most represent contraindications to surgery. Concomitant nonepileptic events, such as stereotypies, breath-holding or hyperventilation spells, self-stimulatory or masturbatory behaviors, staring spells, or even pseudoseizures, are not uncommon in mentally subnormal patients and may have to be clarified by video-EEG monitoring.[73,74]

Mapping of functional cortex presents a number of problems unique to the developmentally disabled. Owing to the complex interplay between developmental lesions and plasticity, localization based on anatomic landmarks is particularly unreliable. Localization of language function in patients with cortical lesions, for example, has been found to depend on the type and timing of the lesions. Specifically, developmental tumors or cortical dysplasias do not displace language cortex, whereas destructive lesions acquired before age 5 may force relocation of function.[75] Problems of localization are compounded by the often poor cooperation of patients during functional studies, such as intra-arterial amobarbital testing or functional magnetic resonance imaging. Despite these difficulties, extraoperative mapping with invasive electrodes often is unnecessary. In those younger than age 5, the potential for language relocation obviates the need for language mapping. In addition, the presence of baseline deficits, such as a hemiparesis, renders mapping of the motor cortex moot. In rare circumstances, however, motor or language deficits are fully reversible, as they result from frequent epileptiform activity. This possibility should be suspected when the deficit fluctuates with the severity of the seizures.

Impact of Developmental Disabilities on the Surgical Procedure

A number of special considerations must be made in planning epilepsy surgery for individuals with developmental disabilities. Because epileptogenic zones frequently are widespread, resections often are more extensive than in other patient populations—a point emphasized by the fact that hemispherectomies are restricted almost exclusively to this patient group. This may force a decision regarding whether to sacrifice functional cortex or to perform an incomplete resection.

Multiple subpial transection offers an alternative option for epileptogenic regions that overlap sensorimotor or language cortex.[76–81] This technique has found a particular niche in the surgical treatment of children with severe communicative disorders resulting from frequent epileptiform activity, such as occurs in Landau-Kleffner syndrome or continuous spike and wave activity during slow-wave sleep.[82,83] Corpus callosotomy may be considered when diffuse or rapid secondarily generalized tonic or atonic seizures are present.

The issue of the timing is particularly germane to epilepsy surgery in the developmentally disabled. Because seizures present earlier in this population and are more severe and refractory, surgical intervention often is contemplated during the first year of life. Surgery at this age, however—particularly large resections or hemispherectomies—is technically demanding and carries a greater risk of complication. Localization of the focus, both electrographically and radiologically, also is challenging. Focal abnormalities frequently manifest electrographically as diffuse or hypsarrhythmic patterns. Radiographic findings in lesions, such as cortical dysplasias, often are subtle or absent in the first few months of life when myelinization still is largely incomplete.[84]

Balancing the disadvantages of early surgical intervention are issues of plasticity and development. The degree of recovery of cortical functions after postnatal insults is greater when the insult occurs at a young age, a finding attributed to a greater plasticity of the immature brain.[85] Thus, functional deficits after cortical resections may be minimized if performed earlier. In addition, early seizures may have adverse consequences on brain development. Because synaptogenesis and synaptic pruning continue well into the first year of postnatal life,[86] frequent seizure activity during this period may disrupt these processes and result in the formation of aberrant cortical circuitry. Possible evidence for this includes the high incidence of poor developmental outcomes after infantile spasms.[29,30,87] The small minority of children with normal outcomes after infantile spasms invariably prove to have spasms that were treated quickly and resolved rapidly.[87]

On the basis of these observations, earlier referral for epilepsy surgery in infants who fail to respond to medical therapy may improve developmental outcomes. In their study of infants undergoing hemispherectomy for intractable infantile spasms, for example, Asarnow et al.[36] found a significant increase in developmental levels at 2-year follow-up as compared to preoperative testing. These authors noted also a trend for better outcomes among those operated on at an earlier age. Studies such as these, however, are significantly constrained by the difficulties involved in identifying both adequate controls and appropriate testing instruments. Further studies are required before these conclusions can be accepted widely.

Conclusion

A high incidence of developmental disabilities is seen among children with epilepsy and, in particular, in those who have medically refractory seizures and are considered for epilepsy surgery. When coexistent, seizures and disabilities typically are more severe and thus may have a considerable impact on quality of life. Recognition of these factors has superseded historical concerns regarding candidacy of severely disabled patients for epilepsy surgery. This change has brought to the fore the important question of whether timely surgical intervention also may alter the natural history of developmental outcomes. The positive experience with early epilepsy surgery in the catastrophic childhood epilepsies has yielded tantalizing results, although further data clearly are needed.

References

1. Coulter DL. Comprehensive management of epilepsy in persons with mental retardation. Epilepsia 1997;38[Suppl 4]:S24–S31.
2. Sunder TR. Meeting the challenge of epilepsy in persons with multiple handicaps. J Child Neurol 1997;12[Suppl 1]:S38–S43.
3. Steffenburg U, Hagberg G, Kyllerman M. Active epilepsy in mentally retarded children: II. Etiology and

reduced pre- and perinatal optimality. Acta Paediatr 1995;84(10):1153–1159.

4. Chevrie JJ, Aicardi J. Convulsive disorders in the first year of life: etiologic factors. Epilepsia 1977;18(4):489–498.

5. Ohtahara S, Ohtsuka Y, Yamatogi Y, et al. Early-Infantile Epileptic Encephalopathy with Suppression-Bursts. In J Roger, M Bureau, CH Dravet, et al. (eds), Epileptic Syndromes in Infancy, Childhood, and Adolescence (2nd ed). London: John Libbey, 1992;25–34

6. Murphy CC, Trevathan E, Yeargin-Allsopp M. Prevalence of epilepsy and epileptic seizures in 10-year-old children: results from the Metropolitan Atlanta Developmental Disabilities Study. Epilepsia 1995;36(9):866–872.

7. von Wendt L, Rantakallio P, Saukkonen AL, Makinen H. Epilepsy and associated handicaps in a 1 year birth cohort in northern Finland. Eur J Pediatr 1985;144(2):149–151.

8. Sillanpaa M. Medico-social prognosis of children with epilepsy. Epidemiological study and analysis of 245 patients. Acta Paediatr Scand Suppl 1973;237:3–104.

9. Huttenlocher PR, Hapke RJ. A follow-up study of intractable seizures in childhood (see comments). Ann Neurol 1990;28(5):699–705.

10. Steffenburg U, Hagberg G, Kyllerman M. Characteristics of seizures in a population-based series of mentally retarded children with active epilepsy. Epilepsia 1996;37(9):850–856.

11. Aksu F. Nature and prognosis of seizures in patients with cerebral palsy. Dev Med Child Neurol 1990;32(8):661–668.

12. Brorson LO, Wranne L. Long-term prognosis in childhood epilepsy: survival and seizure prognosis. Epilepsia 1987;28(4):324–330.

13. Roger J, Dravet C, Menendez P, Bureau M. [The partial epilepsies in childhood—evolution and prognosis factors.] Rev Electroencephalogr Neurophysiol Clin 1981;11(3–4):431–437.

14. Shafer SQ, Hauser WA, Annegers JF, Klass DW. EEG and other early predictors of epilepsy remission: a community study. Epilepsia 1988;29(5):590–600.

15. Annegers JF, Hauser WA, Elveback LR. Remission of seizures and relapse in patients with epilepsy. Epilepsia 1979;20(6):729–737.

16. Matricardi M, Brinciotti M, Benedetti P. Outcome after discontinuation of antiepileptic drug therapy in children with epilepsy. Epilepsia 1989;30(5):582–589.

17. Todt H. The late prognosis of epilepsy in childhood: results of a prospective follow-up study. Epilepsia 1984;25(2):137–144.

18. Matsumoto A, Watanabe K, Sugiura M, et al. Etiologic factors and long-term prognosis of convulsive disorders in the first year of life. Neuropediatrics 1983;14(4):231–234.

19. Thurston JH, Thurston DL, Hixon BB, Keller AJ. Prognosis in childhood epilepsy: additional follow-up of 148 children 15 to 23 years after withdrawal of anticonvulsant therapy. N Engl J Med 1982;306(14):831–836.

20. Trevathan E, Yeargin-Allsop M, Murphy CC, Ding G. Epilepsy among children with mental retardation. Ann Neurol 1988;24:321.

21. Sillanpaa M. The significance of motor handicap in the prognosis of childhood epilepsy. Dev Med Child Neurol 1975;17(1):52–57.

22. Richardson SA, Koller H, Katz M, McLaren J. Seizures and epilepsy in a mentally retarded population over the first 22 years of life. Appl Res Ment Retard 1980;1(1–2):123–138.

23. Steffenburg U, Hagberg G, Viggedal G, Kyllerman M. Active epilepsy in mentally retarded children: I. Prevalence and additional neuro-impairments. Acta Paediatr 1995;84(10):1147–1152.

24. Steffenburg S, Gillberg C, Steffenburg U. Psychiatric disorders in children and adolescents with mental retardation and active epilepsy. Arch Neurol 1996;53(9):904–912.

25. Aicardi J. Epilepsy in brain-injured children. Dev Med Child Neurol 1990;32(3):191–202.

26. Zafeiriou DI, Kontopoulos EE, Tsikoulas I. Characteristics and prognosis of epilepsy in children with cerebral palsy. J Child Neurol 1999;14(5):289–294.

27. Heiskala H, Riikonen R, Santavuori P, et al. West syndrome: individualized ACTH therapy. Brain Dev 1996;18(6):456–460.

28. Riikonen R. Long-term outcome of West syndrome: a study of adults with a history of infantile spasms. Epilepsia 1996;37(4):367–372.

29. Koo B, Hwang PA, Logan WJ. Infantile spasms: outcome and prognostic factors of cryptogenic and symptomatic groups. Neurology 1993;43(11):2322–2327.

30. Matsumoto A, Watanabe K, Negoro T, et al. Long-term prognosis after infantile spasms: a statistical study of prognostic factors in 200 cases. Dev Med Child Neurol 1981;23(1):51–65.

31. Holmes GL. Do seizures cause brain damage? Epilepsia 1991;32[Suppl 5]:S14–S28.

32. Wolraich ML, Siperstein GN, O'Keefe P. Pediatricians' perceptions of mentally retarded individuals. Pediatrics 1987;80(5):643–649.

33. Todres ID, Krane D, Howell MC, Shannon DC. Pediatricians' attitudes affecting decision-making in defective newborns. Pediatrics 1977;60(2):197–201.

34. Duchowny MS, Resnick TJ, Alvarez LA, Morrison G. Focal resection for malignant partial seizures in infancy. Neurology 1990;40(6):980–984.

35. Wyllie E. Surgery for catastrophic localization-related epilepsy in infants. Epilepsia 1996;37[Suppl 1]:S22–S25.

36. Asarnow RF, LoPresti C, Guthrie D, et al. Developmental outcomes in children receiving resection surgery for medically intractable infantile spasms. Dev Med Child Neurol 1997;39(7):430–440.

37. Falconer MA. Reversibility by temporal-lobe resection of the behavioral abnormalities of temporal-lobe epilepsy. N Engl J Med 1973;289(9):451–455.

38. Rasmussen T. Surgical treatment of patients with complex partial seizures. Adv Neurol 1975;11:415–449.

39. Chelune GJ, Naugle RI, Hermann BP, et al. Does presurgical IQ predict seizure outcome after temporal lobectomy? Evidence from the Bozeman Epilepsy Consortium. Epilepsia 1998;39(3):314–318.

40. Dodrill CB, Wilkus RJ, Ojemann GA, et al. Multidisciplinary prediction of seizure relief from cortical resection surgery. Ann Neurol 1986;20(1):2–12.

41. Gleissner U, Johanson K, Helmstaedter C, Elger CE. Surgical outcome in a group of low-IQ patients with focal epilepsy. Epilepsia 1999;40(5):553–559.

42. Paolicchi JM, Jayakar P, Dean P, et al. Predictors of outcome in pediatric epilepsy surgery. Neurology 2000;54(3):642–647.

43. Chugani HT, Shields WD, Shewmon DA, et al. Infantile spasms: I. PET identifies focal cortical dysgenesis in cryptogenic cases for surgical treatment. Ann Neurol 1990;27(4):406–413.

44. Pedespan JM, Loiseau H, Vital A, et al. Surgical treatment of an early epileptic encephalopathy with suppression-bursts and focal cortical dysplasia. Epilepsia 1995;36(1):37–40.

45. Guerreiro MM, Andermann F, Andermann E, et al. Surgical treatment of epilepsy in tuberous sclerosis: strategies and results in 18 patients. Neurology 1998;51(5):1263–1269.

46. Bebin EM, Kelly PJ, Gomez MR. Surgical treatment for epilepsy in cerebral tuberous sclerosis. Epilepsia 1993;34(4):651–657.

47. Wyllie E, Comair Y, Ruggieri P, et al. Epilepsy surgery in the setting of periventricular leukomalacia and focal cortical dysplasia. Neurology 1996;46(3):839–841.

48. Carmant L, Holmes GL. Commissurotomies in children. J Child Neurol 1994;9[Suppl 2]:50–60.

49. Serratosa JM, Gardiner RM, Lehesjoki AE, et al. The molecular genetic bases of the progressive myoclonus epilepsies. Adv Neurol 1999;79:383–398.

50. Dyken PR. The neuronal ceroid lipofuscinoses. J Child Neurol 1989;4(3):165–174.

51. Moser HW. Peroxisomal disorders. Semin Pediatr Neurol 1996;3(4):298–304.

52. DiMauro S, Ricci E, Hirano M, DeVivo DC. Epilepsy in mitochondrial encephalomyopathies. Epilepsy Res Suppl 1991;4:173–180.

53. Harding BN. Progressive neuronal degeneration of childhood with liver disease (Alpers-Huttenlocher syndrome): a personal review. J Child Neurol 1990;5(4):273–287.

54. Laan LA, Renier WO, Arts WF, et al. Evolution of epilepsy and EEG findings in Angelman syndrome. Epilepsia 1997;38(2):195–199.

55. Percy AK. Rett syndrome. Curr Opin Neurol 1995;8(2):156–160.

56. Slot HM, Overweg-Plandsoen WC, Bakker HD, et al. Molybdenum-cofactor deficiency: an easily missed cause of neonatal convulsions. Neuropediatrics 1993;24(3):139–142.

57. Goutieres F, Aicardi J. Atypical presentations of pyridoxine-dependent seizures: a treatable cause of intractable epilepsy in infants. Ann Neurol 1985;17(2):117–120.

58. De Vivo DC, Trifiletti RR, Jacobson RI, et al. Defective glucose transport across the blood-brain barrier as a cause of persistent hypoglycorrhachia, seizures, and developmental delay. N Engl J Med 1991;325(10):703–709.

59. Hawkins EP, Hawkins HK, Armstrong D. Lymphocyte autofluorescence: a screening procedure for neurodegenerative diseases. Pediatr Neurol 1986;2(3):160–166.

60. Koh-S, Jayakar P, Resnick T, et al. The localizing value of ictal SPECT in children with tuberous sclerosis complex and refractory partial epilepsy. Epileptic Disord 1999;1:41–46.

61. Watanabe Y, Hashikawa K, Moriwaki H, et al. SPECT findings in mitochondrial encephalomyopathy. J Nucl Med 1998;39(6):961–964.

62. Maehara T, Shimizu H, Yagishita A, et al. Interictal hyperperfusion observed in infants with cortical dysgenesis. Brain Dev 1999;21(6):407–412.

63. Carrazana EJ, Lombroso CT, Mikati M, et al. Facilitation of infantile spasms by partial seizures. Epilepsia 1993;34(1):97–109.

64. Yamamoto N, Watanabe K, Negoro T, et al. Partial seizures evolving to infantile spasms. Epilepsia 1988;29(1):34–40.

65. Donat JF, Wright FS. Simultaneous infantile spasms and partial seizures. J Child Neurol 1991;6(3):246–250.

66. Kramer U, Sue WC, Mikati MA. Focal features in West syndrome indicating candidacy for surgery. Pediatr Neurol 1997;16(3):213–217.

67. Gambardella A, Palmini A, Andermann F, et al. Usefulness of focal rhythmic discharges on scalp EEG of patients with focal cortical dysplasia and intractable epilepsy. Electroencephalogr Clin Neurophysiol 1996;98(4):243–249.

68. Minassian BA, DeLorey TM, Olsen RW, et al. Angelman syndrome: correlations between epilepsy phenotypes and genotypes. Ann Neurol 1998;43(4):485–493.

69. Robb SA, Harden A, Boyd SG. Rett syndrome: an EEG study in 52 girls. Neuropediatrics 1989;20(4):192–195.

70. Boyd SG, Harden A, Egger J, Pampiglione G. Progressive neuronal degeneration of childhood with liver disease ("Alpers' disease"): characteristic neurophysiological features. Neuropediatrics 1986;17(2):75–80.

71. Vanhanen SL, Sainio K, Lappi M, Santavuori P. EEG and evoked potentials in infantile neuronal ceroid-lipofuscinosis. Dev Med Child Neurol 1997;39(7):456–463.

72. Naqvi SZ, Beach RL, Armao DM, Greenwood RS. Photoparoxysmal response in late infantile neuronal ceroid-lipofuscinosis. Pediatr Neurol 1998;19(5):395–398.

73. Bare MA, Glauser TA, Strawsburg RH. Need for electroencephalogram video confirmation of atypical absence seizures in children with Lennox-Gastaut syndrome. J Child Neurol 1998;13(10):498–500.

74. Glaze DG, Schultz RJ, Frost JD. Rett syndrome: characterization of seizures versus non-seizures. Electroencephalogr Clin Neurophysiol 1998;106(1):79–83.

75. Duchowny M, Jayakar P, Harvey AS, et al. Language cortex representation: effects of developmental versus acquired pathology. Ann Neurol 1996;40(1):31–38.

76. Morrell F, Whisler WW, Bleck TP. Multiple subpial transection: a new approach to the surgical treatment of focal epilepsy. J Neurosurg 1989;70(2):231–239.

77. Devinsky O, Perrine K, Vazquez B, et al. Multiple subpial transections in the language cortex. Brain 1994; 117:255–265.

78. Sawhney IM, Robertson IJ, Polkey CE, et al. Multiple subpial transection: a review of 21 cases. J Neurol Neurosurg Psychiatry 1995;58(3):344–349.

79. Wyler AR, Wilkus RJ, Rostad SW, Vossler DG. Multiple subpial transections for partial seizures in sensorimotor cortex. Neurosurgery 1995;37(6):1122–1127.

80. Hufnagel A, Zentner J, Fernandez G, et al. Multiple subpial transection for control of epileptic seizures: effectiveness and safety. Epilepsia 1997;38(6):678–688.

81. Smith MC. Multiple subpial transection in patients with extratemporal epilepsy. Epilepsia 1998;39[Suppl 4]:S81–S89.

82. Morrell F, Whisler WW, Smith MC, et al. Landau-Kleffner syndrome. Treatment with subpial intracortical transection. Brain 1995;118:1529–1546.

83. Grote CL, Van Slyke P, Hoeppner JA. Language outcome following multiple subpial transection for Landau-Kleffner syndrome. Brain 1999;122:561–566.

84. Sankar R, Curran JG, Kevill JW, et al. Microscopic cortical dysplasia in infantile spasms: evolution of white matter abnormalities. AJNR Am J Neuroradiol 1995;16(6):1265–1272.

85. Aram D, Eisele J. Plasticity and Recovery of Higher Cognitive Functions Following Early Brain Injury. In I Rapin, S Segalowitz (eds), Child Neuropsychology, vol 6. Amsterdam: Elsevier Science, 1992;73–92.

86. Volpe J. Neuronal Proliferation, Migration, Organization and Myelination. In J Volpe (ed), Neurology of the Newborn (3rd ed). Philadelphia: Saunders, 1995;43–92.

87. Glaze DG, Hrachovy RA, Frost JD Jr, et al. Prospective study of outcome of infants with infantile spasms treated during controlled studies of ACTH and prednisone. J Pediatr 1988;112(3):389–396.

Chapter 33

Focal Cortical Resection and Cortical Dysplasias

Steven V. Pacia and Anjanette A. Naga

Resection may relieve seizures in carefully selected patients with focal cortical dysplasias and medically intractable epilepsy. Advances in magnetic resonance imaging (MRI) and increasing experience with intracranial electrode placement procedures for seizure localization and functional mapping have made resections safer, more successful, and an acceptable alternative for many patients who have persistent seizures despite numerous antiepileptic medication trials. Cortical dysplasia results from aberrant neuronal migration or cerebral insults occurring soon after neuronal migration along radial glial fibers.[1] In most cases, determining the exact cause of cortical dysplasia is difficult. Although fetal injury is presumed, little direct evidence exists to substantiate this etiology in many cases. In a minority of dysplasias, including band heterotopia, Miller-Dieker syndrome, and some cases of isolated lissencephaly, cortical dysplasias are genetically determined.[2] Some researchers suggest that some cases of focal cortical dysplasia may represent formes frustes of tuberous sclerosis.[3] This assertion is based on the similarity of histopathologic findings in the two disorders, but currently no genetic studies are available to support this theory.[4]

Dysplastic cortex is intrinsically epileptogenic and may occur focally or diffusely. Lesions may be microscopic, as in some focal cortical dyplasias, or gross cortical deformations as in many cases of pachygyria or polymicrogyria. Cortical dysplasia is reported as the etiology of seizures in 3–20% of patients included in epilepsy surgical series.[5] In this chapter, we discuss the current use of resection for focal epilepsy in patients with cortical dysplasia.

Defining Cortical Dysplasia

Disruptions occurring before, during, and after neuronal migration along radial glial fibers may potentially yield malformations of the cortex. Abnormal cell differentiation prior to cell migration may result in malformed neurons and glial cells.[1] Giant neurons with unusual subcellular characteristics may be found in cortical and subcortical regions, along with balloon cells (cells presumed to be of glial origin), which contain enlarged or multiple nuclei.[1] Both types of cells commonly are present in focal cortical dysplasias and hemimegalencephaly. Figure 33-1 illustrates typical pathologic features in a patient with cortical dysplasia.

Disruptions of neuronal migration along radial glial fibers cause neurons either to fail to reach the cortex or to occupy abnormal cortical locations. Collections of neurons in subcortical white matter are referred to as *neuronal heterotopias*. These abnormalities, exhibiting signal characteristics similar to those of cortical gray matter, may be visible on an MRI scan.[6] Subcortical and periventricular heterotopic neurons, like cortically located dysplastic neurons, also possess intrinsic epileptogenic potential.[7]

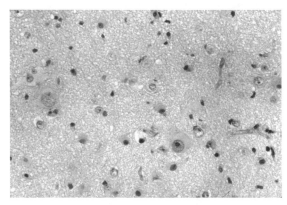

Figure 33-1. A high-powered view of dysplastic neocortex in patient with medically refractory partial epilepsy. Note the lack of radial and laminar organization, as well as the abnormally formed neurons of varying size and shape.

In disorders of abnormal gyration (e.g., pachygyria and polymicrogyria), neurons have reached the cortical mantle but may be found in the wrong cortical layer or may be unusually positioned, disturbing the normal horizontal lamination of the cortex. In other cases, neurons have reached appropriate cortical locations, preserving horizontal lamination, but a cerebral insult (e.g., infection or vascular event) may cause dysplasia, as in the syndrome of four-layered polymicrogyria.[8]

Developmental Disabilities and Cortical Dysplasia

Patients with cortical dysplasia often are developmentally disabled. The exact incidence of cortical dysplasia in developmentally disabled persons is unknown. The degree of cognitive disability has been correlated with the extent of cortical dysplasia and with certain dysplastic syndromes.[9] Of 28 patients with cerebral dysplasia in one study, 27 (93%) had significant cognitive impairments.[9] Profound mental retardation was most common in patients with agyria or pachygyria and was less severe in those with focal cortical dysplastic lesions. Language skills were significantly affected in patients with cortical dysplasia, regardless of the severity of cognitive impairment. In addition to the anatomic extent of dysplasia, seizure frequency and sever-

ity were identified as important factors in determining outcome in patients with cortical dysplasia.[9]

Developmental Disabilities and Tuberous Sclerosis

Similar to cortical dysplasia, tuberous sclerosis is a disorder of cell migration, proliferation, and differentiation. Like those with cortical dysplasia, patients with tuberous sclerosis commonly present with seizures and learning disabilities. It has been suggested that both the number and location of cortical tubers correlate with cognitive performance and severity of seizures.[10] In a large study of 300 cases of tuberous sclerosis, 80% of patients had learning difficulties or were developmentally delayed.[11] Ninety-three percent of all the tuberous sclerosis patients studied experienced at least one seizure during their lifetime, and 63% of patients had chronic seizures.[11]

No large studies of epilepsy surgery in patients with tuberous sclerosis have been conducted. One small series of 18 patients with tuberous sclerosis who had surgery for medically refractory seizures revealed excellent outcomes in those with a single tuber or epileptogenic region identified with both imaging and electroencephalography.[12] In those patients in whom focal resection is not an option because of diffuse onset or multifocal seizures, corpus callosotomy may reduce the frequency and morbidity of generalized seizures in selected patients.[12,13]

Presurgical Evaluation of Patients with Cortical Dysplasia

At most epilepsy centers, surgical candidates suspected of having focal cortical dysplasia undergo the standard battery of presurgical evaluations, including audiovisual electroencephalographic (EEG) study to localize interictal and ictal foci, brain MRI, and functional imaging studies. Scalp EEG studies in patients with cortical dysplastic lesions often reveal multifocal or generalized interictal spikes or seizures, the localization of which is difficult.[14] Although some of these patients may truly have multifocal seizures and, therefore, may not be suitable surgical candidates, many may still have restricted intracranial ictal EEG onsets or focal MRI changes, despite a nonlocalizing scalp EEG study.[14] Therefore, reliance on scalp EEG recordings alone is inadequate to select patients with dysplasia for resection.

High-resolution MRIs have improved our ability to identify some cortical dysplastic lesions. As expected, mild cortical dysplasia with relatively preserved cortical lamination is much less likely to reveal definitive MRI changes than is more profound dysplasia. Subtle MRI findings include changes in gray-white architecture and increased T2-weighted white-matter signal abnormalities (possibly due to heterotopic neurons). More severe dysplastic lesions may be associated with increased cortical thickness and abnormal gyral patterns apparent on T1 and inversion recovery sequences.[15] Figure 33-2 shows a large dysplastic gyrus in the left frontoparietal region of a patient with medically refractory partial epilepsy.

Functional imaging, including positron emission tomography (PET) and single-photon emission computed tomography (SPECT), may help to localize epileptogenic cortical dysplastic lesions when MRI and EEG scans fail to define precisely the epileptogenic zone. The use of PET has been most useful in the evaluation of neonates and infants with cortical dysplasia who may have unremarkable MRI scans despite severe epilepsy. In particular, PET has been used to guide resections in children with infantile spasms, revealing either hypometabolic or hypermetabolic lesions, depending on the timing of the PET tracer injection. In one PET-guided surgical series of children with infantile spasms, only 9 of 23 children had MRIs revealing clear focal abnormalities.[16] Less evidence exists confirming the value of PET for presurgical evaluation of adults with focal cortical dysplasia.

SPECT is more readily available than is PET and therefore is more widely used for presurgical evaluation of both children and adults. Stable tracers that can be administered at the bedside, allowing an interval between the injection and scanning, also allow ictal studies to be performed. Additionally, the coregistration of SPECT and MRI images, along with the ability to subtract interictal and ictal scans digitally, has further enhanced the resolution and reliability of SPECT.[17] This technique holds promise for localizing

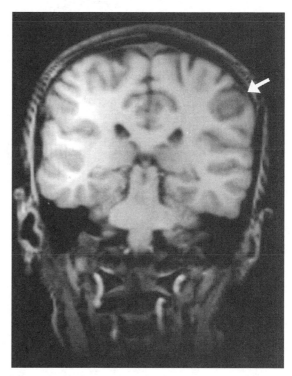

Figure 33-2. A coronal T1-weighted magnetic resonance imaging scan from a patient with partial epilepsy, revealing a large dysplastic gyrus (*arrow*) in the left frontoparietal region.

extratemporal seizures owing to focal cortical dysplasias, as such seizures recorded by scalp EEG tracings often are poorly localized.

Intracranial Electroencephalography and Cortical Dysplasia

Most centers employ chronic intracranial EEG recording or intraoperative electrocorticography (ECoG) of interictal and ictal abnormalities to define the epileptogenic zone in patients suspected of having cortical dysplasia. These studies are guided either by a well-localized scalp EEG study or the presence of an MRI or functional imaging abnormality. When presurgical evaluations are inconclusive, a survey study using a bilateral subdural strip or a subdural strip combined with depth electrodes may be useful in lateralizing or localizing the epileptogenic zone. Intracranial EEG studies are most useful when a restricted ictal focus is identified, confirming that

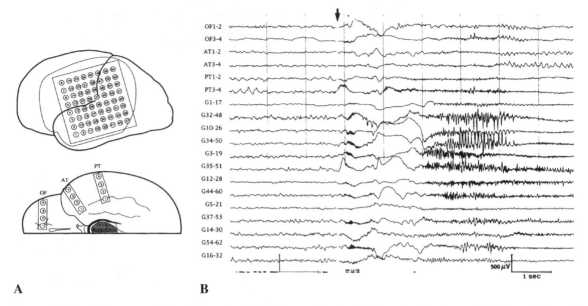

A   **B**

Figure 33-3. A. A 64-contact subdural electrode grid and three subdural strip electrodes placed over the left hemisphere of a patient with medically refractory partial epilepsy and cortical dysplasia. **B.** A left parietotemporal seizure with low-voltage, high-frequency activity at ictal onset (*arrow*) is shown. (AT = anterior temporal; OF = orbitofrontal; PT = posterior temporal.)

seizures arise from a localized imaging abnormality. However, well-localized seizures on intracranial EEG studies may guide successful surgical resections even when all imaging studies are normal.[18] This may be more true of neocortical temporal lobe epilepsy than for epilepsies arising extratemporally.[19] Figure 33-3 illustrates a typical intracranial grid and subdural strip electrode placement and low-voltage, high-frequency ictal discharge over the left parietotemporal region in a patient with cortical dysplasia.

Studies of the value of chronic intracranial EEG specifically for focal cortical dysplasias are limited and offer conflicting recommendations. Hirabayashi et al.[20] concluded that ictal intracranial EEG studies were not useful in the presurgical evaluation of patients with cortical dysplasia. However, only three patients actually underwent intracranial EEG study. In contrast, Bautista et al.[21] point out that intracranial EEG studies often reveal functional or structural pathology that imaging studies may underestimate.[21] Our surgical study of neocortical temporal lobe epilepsy with resections guided by intracranial ictal recordings revealed excellent outcomes in four patients who had unremarkable

MRI scans but in whom pathologic workup revealed cortical dysplasia.[22]

The value of intraoperative ECoG used to localize interictal foci prior to resection is controversial in patients with cortical dysplasia, just as it is for epilepsy due to other etiologies. Some authors concluded that ECoG often gives misleading information.[4] Others believe that in selected cases, especially in those revealing continuous epileptiform discharges, ECoG plays a valuable role in localizing dysplastic tissue for resection.[23]

Surgical Outcome

A recent review of the available literature on surgical outcome for cases of cortical dysplasia concluded that approximately 40% of patients are seizure-free at 2 years postoperatively.[24] This stands in sharp contrast to the 70–80% seizure-free outcomes reported with anterior temporal resections for mesial temporal sclerosis.[25] Not known is whether advances in MRI and functional MRI, which was unavailable in many of the reported cases, are improving these outcome figures. Interestingly, this same cortical dysplasia review found no difference in outcome between the temporal lobe and extratemporal dysplasia groups. In contrast, a prior small series presented by Hirabayashi et al.[20] implied better outcome for those with temporal lobe or restricted frontal lesions as compared with those having widespread frontal, parietal, or occipital lobe foci.

The extent of resection as a predictor of outcome has been examined in several small clinical studies. Palmini et al.[4] reported that in patients in whom at least 50% of the lesion was resected, a good surgical outcome was achieved. The completeness of resection was determined by computed tomography, MRI, or visual inspection. This study also concluded that the extent of excision of the electrophysiologic abnormality did not correlate with outcome. However, this determination was made by interictal EEG abnormalities on scalp or intraoperative EEG studies only. A more recent report from the same authors describes a phenomenon of ictal or continuous epileptogenic discharges recorded with ECoG in some patients with cortical dysplasia.[23] The presence of these discharges postoperatively was negatively correlated with outcome.[26]

Developmental disabilities are not uncommon in patients with cortical dysplasia. The degree of impairment depends on the localization and extent of the dysplasia.[9] In one study, cortical dysplasia patients had lower intelligence quotients than did a control group of mesial temporal sclerosis patients.[20] The degree of cognitive impairment was greater in patients with extratemporal lesions. Additionally, patients with extratemporal cortical dysplasia had poorer surgical outcomes than did those with temporal lobe lesions. These data are consistent with other surgical series that indicate poorer outcome for all patients with extratemporal epilepsy and lower baseline intelligence scores.[27]

Resection for infants with cortical dysplasia is being performed with increasing frequency. For these cases, the convergence of EEG and imaging data may be the most important determinant for successful surgical outcome.[14] This is particularly true for children younger than 3 years because MRI scans in cases of focal dysplasia are frequently unremarkable owing to incomplete myelination.[28] Additionally, imaging abnormalities, when present, may not predict the complete extent of dysplasia.

Dual Pathology: Cortical Dysplasia and Mesial Temporal Sclerosis

Many studies have explored the coexistence of focal cortical dysplasia and mesial temporal sclerosis, but the true incidence of this dual pathology is unknown. Much of this uncertainty results from the lack of agreement among pathologists about which abnormalities truly constitute microdysplasia. Ho et al.[29] reported an 87% incidence of amygdalohippocampal atrophy in patients with temporal lobe cortical dysplasia, with many patients having bilateral mesial temporal atrophy. Conversely, in a clinicopathologic study of 27 patients with mesial temporal sclerosis, 5 patients (24%) were diagnosed as having coexistent cortical dysplasia.[30] Not known is whether cortical dysplasia is the primary abnormality, resulting in seizures and subsequent mesial temporal sclerosis, or whether both abnormalities may be the result of a common etiology.

Conclusion

Cortical dysplasia is a frequent cause of medically refractory partial epilepsy that may occur focally or diffusely. Focal cortical dysplasia may be amenable to surgical resection if localized outside of eloquent cortex and identified with MRI, EEG studies, or functional imaging. High-resolution MRI has greatly improved our ability to localize these lesions preoperatively, and most studies suggest that patients who undergo more complete resections of the abnormalities apparent on imaging have the highest rates of seizure-free outcome. The reliance on scalp and intracranial EEG studies to guide cortical resections is somewhat controversial, although many cases have been reported of MRI-negative cortical dysplastic lesions that were successfully resected under the guidance of intracranial EEG recording of interictal and ictal data. Well-controlled studies are needed to improve our ability to select patients with cortical dysplasia who will benefit from focal resections.

References

1. Robain O. Introduction to the Pathology of Cerebral Cortical Dysplasia. In R Guerrini, F Andermann, R Canapicchi, et al. (eds), Dysplasias of the Cerebral Cortex and Epilepsy. Philadelphia: Lippincott–Raven, 1996;1–9.

2. Reiner O, Carrozo R, Shen Y, et al. Isolation of a Miller-Dieker lissencephaly gene containing G protein, beta-subunit-like repeats. Nature 1993;364:717–721.

3. Palmini A, Andermann F, Olivier A, et al. Focal neuronal migration disorders and intractable partial epilepsy: a study of 30 patients. Ann Neurol 1991;30:741–749.

4. Palmini A, Andermann F, Olivier A, et al. Focal neuronal migration disorders and intractable partial epilepsy: results of surgical treatment. Ann Neurol 1991;30(6):750–757.

5. Kuzniecky R, Murro A, King D, et al. Magnetic resonance imaging in childhood intractable partial epilepsies: pathologic correlations. Neurology 1993;43:681–687.

6. Kuzniecky R, Garcia J, Faught E, Morawetz R. Cortical dysplasia in TLE: MRI correlations. Ann Neurol 1991;29:293–298.

7. Mattia D, Olivier A, Avoli M. Seizure-like discharges recorded in human dysplastic neocortex maintained in vitro. Neurology 1995;45:1391–1395.

8. Richman DP, Stewart RM, Caviness VS Jr. Cerebral microgyria in a 27 week fetus: an architectonic and topographic analysis. J Neuropathol Exp Neurol 1974;33:374–384.

9. Rossi PG, Parmeggiani A, Santucci M, et al. Neuropsychological and Psychiatric Findings in Cerebral Cortex Dysplasias. In R Guerrini, F Andermann, R Canapicchi, et al. (eds), Dysplasias of the Cerebral Cortex and Epilepsy. Philadelphia: Lippincott–Raven, 1996;345–350.

10. Curatolo P. Tuberous Sclerosis: Relationships Between Clinical and EEG Findings and Magnetic Resonance Imaging. In R Guerrini, F Andermann, R Canapicchi, et al. (eds), Dysplasias of the Cerebral Cortex and Epilepsy. Philadelphia: Lippincott–Raven, 1996;191–197.

11. Hunt A. Development, behaviour and seizures in 300 cases of tuberous sclerosis. J Intellect Disabil Res 1993; 37:41–51.

12. Guerreiro MM, Andermann F, Andermann E, et al. Surgical treatment of epilepsy in tuberous sclerosis: strategies and results in 18 patients. Neurology 1998;51:1263–1269.

13. Andermann F, Freeman JM, Vigevano F, Hwang P. Surgically Remediable Diffuse Hemispheric Syndromes. In J Engel Jr (ed), Surgical Treatment of the Epilepsies (2nd ed). New York: Raven Press, 1993;609–621.

14. Wyllie E. Surgery for catastrophic localization-related epilepsy in infants. Epilepsia 1996;37(1):S22–S25.

15. Kuzniecky R. MRI in Focal Cortical Dysplasia: Introduction to the Pathology of Cerebral Cortical Dysplasia. In R Guerrini, F Andermann, R Canapicchi, et al. (eds), Dysplasias of the Cerebral Cortex and Epilepsy. Philadelphia: Lippincott–Raven, 1996;145–150.

16. Chugani HT, Shewmon DA, Peacock WJ, et al. Surgical treatment of intractable neonatal-onset seizures:
the role of positron emission tomography. Neurology 1988;38:1178–1188.

17. O'Brien TJ, So EL, Mullan BP, et al. Subtraction ictal SPECT co-registered to MRI improves clinical usefulness of SPECT in localizing the surgical seizure focus. Neurology 1998;50:445–454.

18. Pacia SV, Ebersole JS. Intracranial EEG in temporal lobe epilepsy. J Clin Neurophysiol 1999;16(5):399–407.

19. Jung WY, Pacia SV, Devinsky O. Neocortical temporal lobe epilepsy: intracranial EEG features and surgical outcome. J Clin Neurophysiol 1999;16(5):419–425.

20. Hirabayashi S, Binnie CD, Janota I, Polkey CE. Surgical treatment of epilepsy due to cortical dysplasia: clinical and EEG findings. J Neurol Neurosurg Psychiatry 1993;56:765–770.

21. Bautista RE, Cobbs MA, Spencer DD, Spencer SS. Predication of surgical outcome by interictal epileptiform abnormalities during intracranial EEG monitoring in patients with extrahippocampal seizures. Epilepsia 1999;40:880–890.

22. Pacia SV, Devinsky O, Perrine K, et al. Clinical features of neocortical temporal lobe epilepsy. Ann Neurol 1996;40(5):724–730.

23. Palmini A, Gambardella A, Andermann F, et al. Intrinsic epileptogenicity of human dysplastic cortex as suggested by corticography and surgical results. Ann Neurol 1995;37:476–487.

24. Sisodiya SM. Surgery for malformations of cortical development causing epilepsy. Brain 2000;123:1075–1091.

25. Engel J Jr, Van Ness PC, Rasmussen TB, Ojemann LM. Outcome with Respect to Epileptic Seizures. In J Engel Jr (ed), Surgical Treatment of the Epilepsies (2nd ed). New York: Raven Press, 1993;609–621.

26. Palmini A, Gambardella A, Andermann F, et al. Outcome of Surgical Treatment in Patients with Localized Cortical Dysplasia and Intractable Epilepsy. In R Guerrini, F Andermann, R Canapicchi, et al. (eds), Dysplasias of the Cerebral Cortex and Epilepsy. Philadelphia: Lippincott–Raven, 1996;367–374.

27. Strauss E, Loring D, Chelune G, et al. Predicting cognitive impairment in epilepsy: findings from the Bozeman Epilepsy Consortium. J Clin Exp Neuropsychol 1995;17(6):909–917.

28. Sugimoto T, Otsubo H, Hwang PA, et al. Outcome of epilepsy surgery in the first three years of life. Epilepsia 1999;40(5):560–565.

29. Ho SS, Kuzniecky RI, Gilliam F, et al. Temporal lobe developmental malformations and epilepsy: dual pathology and bilateral hippocampal abnormalities. Neurology 1998;50:748–754.

30. Prayson RA, Reith JD, Najm IM. Mesial temporal sclerosis: a clinicopathologic study of 27 patients, including 5 with coexistent cortical dysplasia. Arch Pathol Lab Med 1996;120:532–536.

Chapter 34

Hemispherectomy

Eileen P. G. Vining

Hemispherectomy is the most radical neurosurgical procedure that can be performed. It has been available for more than 70 years and is used primarily to relieve unihemispheric, intractable epilepsy in such settings as congenital strokes, major brain malformations and migrational disorders, Rasmussen's syndrome, and Sturge-Weber syndrome. The decision-making process involved in recommending or agreeing to the procedure is sometimes difficult for affected physicians, patients, and families. Multiple surgical techniques that have been described use various degrees of tissue removal and disconnection to minimize long-term sequelae. Outcome for children generally is excellent, particularly with respect to seizure control. This outcome obviously depends on how normally the remaining hemisphere functions, whether all epileptogenic tissue was removed or disconnected completely, and whether postoperative problems remained. All children will be left with a significant hemiparesis or hemiplegia and with a homonymous hemianopia. However, the vast majority will have had the burden of their disability minimized considerably.

History of Hemispherectomy

Two surgeons conceived the procedure of hemispherectomy and performed it in 1928. Both Dandy and L'Hermitte believed that it was a rational approach for trying to eliminate malignant gliomas.[1] However, both surgeons ultimately realized its futility, and the procedure was abandoned for

that indication. A decade later, McKenzie[2] used a similar procedure successfully to treat adult hemiplegic patients who had intractable seizures. In 1950, Krynauw[3] elegantly described the success of the procedure in 12 children. In addition to noting markedly improved seizure control, he recorded a marked improvement in function and behavior. Encouraged by these results, surgeons around the world began performing hemispherectomies to relieve intractable seizures in patients who already had experienced significant hemispheric damage, often owing to vascular events. In addition, Rasmussen advocated its use in the hemispheric inflammatory epilepsy that ultimately came to be known as *Rasmussen's syndrome*.[4] However, this era came to an abrupt halt in the middle to late 1960s after observations by Laine and Gros[5] and then Oppenheimer and Griffith,[6] who described persistent intracranial bleeding as a late complication of hemispherectomy. Surgeons, including Rasmussen, examined alternatives such as partial hemispherectomy, but this did not yield as much improvement in seizure control. Ultimately, Rasmussen's group developed an approach that became known as a *functional hemispherectomy*.[7] By the early 1980s, it had become increasingly clear that hemispherectomy, in one form or another, had to be made available to the numerous children (and less frequently, adults) who could not be helped by less drastic procedures. Since then, suggestions for further modifications in the procedure have continued, and many centers have developed excellent pro-

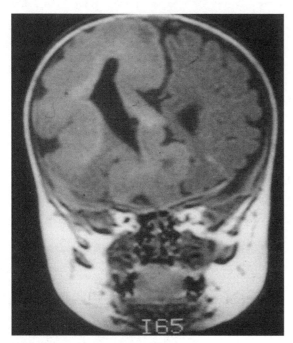

Figure 34-1. Magnetic resonance imaging scan of patient with right-hemisphere neuronal migration disorder and hamartomatous abnormalities of the cortex.

grams to provide this procedure and to evaluate the outcomes of their approaches.[8–10]

Surgery

Hemispherectomy has come to mean a wide variety of procedures. It includes the classic anatomic hemispherectomy that would have been performed by Dandy and other surgeons into the 1960s. It includes variations, such as those proposed by Adams,[11] which involved performing an anatomic hemispherectomy and then reducing the subdural space by suturing the dura to the falx and other fixed structures, blocking the subdural cavity from the ventricular system. Hemidecortication is a variation on the anatomic procedure and involves removing the gray matter and protecting the white matter so that the ventricular system is not breeched.[9,12] Hemidecortication is the procedure employed most frequently at Johns Hopkins Medical Institution. Functional hemispherectomy— in which the central region of the hemisphere is resected, and the rest of the hemisphere is disconnected from the other hemisphere—was developed by Rasmussen and was advanced further by his Montreal colleagues.[7] Modifications of this approach have been made by a number of centers and include techniques using ultrasonographic identification of the ventricular structures to guide resection and peri-insular hemispherotomy.[10,13]

Patient Selection

Convergence of data is a guiding principle in selecting patients for all forms of epilepsy surgery. Sometimes patient selection appears to be an easy prospect when considering hemispherectomy because there may be overwhelming evidence of anatomic abnormality in one hemisphere). However, in many instances, one must try also to determine how normal the other hemisphere is, from both an anatomic and a functional perspective.

A child is considered a candidate for hemispherectomy in the presence of unilateral, intractable seizures. The determination of unilaterality is based on a number of factors, including clinical description of the seizures, unilateral neurologic findings (hand preference at an early age, evidence of hemiparesis-hemisensory deficits), and anatomic and functional test results.

Magnetic resonance imaging might demonstrate a grossly malformed hemisphere, as it did in a child with a neuronal migration disorder and hamartomatous abnormalities of the cortex (Figure 34-1), or it might demonstrate the classic findings of Rasmussen's syndrome, which results in hemispheric atrophy (Figure 34-2). In general, these findings are not subtle and can be detected with any modern, thorough study. However, some of the newer techniques, such as flare imaging and proton-specific inversion recovery, may help to identify additional migrational or cortical abnormalities in the other hemisphere. Other imaging strategies (e.g., positron emission tomography scans, magnetic resonance spectroscopy, and single-photon emission computed tomography scans) usually are not necessary in considering hemispherectomy. These tools, however, may give additional confirmation of the extent of hemispheric abnormality.[14] Electroencephalography is an important test because it is readily available, is easily performed, and provides valuable information. In most instances in which hemispherectomy is being considered, electroencephalographic (EEG) recording helps to confirm unilaterality, with both slowing and epileptiform activity over the involved hemisphere. It often is helpful, especially in cases of migrational disorders, to obtain video monitoring of the seizures. Video-EEG monitoring can help to clarify the clinical elements of the seizure and to identify whether the seizure onset is from the abnormal hemisphere and is multifocal. However, EEG monitoring can be misleading at times, particularly in very young children, and bilateral EEG abnormalities can be found in patients who are otherwise good candidates for hemispherectomy.[15]

Clinicians must continue to manage the information and form a cohesive construct. Is it likely that the other hemisphere is simply a site of rapid spread? Is the slowing simply a response to continuous seizures? Can the activity in the "good" hemisphere be suppressed with benzodiazepines while the source of the primary epileptogenic activity in the abnormal hemisphere continues? Another important indicator of more normal activity in one hemisphere is the overall function of the child. Are they very interactive? Are they achieving many milestones despite numerous seizures and multiple medications? Positive responses to these questions would suggest that the good hemisphere is healthy and resilient.

The question of the timing for operation relates to several factors. First, the nature and the course of the disorder must be clear. This often is not problematic in the case of an infant who begins to have seizures in the neonatal period and in whom magnetic resonance imaging demonstrates hemimegalencephaly. In such a situation, infants are nurtured until they have grown sufficiently and present less of an anesthetic and surgical risk. Determining the nature and course of the disorder also is not problematic in the case of children who have Sturge-Weber syndrome and begin to have seizures in the first months of life; those with seizures that are difficult to control; and those who begin to show evidence of a hemiparesis. Some data suggests that operating very early (prior to age 2) in these children is preferable.[12] In other children who may have experienced a vascular event and are left with significant tissue damage, persisting with medication trials is common until it becomes clear that the seizures and medications are exceedingly disruptive and that proceeding with a surgical remedy would be more prudent. Abandoning the hope of remission is difficult for all parties involved, but the odds against such an outcome are high.

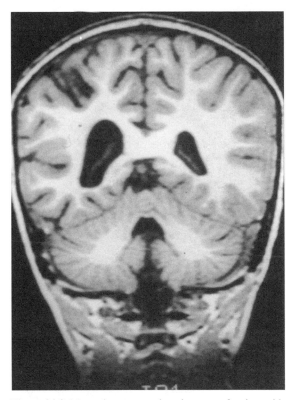

Figure 34-2. Magnetic resonance imaging scan of patient with right-hemisphere diffuse atrophy in Rasmussen's syndrome.

The decision to proceed with a hemispherectomy sometimes is even more difficult for children with Rasmussen's syndrome than for other children, for these are children who had been perfectly normal and suddenly are devastated by seizures. Families seek all possible alternatives before recognizing that hemispherectomy is inevitable. These alternatives include various immunologic therapies (e.g., plasmapheresis, intravenous gamma globulin, or steroids). Parents remain hopeful that the inflammation will disappear as quickly and as completely as it appeared. Affected families and their children must be able to accept the finality of the surgery: the hemiparesis and the homonymous hemianopia. Older children with left-hemispheric abnormality face a greater risk. Their language has become dysfunctional, yet they must risk losing it to regain it. Such patients must face the long road of rehabilitation and therapy. Even older teenagers can undergo a left hemispherectomy and regain fluent and functional speech.[16,17] Decision making must be guided by the realization that surgery is being performed to

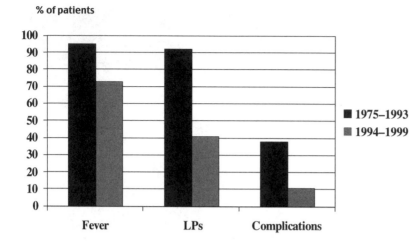

% of patients

■ 1975–1993
■ 1994–1999

Fever   LPs   Complications

Figure 34-3. Complications after hemispherectomy: Effect of time. The percentage of patients with various morbidities (e.g., fever, need for lumbar puncture [LP]) has decreased over time when the period prior to 1994 is compared with the period after 1994.

relieve the burden of the seizures and also to prevent the long-term impact of medication; it is being performed to allow the normal brain to function without the influence of both seizures and medication.

Hemispherectomies should be performed at centers with staff trained to deal with all the facets of the procedure. First, experienced epileptologists must be available to determine that the procedure is appropriate. As the decision making, surgery, and rehabilitation proceed, the center should provide appropriate counseling and support through a parents' network. Obviously, an experienced surgeon and anesthesia team must be available. Because these procedures can be lengthy and entail considerable blood loss, a skilled pediatric intensive care unit staff must recognize and be prepared to correct the many problems of fluid dynamics that can occur, particularly in very young children. Finally, access to excellent rehabilitation services must be available; such a service should be able to deal with the wide range of needs of this patient population, including physical therapy, occupational therapy, speech and language therapy, and sometimes behavioral psychology. Affected children and their families will have been through a grueling experience, both in the seizure disorder and the operation. To adjust to these events and to maintain normal behavioral patterns is difficult. A medical team's expertise in dealing with such matters often is crucial to optimizing other interventions that become necessary. Finally, centers performing hemispherectomies should be involved in protocols and clinical research that will improve the diagnostic strate-

gies, the operative procedures, the habilitation process, and our knowledge base.

Complications

The hemispherectomy procedure is fraught with risk. Resultant deaths have been reported by all centers that perform this surgery routinely. In the Hopkins series of 58 procedures, 4 children died—3 children in the immediate operative and postoperative phase and 1 child 3 years later.[18] The latter was a child with developmental abnormalities of both hemispheres.

The immediate risks appear to be manageable with very aggressive and careful intensive care and attention to fluid management. Complications are significant and can include excessive bleeding (5 of 58 in the Hopkins series), which tends to be seen in younger patients; fluid and electrolyte problems (4 of 58); coma (3 of 58), from which 2 children recovered completely; and hydrocephalus (16 of 58), only one case of which occurred years postoperatively. Other immediate problems include infection, fever, and aseptic meningitis. A recent review of our data suggest that these problems may be decreasing over time with experience in managing such children (Figure 34-3).

Outcomes

The outcomes for children subjected to the hemispherectomy procedure must be viewed from a variety of parameters: seizure control, short- and

Figure 34-4. Seizure outcome after hemispherectomy, on the basis of etiology. The population after hemispherectomy is divided into those who are seizure-free and those who have insignificant seizures (auras), a moderate number of seizures, and ongoing severe seizures. The percentage in each of these categories is plotted according to the etiology of the seizures—Rasmussen's syndrome, dysplasias, vascular abnormalities—and for the overall group.

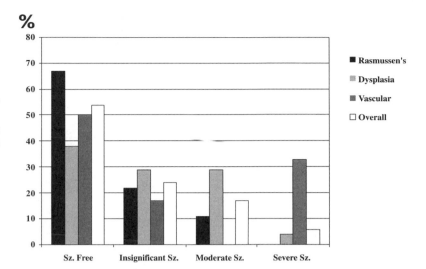

long-term surgical morbidity, intellectual function, motor function, language function and, finally, the ability to lead an independent life. The outcomes clearly depend on a variety of factors, among which are etiology, normalcy of the remaining hemisphere, surgical procedure and associated morbidity, availability and nature of rehabilitation, and perhaps age at surgery and duration of epilepsy.

Overall, the outcome concerning seizures is excellent. Studies generally report that approximately 75% of hemispherectomy patients are seizure-free and perhaps another 20% are considerably improved.[19] This outcome is much better than that for any other form of epilepsy surgery. In an attempt to provide a comprehensive summary of outcomes, Holthausen et al.[20] surveyed a large number of major epilepsy centers and compiled statistics of outcomes, focusing particularly on the relationship to surgical technique employed. These authors found that the outcome for being seizure-free was poorest for hemidecorticectomy (61%) and best for hemispherotomy (86%).[20] Anatomic hemispherectomies yield 64% of patients seizure-free, the Adams modification results in 78% seizure-free, and functional hemispherectomy produces 66% seizure-free. In examining etiology, those authors found that the following proportions of patients achieved seizure-free status: Sturge-Weber syndrome, 82%; hemiatrophy, 77%; Rasmussen's syndrome, 77%; vascular etiologies, 76%; dysplasia, 57%; and all others, 68%.[20] Although this type of survey provides a broad picture of the efficacy of the procedure, it does not account for the biases inherent

in patient selection and referral and for the fact that certain centers that advocate particular procedures may tend to see a particular subset of patients. These outcomes also do not look at the total picture of the results of hemispherectomy.

The Hopkins experience after hemispherectomy is similar. Fifty-eight patients were followed up after surgery for a mean of 6.2 years (0.5–27.3 years). The outcomes, classified by etiology (dysplasia, Rasmussen's syndrome, vascular abnormalities), are shown in Figure 34-4. In an attempt to look more broadly at the effect of hemispherectomy, the Hopkins group devised a method by which to evaluate the success of the procedure by examining the operation's impact on the burden of the disability.[18] In this evaluation, three spheres were considered: seizures, motor function, and intellectual function. We estimated the degree of dysfunction in each of these categories (none, mild, moderate, severe) before and after surgery and created a score ranging from 0 to 9. We found that the burden of disability after hemispherectomy was reduced considerably, even in children who had dysplasia and in whom freedom from seizures was less common. These results are shown in Figure 34-5.

The ability to evaluate the overall impact of this type of surgery obviously is difficult: These children had significant motor handicaps; in many tests of intellectual function, they are penalized by their motor dysfunction. We find that the test scores reported do not appear to be representative of the

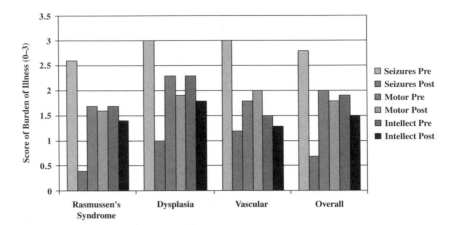

Figure 34-5. Burden of illness before and after hemispherectomy. The burden to the patient of seizures, motor handicap, and intellectual impairment was estimated before hemispherectomy and after recovery. The scores, ranging from 0 (no burden/impairment) to 3 (maximal burden/impairment) were calculated for each patient before and after surgery. The patients were then grouped by etiology, and the averages were calculated for each group. The average burden of illness decreased in most groups after surgery.

young patients' ability to function and learn. Hence, new techniques in assessing intellectual ability will have to be devised.

Language function after hemispherectomy, particularly after dominant hemisphere removal in older children, is a subject of much interest. The capacity and resiliency of the remaining hemisphere often appear excellent. Boatman et al.[17] are involved in studies of this area and recently published their observations of six children who had Rasmussen's syndrome and underwent hemispherectomy between the ages of 7 and 14 years. At 4–16 days postoperatively, the children showed improved phoneme discrimination over baseline and, at 1-year follow-up, receptive language was at or better than baseline. The patients' expressive abilities did not recover as well at that point, and some naming and fluency difficulties persisted. Overall, though, the right hemisphere demonstrates considerable plasticity in the redevelopment of language in such children.

Summary

Hemispherectomy, in its various forms, continues to play a critical role in the relief of intractable unihemispheric epilepsy in children. The process of selecting appropriate candidates sometimes is difficult. The dilemma of whether to proceed in the face of uncertainty about the normalcy of the other hemisphere remains a lingering issue as risk-bene-

fit analysis becomes more sophisticated. This surgery is difficult, with considerable postoperative morbidity in many patients. However, the overall outcomes, both in terms of relief from seizures and improved (or at least stabilized) function, is considerable. Further research to enhance our understanding of whether certain procedures are better suited for certain children and etiologies is necessary. Improved postoperative management and rehabilitation should be sought. Future advances in technology, surgery, and understanding of the plasticity of the nervous system also might enable some of these children to regain some function of the hemiplegic side.

References

1. Dandy W. Removal of right cerebral hemisphere for certain tumors with hemiplegia: preliminary report (abstract). JAMA 1928;90:823–825.
2. McKenzie KC. The present status of a patient who had the right cerebral hemisphere removed. JAMA 1938;111:168.
3. Krynauw RA. Infantile hemiplegia treated by removing one cerebral hemisphere. J Neurol Neurosurg Psychiatry 1950;13:243–267.
4. Aguilar MJ, Rasmussen T. Role of encephalitis in pathogenesis of epilepsy. Arch Neurol 1960;2:663–676.
5. Laine E, Gros C. L'hemispherectomie. Paris: Masson et Cie, 1956.

6. Oppenheimer DR, Griffith HB. Persistent intracranial bleeding as a complication of hemispherectomy. J Neurol Neurosurg Psychiatry 1966;29:229–240.

7. Villemure JG, Rasmussen T. Functional hemispherectomy in children. Neuropediatrics 1993;24:53–55.

8. Peacock WJ. The role of hemispherectomy in the treatment of intractable seizures in childhood. Int Pediatr 1992;7:291–293.

9. Carson BS, Javedan SP, Freeman JM, et al. Hemispherectomy: a hemidecortication approach and review of 52 cases (abstract). J Neurosurg 1996;84:903–911.

10. Schramm J, Behrens E, Entzian W. Hemispherical deafferentation: an alternative to functional hemispherectomy. Neurosurgery 1995;36:509–516.

11. Adams CBT. Hemispherectomy—a modification (abstract). J Neurol Neurosurg Psychiatry 1983;46:617–619.

12. Hoffman HJ, Hendrick EB, Dennis M, et al. Hemispherectomy for Sturge-Weber syndrome. Childs Brain 1979;5:233–248.

13. Villemure JG, Mascott CR. Peri-insular hemispherotomy: surgical principles and anatomy. Neurosurgery 1995;37:975–981.

14. Vining EPG, Arroyo S, Breiter SN, et al. Magnetic resonance (MR) and MR spectroscopy (MRS) findings in children with Rasmussen's syndrome (abstract). Epilepsia 1994;35:146.

15. Vining EPG, Carson BC, Freeman JMF, et al. "Bilateral" epileptic abnormalities: a unilateral cure (abstract). Epilepsia 1987;28:591.

16. Boatman D, Freeman JM, Vining E, Gordon B. Recovery of speech functions following hemispherectomy: prospective, longitudinal studies (abstract). Epilepsia 1994;35:35.

17. Boatman D, Freeman J, Vining E, et al. Language recovery after left hemispherectomy in children with late-onset seizures. Ann Neurol 1999;46:579–586.

18. Vining EPG, Freeman JM, Pillas DJ, et al. Why would you remove half a brain? The outcome of 58 children after hemispherectomy—the Johns Hopkins experience 1968–1996. Pediatrics 1997;100:163–171.

19. Holthausen H, May TW, Adams CTB, et al. Seizures Post Hemispherectomy. In I Tuxhorn, H Holthausen, H Boenigk (eds), Paediatric Epilepsy Syndromes and Their Surgical Treatment. London: John Libbey, 1997;749.

Chapter 35

Corpus Callosotomy in the Developmentally Disabled with Epilepsy

Werner K. Doyle

Medically refractory seizures commonly are seen in the developmentally disabled population. Usually a consequence of the primary developmental pathologic etiology, refractory seizures can have a substantial influence on quality of life of the disabled. When medical management does not control the seizures successfully, surgical options are considered. Corpus callosotomy is one form of surgical management with relatively defined and accepted indications in contemporary surgical management of epilepsy.

Medically intractable seizure disorders in patients in whom a resectable seizure focus cannot be identified are candidates for section of the corpus callosum. Results from a number of institutions generally have been consistent and demonstrate reproducible success in controlling seizures in patients with atonic (drop attacks), tonic, and tonic-clonic generalized seizures. These seizure types are common in the developmentally disabled with epilepsy. Neuropsychological effects resulting from callosotomy generally are outweighed by the concomitant improvement in seizure control.

The objective of this operation is to disrupt the major central nervous system pathway involved in seizure propagation that causes a generalized seizure. The assumption is that disruption of pathways for generalization reduces the frequency and severity of primary and secondary generalized seizures. The operative indications for callosal sectioning are seizure disorders that are uncontrolled with anticonvulsant medication and that are not focal or localized to just one region of the brain (i.e., they are diffuse or multifocal). Callosotomy can be considered for any form of refractory epilepsy that cannot be treated with focal resection, but it generally is reserved for more well-defined situations of atonic seizures. Neuropsychological effects resulting from callosotomy are due to the interruption of interhemispheric information and control, causing varying degrees of disconnection syndromes. These neuropsychological and cognitive effects generally are outweighed by the improvement in seizure control that callosotomy provides. However, callosotomy most often is reserved for the most severe cases in which derangement of quality of life caused by the recurrent seizures is most dramatic.

History

In 1931, Walter Dandy[1] described surgical fenestration of a cavum septi pellucidum cyst in a pediatric patient. The procedure required division of the corpus callosum to approach the cyst. An incidental consequence of the procedure was to control effectively the patient's frequent seizures. Another report by Van Wagenen and Herren[2] several years later described control of intractable seizures in 10 patients with corpus callosum division. The rationale for their surgery was based on these authors' observation that patients with corpus callosum tumors usually would present early in their course with generalized seizures but that as the tumor grew, their seizures became less common, often becoming unilateral without generalization. These authors observed that as the corpus callosum was destroyed progressively by the growing tumor, the seizures diminished. In the 1960s, Bogen[3–5] and Luessenhop[6,7] cited isolated reports of callosum division. These early experiences led to acceptance of corpus callosotomy.[8–13] As the number of surgical cases and literature reports grew, the contemporary view of corpus callosotomy evolved to become an accepted option for specific cases of medically intractable epilepsy. Recently, vagus nerve stimulation (VNS) has influenced the indications for callosotomy, rendering it a second-tier procedure behind VNS. The trend is to consider callosotomy after VNS.

Indications and Selection Criteria

The indications for corpus callosotomy are not defined precisely other than the requirement for having medically refractory seizures. Identifying clear and consistent indications for candidates who will benefit from this procedure is not straightforward. Although certain seizure types respond more favorably than do others, a particular seizure type does not by itself sufficiently guarantee a good result. Seizures that most likely are helped are those classified as generalized (i.e., tonic, clonic, tonic-clonic, and atonic seizures). Complex partial seizures can be improved, but callosotomy results may be unreliable and, at best, only palliative. Focal resection offers definitive cure and, therefore, is a more appropriate first consideration for these seizure types.

Preoperative evaluation for callosotomy is similar to that for focal resective epilepsy surgery. The first phase of evaluation includes magnetic resonance imaging (MRI) to exclude structural etiologies causing seizures, then long-term video-electroencephalographic (video-EEG) monitoring with scalp electrodes to determine the seizure type (complex partial, atonic, tonic, etc.). A complete neuropsychological test battery is performed when not limited by an affected patient's baseline intellectual abilities. Last, an intracarotid amobarbital study (Wada test) is performed to determine language laterality, which is important in predict-

ing adverse dysfunction from the planned disconnection.

Opinions concerning who should undergo invasive monitoring (intracranial electrodes via burr holes or craniotomy) are based on different rationales particular to each center. At our center, we use the following protocol: If seizures have been recorded by video-EEG monitoring out of wakefulness and are found to be tonic, clonic, tonic-clonic, or akinetic, corpus callosotomy may be considered without invasive monitoring. If, however, the patient has complex partial seizures or the seizures have been recorded only during sleep (thus confounding the distinction between a complex partial seizure with rapid secondary generalization and a primary generalized seizure), the patient may be a candidate for invasive monitoring with either depth or subdural strip electrodes. Noninvasive seizure localization studies, such as subtraction single-photon emission computed tomography may influence the decision for invasive monitoring if a seizure focus is identified.

Special attention is directed to the neuropsychological data. If cerebral dominance is on the same side as preferred handedness, postoperative adverse deficits in communicative abilities may result. This outcome appears to be especially true for patients who are right cerebrum–dominant and right-handed and who undergo complete callosal sectioning.

Video-EEG monitoring is an essential aspect of the preliminary investigation, because it not only identifies the callosotomy candidate but may influence details of the surgical procedure. Its role in documenting generalized seizures or excluding a resectable epileptogenic focus is necessary to define the callosotomy candidate. However, video-EEG monitoring may demonstrate a predominantly posterior location of epileptogenic activity, thereby suggesting either a more extensive than typical anterior section or a partial posterior callosal section. Also, if intraoperative EEG recording is used to determine the extent of section, the preoperative EEG study's degree of interictal abnormality offers a preliminary indication for the feasibility of this operative technique.

Both seizure severity and frequency contribute to diminishing quality of life. Patients who experience frequent injuries secondary to their seizures are considered good candidates for callosotomy, as simply decreasing the number of injuries provides a substantial improvement to such patients' well-being.

Modern selection criteria for corpus callosum section are outlined by the Dartmouth-Hitchcock Medical Center's experience. Corpus callosotomy was indicated for (1) seizure disorders characterized by generalized major motor, tonic, or atonic (drop attack) seizures; (2) absence of an identifiable, resectable seizure focus; and (3) documented medical intractability, including exhaustive anticonvulsant trials with appropriate therapeutic levels. Patients with primarily complex partial seizures that are without a localizable focus also have been operated on with encouraging results.[14] Contemporary indications continue to be refined, especially since the availability of VNS beginning in mid-1997. VNS is an appropriate option for these same patients who, in the pre-VNS era, were solely callosotomy candidates. Selection between VNS and callosotomy is based on risks and potential efficacy to enhancing quality of life in specific circumstances. Generally, as VNS is much less of a surgical risk and is reversible, it usually is the first treatment option offered, followed by callosotomy if necessary. These surgical modalities are considered complementary to each other.

The preoperative neurologic examination plays an important role in the process of selecting patients being evaluated for possible callosotomy versus hemispherectomy. In individuals with a functional hand, callosotomy is a surgical option, as it is without the risk of increased motor deficit that hemispherectomy would produce. In borderline cases of partial but present voluntary hand or leg function, callosotomy is an alternative without precluding the possibility of more extensive surgery in the future, should it be necessary.

Generalized seizures, including atonic seizures (drop attacks), tonic seizures, and tonic-clonic seizures, are recognized as most likely to respond to callosotomy.[15] The majority of patients who have undergone callosal section have multiple seizure types; in those with simple partial seizures, the response has been satisfactory (approximately one-third achieving a reduction of at least 80% in that seizure type's frequency).[15] However, refractory simple partial seizures alone do not represent an indication for callosotomy. Of interest is the greater response of complex partial seizure disorders, with approximately 50% of patients achieving at least 80% reduction in frequency. This reflects the disruption, with corpus callosum section, of the symptomatic seizure propagation and its associated effects.[16,17]

Contraindications

Spencer et al.[18,19] found an increased risk of new or exacerbated lateralized cerebral deficits after callosotomy in individuals with dominant speech representation in the hemisphere opposite from that controlling handedness.[19] Although mixed dominance or crossed dominance may represent an increased risk, it is not viewed generally as an absolute contraindication to surgery when taking into account the possible improvement versus risk in the individual cases considered.

Early reports suggested that moderate to severe mental retardation was associated with poor corpus callosotomy outcome.[8,12,20] This finding has not been substantiated and now is considered only a relative contraindication. The surgery's predicted effect on quality of life is the primary consideration in this population.[21] The majority of patients who will benefit from the procedure have a degree of cognitive impairment as expected, given their diffuse or multifocal disease. Also, no absolute contraindication exists with respect to age, if the prognosis of the refractory seizure disorder favors surgical intervention.[22]

Outcomes

Neurologic Outcome

Adverse permanent neurologic sequelae of partial and complete corpus callosotomy are few, excluding the possible generic operative surgical complications, such as hemorrhage, infarct, infection, and anesthesia-related risks. Degrees of transient left hemiparesis, temporary urinary incontinence associated with cingulate gyrus compromise, mutism and decreased speech spontaneity, and abulia variably are seen after anterior section and typically resolve within days or, less often, within a few weeks after the disconnection.[19,23–25] A multivariable mechanism explaining mutism has been suggested.[26,27]

Sensory disconnection deficits usually manifest from posterior callosotomy, producing an inability to respond verbally to objects presented in the nondominant hemisphere's (contralateral) visual field or tactile sensory space. Such disconnection deficits are functionally tolerated during normal activity, because both hemispheres have access to both hemi–visual fields by natural perceptual strategies, such as scanning. Completion of a partial callosotomy may result also in an inability of the nondominant hand to follow verbal commands. This, too, is not disabling during most daily activities. Although patients generally are maintained on the same anticonvulsant regimen as before surgery, a transient seizure frequency increase in the acute postoperative period has been described. This increase may represent an effect of acute disconnection or is related to perioperative anticonvulsant fluctuations. The occasional callosotomy patient who is seizure-free during the first few weeks after surgery eventually has recurrence of refractory events unrelated to long-term seizure outcome.

Many studies have documented problems with interhemispheric information transfer; however, these alterations generally do not adversely influence the patient's activities of daily living.

Electroencephalographic Outcome

Callosotomy's primary effect on the EEG recording is to disrupt bilateral synchrony, although it does not eliminate the presence of active epileptogenic discharges.[28,29] Some frontal lobe epilepsy cases are believed to have too short an interhemispheric conduction time to allow localization by scalp EEG monitoring, and an anterior corpus callosotomy may permit localization of the focus.[30]

Seizure Outcome

Past callosotomy literature is difficult to summarize for several reasons. The surgery never was standardized, with various combinations of midline structures having been divided, including the fornix, anterior and hippocampal commissures, and massa intermedia. Reported series also have included combinations of partial and complete corpus callosal sectioning. Most series have various mixes of epileptic syndromes and seizure types with different surgical procedures,

further confounding interpretation of the results. Last, presurgical evaluation in these earlier reports had not yet been standardized to contemporary clinical concepts. Still, callosotomy provided patients with a 50–95% seizure reduction, the majority of patients experiencing approximately a 65% reduction.[24,31,32]

The higher success rates associated with resection procedures, particularly complete seizure elimination rates (cure), is the argument for offering resection surgery rather than callosotomy to patients with a localizable seizure focus.[33]

Despite varying degrees of the extent of surgery and differences in selection criteria of patients, the results of a number of institutions performing surgery of the corpus callosum for refractory seizures are fairly consistent and may be summarized with relation to seizure type. Spencer[23] summarized the results of 160 patients reported from various institutions, concluding that all types of generalized seizures were eliminated or decreased markedly in 80–90% after complete section but that fewer patients demonstrated this good outcome after partial section. With regard to partial seizures, fewer than 50% of patients experienced elimination or marked reduction, and approximately 25% of patients exhibited an increase or onset of new focal seizures.[23]

Dartmouth-Hitchcock Medical Center reported that approximately two-thirds of partial or complete callosotomy patients after follow-up at 1 year or more had either elimination or greater than 80% reduction of their seizures.[15] These patients presented with major seizures or absence seizures. A similar outcome was observed in 75% who presented with atonic or akinetic seizures. This group also exhibited a similar reduction in the severity of residual seizures. Simple partial seizures were improved in only one-third of patients. Two patients experienced a long-term increase in overall seizure number, and approximately one-fourth experienced new simple partial seizures. New seizures were described as attenuated expressions of the former generalized seizures. Other reports confirm these observations.[34–37]

Neuropsychological Sequelae of Callosotomy

Knowledge of functions and deficits after callosal destruction come from anatomic studies, experimental animal studies, patients with strokes, and, most important, elective corpus callosum division for seizure control. Because further neuropsychological sequelae in those with a baseline developmental cognitive deficit can create additional disability, understanding the neuropsychological aspects of both callosotomy and normal corpus callosum function is essential.

Anatomy and Function

The corpus callosum is the largest interhemispheric commissure. Callosal fibers interconnect homologous association areas of the two hemispheres, without significant connections between primary motor and sensory areas.[38] Other interhemispheric connections in humans include the hippocampal commissure, which interconnects homologous and nonhomologous hippocampal and entorhinal areas[39]; the anterior commissure, which interconnects the olfactory bulbs, amygdalae, and entorhinal and other temporal areas[40]; the posterior commissure, which interconnects cells involved in pupillary and extraocular muscle control; and the habenular commissure, which transmits fibers from the pallidum to the contralateral habenular nuclei. Also, the two sides of the brainstem reticular formation have extensive connections.

The corpus callosum's relatively large size is disproportional to the difficulties defining its functions after complete transection. The function of the corpus callosum, in addition to providing rapid transfer of data from one hemisphere to the other, is thought to be primarily that of inhibiting contralateral activity.[41,42] It may also play an important role in the development of unilateral hemispheric function.

Behavior, Expression, and Consciousness

Intuitively, one would predict that disconnecting the cerebral hemispheres would profoundly alter personality and behavior and perhaps would affect consciousness. However, after recovering from complete callosotomy, most patients are remarkably unchanged in their personality, humor, language, and verbal intelligence. Analytic studies of verbal output may reveal abnormalities, although they vary in degree among those studied. These can be summarized as follows: Attention becomes unstable and less sustained after callosotomy, contributing to fluctuating neglect and difficulty in completing tasks requiring vigilance, such as reading a book.[43–45] Although many facets of spontaneous behavioral expression and comprehension of observed behavior apparently are unaltered by callosotomy, emotional behavior can change.[46] Callosotomy reduces negative affective range exhibited by lack, or display, of muted reactions to unpleasant stimuli or situations.[47] Alexithymia, characterized by a reduced ability to identify and to describe one's feelings, is associated with right hemisphere dysfunction[48,49] and may occur in callosotomy patients who are unable to report verbally regarding their mood.[47,50] The restricted experience and expressiveness extend from primary emotions (e.g., fear and anger) to social emotions (e.g., hatred and embarrassment). These patients may relate a family member's death in a matter-of-fact, unemotional manner.[50] This also explains a callosotomy patient's complete indifference to such dramatic (albeit transient) effects as mutism and hemiparesis.

Verbal and nonverbal emotional expressions can be biased positively. Verbal humor, a left hemisphere function, remains intact, and patients will be able spontaneously to create and comprehend jokes.[50] An occasional consequence of callosal lesions is the alien hand sign, a dramatic neurobehavioral phenomenon in which one hand interferes with the actions of the other hand. This phenomenon may offer insight into hemispheric consciousness. The "patient" (left hemisphere) often is astonished and frustrated by the discordant actions that are expressed most often by the left hand (right hemisphere). The alien hand sign most commonly follows callosal or medial frontal lesions[2,51,52] and develops from callosotomy, whereby the hand ipsilateral to the language-dominant hemisphere exhibits the "alien" activity.[53]

Motor Function, Attention, Language, and Memory

Postcallosotomy patients have learning deficits for acquiring new tasks involving cooperative interaction between two hands (e.g., drawing with an Etch-a-Sketch).[54] Previously acquired bimanual cooperative tasks (e.g., piano playing and bicycling), including alternating and parallel movements, usually are preserved. An attentional system that focuses predominantly on the opposite half of the sensory field is contained in each hemisphere. Dissociation of selective processing can emerge, exhibited typically with superior left-handed performance on visuospatial tasks and better right-handed performance on verbal tasks.[55] Callosotomy effectively can isolate these systems that normally communicate with each other. Further examples include hemispatial dyscalculia, in which a callosotomy subject solves written arithmetic problems disregarding free-field numeric information presented toward the left, multimodality left-sided extinction, and left-hand superiority with continuous performance tasks despite unilateral callosal apraxia.[55] Studies of spatial attention in callosotomy patients reveal that each hemisphere also can direct some attention toward the ipsilateral spatial field, possibly via noncallosal interhemispheric connections.

Language is essentially lateralized to one hemisphere—usually the left, although primitive language abilities are seen contralaterally. Thus, in postcallosotomy patients, an image projected to the right visual field (left hemisphere) can be recognized and described easily by the intrinsic language function of the left brain. In contrast, when the image is projected to the right hemisphere, postcallosotomy patients will respond verbally that they "saw nothing" or "couldn't describe it." In contrast, when asked, they readily point to the object or provide an accurate nonverbal response. The right hemisphere receives the image, although it cannot mount a verbal response.

Callosotomy may impair nonverbal and verbal learning and memory.[56–58] Topographic memory is particularly impaired, resulting in difficulty in remembering where items had been placed (such as keys) and difficulty with navigation through familiar physical environments. Verbal memory can be affected, causing some patients to abandon reading or watching movies because the plot cannot be retained, rendering such entertainments incomprehensible. The verbal memory tasks affected most commonly are recall of short narratives and word association.[56,59,60] Callosotomy patients may have difficulty also with memory for daily routines, such as medication dosing, recalling the object for which they entered a room, and failing to keep an appointment despite being recently reminded.[60,61] Working memory, defined as the ability simultaneously to hold portions of past and current data, is impaired by callosotomy.[50] Memory processes may be altered with interhemispheric disconnection, because memory retrieval within either hemisphere may require interhemispheric cooperation. So, after callosotomy, impairment in memory retrieval is possible.[62] Remote or long-term memory predating the callosotomy is better preserved, probably because these memories had been rehearsed and already have become verbally encoded.[62]

Patients with mixed limb dominance, as evidenced by limb preference, may be at higher risk for language impairment because of an increased likelihood of bilateral representation of language function typically associated with mixed and left-handed dominance. Another likelihood is that, after callosotomy, some language function will be disconnected from the dominant motor system, causing difficulty with writing.[63,64]

Poor neuropsychological outcome might be expected in patients with other anomalous patterns of cognitive function. For example, callosotomy in a patient whose functional memory is contralateral to the language-dominant hemisphere would be expected to produce a disconnection between the ability to recall information and the area in control of the motor speech system, causing mutism or aphasia.[63] Comprehensive neuropsychological examination and intracarotid amobarbital testing to lateralize language and memory ability may identify patients most at risk for such neuropsychological dysfunction. Ferrell et al.[65] reported an acute disconnection syndrome that in some included mutism, personality regression, apraxia, and agnosia. The symptoms were temporary in all but 1 of 10 patients. Improvements in intellectual function were noted in several patients, perhaps associated with reduced frequency and severity of seizures or subsequent reduction in antiepileptic medications.

Sectioning of only the anterior two-thirds of the corpus callosum and preserving the splenium or modifying the operative technique to section the corpus callosum in a two-stage process[66] purportedly have achieved seizure control without the morbidity associated with more extensive procedures.[67–69] Although clinical evidence suggests that the length and severity of the disconnection syndrome was avoided, follow-up of outcome of the various modifications has not included appropriately objective neuropsychological examinations to substantiate that finding.

Complications and Morbidity

Morbidity from callosotomy surgery is considerably greater than that for typical focal cortical resections or temporal lobectomy. Earlier surgical series have reported deaths from hydrocephalus and meningitis. In his series, Wyler[31] reported two deaths, one from an air embolism secondary to a sagittal sinus injury and the other associated with an acute postoperative seizure. Earlier series reported a 50% incidence of hydrocephalus and chemical or bacterial meningitis. These outcomes may have been in part due to opening of the ventricle, allowing cerebrospinal fluid dissemination of inflammatory substances associated with surgery. Modern technical approaches avoid this by remaining within the separable septum pellucidum for the majority of the callosal dissection. Spencer et al.[70] reported an increase in focal seizures after corpus callosotomy, especially in patients who have asymmetric bilateral epileptogenic foci. Wyler[31] also reported two postoperative epidural hematomas in patients who were taking valproic acid, an agent known to decrease platelet function and serving as a relatively common medication used in this population. Increased intracranial swelling or venous infarction of the frontal lobe may occur due to damage to the sagittal sinus or, more commonly, from sacrificing cortical draining veins during the midline exposure.

Completion of Callosotomy

For patients having undergone partial callosal section without obtaining satisfactory seizure improvement, completion of the callosal section may be appropriate. Comparison of results of partial and complete callosal sections between and within institutions has demonstrated overall better outcome with complete section.[20,71,72]

Yale University Medical School's experience with callosotomy completion is similarly positive, concluding that total callosotomy is beneficial when anterior callosotomy fails—especially for persistent tonic-clonic and tonic seizures—and most often is necessary in the setting of diffuse cerebral abnormalities.[70]

Completion of callosal section does have neuropsychological consequences greater than those of partial section,[73] although the benefits in seizure control usually outweigh any negative effect. Not all families or centers routinely proceed with the second-stage procedure.

Technical Aspects

Since 1962, numerous surgical series have been published, including variations and combinations of disruption of the midline structures (corpus callosum, massa intermedia, anterior commissure, hippocampal commissure, etc.) and including unilateral fornix sectioning. Contemporary corpus callosotomy entails just the division of the corpus callosum proper, including the splenium, up to two-thirds of its length defining an anterior callosotomy.

Anatomic imaging studies are essential for safe surgical intervention. MRI's increased sensitivity and contrast over computed tomography in detecting cerebral structural pathology renders it the method of choice for preoperative planning and surgical navigation. For corpus callosum surgery, imaging of brain structures of the midsagittal plane is essential. Preoperative appreciation of dimension and morphology of the corpus callosum enhances a surgeon's anatomic navigation and skill. Computer-assisted image-guided navigation is used routinely at our center for callosotomy. The study also permits visualization of draining veins in the region of the surgical approach, formerly demonstrated only with angiography.[74] After a callosotomy, MRI is the imaging modality of choice to evaluate the extent of callosal sectioning.[75,76]

Many centers advocate division of the anterior two-thirds or three-fourths at the first surgery, sparing just a portion of the posterior callosum, to avoid producing a full sensory disconnection syndrome. Although early reports endorsed complete corpus callosotomy, limited callosum division became popular in the 1980s and has been preferred since. Staging a complete callosal section is recommended for several reasons. Foremost is limiting the disconnection syndrome characterized by mutism, a left-sided apraxia resembling hemiparesis, and adverse bifrontal lobe reflexes. The second rationale for staging the callosotomy is that the anterior section by itself often provides satisfactory outcome. The first stage entails sectioning of the anterior two-thirds of the callosum or whatever length is approached easily by the usually limited surgical exposure (midline vertex craniotomy). The second stage is performed several months later, after a period has passed for adequately assessing efficacy of the initial disconnection. During completion, the remainder of the corpus callosum is sectioned from a more posterior surgical trajectory. Completion of the corpus callosum section is indicated for continued generalized seizures and is performed a minimum of 2 months (and often 6 months) after the original partial disconnection.

Two groups have described intraoperative EEG recording to guide the extent of initial callosal section.[77,78] If intraoperative EEG studies demonstrate sufficiently frequent generalized discharges, section is continued until bilateral synchrony is disrupted significantly.[77,79–81] These authors' most recent report suggests that this technique is not helpful.[82]

At our center, we often combine callosotomy with invasive monitoring as a two-stage operation. This strategy permits identification and treatment of important cortical seizure foci that, when resected, can augment the efficacy of callosotomy, thereby improving overall seizure control. Insufficient experience with this approach precludes detailed discussion of our results, although our preliminary experience is encouraging.

Summary

Candidates for corpus callosotomy have medically intractable seizure disorders without an identified resectable seizure focus. An important selection criterion is refractory atonic seizures (drop attacks) causing repeated physical injury. Reported seizure results have been described broadly. Some series have noted complete control of severe, frequent atonic, tonic, or generalized tonic-clonic seizures in the majority of patients; other series have noted only worthwhile improvement in fewer than 50% of operated patients. Differences in outcome may be due partly to differences in patient selection and extent of callosal section. Although the operation usually is well tolerated, it carries greater risk than resective surgery. Complications include infection, infarction, hemorrhage, and death. Common sequelae are the transient syndrome of mutism and left arm and leg apraxia. Nonetheless, neuropsychological effects resulting from callosotomy generally are outweighed by the improvement in seizure control and patients' improved quality of life.

Further prospective, controlled studies are needed to clarify the role of corpus callosotomy in treating patients with intractable secondary generalized epilepsy and the Lennox-Gastaut syndrome and to define optimal selection criteria and the likelihood of good outcome. However, with the plethora of new anticonvulsant drugs and especially VNS often displacing callosotomy as the first line of surgical management, callosotomy is performed less often and generally is considered a last measure in the most severe cases, in which risks and partial efficacy are acceptable.

VNS, a new surgical modality, shares with callosotomy the same indications and selection criteria. Being reversible and much less invasive and carrying with it significantly less associated morbidity, it is now considered more often before callosotomy in managing refractory seizures not amenable to focal resection. (This important therapeutic modality is discussed in detail in Chapter 31.)

References

1. Dandy WE. Congenital cerebral cysts of the cavum septi pellucidi (fifth ventricle) and cavum vergae (sixth ventricle): diagnosis and treatment. Arch Neurol Psychiatry 1931;25:44–66.
2. Van Wagenen WP, Herren RY. Surgical division of the commissural pathways in the corpus callosum: relation to spread of an epileptic attack. Arch Neurol Psychiatry 1940;44:740–759.
3. Bogen, JE, Fisher ED, Vogel PJ. Cerebral commissurotomy: a second case report. JAMA 1965;194(12):1328–1329.
4. Bogen JE, Sperry RW, Vogel PJ. Addendum: Commissural Section and Propagation of Seizures. In HH Jasper, AA Ward, A Pope (eds), Basic Mechanisms of the Epilepsies. Boston: Little, Brown, 1969;439.
5. Bogen JE, Vogel PJ. Cerebral commissurotomy in man: preliminary case report. Bull Los Angeles Neurol Soc 1962;27:169–172.
6. Luessenhop AJ. Interhemispheric commissurotomy (the split brain operation) as an alternative to hemispherectomy for control of intractable seizures. Am Surg 1970;36:265–268.
7. Luessenhop AJ, Dela Cruz TC, Fenichel GM. Surgical disconnection of the cerebral hemispheres for

intractable seizures. JAMA 1970;213(10):1630–1636.

8. Harbaugh RE, Wilson DH, Reeves AG, Gazzaniga MS. Forebrain commissurotomy for epilepsy: review of 20 consecutive cases. Acta Neurochir (Wien) 1983;68:263–275.

9. Wilson DH, Culver C, Waddington M, Gazzaniga M. Disconnection of the cerebral hemispheres: an alternative to hemispherectomy for the control of intractable seizures. Neurology 1975;25(12):1149–1153.

10. Wilson DH, Reeves A, Gazzaniga M. Division of the corpus callosum for uncontrollable seizures. Neurology 1978;28:649–653.

11. Wilson DH, Reeves A, Gazzaniga M. Corpus Callosotomy for Control of Intractable Seizures. In JA Wada, JK Penry (eds), Advances in Epileptology: the Tenth Epilepsy International Symposium. New York: Raven Press, 1980;205–213.

12. Wilson DH, Reeves A, Gazzaniga M. "Central" commissurotomy for intractable generalized epilepsy: series two. Neurology 1982;32:687–697.

13. Wilson DH, Reeves A, Gazzaniga M, Culver C. Cerebral commissurotomy for control of intractable seizures. Neurology 1977;27(8):708–715.

14. Roberts DW, Reeves AG. Effects of commissurotomy on complex partial epilepsy in patients without a resectable seizure focus. Appl Neurophysiol 1987;50:398–400.

15. Roberts DW. Section of the Corpus Callosum for Epilepsy. In HH Schmidek, WH Sweet (eds), Operative Neurosurgical Techniques: Indications, Methods and Results. Orlando: Grune & Stratton, 1988;1243–1250.

16. Gates JR, Rosenfeld WE, Maxwell RE, et al. Response of multiple seizure types to corpus callosum section. Epilepsia 1987;28:28–34.

17. Roberts DW, Reeves AG. Effect of commissurotomy on complex partial epilepsy in patients without a resectable seizure focus. Appl Neurophysiol 1987;50:398–400.

18. Sass KJ, Spencer DD, Spencer SS, et al. Corpus callosotomy for epilepsy: II. Neurologic and neuropsychological outcome. Neurology 1988;38:24–28.

19. Spencer SS, Gates JR, Reeves AG, et al. Corpus Callosum Section for Uncontrolled Epilepsy. In J Engle (ed), Surgical Treatment of Epilepsy. New York: Raven Press, 1987;425–444.

20. Spencer SS, Spencer DD, Williamson TPD, et al. Corpus callosotomy for epilepsy: I. Seizure effects. Neurology 1988;38:19–24.

21. Lassonde M, Sauerwein C. Neuropsychological outcome of corpus callosotomy in children and adolescents. J Neurosurg Sci 1997;41(1):67–73.

22. Nordgren RE, Reeves AG, Viguera AC, Roberts DW. Corpus callosotomy for intractable seizures in the pediatric age group. Arch Neurol 1991;48:364–372.

23. Spencer SS. Corpus callosum section and other disconnection procedures for medically intractable epilepsy. Epilepsia 1988;29[Suppl 2]:S85–S99.

24. Kwan SY, Wong TT, Chang KP, et al. Seizure outcome after corpus callosotomy: the Taiwan experience. Childs Nerv Syst 2000;16(2):87–92.

25. Quattrini A, Del Pesce M, Provinciali L, et al. Mutism in 36 patients who underwent callosotomy for drug-resistant epilepsy. J Neurosurg Sci 1997;41(1):93–96.

26. Nakasu Y, Isozumi T, Nioka H, Handa J. Mechanism of mutism following the transcallosal approach to the ventricles. Acta Neurochir (Wien) 1991;110(3–4):146–153.

27. Sussman NM, Gur RC, Gur RE, O'Connor MJ. Mutism as a consequence of callosotomy. J Neurosurg 1983;59(3):514–519.

28. Quattrini A, Papo I, Cesarano R, et al. EEG Patterns after callosotomy. J Neurosurg Sci 1997;41(1):85–92.

29. Oguni H, Andermann F, Gotman J, Olivier A. Effect of anterior callosotomy on bilaterally synchronous spike and wave and other EEG discharges. Epilepsia 1994;35(3):505–513.

30. Spencer SS, Katz A, Ebersole J, et al. Ictal EEG changes with corpus callosum section. Epilepsia 1993;34(3):568–573.

31. Fuiks KS, Wyler AR, Hermann BP, Somes G. Seizure outcome from anterior and complete corpus callosotomy. J Neurosurg 1991;74(4):573–578.

32. Sorenson JM, Wheless JW, Baumgartner JE, et al. Corpus callosotomy for medically intractable seizures. Pediatr Neurosurg 1997;27(5):260–267.

33. Engle J Jr. Outcome with Respect to Epileptic Seizures. In J Engle Jr (ed), Surgical Treatment of the Epilepsies. New York: Raven Press, 1987.

34. Gates JR, Rosenfeld WE, Maxwell RE, Lyons RE. Response of multiple seizure types to corpus callosum section. Epilepsia 1987;28(1):28–34.

35. Phillips J, Sakas DE. Anterior callosotomy for intractable epilepsy: outcome in a series of twenty patients. Br J Neurosurg 1996;10(4):351–356.

36. Sakas DE, Phillips J. Anterior callosotomy in the management of intractable epileptic seizures: significance of the extent of resection. Acta Neurochir (Wien) 1996;138(6):700–707.

37. Rossi GF, Colicchio G, Marchese E, Pompucci A. Callosotomy for severe epilepsies with generalized seizures: outcome and prognostic factors. Acta Neurochir (Wien) 1996;138(2):221–227.

38. Welker WI, Seidenstein S. Somatic sensory representation in the cerebral cortex of the raccoon (*Procyon lotor*). J Comp Neurol 1959;111:469–501.

39. Blackstad TW. Commissural connections of the hippocampal region in the rat, with special reference to their mode of termination. J Comp Neurol 1956;105:417–537.

40. Brodal A. Neurological Anatomy. New York: Oxford University Press, 1981;658.

41. Zaidel D. Memory and Spatial Cognition Following Commissurotomy. In F Boller, J Grafman (eds), Handbook of Neuropsychology, vol 4. Amsterdam: Elsevier Science, 1990;151–166.

42. Selnes OA. The corpus callosum: some anatomical and functional considerations with special reference to language. Brain Lang 1974;1:111–139.

43. Dimond SJ, Farrington L, Johnson P. Differing emotional responses from right and left hemispheres. Nature 1976;261:690–692.

44. Ellenberg L, Sperry RW. Capacity for holding sustained attention following commissurotomy. Cortex 1979;15:421–436.

45. Trevarthen C. Integrative Functions of the Cerebral Commissures. In F Boller, J Grafman (eds), Handbook of Neuropsychology, vol 4. New York: Elsevier, 1990;49–83.

46. Gazzaniga MA, Sperry RW. Language after section of the cerebral commissures. Brain 1967;90:131–148.

47. Hoppe KD, Bogen JE. Alexithymia in twelve commissurotimized patients. Psychother Psychosom 1977;28:148–155.

48. Jessimer M, Markham R. Alexithymia: a right hemisphere dysfunction specific to recognition of certain facial expressions? Brain Cogn 1997;34:346–358.

49. Gross-Tsur V, Shalev RS, Manor O, Amin W. Developmental right-hemisphere syndrome: clinical spectrum of the nonverbal learning disability. J Learn Disabil 1995;28:80–86.

50. Zaidel DW. A View of the World from a Split-Brain Perspective. In E Critchley (ed), The Neurological Boundaries of Reality. London: Farracid, 1994;161–174.

51. Akelitis AJ. Studies on the corpus callosum: IV. Diagnostic dyspraxia in epileptics following partial and complete section of the corpus callosum. Am J Psychiatry 1945;101:594–599.

52. Leiguarda R, Starkstein S, Berthier M. Anterior callosal haemorrhage: partial interhemispheric disconnection syndrome. Brain 1989;112:1019–1037.

53. Geschwind DH, Iacoboni M, Mega MS, et al. Alien hand syndrome: interhemispheric motor disconnection due to a lesion in the midbody of the corpus callosum. Neurology 1995;45(4):802–808.

54. Zaidel D, Sperry RW. Some long term motor effects of cerebral commissurotomy in man. Neuropsychologia 1977;15:493–504.

55. Loring DW, Meador KJ, Lee GP. Differential-handed response to verbal and visual spatial stimuli: evidence of specialized hemispheric processing following callosotomy. Neuropsychologia 1989;27(6):811–827.

56. Zaidel D, Sperry RW. Memory impairment after commissurotomy in man. Brain 1974;97:253–272.

57. Huppert FA. Memory in split-brain patients: a comparison with organic amnestic syndromes. Cortex 1981;17:303–312.

58. Zaidel D. Memory and Spatial Cognition Following Commissurotomy. In F Boller, J Grafman (eds), Handbook of Neuropsychology, vol 4. Amsterdam: Elsevier, 1990;51–166.

59. Ledoux JE, Risse GL, Springer SP, et al. Cognition and commissurotomy. Brain 1977;100:87–104.

60. Ferguson SM, Rayport M, Lossie SW. Neuropsychiatric Observations on Behavioral Consequences of Corpus Callosum Section for Seizure Control. In AG Reeves (ed), Epilepsy and the Corpus Callosum. New York: Plenum, 1985.

61. Zaidel E, Clarke JM, Suyenobu B. Hemispheric Independence: A Paradigm Case for Cognitive Neuroscience. In AB Scheibel, AF Wechsler (eds), Neurobiology of Higher Cognitive Function. New York: Guilford Press, 1990;297–352.

62. Zaidel D, Sperry RW. Memory impairment after commissurotomy in man. Brain 1974;97:263–272.

63. Rayport M, Ferguson SM, Corrie WS. Mutism after corpus callosotomy for intractable seizure control. Epilepsia 1984;25:665.

64. Sass KJ, Novelly RA, Spencer DD, Spencer SS. Postcallosotomy language impairments in patients with crossed cerebral dominance. J Neurosurg 1990;72(1):85–90.

65. Ferrel RB, Culver CM, Tucker GJ. Psychosocial and cognitive function after commissurotomy for intractable seizures. J Neurosurg 1983;58:374–380.

66. Harbaugh RE, Wilson DH, Reeves AG, Gazzaniga MS. Forebrain commissurotomy for epilepsy: review of 20 consecutive cases. Acta Neurochir (Wien) 1983;68:263–275.

67. Gordon HW, Bogen JE, Sperry RW. Absence of deconnection syndrome in two patients with partial section of the neocommissures. Brain 1971;94:327–336.

68. Wilson DH, Reeves AG, Gazzaniga MS, Culver C. Cerebral commissurotomy for control of intractable seizures. Neurology 1977;27(8):708–715.

69. Wilson DH, Reeves AG, Gazzaniga MS. Division of the corpus callosum for uncontrolled epilepsy. Neurology 1978;28:649–653.

70. Spencer SS, Spencer DD, Sass K, et al. Anterior, total, and two-stage corpus callosum section: differential and incremental seizure responses. Epilepsia 1993;34(3):561–567.

71. Murro AM, Flanigin HF, Gallagher BB, et al. Corpus callosotomy for the treatment of intractable epilepsy. Epilepsy Res 1988;2(1):44–50.

72. Purves SJ, Wada JA, Woodhurst WB, et al. Results of anterior corpus callosum section in 24 patients with medically intractable seizures. Neurology 1988;38:1194–1201.

73. Gazzaniga MS, Risse GL, Springer SP, et al. Psychologic and neurologic consequences of partial

and complete cerebral commissurotomy. Neurology 1975;25:10–15.

74. Rayport M, Corrie WS, Ferguson SM. Corpus Callosum Section for Control of Clinically and Electroencephalographically Classified Intractable Seizures. In AG Reeves (ed), Epilepsy and Corpus Callosum. New York: Plenum Press, 1985;329–337.

75. Harris RD, Roberts DW, Cromwell LD. MR imaging of corpus callosotomy. AJNR Am J Neuroradiol 1989; 10(4):677–680.

76. Sussman NM, Scanlon M, Garfinkle W, et al. Magnetic resonance imaging after corpus callosotomy. Neurology 1987;37(2):350–354.

77. Maxwell RE, Gates JR, Gumnit RJ. Corpus Callosotomy at the University of Minnesota. In J Engel Jr (ed), Surgical Treatment of the Epilepsies. New York: Raven Press, 1987;659–666.

78. Marino R Jr, Radvany J, Huck FR, et al. Selective electroencephalograph-guided microsurgical callosotomy for refractory generalized epilepsy. Surg Neurol 1990;34(4):219–228.

79. Gates JR, Leppik IE, Yap J, Gumnit RJ. Corpus callosotomy: clinical and electroencephalographic effects. Epilepsia 1984;25:308–316.

80. Gates JR, Maxwell R, Leppik IE, et al. Electroencephalographic and Clinical Effects of Total Corpus Callosotomy. In AG Reeves (ed), Epilepsy and the Corpus Callosum. New York: Plenum Press, 1985;315–328.

81. Gates JR, Rosenfeld WE, Maxwell RE, Lyons RE. Response of multiple seizure types to corpus callosum section. Epilepsia 1987;28:28–34.

82. Fiol ME, Gates JR, Mireles R, et al. Value of intraoperative EEG changes during corpus callosotomy in predicting surgical results. Epilepsia 1993;34(1):74–78.

Index

Note: Page numbers followed by *f* indicate figures; numbers followed by *t* indicate tables.